Drug Discovery and Development

Senior Content Strategist: *Pauline Graham*
Content Development Specialist: *Carole McMurray*
Senior Project Manager: *Beula Christopher*
Designer: *Miles Hitchen*
Illustration Manager: *Jennifer Rose*

Drug Discovery and Development

Technology in Transition

Edited by

RG Hill BPharm PhD DSc (Hon) FMedSci

President Emeritus, British Pharmacological Society; Visiting Professor of Pharmacology, Department of Medicine, Imperial College, London; Formerly, Executive Director and Head, Licensing and External Research, Europe, MSD/Merck Research Laboratories

HP Rang MB BS MA DPhil FMedSci FRS

President-Elect British Pharmacological Society, Emeritus Professor of Pharmacology, University College, London; Formerly Director, Novartis Institute for Medical Sciences, London

Foreword by

Patrick Vallance BSc MBBS FRCP FMedSci

President, Pharmaceuticals Research and Development, GlaxoSmithKline, Brentford, UK

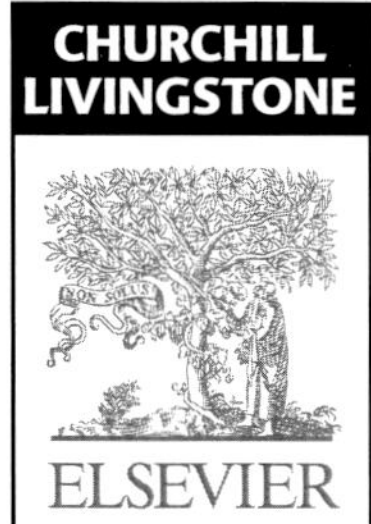

Edinburgh London New York Oxford Philadelphia St Louis Sydney Toronto 2013

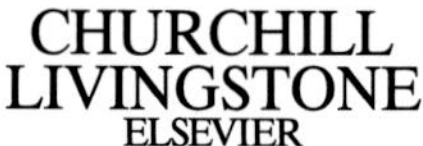

First edition 2006
Second edition 2013

ISBN 978-0-7020-4299-7

British Library Cataloguing in Publication Data
A catalogue record for this book is available from the British Library

Library of Congress Cataloging in Publication Data
A catalog record for this book is available from the Library of Congress

Notices

Knowledge and best practice in this field are constantly changing. As new research and experience broaden our understanding, changes in research methods, professional practices, or medical treatment may become necessary.

Practitioners and researchers must always rely on their own experience and knowledge in evaluating and using any information, methods, compounds, or experiments described herein. In using such information or methods they should be mindful of their own safety and the safety of others, including parties for whom they have a professional responsibility.

With respect to any drug or pharmaceutical products identified, readers are advised to check the most current information provided (i) on procedures featured or (ii) by the manufacturer of each product to be administered, to verify the recommended dose or formula, the method and duration of administration, and contraindications. It is the responsibility of practitioners, relying on their own experience and knowledge of their patients, to make diagnoses, to determine dosages and the best treatment for each individual patient, and to take all appropriate safety precautions.

To the fullest extent of the law, neither the Publisher nor the authors, contributors, or editors, assume any liability for any injury and/or damage to persons or property as a matter of products liability, negligence or otherwise, or from any use or operation of any methods, products, instructions, or ideas contained in the material herein.

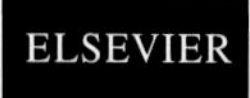

Printed in China

Foreword

Medicines have done more to alter the practice of medicine and improve the outlook for patients than any other intervention. HIV infection has been transformed from a death sentence to a chronic managed disorder, many childhood leukaemias can be cured, surgery for peptic ulcers is a thing of the past, treatment of high blood pressure and the introduction of statins has dramatically reduced cardiovascular disease burden. Despite these and many other examples, the pharmaceutical industry has been in a crisis. The number of new medicines approved each year has not kept pace with either the rate of scientific discovery or the huge investment made in R&D. There appears to be a discrepancy between the ability to make biological discoveries and ability to translate these into meaningful inventions – the new medicines that will improve the health of this and future generations. There have been gloom and doom headlines for the past decade or more and an erosion of trust in the industry. Many will argue that the low hanging fruit has been picked and that we are now in a period where we are left with the more difficult problems to solve. I do not accept this argument.

This new edition comes at a time when I believe the tide has turned and that the opportunity is in fact greater than it has ever been. Witness the number of new oncology medicines making it through the pipeline of discovery and development. Here we have new treatments, some of which have a dramatic effect and many of which are true exemplars of what we mean by stratified treatments targeted towards specific patient populations or specific subsets of tumours. Look also at the rise in antibody treatments and the impact being made in auto-immune and inflammatory disorders. Many pipelines are beginning to fill up and with a different type of medicine. Medicines that aren't just small molecules but include antibodies, nucleic acid based treatments and even cell-based therapies. Medicines that do not target all-comers across an entire broad disease but rather aim to treat where the mechanism can have the biggest impact, whether that be in a smaller disease market or in segments of one or more larger disease area. These changes are not surprising and reflect the evolution of understanding as traditional definitions of disease based on clinical observation become more refined by modern biology. There is, I believe a convergence of interests in these changes. Scientists want to make a medicine that has a big impact on a specific disease area. This of course is also what patients and doctors want. It is also what underlies the process of health technology assessment, health economics and the various forms of reimbursement and market access panels that have emerged across the globe. We will see many more medicines emerging over the next few decades and many will have bigger effects in smaller populations.

This book tackles these issues head on and in an accessible and authoritative manner. It is written by experts and has something for everyone, from the beginner to the seasoned professional. There is one common theme running through the book that I hope will be heeded. Drug discovery and development is about judgement and about integration of disciplines. There are still too many unknowns for this to be a routine process. Making a medicine requires that the disciplines from genetics, chemistry, biology, protein engineering, pharmacology, experimental medicine, clinical medicine, modelling and simulation, epidemiology and many others come together in an integrated way and that bold decisions are made on the basis of what is inevitably incomplete information. I think this book will help those aiming to be part of this exciting and challenging mission.

Patrick Vallance BSc MBBS FRCP FMedSci

Preface

to 2nd Edition

The intention that we set out with when starting the task of editing this new edition was to bring the book fully up to date but to try to keep the style and ethos of the original. All of the chapters have been updated and many have been extensively revised or completely rewritten by new authors. There are two completely novel topics given chapters of their own (Protein Scaffolds as Antibody Replacements; Imaging in Clinical Drug Development) as these topics were judged to be of increasing importance for the future. There are a greater number of authors contributing to this new edition and an attempt has been made to recruit some of our new authors from the traditional stronghold of our subject in the large pharmaceutical companies but also to have contributions from individuals who work in biotechnology companies, academic institutions and CROs. These segments of the industry are of increasing importance in sustaining the flow of new drugs yet have a different culture and different needs to those of the bigger companies. We are living in turbulent times and the traditional models of drug discovery and development are being questioned. Rather than the leadership position in research being automatically held by traditional large pharmaceutical companies we now have the creative mixture of a small number of very large companies (often with a focus on outsourcing a large part of their research activities), a vigorous and growing biotechnology / small specialty pharmaceutical company sector and a significant number of academic institutions engaged in drug discovery. It is interesting to speculate on how the face of drug discovery may look 5 years from now but it will certainly be different with movement of significant research investment to growth economies such as China and a reduction in such investment being made in the US and Western Europe. We hope that this new edition continues to fill the need for a general guide and primer to drug discovery and development and has moved with the times to reflect the changing face of our industry.

RG Hill
HP Rang

Preface

to 1st edition

A large pharmaceutical company is an exceptionally complex organization. Several features stand out. First, like any company, it must make a profit, and handle its finances efficiently in order to survive. Modern pharmaceutical companies are so large that they are financially comparable to a small nation, and the average cost of bringing a new drug to market – about $800m – is a sum that any government would think twice about committing.

Second, there is an underlying altruism in the mission of a pharmaceutical company, in the sense that its aim is to provide therapies that meet a significant medical need, and thereby relieve human suffering. Though cynics will point to examples where the profit motive seems to have prevailed over ethical and altruistic concerns, the fact remains that the modern pharmacopeia has enormous power to alleviate disease, and owes its existence almost entirely to the work of the pharmaceutical industry.

Third, the industry is research-based to an unusual extent. Biomedical science has arguably advanced more rapidly than any other domain of science in the last few decades, and new discoveries naturally create expectations that they will lead on improved therapies. Though discoveries in other fields may have profound implications for our understanding of the natural world, their relevance for improving the human condition is generally much less direct. For this reason, the pharmaceutical industry has to stay abreast of leading-edge scientific progress to a greater extent than most industries.

Finally, the products of the pharmaceutical industry have considerable social impact, producing benefits in terms of life expectancy and relief of disability, risks of adverse effects, changes in lifestyle – for example, the contraceptive pill – and financial pressures which affect healthcare policy on a national and international scale. In consequence, an elaborate, and constantly changing, regulatory system exists to control the approval of new drugs, and companies need to devote considerable resources to negotiating this tricky interface.

This book provides an introduction to the way a pharmaceutical company goes about its business of discovering and developing new drugs. The first part gives a brief historical account of the evolution of the industry from its origins in the mediaeval apothecaries' trade, and discusses the changing understanding of what we mean by disease, and what therapy aims to achieve, as well as summarizing case histories of the discovery and development of some important drugs.

The second part focuses on the science and technology involved in the discovery process, that is the stages by which a promising new chemical entity is identified, from the starting point of a medical need and an idea for addressing it. A chapter on biopharmaceuticals, whose discovery and development tend to follow routes somewhat different from synthetic compounds, is included here, as well as accounts of patent issues that arise in the discovery phase, and a chapter on research management in this environment. Managing drug discovery scientists can be likened in some ways to managing a team of huskies on a polar journey. Huskies provide the essential driving force, but are somewhat wayward and unpredictable creatures, prone to fighting each other, occasionally running off on their own, and inclined to bite the expedition leader. Success in husky terms means gaining the respect of other huskies, not of humans. (We must not, of course, push the analogy too far. Scientists, unlike huskies, do care about reaching the goal, and the project management plan – in my experience at least – does not involve killing them to feed their colleagues.)

The third section of the book deals with drug development, that is the work that has to be undertaken to turn the drug candidate that emerges from the discovery process into a product on the market, and a final chapter presents some facts and figures about the way the whole process operates in practice.

No small group on its own can produce a drug, and throughout the book there is strong emphasis on the need for interdisciplinary team-work. The main reason for writing it was to help individual specialists to understand better the work of colleagues who address different aspects of the problem. The incentive came from my own experience when, after a career in academic pharmacology, I joined Sandoz as a research director in 1985, motivated by a wish to see whether my knowledge of pharmacology could be put to use in developing useful new medicines. It was a world startlingly different from what I was used to, full of people – mostly very friendly and forthcoming – whose work I really did not understand. Even the research laboratories worked in a different way. Enjoyable though it was to explore this new territory, and to come to understand the language and preoccupations of colleagues in other disciplines, it would have been a lot quicker and more painless had I been able to read a book about it first! No such book existed, nor has any appeared since. Hence this book, which is aimed not only at scientists who want to understand better the broad range of activities involved in producing a new drug, but also non-scientists who want to understand the realities of drug discovery research. Inevitably, in covering such a broad range, the treatment has to be superficial, concentrating on general principles rather than technical details, but further reading is suggested for those seeking more detail. I am much indebted to my many friends and colleagues, especially to those who have taken the time to write chapters, but also to those with whom I have worked over the years and who taught me many valuable lessons.

It is hoped that those seeking a general guide to pharmaceutical R & D will find the book helpful.

H P Rang

Contributors

Peter Ballard, PhD
AstraZeneca R&D, Alderley Park, Cheshire, UK

Julian Bertschinger-Ehrler, PhD
CEO, Covagen AG, Zurich-Schlieren, Switzerland

Paul Beswick, BSc, PhD, FRSC
Head, Department of Medicinal Chemistry, Almirall S.A., Barcelona, Spain

Patrick Brassil, PhD
Theravance Inc, South San Francisco, California, USA

Susanne Bredenberg, BSc (Pharm), PhD
Pharmaceutical Science Director, Orexo AB, Uppsala, Sweden

Khanh H Bui, PhD
AstraZeneca R&D, Wilmington, Delaware, USA

David Cronk, CBiol MSB
Senior Director, Biology, BioFocus, Saffron Walden, Essex, UK

Hugues Dolgos, PhD
Global head of DMPK, Merck-Serono R&D, Geneva, Switzerland

Dragan Grabulovski, PhD
CSO, Covagen AG, Zurich-Schlieren, Switzerland

Philip Grubb, MA, BSc, DPhil
Chartered Patent Attorney (UK), European Patent Attorney, Formerly Intellectual Property Counsel, Novartis International, Basel, Switzerland

Inger Hägglöf, MSc (Pharm)
Regulatory Affairs Manager, AstraZeneca AB, Södertälje, Sweden

Raymond G Hill, BPharm, PhD, DSc (Hon), FMedSci
President Emeritus, British Pharmacological Society; Visiting Professor of Pharmacology, Department of Medicine, Imperial College, London; Formerly, Executive Director and Head, Licensing and External Research, Europe, MSD/Merck Research Laboratories

Åsa Holmgren, MSc (Pharm)
Senior Vice President Regulatory Affairs, Orexo AB, Uppsala, Sweden

Charlotte Keywood, MBBS, MRCP, FFPM
Chief Medical Officer, Addex Pharma SA, Plan les Ouates, Switzerland

Vincent Lawton, PhD
Chairman, Aqix Limited, London, UK

Harry LeVine, III, PhD
Associate Professor, Center on Aging, Center for Structural Biology, Department of Molecular and Cellular Biochemistry, University of Kentucky, Lexington, Kentucky, USA

Thomas Lundqvist, MSc (Pharm)
EVP, Orexo AB, Uppsala, Sweden

Paul M Matthews, MA, MD, DPhil, FRCP
Head, Division of Brain Sciences and Professor, Imperial College; Vice President, GlaxoSmithKline Research and Development, Ltd., London, UK

Alan Naylor, BSc, PhD, FRSC
Independent Consultant, Alan Naylor Consultancy Ltd., Royston, UK

Robert McBurney, PhD
Chief Executive Officer, Accelerated Cure Project for Multiple Sclerosis, Waltham, Massachusetts, USA

Carl Petersson, PhD
Principal Scientist, Medicinal Chemistry, CNSP iMed Science Södertälje, AstraZeneca Research and Development, Innovative Medicines, Södertälje, Sweden

Humphrey P Rang, MB BS, MA, DPhil, FMedSci, FRS
President-Elect British Pharmacological Society, Emeritus Professor of Pharmacology, University College, London; Formerly Director, Novartis Institute for Medical Sciences, London

Barry Robson, BSc Hons, PhD, DSc
University Director of Research and Professor of Biostatistics, Epidemiology and Evidence Based Medicine, St. Matthew's University Grand Cayman, Cayman Islands; Distinguished Scientist, Mathematics and Computer Science, University of Wisconsin-Stout, Wisconsin, USA; Chief Scientific Officer, Quantal Semantics Inc., Raleigh, North Carolina, USA; Chief Executive Officer, The Dirac Foundation, Oxfordshire, UK

Anders Tunek, PhD
Senior Principal Scientist, AstraZeneca, Mölndal, Sweden

Peter J H Webborn, PhD
AstraZeneca R&D, Macclesfield, UK

Contents

Section 4: Facts and figures

Section 1

Introduction and background

Chapter 1

The development of the pharmaceutical industry

H P Rang

ANTECEDENTS AND ORIGINS

Our task in this book is to give an account of the principles underlying drug discovery as it happens today, and to provide pointers to the future. The present situation, of course, represents merely the current frame of a long-running movie. To understand the significance of the different elements that appear in the frame, and to predict what is likely to change in the next few frames, we need to know something about what has gone before. In this chapter we give a brief and selective account of some of the events and trends that have shaped the pharmaceutical industry. Most of the action in our metaphorical movie happened in the last century, despite the film having started at the birth of civilization, some 10 000 years ago. The next decade or two will certainly see at least as much change as the past century.

Many excellent and extensive histories of medicine and the pharmaceutical industry have been published, to which readers seeking more detailed information are referred (Mann, 1984; Sneader, 1985; Weatherall, 1990; Porter, 1997; see also Drews, 2000, 2003).

Disease has been recognized as an enemy of humankind since civilization began, and plagues of infectious diseases arrived as soon as humans began to congregate in settlements about 5000 years ago. Early writings on papyrus and clay tablets describe many kinds of disease, and list a wide variety of herbal and other remedies used to treat them. The earliest such document, the famous Ebers papyrus, dating from around 1550BC, describes more than 800 such remedies. Disease was in those times regarded as an affliction sent by the gods; consequently, the remedies were aimed partly at neutralizing or purging the affliction, and partly at appeasing the deities. Despite its essentially theistic basis, early medicine nevertheless discovered, through empiricism and common sense, many plant extracts whose pharmacological properties we recognize and still use today; their active principles include opium alkaloids, ephedrine, emetine, cannabis, senna and many others[1].

In contrast to the ancient Egyptians, who would, one feels, have been completely unsympathetic to medical science had they been time-warped into the 21st century, the ancient Greeks might have felt much more at home in the present era. They sought to understand nature, work out its rules and apply them to alleviate disease, just as we aim to do today. The Hippocratic tradition had little time for theistic explanations. However, the Greeks were not experimenters, and so the basis of Greek medicine remained essentially theoretical. Their theories were philosophical constructs, whose perceived validity rested on their elegance and logical consistency; the idea of testing theory by experiment came much later, and this aspect of present-day science would have found no resonance in ancient Greece. The basic concept of four humours – black bile, yellow bile, blood and phlegm – proved, with the help of Greek reasoning, to be an extremely versatile framework for explaining health and disease. Given the right starting point – cells, molecules and tissues instead of humours – they would quickly have come to terms with modern medicine. From a therapeutic perspective, Greek medicine placed rather little emphasis on herbal remedies; they incorporated earlier teachings on the subject, but made few advances of their own. The Greek traditions formed the basis of the prolific writings of Galen in the 2nd century AD, whose influence dominated the practice of medicine in Europe well into the Renaissance. Other

[1]There were, it should be added, far more – such as extracts of asses' testicles, bats' eyes and crocodile dung – that never found their way into modern pharmacology.

civilizations, notably Indian, Arabic and Chinese, similarly developed their own medical traditions, which – unlike those of the Greeks – still flourish independently of the Western ones.

Despite the emphasis on herbal remedies in these early medical concepts, and growing scientific interest in their use as medicines from the 18th century onwards, it was only in the mid-19th century that chemistry and biology advanced sufficiently to give a scientific basis to drug therapy, and it was not until the beginning of the 20th century that this knowledge actually began to be applied to the discovery of new drugs. In the long interim, the apothecary's trade flourished; closely controlled by guilds and apprenticeship schemes, it formed the supply route for the exotic preparations that were used in treatment. The early development of therapeutics – based, as we have seen, mainly on superstition and on theories that have been swept away by scientific advances – represents prehistory as far as the development of the pharmaceutical industry is concerned, and there are few, if any, traces of it remaining[2].

THERAPEUTICS IN THE 19TH CENTURY

Although preventive medicine had made some spectacular advances, for example in controlling scurvy (Lind, 1763) and in the area of infectious diseases, vaccination (Jenner, 1798), curtailment of the London cholera epidemic of 1854 by turning off the Broad Street Pump (Snow), and control of childbirth fever and surgical infections using antiseptic techniques (Semmelweis, 1861; Lister, 1867), therapeutic medicine was virtually non-existent until the end of the 19th century.

Oliver Wendell Holmes – a pillar of the medical establishment – wrote in 1860: 'I firmly believe that if the whole materia medica, as now used, could be sunk to the bottom of the sea, it would be all the better for mankind – and the worse for the fishes' (see Porter, 1997). This may have been a somewhat ungenerous appraisal, for some contemporary medicines – notably digitalis, famously described by Withering in 1785, extract of willow bark (salicylic acid), and *Cinchona* extract (quinine) – had beneficial effects that were well documented. But on balance, Holmes was right – medicines did more harm than good.

[2]Plenty of traces remain outside the pharmaceutical industry, in the form of a wide variety of 'alternative' and 'complementary' therapeutic procedures, such as herbalism, moxibustion, reflexology and acupuncture, whose underlying principles originated in the prescientific era and remain largely beyond the boundaries of science. It may not be long, given the growing appeal of such approaches in the public's eye, before the mainstream pharmaceutical industry decides that it must follow this trend. That will indeed be a challenge for drug discovery research.

We can obtain an idea of the state of therapeutics at the time from the first edition of the *British Pharmacopoeia*, published in 1864, which lists 311 preparations. Of these, 187 were plant-derived materials, only nine of which were purified substances. Most of the plant products – lemon juice, rose hips, yeast, etc. – lacked any components we would now regard as therapeutically relevant, but some – digitalis, castor oil, ergot, colchicum – were pharmacologically active. Of the 311 preparations, 103 were 'chemicals', mainly inorganic – iodine, ferrous sulfate, sodium bicarbonate, and many toxic salts of bismuth, arsenic, lead and mercury – but also a few synthetic chemicals, such as diethyl ether and chloroform. The remainder comprised miscellaneous materials and a few animal products, such as lard, cantharidin and cochineal.

AN INDUSTRY BEGINS TO EMERGE

For the pharmaceutical industry, the transition from prehistory to actual history occurred late in the 19th century (3Q19C, as managers of today might like to call it), when three essential strands came together. These were: the evolving science of biomedicine (and especially pharmacology); the emergence of synthetic organic chemistry; and the development of a chemical industry in Europe, coupled with a medical supplies trade – the result of buoyant entrepreneurship, mainly in America.

Developments in biomedicine

Science began to be applied wholeheartedly to medicine – as to almost every other aspect of life – in the 19th century. Among the most important milestones from the point of view of drug discovery was the elaboration in 1858 of cell theory, by the German pathologist Rudolf Virchow. Virchow was a remarkable man: pre-eminent as a pathologist, he also designed the Berlin sewage system and instituted hygiene inspections in schools, and later became an active member of the Reichstag. The tremendous reductionist leap of the cell theory gave biology – and the pharmaceutical industry – the scientific foundation it needed. It is only by thinking of living systems in terms of the function of their cells that one can begin to understand how molecules affect them.

A second milestone was the birth of pharmacology as a scientific discipline when the world's first Pharmacological Institute was set up in 1847 at Dorpat by Rudolf Buchheim – literally by Buchheim himself, as the Institute was in his own house and funded by him personally. It gained such recognition that the university built him a new one 13 years later. Buchheim foresaw that pharmacology as a science was needed to exploit the knowledge of physiology, which was being advanced by pioneers such as Magendie and Claude Bernard, and link it to therapeutics.

When one remembers that this was at a time when organic chemistry and physiology were both in their cradles, and therapeutics was ineffectual, Buchheim's vision seems bold, if not slightly crazy. Nevertheless, his Institute was a spectacular success. Although he made no truly seminal discoveries, Buchheim imposed on himself and his staff extremely high standards of experimentation and argument, which eclipsed the empiricism of the old therapeutic principles and attracted some exceptionally gifted students. Among these was the legendary Oswald Schmiedeberg, who later moved to Strasbourg, where he set up an Institute of Pharmacology of unrivalled size and grandeur, which soon became the Mecca for would-be pharmacologists all over the world.

A third milestone came with Louis Pasteur's germ theory of disease, proposed in Paris in 1878. A chemist by training, Pasteur's initial interest was in the process of fermentation of wine and beer, and the souring of milk. He showed, famously, that airborne infection was the underlying cause, and concluded that the air was actually alive with microorganisms. Particular types, he argued, were pathogenic to humans, and accounted for many forms of disease, including anthrax, cholera and rabies. Pasteur successfully introduced several specific immunization procedures to give protection against infectious diseases. Robert Koch, Pasteur's rival and near-contemporary, clinched the infection theory by observing anthrax and other bacilli in the blood of infected animals.

The founder of chemotherapy – some would say the founder of molecular pharmacology – was Paul Ehrlich (see Drews, 2004 for a brief biography). Born in 1854 and trained in pathology, Ehrlich became interested in histological stains and tested a wide range of synthetic chemical dyes that were being produced at that time. He invented 'vital staining' – staining by dyes injected into living animals – and described how the chemical properties of the dyes, particularly their acidity and lipid solubility, influenced the distribution of dye to particular tissues and cellular structures. Thence came the idea of specific binding of molecules to particular cellular components, which directed not only Ehrlich's study of chemotherapeutic agents, but much of pharmacological thinking ever since. 'Receptor' and 'magic bullets' are Ehrlich's terms, though he envisaged receptors as targets for toxins, rather than physiological mediators. Working in Koch's Institute, Ehrlich developed diphtheria antitoxin for clinical use, and put forward a theory of antibody action based on specific chemical recognition of microbial macromolecules, work for which he won the 1908 Nobel Prize. Ehrlich became director of his own Institute in Frankfurt, close to a large dye works, and returned to his idea of using the specific binding properties of synthetic dyes to develop selective antimicrobial drugs.

At this point, we interrupt the biological theme at the end of the 19th century, with Ehrlich in full flood, on the verge of introducing the first designer drugs, and turn to the chemical and commercial developments that were going on simultaneously.

Developments in chemistry

The first synthetic chemicals to be used for medical purposes were, ironically, not therapeutic agents at all, but anaesthetics. Diethyl ether ('sweet oil of vitriol') was first made and described in 1540. Early in the 19th century, it and nitrous oxide (prepared by Humphrey Davy in 1799 and found – by experiments on himself – to have stupefying properties) were used to liven up parties and sideshows; their usefulness as surgical anaesthetics was demonstrated, amid much controversy, only in the 1840s[3], by which time chloroform had also made its appearance. Synthetic chemistry at the time could deal only with very simple molecules, made by recipe rather than reason, as our understanding of molecular structure was still in its infancy. The first therapeutic drug to come from synthetic chemistry was amyl nitrite, prepared in 1859 by Guthrie and introduced, on the basis of its vasodilator activity, for treating angina by Brunton in 1864 – the first example of a drug born in a recognizably 'modern' way, through the application of synthetic chemistry, physiology and clinical medicine. This was a landmark indeed, for it was nearly 40 years before synthetic chemistry made any further significant contribution to therapeutics, and not until well into the 20th century that physiological and pharmacological knowledge began to be applied to the invention of new drugs.

It was during the latter half of the 19th century that the foundations of synthetic organic chemistry were laid, the impetus coming from work on aniline, a copious byproduct of the coal-tar industry. An English chemist, Perkin, who in 1856 succeeded in preparing from aniline a vivid purple compound, *mauvein*, laid the foundations. This was actually a chemical accident, as Perkin's aim had been to synthesize quinine. Nevertheless, the discovery gave birth to the synthetic dyestuffs industry, which played a major part in establishing the commercial potential of synthetic organic chemistry – a technology which later became a lynchpin of the evolving pharmaceutical industry. A systematic approach to organic synthesis went hand in hand with improved understanding of chemical structure. Crucial steps were the establishment of the rules of chemical equivalence (valency), and the elucidation of the structure of benzene by Von Kekulé in 1865. The first representation of a structural formula depicting the bonds

[3]An event welcomed, in his inimitable prose style, by Oliver Wendell Holmes in 1847: 'The knife is searching for disease, the pulleys are dragging back dislocated limbs – Nature herself is working out the primal curse which doomed the tenderest of her creatures to the sharpest of her trials, but the fierce extremity of suffering has been steeped in the waters of forgetfulness, and the deepest furrow in the knotted brow of agony has been smoothed forever'.

between atoms in two dimensions, based on valency rules, also appeared in 1865[4].

The reason why Perkin had sought to synthesize quinine was that the drug, prepared from *Cinchona* bark, was much in demand for the treatment of malaria, one of whose effects is to cause high fever. So quinine was (wrongly, as it turned out) designated as an antipyretic drug, and used to treat fevers of all kinds. Because quinine itself could not be synthesized, fragments of the molecule were made instead; these included antipyrine, phenacetin and various others, which were introduced with great success in the 1880s and 1890s. These were the first drugs to be 'designed' on chemical principles[5].

The apothecaries' trade

Despite the lack of efficacy of the pharmaceutical preparations that were available in the 19th century, the apothecary's trade flourished; then, as now, physicians felt themselves obliged to issue prescriptions to satisfy the expectations of their patients for some token of remedial intent. Early in the 19th century, when many small apothecary businesses existed to satisfy the demand on a local basis, a few enterprising chemists undertook the task of isolating the active substances from these plant extracts. This was a bold and inspired leap, and one that attracted a good deal of ridicule. Although the old idea of 'signatures', which held that plants owed their medicinal properties to their biological characteristics[6], was falling into disrepute, few were willing to accept that individual chemical substances could be responsible for the effects these plants produced, such as emesis, narcosis, purgation or fever. The trend began with Friedrich Sertürner, a junior apothecary in Westphalia, who in 1805 isolated and purified morphine, barely surviving a test of its potency on himself. This was the first 'alkaloid', so named because of its ability to neutralize acids and form salts. This discovery led to the isolation of several more plant alkaloids, including emetine, strychnine, caffeine and quinine, mainly by two remarkably prolific chemists, Caventou and Pelletier, working in Paris in the period 1810–1825. The recognition that medicinal plants owed their properties to their individual chemical constituents, rather than to some intangible property associated with their living nature, marks a critical point in the history of the pharmaceutical industry. It can be seen as the point of origin of two of the three strands from which the industry grew – namely the beginnings of the 'industrialization' of the apothecary's trade, and the emergence of the science of pharmacology. And by revealing the chemical nature of medicinal preparations, it hinted at the future possibility of making medicines artificially. Even though, at that time, synthetic organic chemistry was barely out of its cradle, these discoveries provided the impetus that later caused the chemical industry to turn, at a very early stage in its history, to making drugs.

The first local apothecary business to move into large-scale production and marketing of pharmaceuticals was the old-established Darmstadt firm Merck, founded in 1668. This development, in 1827, was stimulated by the advances in purification of natural products. Merck was closely followed in this astute business move by other German- and Swiss-based apothecary businesses, giving rise to some which later also became giant pharmaceutical companies, such as Schering and Boehringer. The American pharmaceutical industry emerged in the middle of the 19th century. Squibb began in 1858, with ether as its main product. Soon after came Parke Davis (1866) and Eli Lilly (1876); both had a broader franchise as manufacturing chemists. In the 1890s Parke Davis became the world's largest pharmaceutical company, one of whose early successes was to purify crystalline adrenaline from adrenal glands and sell it in ampoules for injection. The US scientific community contested the adoption of the word 'adrenaline' as a trade name, but industry won the day and the scientists were forced to call the hormone 'epinephrine'.

The move into pharmaceuticals was also followed by several chemical companies such as Bayer, Hoechst, Agfa, Sandoz, Geigy and others, which began, not as apothecaries, but as dyestuffs manufacturers. The dyestuffs industry at that time was also based largely on plant products, which had to be refined, and were sold in relatively small quantities, so the commercial parallels with the pharmaceutical industry were plain. Dye factories, for obvious reasons, were usually located close to large rivers, a fact that accounts for the present-day location of many large pharmaceutical companies in Europe. As we shall see, the link with the dyestuffs industry later came to have much more profound implications for drug discovery.

From about 1870 onwards – following the crucial discovery by Kekulé of the structure of benzene – the dyestuffs industry turned increasingly to synthetic chemistry as a source of new compounds, starting with aniline-based dyes. A glance through any modern pharmacopoeia will show the overwhelming preponderance of synthetic

---

[4]Its author, the Edinburgh chemist Alexander Crum Brown, was also a pioneer of pharmacology, and was the first person to use a chemical reaction – quaternization of amines – to modify naturally occurring substances such as strychnine and morphine. With Thomas Fraser, in 1868, he found that this drastically altered their pharmacological properties, changing strychnine, for example, from a convulsant to a paralysing agent. Although they knew neither the structures of these molecules nor the mechanisms by which they acted, theirs was the first systematic study of structure–activity relationships.
[5]These drugs belong pharmacologically to the class of non-steroidal anti-inflammatories (NSAIDs), the most important of which is aspirin (acetylsalicylic acid). Ironically, aspirin itself had been synthesized many years earlier, in 1855, with no pharmacological purpose in mind. Aspirin was not developed commercially until 1899, subsequently generating huge revenues for Bayer, the company responsible.
[6]According to this principle, pulmonaria (lungwort) was used to treat respiratory disorders because its leaves resembled lungs, saffron to treat jaundice, and so on.

aromatic compounds, based on the benzene ring structure, among the list of useful drugs. Understanding the nature of aromaticity was critical. Though we might be able to dispense with the benzene ring in some fields of applied chemistry, such as fuels, lubricants, plastics or detergents, its exclusion would leave the pharmacopoeia bankrupt. Many of these dyestuffs companies saw the potential of the medicines business from 1880 onwards, and moved into the area hitherto occupied by the apothecaries. The result was the first wave of companies ready to apply chemical technology to the production of medicines. Many of these founder companies remained in business for years. It was only recently, when their cannibalistic urges took over in the race to become large, that mergers and takeovers caused many names to disappear.

Thus the beginnings of a recognizable pharmaceutical industry date from about 1860–1880, its origins being in the apothecaries and medical supplies trades on the one hand, and the dyestuffs industry on the other. In those early days, however, they had rather few products to sell; these were mainly inorganic compounds of varying degrees of toxicity and others best described as concoctions. Holmes (see above) dismissed the pharmacopoeia in 1860 as worse than useless.

To turn this ambitious new industry into a source of human benefit, rather than just corporate profit, required two things. First, it had to embrace the principles of biomedicine, and in particular pharmacology, which provided a basis for understanding how disease and drugs, respectively, affect the function of living organisms. Second, it had to embrace the principles of chemistry, going beyond the descriptors of colour, crystallinity taste, volatility, etc., towards an understanding of the structure and properties of molecules, and how to make them in the laboratory. As we have seen, both of these fields had made tremendous progress towards the end of the 19th century, so at the start of the 20th century the time was right for the industry to seize its chance. Nevertheless, several decades passed before the inventions coming from the industry began to make a major impact on the treatment of disease.

The industry enters the 20th century

By the end of the 19th century various synthetic drugs had been made and tested, including the 'antipyretics' (see above) and also various central nervous system depressants. Chemical developments based on chloroform had produced chloral hydrate, the first non-volatile CNS depressant, which was in clinical use for many years as a hypnotic drug. Independently, various compounds based on urea were found to act similarly, and von Mering followed this lead to produce the first barbiturate, *barbitone* (since renamed barbital), which was introduced in 1903 by Bayer and gained widespread clinical use as a hypnotic, tranquillizer and antiepileptic drug – the first blockbuster. Almost simultaneously, Einthorn in Munich synthesized *procaine*, the first synthetic local anaesthetic drug, which followed the naturally occurring alkaloid cocaine. The local anaesthetic action of cocaine on the eye was discovered by Sigmund Freud and his ophthalmologist colleague Koeller in the late 19th century, and was heralded as a major advance for ophthalmic surgery. After several chemists had tried, with limited success, to make synthetic compounds with the same actions, procaine was finally produced and introduced commercially in 1905 by Hoechst. Barbitone and procaine were triumphs for chemical ingenuity, but owed little or nothing to physiology, or, indeed, to pharmacology. The physiological site or sites of action of barbiturates remain unclear to this day, and their mechanism of action at the molecular level was unknown until the 1980s.

From this stage, where chemistry began to make an impact on drug discovery, up to the last quarter of the 20th century, when molecular biology began to emerge as a dominant technology, we can discern three main routes by which new drugs were discovered, namely chemistry-driven approaches, target-directed approaches, and accidental clinical discoveries. In many of the most successful case histories, graphically described by Weatherall (1990), the three were closely interwoven. The remarkable family of diverse and important drugs that came from the original sulfonamide, lead, described below, exemplifies this pattern very well.

Chemistry-driven drug discovery

Synthetic chemistry

The pattern of drug discovery driven by synthetic chemistry – with biology often struggling to keep up – became the established model in the early part of the 20th century, and prevailed for at least 50 years. The balance of research in the pharmaceutical industry up to the 1970s placed chemistry clearly as the key discipline in drug discovery, the task of biologists being mainly to devise and perform assays capable of revealing possible useful therapeutic activity among the many anonymous white powders that arrived for testing. Research management in the industry was largely in the hands of chemists. This strategy produced many successes, including benzodiazepine tranquillizers, several antiepileptic drugs, antihypertensive drugs, antidepressants and antipsychotic drugs. The surviving practice of classifying many drugs on the basis of their chemical structure (e.g. phenothiazines, benzodiazepines, thiazides, etc.), rather than on the more logical basis of their site or mode of action, stems from this era. The development of antiepileptic drugs exemplifies this approach well. Following the success of barbital (see above) several related compounds were made, including the phenyl derivative *phenobarbital*, first made in 1911. This proved to be an effective hypnotic (i.e. sleep-inducing) drug, helpful in allowing peaceful nights in a ward full of restive patients. By chance, it was found by a German doctor also to reduce the frequency of seizures when tested in epileptic patients – an example of clinical serendipity (see below) – and it became widely used for this purpose, being much more effective in this regard than barbital itself. About 20 years later, Putnam, working in Boston, developed an animal model whereby epilepsy-like seizures could be induced in mice by electrical stimulation of the brain via extracranial electrodes. This simple model allowed hundreds of compounds to be tested for potential antiepileptic activity. *Phenytoin* was an early success of this programme, and several more compounds followed, as chemists from several companies embarked on synthetic programmes. None of this relied at all on an understanding of the mechanism of action of these compounds – which is still controversial; all that was needed were teams of green-fingered chemists, and a robust assay that predicted efficacy in the clinic.

Natural product chemistry

We have mentioned the early days of pharmacology, with its focus on plant-derived materials, such as *atropine, tubocurarine, strychnine, digitalis* and *ergot alkaloids*, which were almost the only drugs that existed until well into the 20th century. Despite the rise of synthetic chemistry, natural products remain a significant source of new drugs, particularly in the field of chemotherapy, but also in other applications. Following the discovery of *penicillin* by Fleming in 1929 – described by Mann (1984) as 'the most important medical discovery of all time' – and its development as an antibiotic for clinical use by Chain and Florey in 1938, an intense search was undertaken for antibacterial compounds produced by fungi and other microorganisms, which yielded many useful antibiotics, including *chloramphenicol* (1947), *tetracyclines* (1948), *streptomycin* (1949) and others. The same fungal source that yielded streptomycin also produced *actinomycin D*, used in cancer chemotherapy. Higher plants have continued to yield useful drugs, including *vincristine* and *vinblastine* (1958), and *paclitaxel* (Taxol, 1971).

Outside the field of chemotherapy, successful drugs derived from natural products include *ciclosporin* (1972) and *tacrolimus* (1993), both of which come from fungi and are used to prevent transplant rejection. Soon after came *mevastatin* (1976), another fungal metabolite, which was the first of the 'statin' series of cholesterol-lowering drugs that act by inhibiting the enzyme HMG CoA reductase.

Overall, the pharmaceutical industry continues to have something of a love–hate relationship with natural products. They often have weird and wonderful structures that cause hardened chemists to turn pale; they are often near-impossible to synthesize, troublesome to produce from natural sources, and 'optimizing' such molecules to make them suitable for therapeutic use is akin to remodelling Westminster Abbey to improve its acoustics. But the fact remains that Nature unexpectedly provides some of our most useful drugs, and most of its potential remains untapped.

Target-directed drug discovery

Although chemistry was the pre-eminent discipline in drug discovery until the 1970s, the seeds of the biological revolution had long since been sown, and within the chemistry-led culture of the pharmaceutical industry these developments began to bear fruit in certain areas. This happened most notably in the field of chemotherapy, where Ehrlich played such an important role as the first 'modernist' who defined the principles of drug specificity in terms of a specific interaction between the drug molecule and a target molecule – the 'receptive substance' – in the organism, an idea summarized in his famous Latin catchphrase *Corpora non agunt nisi fixata*. Although we now take it for granted that the chemical nature of the target molecule, as well as that of the drug molecule, determines what effects a drug will produce, nobody before Ehrlich had envisaged drug action in this way[7]. By linking chemistry and biology, Ehrlich effectively set the stage for drug discovery in the modern style. But despite Ehrlich's seminal role in the evolution of the pharmaceutical industry, discoveries in his favourite field of endeavour, chemotherapy, remained for many years empirical rather than target directed[8].

The fact is that Ehrlich's preoccupation with the binding of chemical dyes, as exemplified by biological stains, for specific constituents of cells and tissues, turned out to be misplaced, and not applicable to the problem of achieving selective toxicity. Although he soon came to realize that the dye-binding moieties of cells were not equivalent to the supposed drug-binding moieties, neither he nor anyone else succeeded in identifying the latter and using them as defined targets for new compounds. The history of successes in the field of chemotherapy prior to the antibiotic era, some of which are listed in Table 1.1,

---

[7]Others came close at around the same time, particularly the British physiologist J. N. Langley (1905), who interpreted the neuromuscular blocking effect of 'curari' in terms of its interaction with a specific 'receptive substance' at the junction between the nerve terminal and the muscle fibre. This was many years before chemical transmission at this junction was discovered. Langley's student, A. V. Hill (1909), first derived the equations based on the Law of Mass Action, which describe how binding varies with drug concentration. Hill's quantitative theory later formed the basis of 'receptor theory', elaborated by pharmacologists from A. J. Clark (1926) onwards. Although this quantitative approach underlies much of our current thinking about drug–receptor interactions, it was Ehrlich's more intuitive approach that played the major part in shaping drug discovery in the early days.

[8]Even now, important new chemotherapeutic drugs, such as the taxanes, continue to emerge through a combination of a chance biological discovery and high-level chemistry.

Table 1.1 Examples of drugs from different sources: natural products, synthetic chemistry and biopharmaceuticals

Natural products	Synthetic chemistry	Biopharmaceuticals produced by recombinant DNA technology
Antibiotics (penicillin, streptomycin, tetracyclines, cephalosporins, etc.)	Early successes include: Antiepileptic drugs	Human insulin (the first biotech product, registered 1982)
Anticancer drugs (doxorubicin, bleomycin, actinomycin, vincristine, vinblastine, paclitaxel (Taxol), etc.)	Antihypertensive drugs Antimetabolites Barbiturates	Human growth hormone α-interferon, γ-interferon Hepatitis B vaccine
Atropine, hyoscine	Bronchodilators	Tissue plasminogen activator (t-PA)
Ciclosporin	Diuretics	Hirudin
Cocaine	Local anaesthetics	Blood clotting factors
Colchicine	Sulfonamides	Erythropoietin
Digitalis (digoxin)	*[Since c.1950, synthetic chemistry has accounted for the great majority of new drugs]*	G-CSF, GM-CSF
Ephedrine		
Heparin		
Human growth hormone*		
Insulin (porcine, bovine)*		
Opium alkaloids (morphine, papaverine)		
Physostigmine		
Rauwolfia alkaloids (reserpine)		
Statins		
Streptokinase		
Tubocurarine		
Vaccines		

*Now replaced by material prepared by recombinant DNA technology.
G-CSF, granulocyte colony-stimulating factor; GM-CSF, granulocyte macrophage colony-stimulating factor.

actually represents a series of striking achievements in synthetic chemistry, coupled to the development of assay systems in animals, according to the chemistry-led model that we have already discussed. The popular image of 'magic bullets' – a phrase famously coined by Ehrlich – designed to home in, like cruise missiles, on defined targets is actually a misleading one in the context of the early days of chemotherapy, but there is no doubt that Ehrlich's thinking prepared the ground for the steady advance of target-directed approaches to drug discovery, a trend that, from the 1950s onwards, steadily shifted the industry's focus from chemistry to biology (Maxwell and Eckhardt, 1990; Lednicer, 1993). A few selected case histories exemplify this general trend.

The sulfonamide story

Ehrlich's major triumph was the discovery in 1910 of *Salvarsan* (Compound 606), the first compound to treat syphilis effectively, which remained in use for 40 years. Still, bacterial infections, such as pneumonia and wound infections, proved resistant to chemical treatments for many years, despite strenuous effort on the part of the pharmaceutical industry. In 1927, IG Farbenindustrie,

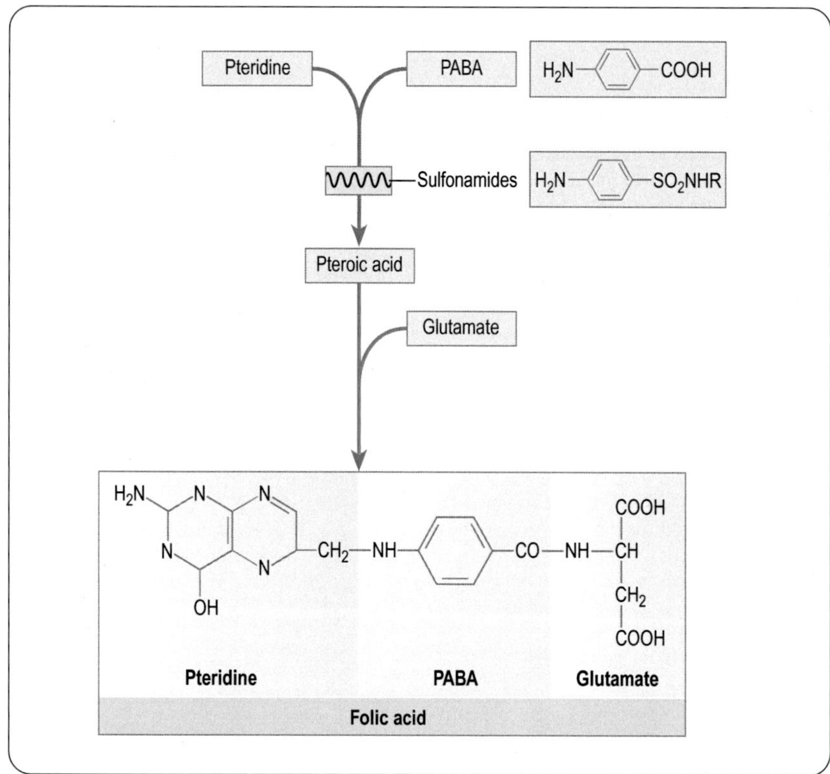

Fig. 1.1 Folic acid synthesis and PABA.

which had a long-standing interest in discovering antimicrobial drugs, appointed Gerhard Domagk to direct their research. Among the various leads that he followed was a series of azo dyes, included among which were some sulfonamide derivatives (a modification introduced earlier into dyestuffs to improve their affinity for certain fibres). These were much more effective in animals, and less toxic, than anything that had gone before, and *Prontosil* – a dark-red azo dye – was introduced in 1935. In the same year, it saved the life of Domagk's daughter, who developed septicaemia after a needle prick. It was soon discovered that the azo linkage in the Prontosil molecule was rapidly cleaved in the body, yielding the colourless compound *sulfanilamide*, which accounted for the antibacterial effect of Prontosil[9].

With chemistry still firmly in the driving seat, and little concern about mechanisms or targets, many sulfonamides were made in the next few years and they dramatically improved the prognosis of patients suffering from infectious diseases.

The mechanistic light began to dawn in 1940, when D. D. Woods, a microbiologist in Oxford, discovered that the antibacterial effect of sulfonamides was antagonized by *p*-aminobenzoic acid (PABA), a closely related compound and a precursor in the biosynthesis of folic acid (Figure 1.1). Bacteria, but not eukaryotic cells, have to synthesize their own folic acid to support DNA synthesis. Woods deduced that sulfonamides compete with PABA for a target enzyme, now known to be dihydropteroate synthase, and thus prevent folic acid synthesis.

The discovery of sulfonamides and the elucidation of their mechanism of action had great repercussions, scientifically as well as clinically. In the drug discovery field, it set off two major lines of inquiry. First, the sulfonamide structure proved to be a rich source of molecules with many different, and useful, pharmacological properties – an exuberant vindication of the chemistry-led approach to drug discovery. Second, attacking the folic acid pathway proved to be a highly successful strategy for producing therapeutically useful drugs – a powerful boost for the 'targeteers', who were still few in number at this time.

[9]Sulfanilamide, a known compound, could not be patented, and so many companies soon began to make and sell it in various formulations. In 1937 about 80 people who took the drug died as a result of solvent-induced liver and kidney damage. It was this accident that led to the US Food and Drug Act, with the Food & Drug Administration (FDA) to oversee it (see Chapter 20).

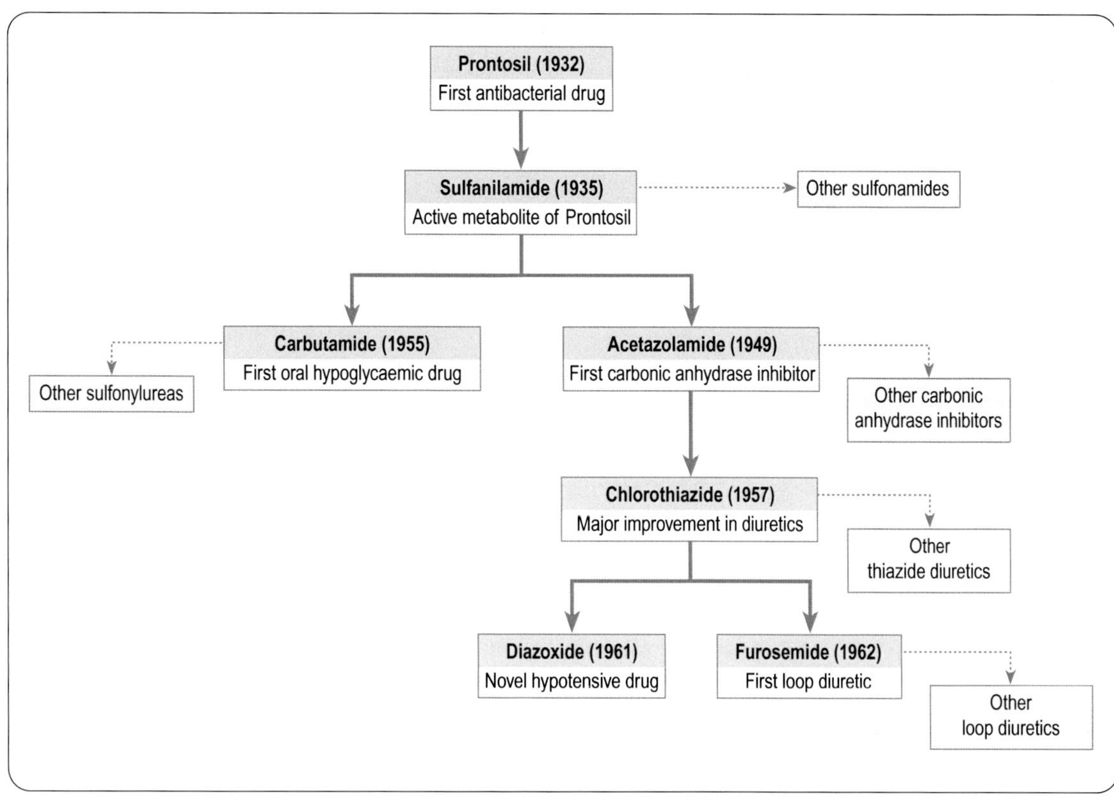

Fig. 1.2 Sulfonamide dynasty.

The chemical dynasty originating with sulfanilamide is shown in Figure 1.2. An early spin-off came from the clinical observation that some sulfonamides produced an alkaline diuresis, associated with an increased excretion of sodium bicarbonate in the urine. Carbonic anhydrase, an enzyme which catalyses the interconversion of carbon dioxide and carbonic acid, was described in 1940, and its role in renal bicarbonate excretion was discovered a few years later, which prompted the finding that some, but not all, sulfonamides inhibit this enzyme. Modification of the sulfonamide structure led eventually to *acetazolamide* the first commercially available carbonic anhydrase inhibitor, as a diuretic in 1952. Following the diuretic trail led in turn to *chlorothiazide* (1957), the first of the thiazide diuretics, which, though devoid of carbonic anhydrase inhibitory activity, was much more effective than acetazolamide in increasing sodium excretion, and much safer than the earlier mercurial diuretics, which had until then been the best drugs available for treating oedema associated with heart failure and other conditions. Still further modifications led first to *furosemide* (1962) and later to *bumetanide* (1984), which were even more effective than the thiazides in producing a rapid diuresis – 'torrential' being the adjective applied by clinicians with vivid imaginations. Other modifications of the thiazide structures led to the accidental but important discovery of a series of hypotensive vasodilator drugs, such as *hydralazine* and *diazoxide*. In yet another development, *carbutamide*, one of the sulfonamides synthesized by Boehringer in 1954 as part of an antibacterial drug programme, was found accidentally to cause hypoglycaemia. This drug was the first of the sulfonylurea series, from which many further derivatives, such as *tolbutamide* and *glibenclamide*, were produced and used successfully to treat diabetes. All of these products of the sulfonamide dynasty are widely used today. Their chemical relationship to sulfonamides is clear, though none of them has antibacterial activity. Their biochemical targets in smooth muscle, the kidney, the pancreas and elsewhere, are all different. Chemistry, not biology, was the guiding principle in their discovery and synthesis.

Target-directed approaches to drug design have played a much more significant role in areas other than antibacterial chemotherapy, the approaches being made possible by advances on two important fronts, separated, as it happens, by the Atlantic Ocean. In the United States, the antimetabolite principle, based on interfering with defined metabolic pathways, proved to be highly successful, due largely to the efforts of George Hitchings and Gertrude Elion at

Burroughs Wellcome. In Europe, drug discovery took its lead more from physiology than biochemistry, and sprung from advances in knowledge of chemical transmitters and their receptors. The names of Henry Dale and James Black deserve special mention here.

Hitchings and Elion and the antimetabolite principle

George Hitchings and Gertrude Elion came together in 1944 in the biochemistry department of Burroughs Wellcome in Tuckahoe, New York. Their biochemical interest lay in the synthesis of folic acid, based on the importance of this pathway for the action of sulfonamides, and they set about synthesizing potential 'antimetabolites' of purines and pyrimidines as chemotherapeutic agents. At the time, it was known that this pathway was important for DNA synthesis, but the role of DNA in cell function was uncertain. It turned out to be an inspired choice, and theirs was one of the first drug discovery programmes to focus on a biochemical pathway, rather than on a series of chemical compounds[10].

Starting from a series of purine and pyrimidine analogues, which had antibacterial activity, Hitchings and Elion identified a key enzyme in the folic acid pathway, namely dihydrofolate reductase, which was necessary for DNA synthesis and was inhibited by many of their antibacterial pyrimidine analogues. Because all cells, not just bacteria, use this reaction to make DNA, they wondered why the drugs showed selectivity in their ability to block cell division, and found that the enzyme showed considerable species variation in its susceptibility to inhibitors. This led them to seek inhibitors that would selectively attack bacteria, protozoa and human neoplasms, which they achieved with great success. Drugs to emerge from this programme included the antituberculosis drug *pyrimethamine*, the antibacterial *trimethoprim*, and the anticancer drug *6-mercaptopurine*, as well as *azathioprine*, an immunosuppressant drug that was later widely used to prevent transplant rejection. Another spin-off from the work of Hitchings and Elion was *allopurinol*, an inhibitor of purine synthesis that is used in the treatment of gout. Later on, Elion – her enthusiasm for purines and pyrimidines undiminished – led the research group which in 1977 discovered one of the first effective antiviral drugs, *aciclovir*, an inhibitor of DNA polymerase, and later the first antiretroviral drug, *zidovudine* (AZT), which inhibits reverse transcriptase. Hitchings and Elion, by focusing on the metabolic pathways involved in DNA synthesis, invented an extraordinary range of valuable therapeutic drugs, an achievement unsurpassed in the history of drug discovery.

[10]They were not alone. In the 1940s, a group at Lederle laboratories made *aminopterin* and *methotrexate*, folic acid antagonists which proved effective in treating leukaemia.

James Black and receptor-targeted drugs

As already mentioned, the concept of 'receptors' as recognition sites for hormones and other physiological mediators came from J. N. Langley's analysis of the mechanism of action of 'curari'. Henry Dale's work on the distinct 'muscarinic' and 'nicotinic' actions of acetylcholine also pointed to the existence of two distinct types of cholinergic receptor, though Dale himself dismissed the receptor concept as an abstract and unhelpful cloak for ignorance. During the 1920s and 1930s, major discoveries highlighting the role of chemical mediators were made by physiologists, including the discovery of insulin, adrenal steroids and several neurotransmitters, and the realization that chemical signalling was crucial for normal function focused attention on the receptor mechanisms needed to decode these signals. Pharmacologists, particularly A. J. Clark, J. H. Gaddum and H. O. Schild, applied the Law of Mass Action to put ligand–receptor interactions on a quantitative basis. Schild's studies on drug antagonism in particular, which allowed the binding affinity of competitive antagonists to receptors to be estimated from pharmacological experiments, were an important step forward, which provided the first – and still widely used – quantitative basis for classifying drug receptors. On the basis of such quantitative principles, R. P. Ahlquist in 1948 proposed the existence of two distinct classes of adrenergic receptor, α and β, which accounted for the varied effects of epinephrine and norepinephrine on the cardiovascular system. This discovery inspired James Black, working in the research laboratories of Imperial Chemical Industries in the UK, to seek antagonists that would act selectively on β-adrenoceptors and thus block the effects of epinephrine on the heart, which were thought to be harmful in patients with coronary disease. His chemical starting point was *dichloroisoprenaline*, which had been found by Slater in 1957 to block the relaxant effects of epinephrine on bronchial smooth muscle – of no interest to Slater at the time, as he was looking for compounds with the opposite effect. The result of Black's efforts was the first β-adrenoceptor blocking drug, *pronethalol* (1960), which had the desired effects in humans but was toxic. It was quickly followed by *propranolol* (registered in 1964[11]) – one of the earliest blockbusters, which found many important applications in cardiovascular medicine. This was the first time that a receptor, identified pharmacologically, had been deliberately targeted in a drug discovery project.

Black, after moving to Smith Kline and French, went on from this success to look for novel histamine antagonists

[11]Ironically, propranolol had been made in 1959 in the laboratories of Boehringer Ingelheim, as part of a different, chemistry-led project. Only when linked to its target could the clinical potential of propranolol be revealed – chemistry alone was not enough!

that would block the stimulatory effect of histamine on gastric acid secretion, this effect being resistant to the then-known antihistamine drugs. The result of this project, in which the chemistry effort proved much tougher than the β-adrenoceptor antagonist project, was the first H_2-receptor antagonist, *burimamide* (1972). This compound was a major clinical advance, being the first effective drug for treating peptic ulcers, but (like pronethalol) was quickly withdrawn because of toxicity to be replaced by *cimetidine* (1976). In 1988 Black, along with Hitchings and Elion, was awarded the Nobel Prize.

Black's work effectively opened up the field of receptor pharmacology as an approach to drug discovery, and the pharmaceutical industry quickly moved in to follow his example. Lookalike β-adrenoceptor antagonists and H_2-receptor antagonists followed rapidly during the 1970s and 1980s, and many other receptors were set up as targets for potential therapeutic agents, based on essentially the same approach – though with updated technology – that Black and his colleagues had introduced (Page et al., 2011; Walker, 2011).

Drews (2000) estimated that of 483 identified targets on which the current set of approved drugs act, G-protein-coupled receptors – of which β-adrenoceptors and H_2-receptors are typical examples – account for 45%. Many other successful drugs have resulted from target-directed projects along the lines pioneered by Black and his colleagues. In recent years, of course, receptors have changed from being essentially figments in an operational scheme devised by pharmacologists to explain their findings, to being concrete molecular entities that can be labelled, isolated as proteins, cloned and expressed, just like many other proteins. As we shall see in later chapters, these advances have completely transformed the techniques employed in drug discovery research.

Accidental clinical discoveries

Another successful route to the discovery of new drugs has been through observations made in the clinic. Until drug discovery became an intentional activity, such serendipitous observations were the only source of knowledge. Withering's discovery in 1785 of the efficacy of digitalis in treating dropsy, and Wenkebach's discovery in 1914 of the antidysrhythmic effect of quinine, when he treated a patient with malaria who also happened to suffer from atrial tachycardia, are two of many examples where the clinical efficacy of plant-derived agents has been discovered by highly observant clinicians. More recently, clinical benefit of unexpected kinds has been discovered with synthetic compounds developed for other purposes. In 1937, for example, Bradley tried *amphetamine* as a means of alleviating the severe headache suffered by children after lumbar puncture (spinal tap) on the grounds that the drug's cardiovascular effects might prove beneficial. The headache was not alleviated, but Bradley noticed that the children became much less agitated. From this chance observation he went on to set up one of the first controlled clinical trials, which demonstrated unequivocally that amphetamine had a calming effect – quite unexpected for a drug known to have stimulant effects in other circumstances. From this developed the widespread use, validated by numerous controlled clinical trials, of amphetamine-like drugs, particularly *methylphenidate* (Ritalin) to treat attention deficit hyperactivity disorder (ADHD) in children. Other well-known examples include the discovery of the antipsychotic effects of phenothiazines by Laborit in 1949. Laborit was a naval surgeon, concerned that patients were dying from 'surgical shock' – circulatory collapse resulting in irreversible organ failure – after major operations. Thinking that histamine might be involved, he tested the antihistamine *promethazine* combined with autonomic blocking drugs to prevent this cardiovascular reaction. Although it was ineffective in treating shock, promethazine caused some sedation and Laborit tried some chemically related sedatives, notably *promazine*, which had little antihistamine activity. Patients treated with it fared better during surgery, but Laborit particularly noticed that they appeared much calmer postoperatively He therefore persuaded his psychiatrist colleagues to test the drug on psychotic patients, tests that quickly revealed the drug's antipsychotic effects and led to the development of the antipsychotic *chlorpromazine*. In a sequel, other phenothiazine-like tricyclic compounds were tested for antipsychotic activity but were found accidentally to relieve the symptoms of depression. After Bradley and Laborit, psychiatrists had become alert to looking for the unexpected.

Astute clinical observation has revealed many other unexpected therapeutic effects, for example the efficacy of various antidepressant and antiepileptic drugs in treating certain intractable pain states.

The regulatory process

In the mid-19th century restrictions on the sale of poisonous substances were imposed in the USA and UK, but it was not until the early 1900s that any system of 'prescription-only' medicines was introduced, requiring approval by a medical practitioner. Soon afterwards, restrictions began to be imposed on what 'cures' could be claimed in advertisements for pharmaceutical products and what information had to be given on the label; legislation evolved at a leisurely pace. Most of the concern was with controlling frankly poisonous or addictive substances or contaminants, not with the efficacy and possible harmful effects of new drugs.

In 1937, the use of diethylene glycol as a solvent for a sulfonamide preparation caused 107 deaths in the USA, and a year later the 1906 Food and Drugs Act was revised, requiring safety to be demonstrated before new products could be marketed, and also allowing federal inspection of manufacturing facilities. The requirement for proven efficacy, as well as safety, was added in the Kefauver–Harris amendment in 1962.

In Europe, preoccupied with the political events in the first half of the century, matters of drug safety and efficacy were a minor concern, and it was not until the mid-1960s, in the wake of the thalidomide disaster – a disaster averted in the USA by an assiduous officer, who used the provisions of the 1938 Food and Drugs Act to delay licensing approval – that the UK began to follow the USA's lead in regulatory laws. Until then, the ability of drugs to do harm – short of being frankly poisonous or addictive – was not really appreciated, most of the concern having been about contaminants. In 1959, when thalidomide was first put on the market by the German company Chemie Grünenthal, regulatory controls did not exist in Europe: it was up to the company to decide how much research was needed to satisfy itself that the drug was safe and effective. Grünenthal made a disastrously wrong judgement (see Sjöstrom and Nilsson, 1972, for a full account), which resulted in an estimated 10 000 cases of severe congenital malformation following the company's specific recommendation that the drug was suitable for use by pregnant women. This single event caused an urgent reappraisal, leading to the introduction of much tighter government controls.

In the UK, the Committee on the Safety of Drugs was established in 1963. For the first time, as in the USA, all new drugs (including new mixtures and formulations) had to be submitted for approval before clinical trials could begin, and before they could be marketed. Legally, companies could proceed even if the Committee did not approve, but very few chose to do so. This loophole was closed by the Medicines Act (1968), which made it illegal to proceed with trials or the release of a drug without approval. Initially, safety alone was the criterion for approval; in 1970, under the Medicines Act, evidence of efficacy was added to the criteria for approval. It was the realization that all drugs, not just poisons or contaminants, have the potential to cause harm that made it essential to seek proof of therapeutic efficacy to ensure that the net effect of a new drug was beneficial.

In the decade leading up to 1970, the main planks in the regulatory platform – evidence of safety, efficacy and chemical purity – were in place in most developed countries. Subsequently, the regulations have been adjusted in various minor ways, and adopted with local variations in most countries.

A progressive tightening of the restrictions on the licensing of new drugs continued for about two decades after the initial shock of thalidomide, as public awareness of the harmful effects of drugs became heightened, and the regulatory bodies did their best to respond to public demand for assurance that new drugs were 'completely safe'. The current state of licensing regulations is described in Chapter 20.

CONCLUDING REMARKS

In this chapter we have followed the evolution of ideas and technologies that have led to the state of drug discovery research that existed circa 1970. The main threads, which came together, were:

- Clinical medicine, by far the oldest of the antecedents, which relied largely on herbal remedies right up to the 20th century
- Pharmacy, which began with the apothecary trade in the 17th century, set up to serve the demand for herbal preparations
- Organic chemistry, beginning in the mid-19th century and evolving into medicinal chemistry via dyestuffs
- Pharmacology, also beginning in the mid-19th century and setting out to explain the effects of plant-derived pharmaceutical preparations in physiological terms.

Some of the major milestones are summarized in Table 1.2.

The pharmaceutical industry as big business began around the beginning of the 20th century and for 60 or more years was dominated by chemistry. Gradually, from the middle of the century onwards, the balance shifted towards pharmacology until, by the mid-1970s, chemistry and pharmacology were evenly balanced. This was a highly productive period for the industry, which saw many new drugs introduced; some of them truly novel but also many copycat drugs, which found an adequate market despite their lack of novelty. The maturation of the scientific and technological basis of the discovery process to its 1970s level coincided with the development of much more stringent regulatory controls, which also reached a degree of maturity at this time, and an acceptable balance seemed to be struck between creativity and restraint.

We ended our historical account in the mid-1970s, when drug discovery seemed to have found a fairly serene and successful equilibrium, and products and profits flowed at a healthy rate. Just around the corner, however, lay the arrival on the drug discovery scene of molecular biology and its commercial wing, the biotechnology industry, which over the next 20 years were to transform the process and diversify its products in a dramatic fashion (see Chapters 3, 12 and 13). Starting in 1976, when the first biotechnology companies (Cetus and Genentech) were founded in the USA, there are now about 1300 such companies in the USA and another 900 in Europe, and the products of such enterprises account for a steadily rising proportion – currently about 25% – of new therapeutic agents registered. As well as contributing directly in terms of products, biotechnology is steadily and radically transforming the ways in which conventional drugs are discovered.

Table 1.2 Milestones in the development of the pharmaceutical industry

Year	Event	Notes
c.1550 BC	Ebers papyrus	The earliest known compendium of medical remedies
1540	Diethyl ether synthesized	'Sweet oil of vitriol', arguably the first synthetic drug
1668	Merck (Darmstadt) founded	The apothecary business which later (1827) evolved into the first large-scale pharmaceutical company
1763	Lind shows that lack of fruit causes scurvy	
1775	Nitrous oxide synthesized	
1785	Withering describes use of digitalis extract to treat 'dropsy'	The first demonstration of therapeutic efficacy
1798	Jenner shows that vaccination prevents smallpox	
1799	Humphrey Davy demonstrates anaesthetic effect of nitrous oxide	
1803	Napoleon established examination and licensing scheme for doctors	
1806	Sertürner purifies morphine and shows it to be the active principle of opium	A seminal advance – the first evidence that herbal remedies contain active chemicals. Many other plant alkaloids isolated 1820–1840
1846	Morton administers ether as anaesthetic at Massachusetts General Hospital	The first trial of surgical anaesthesia
1847	Chloroform administered to Queen Victoria to control labour pain	
1847	The first Pharmacological Institute set up by Bucheim	
mid-19C	The first pharmaceutical companies formed:	
	Merck (1827)	
	Squibb (1858)	
	Hoechst (1862)	
	Parke Davis (1866)	
	Lilley (1876)	
	Burroughs Wellcome (1880)	In many cases, pharmaceutical companies evolved from dyestuffs companies or apothecaries
1858	Virchow proposes cell theory	
1859	Amyl nitrite synthesized	
1865	Benzene structure elucidated (Kekule), and first use of structural fromulae to describe organic molecules	Essential foundations for the development of organic synthesis
1867	Brunton demonstrates use of amyl nitrite to relieve anginal pain	
1878	Pasteur proposes germ theory of disease	
1898	Heroin (diacetylmorphine) developed by Bayer	The first synthetic derivative of a natural product. Heroin was marketed as a safe and non-addictive alternative to morphine

Continued

Table 1.2 *Continued*

Year	Event	Notes
1899	Aspirin developed by Bayer	
1903	Barbital developed by Bayer	
1904	Elliott demonstrates biological activity of extracts of adrenal glands, and proposes adrenaline release as a physiological mechanism	The first evidence for a chemical mediator – the basis of much modern pharmacology
1910	Ehrlich discovers Salvarsan	The first antimicrobial drug, which revolutionized the treatment of syphilis
1912	Starling coins the term 'hormone'	
1921	MacLeod, Banting and Best discover insulin	Produced commercially from animal pancreas by Lilly (1925)
1926	Loewi demonstrates release of 'Vagusstoff' from heart	The first clear evidence for chemical neurotransmission
1929	Fleming discovers penicillin	Penicillin was not used clinically until Chain and Florey solved production problems in 1938
1935	Domagk discovers sulfonamides	The first effective antibacterial drugs, and harbingers of the antimetabolite era
1936	Steroid hormones isolated by Upjohn company	
1937	Bovet discovers antihistamines	Subsequently led to discovery of antipsychotic drugs
1946	Gilman and Philips demonstrate anticancer effect of nitrogen mustards	The first anticancer drug
1951	Hitchings and Elion discover mercaptopurine	The first anticancer drug from the antimetabolite approach
1961	Hitchings and Schwartz discover azathioprine	Also from the antimetabolite programme, the first effective immunosuppressant able to prevent transplant rejection
1962	Black and his colleagues discover pronethalol	The first β-adrenoceptor antagonist to be used clinically
1972	Black and his colleagues discover burimamide	The first selective H_2 antagonist
1976	Genentech founded	The first biotech company, based on recombinant DNA technology
c.1990	Introduction of combinatorial chemistry	

The last quarter of the 20th century was a turbulent period which affected quite radically the scientific basis of the development of new medicines, as well as the commercial environment in which the industry operates. The changes that are occurring in the first quarter of the 21st century show no sign of slowing down, and it is too soon to judge which developments will prove genuinely successful in terms of drug discovery, and which will not. In later chapters we discuss in detail the present state of the art with respect to the science and technology of drug discovery. The major discernible trends are as follows:

- Genomics as an approach to identifying new drug targets (Chapters 6 and 7)
- Increasing use of informatics technologies to store and interpret data (Chapter 7)
- High-throughput screening of large compound libraries as a source of chemical leads (Chapter 8)
- Computational and automated chemistry as a means of efficiently and systematically synthesizing collections of related compounds with drug-like properties (Chapter 9)

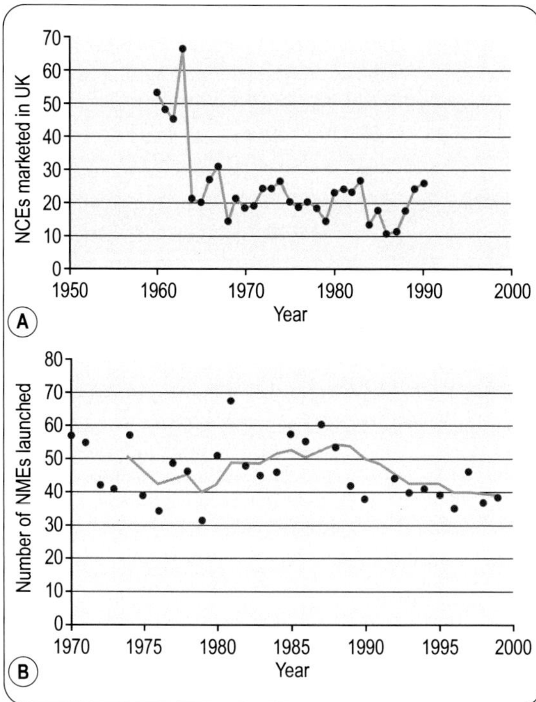

Fig. 1.3 Productivity – new drugs introduced 1970–2000. (a) Number of new chemical entities (NCEs) marketed in the UK 1960–1990 showing the dramatic effect of the thalidomide crisis in 1961. (Data from Griffin (1991) International Journal of Pharmacy 5: 206–209.) (b) Annual number of new molecular entities marketed in 20 countries worldwide 1970–1999. The line represents a 5-year moving average. In the subsequent years up to 2011 the number of new compounds introduced has levelled off to about 24 per year (see Chapter 22).

Data from Centre for Medicines Research Pharma R&D Compendium, 2000.

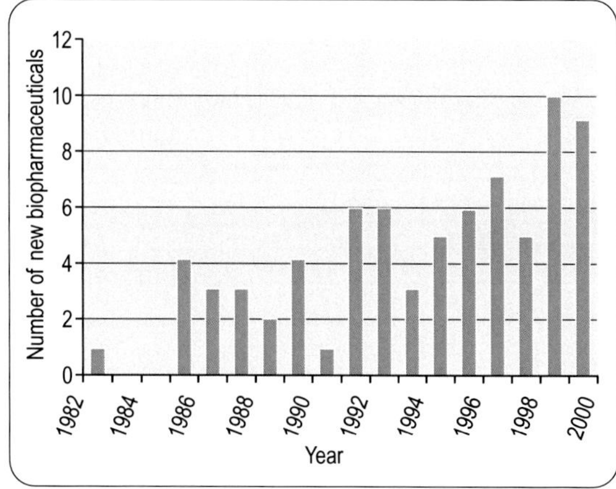

Fig. 1.4 Growth of biopharmaceuticals. Between 2000 and 2010 an average of 4.5 new biopharmaceuticals were introduced each year (see Chapter 22).

- Increased emphasis on 'drugability' – mainly centred on pharmacokinetics and toxicology – in the selection of lead compounds (Chapter 10)
- Increased use of transgenic animals as disease models for drug testing (Chapter 11)
- The growth of biopharmaceuticals (Chapters 12 and 13)
- The use of advanced imaging techniques to aid drug discovery and development (Chapter 18).

What effect are these changes having on the success of the industry in finding new drugs? Despite the difficulty of defining and measuring such success, the answer seems to be 'not much so far'. Productivity, measured by the flow of new drugs (Figure 1.3) seems to have drifted downwards over the last 20 years, and very markedly so since the 1960s, when regulatory controls began to be tightened. This measure, of course, takes no account of whether new drugs have inherent novelty and represent a significant therapeutic advance, or are merely the result of one company copying another. There are reasons for thinking that new drugs are now more innovative than they used to be, as illustrated by the introduction of selective kinase inhibitors for treating particular types of cancer (see Chapter 4). One sign is the rapid growth of biopharmaceuticals relative to conventional drugs (Figure 1.4) – and it has been estimated that by 2014 the top six drugs in terms of sales revenues will all be biologicals (Avastin, Humira, Rituxan, Enbrel, Lantus and Herceptin) and that biotechnology will have been responsible for 50% of all new drug introductions (Reuters Fact Box 2010); see also Chapters 12 and 22). Most biopharmaceuticals represent novel therapeutic strategies, and there may be less scope for copycat projects, which still account for a substantial proportion of new synthetic drugs, although biosimilars are starting to appear. Adding to the disquiet caused by the downward trend in Figure 1.3 is the fact that research and development expenditure has steadily increased over the same period, and that development times – from discovery of a new molecule to market – have remained at 10–12 years since 1982. Costs, times and success rates are discussed in more detail in Chapter 22.

Nobody really understands why the apparent drop in research productivity has occurred, but speculations abound. One factor may be the increasing regulatory hurdles, which mean that development takes longer and costs more than it used to, so that companies have become more selective in choosing which compounds to develop. Another factor may be the trend away from 'me-too' drugs (drugs that differ little, if at all, from those already in use, but which nevertheless in the past have provided the company with a profitable share of the market while providing little or no extra benefit to patients).

The hope is that the downward trend will be reversed as the benefit of new technologies to the drug discovery process works through the system, as long development times mean that novel technologies only make an impact on registrations some 20 years after their introduction.

In the remainder of this book, we describe drug discovery at the time of writing (2011) – a time when the molecular biology revolution is still in full swing. In a few years' time our account will undoubtedly look as dated as the 1970s scenario seems to us today.

REFERENCES

Drews J. Drug discovery: a historical perspective. Science 2000;287:1960–4.

Drews J. In quest of tomorrow's medicines. 2nd ed. New York: Springer; 2003.

Drews J. Paul Ehrlich: magister mundi. Nature Reviews Drug Discovery 2004;3:797–801.

Lednicer D, editor. Chronicles of drug discovery. vol 3. Washington, DC: American Chemical Society; 1993.

Mann RD. Modern drug use: an enquiry on historical principles. Lancaster: MTP Press; 1984.

Maxwell RA, Eckhardt SB. Drug discovery: a casebook and analysis. Clifton, NJ: Humana Press; 1990.

Page C, Schaffhausen J, Shankley NP. The scientific legacy of Sir James W Black. Trends in Pharmacological Science 2011;32:181–2.

Porter R. The greatest benefit to mankind: a medical history of humanity from antiquity to the present. London: Harper Collins; 1997.

Reuters Fact Box. Apr 13th 2010 http://www.reuters.com/article/2010/04/13 (accessed July 7th 2011).

Sjöstrom H, Nilsson R. Thalidomide and the power of the drug companies. Harmondsworth: Penguin; 1972.

Sneader W. Drug discovery: the evolution of modern medicines. Chichester: John Wiley; 1985.

Walker MJA. The major impacts of James Black's drug discoveries on medicine and pharmacology. Trends in Pharmacological Science 2011;32:183–8.

Weatherall M. In search of a cure: a history of pharmaceutical discovery. Oxford: Oxford University Press; 1990.

Chapter | 2 |

The nature of disease and the purpose of therapy

H P Rang, R G Hill

INTRODUCTION

In this book, we are concerned mainly with the drug discovery and development process, proudly regarded as the mainspring of the pharmaceutical industry. In this chapter we consider the broader context of the human environment into which new drugs and medicinal products are launched, and where they must find their proper place. Most pharmaceutical companies place at the top of their basic mission statement a commitment to improve the public's health, to relieve the human burden of disease and to improve the quality of life. Few would argue with the spirit of this commitment. Nevertheless, we need to look more closely at what it means, how disease is defined, what medical therapy aims to alter, and how – and by whom – the effects of therapy are judged and evaluated. Here we outline some of the basic principles underlying these broader issues.

CONCEPTS OF DISEASE

The practice of medicine predates by thousands of years the science of medicine, and the application of 'therapeutic' procedures by professionals similarly predates any scientific understanding of how the human body works, or what happens when it goes wrong. As discussed in Chapter 1, the ancients defined disease not only in very different terms, but also on a quite different basis from what we would recognize today. The origin of disease and the measures needed to counter it were generally seen as manifestations of divine will and retribution, rather than of physical malfunction. The scientific revolution in medicine, which began in earnest during the 19th century and has been steadily accelerating since, has changed our concept of disease quite drastically, and continues to challenge it, raising new ethical problems and thorny discussions of principle. For the centuries of prescientific medicine, codes of practice based on honesty, integrity and professional relationships were quite sufficient: as therapeutic interventions were ineffective anyway, it mattered little to what situations they were applied. Now, quite suddenly, the language of disease has changed and interventions have become effective; not surprisingly, we have to revise our ideas about what constitutes disease, and how medical intervention should be used. In this chapter, we will try to define the scope and purpose of therapeutics in the context of modern biology. In reality, however, those in the science-based drug discovery business have to recognize the strong atavistic leanings of many healthcare professions[1], whose roots go back much further than the age of science.

Therapeutic intervention, including the medical use of drugs, aims to prevent, cure or alleviate disease states. The question of exactly what we mean by disease, and how we distinguish disease from other kinds of human affliction and dysfunction, is of more than academic importance, because policy and practice with respect to healthcare provision depend on where we draw the line between what is an appropriate target for therapeutic intervention and what is not. The issue concerns not only doctors, who have to decide every day what kind of complaints warrant treatment, the patients who receive the treatment and all those involved in the healthcare business – including, of course, the pharmaceutical industry. Much has been

[1]The upsurge of 'alternative' therapies, many of which owe nothing to science – and, indeed, reject the relevance of science to what its practitioners do – perhaps reflects an urge to return to the prescientific era of medical history.

written on the difficult question of how to define health and disease, and what demarcates a proper target for therapeutic intervention (Reznek, 1987; Caplan, 1993; Caplan et al., 2004); nevertheless, the waters remain distinctly murky.

One approach is to define what we mean by health, and to declare the attainment of health as the goal of all healthcare measures, including therapeutics.

What is health?

In everyday parlance we use the words 'health', 'fitness', 'wellbeing' on the one hand, and 'disease', 'illness', 'sickness', 'ill-health', etc., on the other, more or less interchangeably, but these words become slippery and evasive when we try to define them. The World Health Organization (WHO), for example, defines health as 'a state of complete physical, mental and social wellbeing and not merely the absence of sickness or infirmity'. On this basis, few humans could claim to possess health, although the majority may not be in the grip of obvious sickness or infirmity. Who is to say what constitutes 'complete physical, mental and social wellbeing' in a human being? Does physical wellbeing imply an ability to run a marathon? Does a shy and self-effacing person lack social wellbeing?

We also find health defined in functional terms, less idealistically than in the WHO's formulation: '...health consists in our functioning in conformity with our natural design with respect to survival and reproduction, as determined by natural selection...' (Caplan, 1993). Here the implication is that evolution has brought us to an optimal – or at least an acceptable – compromise with our environment, with the corollary that healthcare measures should properly be directed at restoring this level of functionality in individuals who have lost some important element of it. This has a fashionably 'greenish' tinge, and seems more realistic than the WHO's chillingly utopian vision, but there are still difficulties in trying to use it as a guide to the proper application of therapeutics. Environments differ. A black-skinned person is at a disadvantage in sunless climates, where he may suffer from vitamin D deficiency, whereas a white-skinned person is liable to develop skin cancer in the tropics. The possession of a genetic abnormality of haemoglobin, known as sickle-cell trait, is advantageous in its heterozygous form in the tropics, as it confers resistance to malaria, whereas homozygous individuals suffer from a severe form of haemolytic anaemia (sickle-cell disease). Hyperactivity in children could have survival value in less developed societies, whereas in Western countries it disrupts families and compromises education. Obsessionality and compulsive behaviour are quite normal in early motherhood, and may serve a good biological purpose, but in other walks of life can be a severe handicap, warranting medical treatment.

Health cannot, therefore, be regarded as a definable state – a fixed point on the map, representing a destination that all are seeking to reach. Rather, it seems to be a continuum, through which we can move in either direction, becoming more or less well adapted for survival in our particular environment. Perhaps the best current definition is that given by Bircher (2005) who states that 'health is a dynamic state of wellbeing characterized by physical, mental and social potential which satisfies the demands of life commensurate with age, culture and personal responsibility'. Although we could argue that the aim of healthcare measures is simply to improve our state of adaptation to our present environment, this is obviously too broad. Other factors than health – for example wealth, education, peace, and the avoidance of famine – are at least as important, but lie outside the domain of medicine. What actually demarcates the work of doctors and healthcare workers from that of other caring professionals – all of whom may contribute to health in different ways – is that the former focus on *disease*.

What is disease?

Consider the following definitions of disease:

- A condition which alters or interferes with the normal state of an organism and is usually characterized by the abnormal functioning of one or more of the host's systems, parts or organs (*Churchill's Medical Dictionary*, 1989).
- A morbid entity characterized usually by at least two of these criteria: recognized aetiologic agents, identifiable groups of signs and symptoms, or consistent anatomical alterations (elsewhere, 'morbid' is defined as diseased or pathologic) (*Stedman's Medical Dictionary*, 1990).
- 'Potential insufficient to satisfy the demands of life' as outlined by Bircher (2005) in his definition of health above.

We sense the difficulty that these thoughtful authorities found in pinning down the concept. The first definition emphasizes two aspects, namely *deviation from normality*, and *dysfunction;* the second emphasizes *aetiology* (i.e. causative factors) and *phenomenology* (signs, symptoms, etc.), which is essentially the manifestation of dysfunction.

Deviation from normality does not define disease

The criterion of deviation from normality begs many questions. It implies that we know what the 'normal state' is, and can define what constitutes an alteration of it. It suggests that if our observations were searching enough, we could unfailingly distinguish disease from normality. But we know, for example, that the majority of 50-year-olds will have atherosclerotic lesions in their arteries, or that some degree of osteoporosis is normal in postmenopausal women. These are not deviations from normality, nor do they in themselves cause dysfunction, and so they do not fall within these definitions of disease, yet both are seen as pathological and as legitimate – indeed important – targets for therapeutic intervention. Furthermore, as discussed below, deviations from normality are often beneficial and much prized.

Phenomenology and aetiology are important factors – the naturalistic view

Setting aside the normality criterion, the definitions quoted above are examples of the *naturalistic*, or observation-based, view of disease, defined by phenomenology and backed up in many cases by an understanding of aetiology. It is now generally agreed that this by itself is insufficient, for there is no *general* set of observable characteristics that distinguishes disease from health. Although individual diseases of course have their defining characteristics, which may be structural, biochemical or physiological, there is no common feature. Further, there are many conditions, particularly in psychiatry, but also in other branches of medicine, where such physical manifestations are absent, even though their existence as diseases is not questioned. Examples would include obsessive-compulsive disorder, schizophrenia, chronic fatigue syndrome and low back pain. In such cases, of which there are many examples, the disease is defined by symptoms of which only the patient is aware, or altered behaviour of which he and those around him are aware: defining features at the physical, biochemical or physiological level are absent, or at least not yet recognized.

Harm and disvalue – the normative view

The shortcomings of the naturalistic view of disease, which is in principle value free, have led some authors to take the opposite view, to the extent of denying the relevance of any kind of objective criteria to the definition of disease. Crudely stated, this value-based (or *normative*) view holds that disease is simply any condition the individual or society finds disagreeable or harmful (i.e. *disvalues*). Taken to extremes by authors such as Szasz and Illich, this view denies the relevance of the physical manifestations of illness, and focuses instead on illness only as a manifestation of *social* intolerance or malfunction. Although few would go this far – and certainly modern biologists would not be among them – it is clear that value-laden judgements play a significant role in determining what we choose to view as disease. In the mid-19th century masturbation was regarded as a serious disease, to be treated if necessary by surgery, and this view persisted well into the 20th century. 'Drapetomania', defined as a disease of American slaves, was characterized by an obsessional desire for freedom. Homosexuality was seen as pathological, and determined attempts were made to treat it.

A definition of disease which tries to combine the concepts of biological malfunction and harm (or disvalue) was proposed by Caplan et al. (1981):

> *'States of affairs are called diseases when they are due to physiological or psychological processes that typically cause states of disability, pain or deformity, and are generally held to be below acceptable physiological or psychological norms.'*

What is still lacking is any reference to aetiology, yet this can be important in recognizing disease, and, indeed, is increasingly so as we understand more about the underlying biological mechanisms. A patient who complains of feeling depressed may be reacting quite normally to a bereavement, or may come from a suicide-prone family, suggestive of an inherited tendency to depressive illness. The symptoms might be very similar, but the implications, based on aetiology, would be different.

In conclusion, disease proves extremely difficult to define (Scully, 2004). The closest we can get at present to an operational definition of disease rests on a combination of three factors: phenomenology, aetiology and disvalue, as summarized in Figure 2.1.

Labelling human afflictions as diseases (i.e. 'medicalizing' them) has various beneficial and adverse consequences, both for the affected individuals and for healthcare providers. It is of particular relevance to the pharmaceutical industry, which stands to benefit from the labelling of borderline conditions as diseases meriting therapeutic intervention. Strong criticism has been levelled at the pharmaceutical industry for the way in which it uses its resources to promote the recognition of questionable disorders, such as female sexual dysfunction or social phobia, as diseases, and to elevate identified risk factors – asymptomatic in themselves but increasing the likelihood of disease occurring later – to the level of diseases in their own right. A pertinent polemic (Moynihan et al., 2004) starts with the sentence: 'there's a lot of money to be made from telling healthy people they're sick', and emphasizes the thin line that divides medical education from marketing (see Chapter 21).

THE AIMS OF THERAPEUTICS

Components of disvalue

The discussion so far leads us to the proposition that the proper aim of therapeutic intervention is to minimize the disvalue associated with disease. The concept of disvalue is, therefore, central, and we need to consider what comprises it. The disvalue experienced by a sick individual has

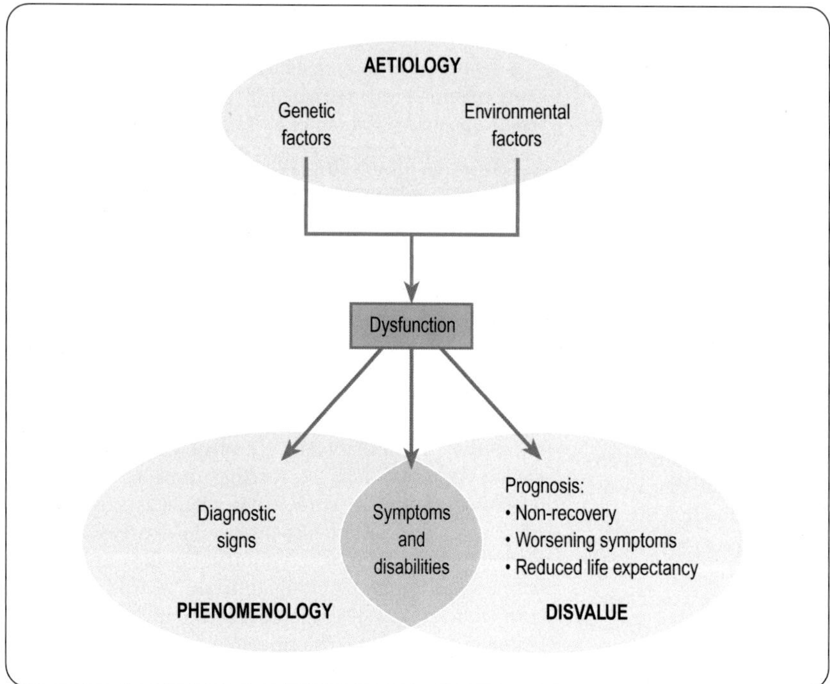

Fig. 2.1 Three components of disease.

two distinct components[2] (Figure 2.1), namely *present symptoms and disabilities* (collectively termed *morbidity*), and future *prognosis* (namely the likelihood of increasing morbidity, or premature death). An individual who is suffering no abnormal symptoms or disabilities, and whose prognosis is that of an average individual of the same age, we call 'healthy'. An individual with a bad cold or a sprained ankle has symptoms and disabilities, but probably has a normal prognosis. An individual with asymptomatic lung cancer or hypertension has no symptoms but a poor prognosis. Either case constitutes disease, and warrants therapeutic intervention. Very commonly, both components of disvalue are present and both need to be addressed with therapeutic measures – different measures may be needed to alleviate morbidity and to improve prognosis. Of course, such measures need not be confined to physical and pharmacological approaches.

The proposition at the beginning of this section sets clear limits to the aims of therapeutic intervention, which encompass the great majority of non-controversial applications. Real life is, of course, not so simple, and in the next section we consider some of the important exceptions and controversies that healthcare professionals and policy-makers are increasingly having to confront.

[2]These concepts apply in a straightforward way to many real-life situations, but there are exceptions and difficulties. For example, in certain psychiatric disorders the patient's judgement of his or her state of morbidity is itself affected by the disease. Patients suffering from mania, paranoid delusions or severe depression may pursue an extremely disordered and self-destructive lifestyle, while denying that they are ill and resisting any intervention. In such cases, society often imposes its own judgement of the individual's morbidity, and may use legal instruments such as the Mental Health Act to apply therapeutic measures against the patient's will.

Vaccination represents another special case. Here, the disvalue being addressed is the theoretical risk that a healthy individual will later contract an infectious disease such as diphtheria or measles. This risk can be regarded as an adverse factor in the prognosis of a perfectly normal individual.

Similarly, a healthy person visiting the tropics will, if he is wise, take antimalarial drugs to avoid infection – in other words, to improve his prognosis.

Therapeutic intervention is not restricted to treatment or prevention of disease

The term 'lifestyle drugs' is a recent invention, but the concept of using drugs, and other types of interventions, in a medical setting for purposes unrelated to the treatment of disease is by no means new.

Pregnancy is not by any definition a disease, nor are skin wrinkles, yet contraception, abortion and plastic surgery are well established practices in the medical domain. Why are we prepared to use drugs as contraceptives or abortifacients, but condemn using them to enhance sporting performance? The basic reason seems to be that we attach disvalue to unwanted pregnancy (i.e. we consider it harmful). We also attach disvalue to alternative means of avoiding unwanted pregnancy, such as sexual abstinence or using condoms. Other examples, however, such as cosmetic surgery to remove wrinkles or reshape breasts, seem to refute the disvalue principle: minor cosmetic imperfections are in no sense harmful, but society nonetheless concedes to the demand of individuals that medical technology should be deployed to enhance their beauty. In other cases, such as the use of sildenafil (Viagra) to improve male sexual performance, there is ambivalence about whether its use should be confined to those with evidence for erectile dysfunction (i.e. in whom disvalue exists) or whether it should also be used in normal men.

It is obvious that departures from normality can bring benefit as well as disadvantage. Individuals with above-average IQs, physical fitness, ball-game skills, artistic talents, physical beauty or charming personalities have an advantage in life. Is it, then, a proper role of the healthcare system to try to enhance these qualities in the average person? Our instinct says not, because the average person cannot be said to be diseased or suffering. There may be value in being a talented footballer, but there is no harm in not being one. Indeed, the value of the special talent lies precisely in the fact that most of us do not possess it. Nevertheless, a magical drug that would turn anyone into a brilliant footballer would certainly sell extremely well; at least until footballing skills became so commonplace that they no longer had any value[3].

Football skills may be a fanciful example; longevity is another matter. The 'normal' human lifespan varies enormously in different countries, and in the West it has increased dramatically during our own lifetime (Figure 2.2). Is lifespan prolongation a legitimate therapeutic aim? Our instinct – and certainly medical tradition – suggests that delaying premature death from disease is one of the most important functions of healthcare, but we are very ambivalent when it comes to prolonging life in the aged. Our ambivalence stems from the fact that the aged are often irremediably infirm, not merely chronologically old. In the future we may understand better why humans become infirm, and hence more vulnerable to the environmental and genetic circumstances that cause them to become ill and die. And beyond that we may discover how to retard or prevent aging, so that the 'normal' lifespan will be much prolonged. Opinions will differ as to whether this will be the ultimate triumph of medical science or the ultimate social disaster[4]. A particular consequence of improved survival into old age is an increased incidence of dementia in the population. It is estimated that some 700 000 people in the UK have dementia and world wide prevalence is thought to be over 24 million. The likelihood of developing dementia becomes greater with age and 1.3% of people in the UK between 65 and 69 suffer from dementia, rising to 20% of those over 85. In the UK alone it has been forecast that the number of individuals with dementia could reach 1.7 million by 2051 (Nuffield Council on Bioethics, 2009).

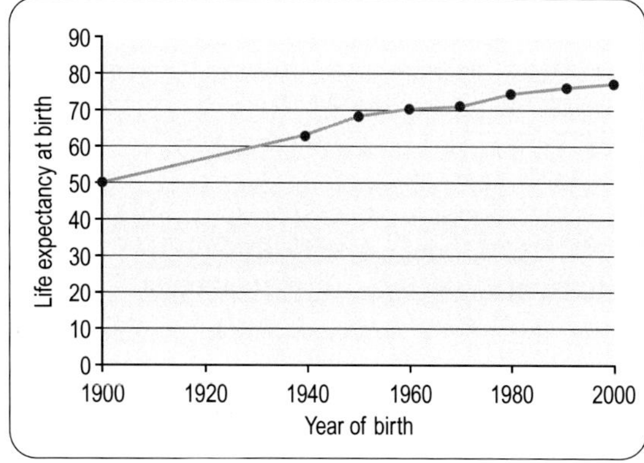

Fig. 2.2 Human lifespan in the USA.
Data from National Centre for Health Statistics, 1998.

Conclusions

We have argued that that disease can best be defined in terms of three components, aetiology, phenomenology and disvalue, and that the element of disvalue is the most important determinant of what is considered appropriate to treat. In the end, though, medical practice evolves in a more pragmatic fashion, and such arguments prove to be of limited relevance to the way in which medicine is actually practised, and hence to the therapeutic goals the drug industry sees as commercially attractive. Politics, economics, and above all, social pressures are the determinants, and the limits are in practice set more by our technical capabilities than by issues of theoretical propriety.

Although the drug industry has so far been able to take a pragmatic view in selecting targets for therapeutic intervention, things are changing as technology advances. The increasing cost and sophistication of what therapeutics can offer mean that healthcare systems the world over are being forced to set limits, and have to go back to the issue of what constitutes disease. Furthermore, by invoking the concept of disease, governments control access to many other social resources (e.g. disability benefits, entry into the armed services, insurance pay-outs, access to life insurance, exemption from legal penalties, etc.).

[3]The use of drugs to improve sporting performance is one of many examples of 'therapeutic' practices that find favour among individuals, yet are strongly condemned by society. We do not, as a society, attach disvalue to the possession of merely average sporting ability, even though the individual athlete may take a different view.
[4]Jonathan Swift, in *Gulliver's Travels*, writes of the misery of the Struldbrugs, rare beings with a mark on their forehead who, as they grew older, lost their youth but never died, and who were declared 'dead in law' at the age of 80.

So far, we have concentrated mainly on the impact of disease on individuals and societies. We now need to adopt a more biological perspective, and attempt to put the concept of disease into the framework of contemporary ideas about how biological systems work.

FUNCTION AND DYSFUNCTION: THE BIOLOGICAL PERSPECTIVE

The dramatic revelations of the last few decades about the molecular basis of living systems have provided a new way of looking at function and dysfunction, and the nature of disease. Needless to say, molecular biology could not have developed without the foundations of scientific biology that were built up in the 19th century. As we saw in Chapter 1, this was the period in which science came to be accepted as the basis on which medical practice had to be built. Particularly significant was cell theory, which established the cell as the basic building block of living organisms. In the words of the pioneering molecular biologist, François Jacob: 'With the cell, biology discovered its atom'. It is by focusing on the instruction sets that define the form and function of cells, and the ways in which these instructions are translated in the process of generating the structural and functional phenotypes of cells, that molecular biology has come to occupy centre stage in modern biology. Genes specify proteins, and the proteins a cell produces determine its structure and function.

From this perspective, deviations from the norm, in terms of structure and function at the cellular level, arise through deviations in the pattern of protein expression by individual cells, and they may arise either through faults in the instruction set itself (genetic mutations) or through environmental factors that alter the way in which the instruction set is translated (i.e. that affect gene expression). We come back to the age-old distinction between inherited and environmental factors (nature and nurture) in the causation of disease, but with a sharper focus: altered gene expression, resulting in altered protein synthesis, is the mechanism through which all these factors operate. Conversely, it can be argued[5] that all therapeutic measures (other than physical procedures, such as surgery) also work at the cellular level, by influencing the same fundamental processes (gene expression and protein synthesis), although the link between a drug's primary target and the relevant effect(s) on gene expression that account for its therapeutic effect may be very indirect. We can see how it has come about that molecular biology, and in particular genomics, has come to figure so largely in the modern drug discovery environment.

[5]This represents the ultimate reductionist view of how living organisms work, and how they respond to external influences. Many still hold out against it, believing that the 'humanity' of man demands a less concrete explanation, and that 'alternative' systems of medicine, not based on our scientific understanding of biological function, have equal validity. Many doctors apparently feel most comfortable somewhere on the middle ground, and society at large tends to fall in behind doctors rather than scientists.

Levels of biological organization

Figure 2.3 shows schematically the way in which the genetic constitution of a human being interacts with his or her environment to control function at many different levels, ranging from protein molecules, through single cells, tissues and integrated physiological systems, to the individual, the family and the population at large. For simplicity, we will call this the *bioaxis*. 'Disease', as we have discussed, consists of alterations of function sufficient to cause disability or impaired prognosis at the level of the individual. It should be noted that the arrows along the bioaxis in Figure 2.3 are bidirectional – that is, disturbances at higher levels of organization will in general affect function at lower levels, and vice versa. Whereas it is obvious that genetic mutations can affect function further up the bioaxis (as in many inherited diseases, such as muscular dystrophy, cystic fibrosis or thalassaemia), we should not forget that environmental influences also affect gene function. Indeed, we can state that any long-term phenotypic change (such as weight gain, muscle weakness or depressed mood) *necessarily* involves alterations of gene expression. For example:

- Exposure to a stressful environment will activate the hypothalamopituitary system and thereby increase adrenal steroid secretion, which in turn affects gene transcription in many different cells and tissues, affecting salt metabolism, immune responses and many other functions.
- Smoking, initiated as result of social factors such as peer pressure or advertising, becomes addictive as a result of changes in brain function, phenotypic changes which are in turn secondary to altered gene expression.
- Exposure to smoke carcinogens then increases the probability of cancer-causing mutations in the DNA of the cells of the lung. The mutations, in turn, result in altered protein synthesis and malignant transformation, eventually producing a localized tumour and, later, disseminated cancer, with damage to the function of tissues and organs leading to symptoms and premature death.

The pathogenesis of any disease state reveals a similar level of complexity of such interactions between different levels of the bioaxis.

There are two important conclusions to be drawn from the bidirectionality of influence between events at different levels of the bioaxis. One is that it is difficult to pinpoint the *cause* of a given disease. Do we regard the cause of lung cancer in an individual patient as the lack

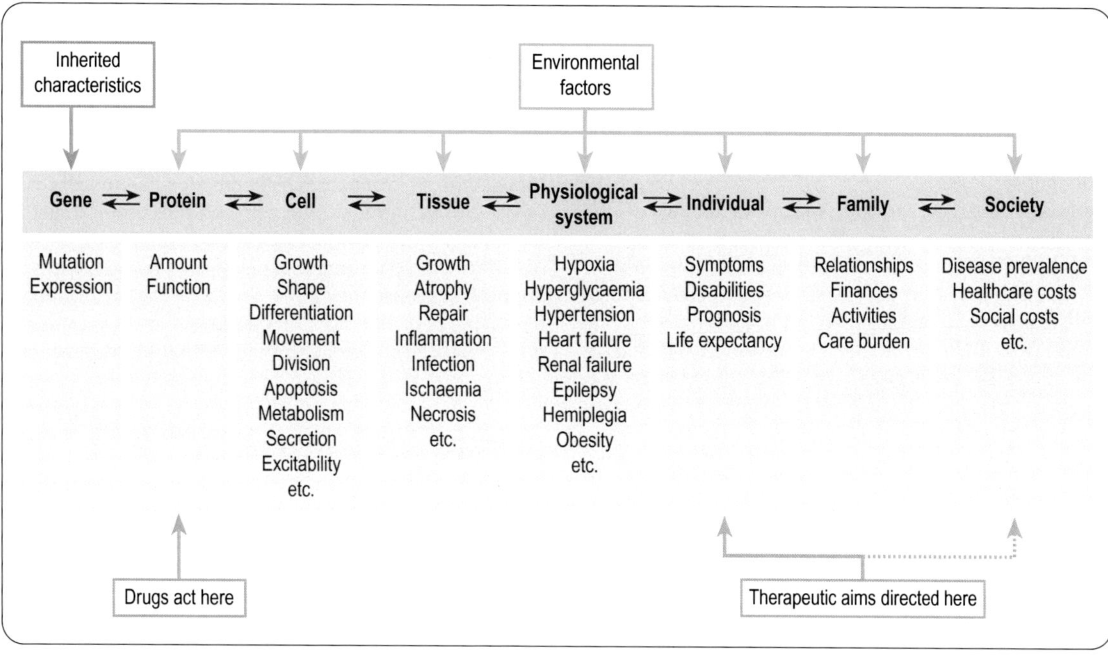

Fig. 2.3 The nature of disease.

of control over tobacco advertising, the individual's susceptibility to advertising and peer pressure, the state of addiction to nicotine, the act of smoking, the mutational event in the lung epithelial cell, or the individual's inherited tendency to lung cancer? There is no single answer, and the uncertainty should make us wary of the stated claim of many pharmaceutical companies that their aim is to correct the causes rather than the symptoms of disease. The truth, more often than not, is that we cannot distinguish them. Rather, the aim should be to intervene in the disease process in such a way as to minimize the disvalue (disability and impaired prognosis) experienced by the patient.

The second conclusion is that altered gene expression plays a crucial role in pathogenesis and the production of any long-term phenotypic change. If we are thinking of timescales beyond, at maximum, a few hours, any change in the structure and function of cells and tissues will be associated with changes in gene expression. These changes will include those responsible for the phenotypic change (e.g. upregulation of cytokine genes in inflammation, leading to leukocyte accumulation), and those that are consequences of it (e.g. loss of bone matrix following muscle paralysis); some of the latter will, in turn, lead to secondary phenotypic changes, and so on. The pattern of genes expressed in a cell or tissue (sometimes called the 'transcriptome', as distinct from the 'genome', which represents all of the genes present, whether expressed or not), together with the 'proteome' (which describes the array of proteins present in a cell or tissue), provides a uniquely detailed description of how the cell or tissue is behaving. Molecular biology is providing us with powerful methods for mapping the changes in gene and protein expression associated with different functional states – including disease states and therapeutic responses – and we discuss in more detail in Chapters 6 and 7 the way these new windows on function are influencing the drug discovery process (see Debouck and Goodfellow, 1999).

Therapeutic targets

Traditionally medicine has regarded the interests of the individual patient as paramount, putting them clearly ahead of those of the community or general population. The primacy of the patient's interests remains the guiding principle for the healthcare professions; in other words, their aim is to address disvalue as experienced by the patient, not to correct biochemical abnormalities, nor to put right the wrongs of society. The principal aim of therapeutic intervention, as shown in Figure 2.3, is therefore to alleviate the condition of the individual patient. Genetic, biochemical or physiological deviations which are not associated with any disvalue for the patient (e.g. possession of a rare blood group, an unusually low heart rate or blood pressure, or blood cholesterol concentration) are not treated as diseases because they neither cause symptoms nor carry an unfavourable prognosis. High blood pressure, or high blood cholesterol, on the other hand, do confer disvalue because they carry a poor prognosis, and are targets for treatment – surrogate targets, in the sense that the actual aim is to remedy the unfavourable prognosis, rather than to correct the physiological abnormality per se.

Although the present and future wellbeing of the individual patient remains the overriding priority for medical care, the impact of disease is felt not only by individuals, but also by society in general, partly for economic reasons, but also for ideological reasons. Reducing the overall burden of disease, as measured by rates of infant mortality, heart disease or AIDS, for example, is a goal for governments throughout the civilized world, akin to the improvement of educational standards. The disease-related disvalue addressed in this case, as shown by the secondary arrow in Figure 2.3, is experienced at the national, rather than the individual level, for individuals will in general be unaware of whether or not they have benefited personally from disease prevention measures. As the therapeutic target has come to embrace the population as a whole, so the financial burden of healthcare has shifted increasingly from individuals to institutional providers of various kinds, mainly national agencies or large-scale commercial healthcare organizations. Associated with this change, there has been a much more systematic focus on assessment in economic terms of the burden of disease (disvalue, to return to our previous terminology) in the community, and the economic cost of healthcare measures. The new and closely related disciplines of *pharmacoeconomics* and *pharmacoepidemiology*, discussed later, reflect the wish (a) to quantify disease-related disvalue and therapeutic benefit in economic terms, and (b) to assess the impact of disease and therapy for the population as a whole, and not just for the individual patient.

The relationship between drug targets and therapeutic targets

There are very few exceptions to the rule, shown in Figure 2.3, that protein molecules are the primary targets of drug molecules. We will come back to this theme repeatedly later, because of its prime importance for the drug discovery process. We should note here that many complex biological steps intervene between the primary drug target and the therapeutic target. Predicting, on the one hand, whether a drug that acts specifically on a particular protein will produce a worthwhile therapeutic effect, and in what disease state, or, on the other hand, what protein we should choose to target in order to elicit a therapeutic effect in a given disease state, are among the thorniest problems for drug discoverers. Molecular biology is providing new insights into the nature of genes and proteins and the relationship between them, whereas time-honoured biochemical and physiological approaches can show how disease affects function at the level of cells, tissues, organs and individuals. The links between the two nevertheless remain tenuous, a fact which greatly limits our ability to relate drug targets to therapeutic effects. Not surprisingly, attempts to bridge this Grand Canyon form a major part of the work of many pharmaceutical and biotechnology companies. Afficionados like to call themselves 'postgenomic' biologists; Luddites argue that they are merely coming down from a genomic 'high' to face once more the daunting complexities of living organisms. We patient realists recognize that a biological revolution has happened, but do not underestimate the time and money needed to bridge the canyon. More of this later.

THERAPEUTIC INTERVENTIONS

Therapeutics in its broadest sense covers all types of intervention aimed at alleviating the effects of disease. The term 'therapeutics' generally relates to procedures based on accepted principles of medical science, that is, on 'conventional' rather than 'alternative' medical practice[6]. The account of drug discovery presented in this book relates exclusively to conventional medicine – and for this we make no apology – but it needs to be realized that the therapeutic landscape is actually much broader, and includes many non-pharmacological procedures in the domain of conventional medicine, as well as quasi-pharmacological practices (e.g. homeopathy and herbalism) in the 'alternative' domain.

As discussed above, the desired effect of any therapeutic interventions is to improve *symptoms* or *prognosis* or both. From a pathological point of view, therapeutic interventions may be directed at *disease prevention*, *alleviation* of the effects of existing disease, or permanent *cure* (i.e. restoration to a state of function and prognosis equivalent to those of a healthy individual of the same age, without the need for continuing therapeutic intervention). In practice, there are relatively few truly curative interventions, and they are mainly confined to certain surgical procedures (e.g. removal of circumscribed tumours, fixing of broken bones) and chemotherapy of some infectious and malignant disorders. Most therapeutic interventions aim to alleviate symptoms and/or improve prognosis, and there is increasing emphasis on disease prevention as an objective.

It is important to realize that many types of interventions are carried out with therapeutic intent whose efficacy has not been rigorously tested. This includes not

[6]Scientific doctors rail against the term 'alternative', arguing that if a therapeutic practice can be shown to work by properly controlled trials, it belongs in mainstream medicine. If such trials fail to show efficacy, the practice should not be adopted. Paradoxically, whereas 'therapeutics' generally connotes conventional medicine, the term 'therapy' tends to be used most often in the 'alternative' field.

only the myriad alternative medical practices, but also many accepted conventional therapies for which a good scientific basis may exist but which have not been subjected to rigorous clinical trials.

MEASURING THERAPEUTIC OUTCOME

Effect, efficacy, effectiveness and benefit

These terms have acquired particular meanings – more limited than their everyday meanings – in the context of therapeutic trials.

Pharmacological *effects* of drugs (i.e. their effects on cells, organs and systems) are, in principle, simple to measure in animals, and often also in humans. We can measure effects on blood pressure, plasma cholesterol concentration, cognitive function, etc., without difficulty. Such measures enable us to describe quantitatively the pharmacological properties of drugs, but say nothing about their usefulness as therapeutic agents.

Efficacy describes the ability of a drug to produce a desired therapeutic effect in patients under carefully controlled conditions. The gold standard for measurements of efficacy is the randomized controlled clinical trial, described in more detail in Chapter 17. The aim is to discover whether, based on a strictly defined outcome measure, the drug is more or less beneficial than a standard treatment or placebo, in a selected group of patients, under conditions which ensure that the patients actually receive the drug in the specified dose. Proof of efficacy, as well as proof of safety, is required by regulatory authorities as a condition for a new drug to be licensed. Efficacy tests what the drug can do under optimal conditions, which is what the prescriber usually wants to know.

Effectiveness describes how well the drug works in real life, where the patients are heterogeneous, are not randomized, are aware of the treatment they are receiving, are prescribed different doses, which they may or may not take, often in combination with other drugs. The desired outcome is generally less well defined than in efficacy trials, related to general health and freedom from symptoms, rather than focusing on a specific measure. The focus is not on the response of individual patients under controlled conditions, but on the overall usefulness of the drug in the population going about its normal business. Studies of effectiveness are of increasing interest to the pharmaceutical companies themselves, because effectiveness rather than efficacy alone ultimately determines how well the drug will sell, and because effectiveness may depend to some extent on the companies' marketing strategies (see Chapter 21). Effectiveness measures are also becoming increasingly important to the many agencies that now regulate the provision of healthcare, such as formulary committees, insurance companies, health management organizations, and bodies such as the grandly titled National Institute for Health and Clinical Excellence (NICE), set up by the UK Government in 1999 to advise, on the basis of cost-effectiveness, which drugs and other therapeutic procedures should be paid for under the National Health Service.

Benefit comprises effectiveness expressed in monetary terms. It is popular with economists, as it allows cost and benefit to be compared directly, but treated with deep suspicion by many who find the idea of assigning monetary value to life and wellbeing fundamentally abhorrent.

Returning to the theme of Figure 2.3, we can see that whereas *effect* and *efficacy* are generally measured at the level of cells, tissues, systems and individuals, *effectiveness* and *benefit* are measures of drug action as it affects populations and society at large. We next consider two growing disciplines that have evolved to meet the need for information at these levels, and some of the methodological problems that they face.

PHARMACOEPIDEMIOLOGY AND PHARMACOECONOMICS

Pharmacoepidemiology (Strom, 2005) is the study of the use and effects of drugs in human populations, as distinct from individuals, the latter being the focus of clinical pharmacology. The subject was born in the early 1960s, when the problem of adverse drug reactions came into prominence, mainly as a result of the infamous thalidomide disaster. The existence of rare but serious adverse drug reactions, which can be detected only by the study of large numbers of subjects, was the initial stimulus for the development of pharmacoepidemiology, and the detection of adverse drug reactions remains an important concern. The identification of Reye's syndrome as a serious, albeit rare, consequence of using aspirin in children is just one example of a successful pharmacoepidemiological study carried out under the auspices of the US Department of Health and published in 1987. The subject has gradually become broader, however, to cover aspects such as the variability of drug responses between individuals and population groups, the level of compliance of individual patients in taking drugs that are prescribed, and the overall impact of drug therapies on the population as a whole, taking all of these factors into account. The widely used antipsychotic drug *clozapine* provides an interesting example of the importance of pharmacoepidemiological issues in drug evaluation. Clozapine, first introduced in the 1970s, differed from its predecessors, such as haloperidol, in several ways, some good and some bad. On the good side, clozapine has a much lower tendency than haloperidol to cause extrapyramidal motor effects (a serious problem with many antipsychotic drugs), and it appeared to have the ability to improve not only the positive symptoms of schizophrenia (hallucinations, delusions, thought disorder, stereotyped behaviour) but also the negative symptoms (social withdrawal, apathy). Compliance is also better with clozapine, because the patient usually has fewer severe side effects. On the bad side, in about 1% of patients clozapine causes a fall in the blood white cell count (leukopenia), which can progress to an irreversible state of agranulocytosis unless the drug is stopped in time. Furthermore, clozapine does not produce benefit in all schizophrenic patients – roughly one-third fail to show improvement, and there is currently no way of knowing in advance which patients will benefit. Clozapine is also more expensive than haloperidol. Considered from the perspective of an individual patient, and with hindsight, it is straightforward to balance the pros and cons of using clozapine rather than haloperidol, based on the severity of the extrapyramidal side effects, the balance of positive and negative symptoms that the patient has, whether clozapine is affecting the white cell count, and whether the patient is a responder or a non-responder. From the perspective of the overall population, evaluating the pros and cons of clozapine and haloperidol (or indeed of any two therapies) requires epidemiological data: how frequent are extrapyramidal side effects with haloperidol, what is the relative incidence of positive and negative symptoms, what is the incidence of agranulocytosis with clozapine, what proportion of patients are non-responders, what is the level of patient compliance with haloperidol and clozapine?

In summary, pharmacoepidemiology is a special area of clinical pharmacology which deals with population, rather than individual, aspects of drug action, and provides the means of quantifying *variability* in the response to drugs. Its importance for the drug discovery process is felt mainly at the level of clinical trials and regulatory affairs, for two reasons (Dieck et al., 1994). First, allowing for variability is essential in drawing correct inferences from clinical trials (see Chapter 17). Second, variability in response to a drug is per se disadvantageous, as drug A, whose effects are unpredictable, is less useful than drug B which acts consistently, even though the mean balance between beneficial and unwanted effects may be the same for both. From the population perspective, drug B looks better than drug A, even though for many individual patients the reverse may be true.

Pharmacoeconomics, a branch of health economics, is a subject that grew up around the need for healthcare providers to balance the ever-growing costs of healthcare against limited resources. The arrival of the welfare state, which took on healthcare provision as a national rather than an individual responsibility, was the signal for economists to move in. Good accounts of the basic principles and their application to pharmaceuticals are given by Gold et al. (1996), Johannesson (1996) and McCombs (1998). The aim of pharmacoeconomics is to measure the benefits and costs of drug treatments, and in the end to provide a sound basis for comparing the value for money of different treatments. As might be expected, the subject arouses fierce controversy. Economics in general is often criticized for defining the price of everything but appreciating the value of nothing, and health economics particularly tends to evoke this reaction, as health and quality of life are such ill-defined and subjective, yet highly emotive, concepts. Nevertheless, pharmacoeconomics is a rapidly growing discipline and will undoubtedly have an increasing influence on healthcare provision.

Pharmacoeconomic evaluation of new drugs is often required by regulatory authorities, and is increasingly being used by healthcare providers as a basis for choosing how to spend their money. Consequently, pharmaceutical companies now incorporate such studies into the clinical trials programmes of new drugs. The trend can be seen as a gradual progression towards the right-hand end of the bioaxis in Figure 2.3 in our frame of reference for assessing the usefulness of a new drug. Before 1950, new drugs were often introduced into clinical practice on the basis of studies in animals and a few human volunteers; later, formal randomized controlled clinical trials on carefully selected patient populations, with defined outcome measures, became the accepted standard, along with postmarketing pharmacoepidemiological studies to detect adverse reactions. Pharmacoeconomics represents the further shift of focus to include society in general and its provisions for healthcare. A brief outline of the main approaches used in pharmacoeconomic analysis follows.

Pharmacoeconomics covers four levels of analysis:

- Cost identification
- Cost-effectiveness analysis
- Cost-utility analysis
- Cost–benefit analysis.

Cost identification consists of determining the full cost in monetary units of a particular therapeutic intervention, including hospitalization, working days lost, etc., as well as direct drug costs. It pays no attention to outcome, and its purpose is merely to allow the costs of different procedures to be compared. The calculation is straightforward, but deciding exactly where to draw the line (e.g. whether to include indirect costs, such as loss of income by patients and carers) is somewhat arbitrary. Nevertheless, cost identification is the least problematic part of pharmacoeconomics.

Cost-effectiveness analysis aims to quantify outcome as well as cost. This is where the real problems begin. The outcome measure most often used in cost-effectiveness analysis is based on prolongation of life, expressed as *life-years saved per patient treated*. Thus if treatment prolongs the life expectancy of patients, on average, from 3 years to 5 years, the number of life-years gained per patient is 2.

Comparing cost and outcome for different treatments then allows the cost per life-year saved to be determined for each. For example, a study of various interventions in coronary heart disease, cited by McCombs (1998), showed that the cost per life-year saved was $5900 for use of a β-adrenoceptor blocker in patients who had suffered a heart attack, the corresponding figure for use of a cholesterol-lowering drug in patients with coronary heart disease was $7200, while coronary artery bypass surgery cost $34 000 per life-year saved. As these drugs have reached the end of their patent life and become low-priced generic medicines, the cost difference changes in favour of their use. Any kind of all-or-nothing event, such as premature births prevented, hospital admissions avoided, etc., can be used for this kind of analysis. Its weakness is that it is a very crude measure, making no distinction between years of life spent in a healthy and productive mode and years of life spent in a state of chronic illness.

Cost-utility analysis is designed to include allowance for quality of life, as well as survival, in the calculation, and is yet more controversial, for it becomes necessary somehow to quantify quality – not an endeavour for the faint-hearted. What the analysis seeks to arrive at is an estimate known as *quality-adjusted life-years (QALYs)*. Thus if the quality of life for a given year, based on the results of the questionnaire, comes out at 70% of the value for an average healthy person of the same age, that year represents 0.7 QALYs, compared with 1 QALY for a year spent in perfect health, the assumption being that 1 year spent at this level of illness is 'worth' 0.7 years spent in perfect health.

Many different questionnaire-based rating scales have been devised to reflect different aspects of an individual's state of health or disability, such as ability to work, mobility, mental state, pain, etc. Some relate to specific disease conditions, whereas others aim to provide a general 'quality-of-life' estimate (Jaeschke and Guyatt, 1994), some of the best-known being the *Sickness Impact Profile*, the *Nottingham Health Profile*, the *McMaster Health Index*, and a 36-item questionnaire known as *SF-36*. In addition to these general quality-of-life measures, a range of disease-specific questionnaires have been devised which give greater sensitivity in measuring the specific deficits associated with particular diseases. Standard instruments of this kind are now widely used in pharmacoeconomic studies.

To use such ratings in estimating QALYs it is necessary to position particular levels of disability on a life/death scale, such that 1 represents alive and in perfect health and 0 represents dead. This is where the problems begin in earnest. How can we possibly say what degree of pain is equivalent to what degree of memory loss, for example, or how either compares with premature death? This problem has, of course, received a lot of expert attention (Gold et al., 1996; Johannesson, 1996; Drummond et al., 1997) and various solutions have been proposed, some of

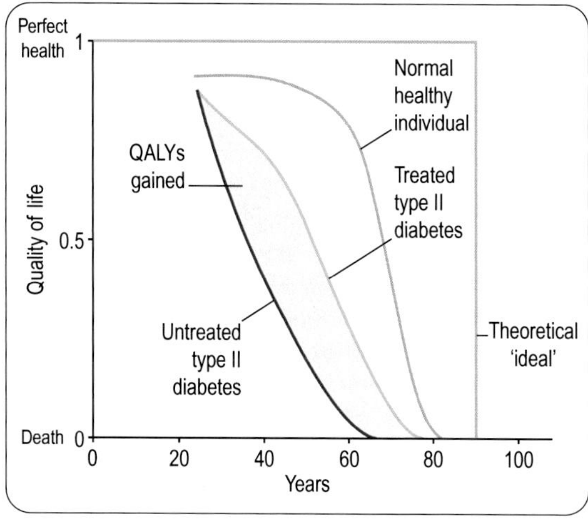

Fig. 2.4 Quality of life affected by disease and treatment.

which, to the untrained observer, have a distinctly chilling and surreal quality. For example, the standard gamble approach, which is well grounded in the theory of welfare economics, involves asking the individual a question of the following kind:

> ***Imagine you have the choice of remaining in your present state of health for 1 year or taking a gamble between dying now and living in perfect health for 1 year. What odds would you need to persuade you to take the gamble?***[7]

If the subject says 50:50, the implication is that he values a year of life in his present state of health at 0.5 QALYs. An alternative method involves asking the patient how many years of life in their present condition he or she would be prepared to forfeit in exchange for enjoying good health until they die. Although there are subtle ways of posing this sort of question, such an evaluation, which most ordinary people find unreal, is implicit in the QALY concept. Figure 2.4 shows schematically the way in which quality of life, as a function of age, may be affected by disease and treatment, the area between the curves for untreated and treated patients representing the QALYs saved by the treatment. In reality, of course, continuous measurements spanning several decades are not possible, so the actual data on which QALY estimates are based in practice are much less than is implied by the idealized diagram in Figure 2.4. Cost-utility analysis results in an estimate of monetary cost per QALY gained and it is becoming widely accepted as a standard method for pharmacoeconomic analysis. Examples of cost per QALY

[7]Imagine being asked this by your doctor! 'But I only wanted something for my sore throat', you protest weakly.

gained range from £3700 for the use of sildenafil (Viagra) in treating erectile dysfunction (Stolk et al., 2000) to £328 000 for the treatment of multiple sclerosis with β-interferon (Parkin et al., 2000), this high value being accounted for by the high cost and limited therapeutic efficacy of the drug. 'Acceptable' thresholds for cost-effectiveness are suggested to be in the range of £8000–£30 000 per QALY gained (Hunter and Wilson, 2011). It is hard, if not impossible, to make sure that available funds are spent in the most appropriate way. For example, Avastin (bevacizumab) is a monoclonal antibody used in the treatment of colorectal cancer and NICE estimate that some 6500 patients per year would be eligible for treatment with this drug. The cost of a course of treatment is £20 800 per patient and overall average survival is increased by between 1.4 and 2.2 months depending on whether it is being used for first- or second-line therapy. Funding the use of Avastin in this way would cost £135 million per year or >1% of the total NHS drugs budget of £11 billion per year (Hunter and Wilson, 2011). In principle, cost-utility analysis allows comparison of one form of treatment against another, and this explains its appeal to those who must make decisions about the allocation of healthcare resources. It has been adopted as the method of choice for pharmacoeconomic analysis of new medicines by several agencies, such as the US Public Health Service and the Australian Pharmaceutical Benefits Advisory Committee.

Hardline economists strive for an absolute scale by which to judge the value of healthcare measures compared with other resource-consuming initiatives that societies choose to support. *Cost–benefit* analysis fulfils this need in principle, by translating healthcare improvements into monetary units that can be directly balanced against costs, to assess whether any given procedure is, on balance, 'profitable'. The science of welfare economics has provided various tools for placing a monetary value on different experiences human beings find agreeable or disagreeable, based generally on the 'willingness-to-pay' principle. Not surprisingly, attempts to value human life and health in cash terms lead rapidly into an ethical and moral minefield, dangerous enough in the context of a single nation and its economy, but much more so in the global context. As a result, cost–benefit analysis has been largely shunned as a practical approach for evaluating medicines, but may be unavoidable as more personalized and expensive medicines become available (Hunter and Wilson, 2011 and Chapter 22).

SUMMARY

In this chapter we have discussed concepts of disease and the aims of therapeutics, the needs newly introduced drugs have to satisfy, and the ways in which their ability to satisfy those needs are judged in practice. There are many uncertainties and ambiguities surrounding the definition of disease, and ideas are constantly shifting, but the two components that most satisfactorily define it are *dysfunction* and *disvalue*. Disvalue, which therapeutic interventions aim to mitigate, in turn has two main components, namely *morbidity* and *prognosis*.

We have described the bioaxis, which represents the various levels in the organizational heirarchy of living systems in general, and human beings in particular, and emphasized that disease inevitably affects all levels on the bioaxis. The drugs that we invent home in very specifically on one level, namely proteins, although the effects we want to produce are at another level, namely individuals. Furthermore, we emphasize that healthcare issues are increasingly being viewed from the perspective of populations and societies, and so the impact of drugs at these levels – even further removed from their primary targets – has to be evaluated. Evaluation of drug effects from these rather lofty perspectives, through the application of the emerging disciplines of pharmacoepidemiology and pharmacoeconomics, although fraught with problems, is an important trend the pharmaceutical industry cannot ignore.

Having taken this rather nervy look at the world about us, we turn in the next chapter to discuss the different therapeutic modalities on which the pharmaceutical and biotechnology industries have focused, before retreating to the safer ground at the left-hand end of the bioaxis, where the modern-day drug discovery business begins.

REFERENCES

Bircher J. Towards a dynamic definition of health and disease. Medical Health Care and Philosophy 2005;8:335–41.

Caplan AL, Engelhardt Jr HT, McCartney JJ, editors. Concepts of health and disease: interdisciplinary perspectives. London: Addison-Wesley; 1981.

Caplan AL. The concepts of health, illness, and disease. In: Bynum WF, Porter R, editors. Companion encyclopedia of the history of medicine. vol. 1. London: Routledge; 1993.

Caplan AL, McCartney JJ, Sisti DA, editors. Health, disease, and illness: concepts in medicine. Washington, DC: Georgetown University Press; 2004.

Debouck C, Goodfellow PN. DNA microarrays in drug discovery and development. Nature Genetics 1999;(Suppl. 21):48–50.

Dieck GS, Glasser DB, Sachs RM. Pharmacoepidemiology: a view from industry. In: Strom BL, editor.

Pharmacoepidemiology. Chichester: John Wiley; 1994. p. 73–85.

Drummond MF, O'Brien B, Stoddart GI, et al. Methods for the economic evaluation of healthcare programmes. Oxford: Oxford University Press; 1997.

Gold MR, Siegel JE, Russell LB, et al, editors. Cost-effectiveness in health and medicine. New York: Oxford University Press; 1996.

Hunter D, Wilson J. Hyper-expensive treatments. Background paper for Forward Look 2011. London: Nuffield Council on Bioethics; 2011. p. 23.

Jaeschke R, Guyatt GH. Using quality-of-life measurements in pharmacoepidemiology research. In: Strom BL, editor. Pharmacoepidemiology. Chichester: John Wiley; 1994. p. 495–505.

Johannesson M. Theory and methods of economic evaluation of health care. Dordrecht: Kluwer Academic; 1996.

McCombs JS. Pharmacoeconomics: what is it and where is it going? American Journal of Hypertension 1998;11:112S–9S.

Moynihan R, Heath I, Henry D. Selling sickness: the pharmaceutical industry and disease mongering. British Medical Journal 2004;324:886–91.

Nuffield Council on Bioethics. Dementia – ethical issues. London: NCOB; 2009. p. 172.

Parkin D, Jacoby A, McNamee P, et al. Treatment of multiple sclerosis with interferon beta: an appraisal of cost-effectiveness and quality of life. Journal of Neurology, Neurosurgery and Psychiatry 2000;68:144–9.

Reznek L. The nature of disease. New York: Routledge & Kegan Paul; 1987.

Scully JL. What is a disease? EMBO Reports 2004;5:650–3.

Stolk EA, Busschbach JJ, Caffa M, et al. Cost utility analysis of sildenafil compared with papaverine-phentolamine injections. British Medical Journal 2000;320:1156–7.

Strom BL, editor. Pharmacoepidemiology 4th Edition. Chichester: John Wiley; 2005.

Chapter 3

Therapeutic modalities

H P Rang, H LeVine, R G Hill

INTRODUCTION

Therapeutics in its broadest sense covers all types of intervention aimed at alleviating the effects of disease. The term 'therapeutics' generally relates to procedures based on accepted principles of medical science, that is, on 'conventional' rather than 'alternative' medical practice.

The account of drug discovery presented in this book relates exclusively to conventional medicine – and for this we make no apology – but it needs to be realized that the therapeutic landscape is actually much broader, and includes many non-pharmacological procedures in the domain of conventional medicine, as well as quasi-pharmacological practices in the 'alternative' domain.

As discussed in Chapter 2, the desired effect of any therapeutic intervention is to improve *symptoms* or *prognosis* or both. From a pathological point of view, therapeutic interventions may be directed at *disease prevention, alleviation* of the effects of existing disease, or permanent *cure* (i.e. restoration to a state of function and prognosis equivalent to those of a healthy individual of the same age, without the need for continuing therapeutic intervention). In practice, there are relatively few truly curative interventions, and they are mainly confined to certain surgical procedures (e.g. removal of circumscribed tumours, fixing of broken bones) and chemotherapy of some infectious and malignant disorders. Most therapeutic interventions aim to alleviate symptoms and/or improve prognosis, and there is increasing emphasis on disease prevention as an objective.

It is important to realize that many types of intervention are carried out with therapeutic intent whose efficacy has not been rigorously tested. This includes not only the myriad alternative medical practices, but also many accepted conventional therapies for which a sound scientific basis may exist but which have not been subjected to rigorous clinical trials.

Therapeutic interventions that lie within the field of conventional medicine can be divided into the following broad categories:

- Advice and counselling (e.g. genetic counselling)
- Psychological treatments (e.g. cognitive therapies for anxiety disorders, depression, etc.)
- Dietary and nutritional treatments (e.g. gluten-free diets for coeliac disease, diabetic diets, etc.)
- Physical treatments, including surgery, radiotherapy
- Pharmacological treatments – encompassing the whole of conventional drug therapy
- Biological and biopharmaceutical treatments, a broad category including vaccination, transplantation, blood transfusion, biopharmaceuticals (see Chapters 12 and 13), in vitro fertilization, etc.

On the fringe of conventional medicine are preparations that fall into the category of 'nutriceuticals' or 'cosmeceuticals'. Nutriceuticals include a range of dietary preparations, such as slimming diets, and diets supplemented with vitamins, minerals, antioxidants, unsaturated fatty acids, fibre, etc. These preparations generally have some scientific rationale, although their efficacy has not, in most cases, been established by controlled trials. They are not subject to formal regulatory approval, so long as they do not contain artificial additives other than those that have been approved for use in foods. Cosmeceuticals is a fancy name for cosmetic products similarly supplemented with substances claimed to reduce skin wrinkles, promote hair growth, etc. These products achieve very large sales, and some pharmaceutical companies have expanded their business in this direction. We do not discuss these fringe 'ceuticals' in this book.

Within each of the medical categories listed above lies a range of procedures: at one end of the spectrum are procedures that have been fully tried and tested and are recognized by medical authorities; at the other is outright quackery of all kinds. Somewhere between lie widely used 'complementary' procedures, practised in some cases under the auspices of officially recognized bodies, which have no firm scientific foundation. Here we find, among psychological treatments, hypnotherapy and analytical psychotherapy; among nutritional treatments, 'health foods', added vitamins, and diets claimed to avoid ill-defined food allergies; among physical treatments, acupuncture and osteopathy; among chemical treatments, homeopathy, herbalism and aromatherapy. Biological procedures lying in this grey area between scientific medicine and quackery are uncommon (and we should probably be grateful for this) – unless one counts colonic irrigation and swimming with dolphins.

In this book we are concerned with the last two treatment categories on the list, summarized in Table 3.1, and in this chapter we consider the current status and future prospects of the three main fields; namely, 'conventional' therapeutic drugs, biopharmaceuticals and various biological therapies.

CONVENTIONAL THERAPEUTIC DRUGS

Small-molecule drugs, either synthetic compounds or natural products, have for a long time been the mainstay of therapeutics and are likely to remain so, despite the rapid growth of biopharmaceuticals in recent years. For their advantages and disadvantages see Box 3.1.

Although the pre-eminent role of conventional small-molecule drugs may decline as biopharmaceutical products grow in importance, few doubt that they will continue to play a major role in medical treatment. New technologies described in Section 2, particularly automated chemistry, high-throughput screening and genomic approaches to target identification, have already brought about an acceleration of drug discovery, the fruits of which are only just beginning to appear. There are also high expectations that more sophisticated drug delivery systems (see Chapter 16) will allow drugs to act much more selectively where they are needed, and thus reduce the burden of side effects.

Box 3.1 Advantages and disadvantages of small-molecule drugs

Advantages

- 'Chemical space' is so vast that synthetic chemicals, according to many experts, have the potential to bind specifically to any chosen biological target: the right molecule exists; it is just a matter of finding it.
- Doctors and patients are thoroughly familiar with conventional drugs as medicines, and the many different routes of administration that are available. Clinical pharmacology in its broadest sense has become part of the knowledge base of every practising doctor, and indeed, part of everyday culture. Although sections of the public may remain suspicious of drugs, there are few who will refuse to use them when the need arises.
- Oral administration is often possible, as well as other routes where appropriate.
- From the industry perspective, small-molecule drugs make up more than three-quarters of new products registered over the past decade. Pharmaceutical companies have long experience in developing, registering, producing, packaging and marketing such products.
- Therapeutic peptides are generally straightforward to design (as Nature has done the job), and are usually non-toxic.

Disadvantages

- As emphasized elsewhere in this book, the flow of new small-molecule drugs seems to be diminishing, despite increasing R&D expenditure.
- Side effects and toxicity remain a serious and unpredictable problem, causing failures in late development, or even after registration. One reason for this is that the selectivity of drug molecules with respect to biological targets is by no means perfect, and is in general less good than with biopharmaceuticals.
- Humans and other animals have highly developed mechanisms for eliminating foreign molecules, so drug design often has to contend with pharmacokinetic problems.
- Oral absorption is poor for many compounds. Peptides cannot be given orally.

BIOPHARMACEUTICALS

For the purposes of this book, biopharmaceuticals are therapeutic protein or nucleic acid preparations made by techniques involving recombinant DNA technology (Walsh, 2003), although smaller nucleotide assemblies are now being made using a chemical approach. Although proteins such as insulin and growth hormone, extracted from human or animal tissues, have long been used therapeutically, the era of biopharmaceuticals began in 1982 with the development by Eli Lilly of recombinant human insulin (Humulin), made by genetically engineered *Escherichia coli*. Recombinant human growth hormone (also produced in *E. coli*), erythropoietin (Epogen) and

Table 3.1 The main types of chemical therapeutic agent

Type	Source	Examples	Notes
Conventional small-molecule drugs	Synthetic organic compounds*	Most of the pharmacopoeia	The largest category of drugs in use, and of new registrations
	Natural products	Paclitaxel (Taxol), many antibiotics and anticancer drugs (e.g. penicillins, aminoglycosides, erythromycin), opiates (e.g. morphine), statins (e.g. lovastatin), ciclosporin, fujimycin	Continues to be an important source of new therapeutic drugs
	Semisynthetic compounds (i.e. compounds made by derivatizing natural products)	Penicillin derivatives (e.g. ampicillin), second-generation statins (e.g. simvastatin)	Strategy for generating improved 'second-generation' drugs from natural products
Peptide and protein mediators	Synthetic	Somatostatin, calcitonin, vasopressin	Peptides up to approximately 20 residues can be reliably made by solid-phase synthesis
	Extracted from natural sources (human, animal, microbial)	Insulin, growth hormone, human γ-globulins, botulinum toxin	At one time the only source of such hormones. Now largely replaced by recombinant biotechnology products. γ-globulins still obtained from human blood
	Recombinant DNA technology	Human insulin, erythropoietin, human growth hormone, GM-CSF TNF-α, hirudin	Many different expression systems in use and in development
Antibodies	Animal antisera, human immunoglobulins	Antisera used to treat infections such as hepatitis A and B, diphtheria, rabies, tetanus. Also poisoning by botulinum, snake and spider venoms, etc.	
	Monoclonal antibodies	Trastuzumab (directed against epidermal growth factor receptor), rituximab (directed against B-cell surface antigen)	A rapidly growing class of biopharmaceuticals, with many products in development
Enzymes	Recombinant DNA technology	Cerebrosidase, dornase, galactosidase	
Vaccines	Infecting organism (killed, attenuated or non-pathogenic strains)	Smallpox, diphtheria, measles, tuberculosis, tetanus, influenza and many others	The conventional approach, still widely used. Some risk of introducing viable pathogens
	Antigens produced by recombinant DNA technology	Many of the above vaccines now available as recombinant antigens	Advantages are greater consistency and elimination of risk of introducing pathogens
DNA products	Recombinant DNA technology	Antisense and siRNA oligonucleotides (e.g. Vitravene)	Many products in clinical development. Vitravene (for treating cytomegalovirus infection) is the only marketed product so far

Continued

Table 3.1 *Continued*

Type	Source	Examples	Notes
Cells	Human donors, engineered cell lines	Various stem cell therapies in development	
Tissues	Human donors, animal tissues, engineered tissues	Apligraf	Bilayer of human skin cells
Organs	Human donors	Transplant surgery	

*Not considered here are many 'adjunct' therapies, such as oxygen, antiseptic agents, anaesthetic agents, intravenous salts, etc., which are outside the scope of this book.

tissue plasminogen activator (tPA) made by engineered mammalian cells followed during the 1980s. This was the birth of the biopharmaceutical industry, and since then new bioengineered proteins have contributed an increasing proportion of new medicines to be registered (see Table 3.1 for some examples, and Chapters 12 and 22 for more details). The scope of protein biopharmaceuticals includes copies of endogenous mediators, blood clotting factors, enzyme preparations and monoclonal antibodies, as well as vaccines. See Box 3.2 for their advantages and disadvantages. This field has now matured to the point that we are now facing the prospect of biosimilars consequent on the expiry of the first set of important patents in 2004 and notwithstanding the difficulty of defining 'difference' in the biologicals space (Covic and Kuhlmann 2007).

Immunization against infectious diseases dates from 1796, when Jenner first immunized patients against smallpox by infecting them with the relatively harmless cowpox. Many other immunization procedures were developed in the 19th century, and from the 20th century onwards pharmaceutical companies began producing standardized versions of the antigens, often the attenuated or modified organisms themselves, as well as antisera which would give immediate passive protection against disease organisms. Vaccines and immune approaches to controlling disease are still a major concern, and increasingly biotechnology-derived vaccines are being developed to improve the efficacy of, and reduce the risks associated with, preparations made from infectious material.

Overall, biopharmaceuticals offer great promise for the future, and rapid progress is being made in the technologies used to produce them (Scrip Report, 2001; Covic and Kuhlmann 2007). Currently, nearly all approved biopharmaceuticals are proteins, the majority being copies of endogenous mediators, monoclonal antibodies or vaccines. Many of the clinically useful hormones and mediators that we currently know about have already been produced as biopharmaceuticals, but future advances are rapidly being made as basic research discovers new protein signalling mechanisms. Monoclonal antibodies and antibody mimicking scaffold proteins (see Chapter 13) offer much broader possibilities, and progress is being facilitated by identifying the genes for important functional proteins, such as key enzymes, transporters, etc. Once the DNA sequence of a putative target is known, its amino acid sequence can be inferred and an antibody or antibody-mimetic protein can be produced, even if the target protein

Box 3.2 **Advantages and disadvantages of biopharmaceuticals**

Advantages

- The main benefit offered by biopharmaceutical products is that they open up the scope of protein therapeutics, which was previously limited to proteins that could be extracted from animal or human sources.
- The discovery process for new biopharmaceuticals is often quicker and more straightforward than with synthetic compounds, as screening and lead optimization are not required.
- Unexpected toxicity is less common than with synthetic molecules.
- The risk of immune responses to non-human proteins – a problem with porcine or bovine insulins – is avoided by expressing the human sequence.
- The risk of transmitting virus or prion infections is avoided.

Disadvantages

- Producing biopharmaceuticals on a commercial scale is expensive, requiring complex purification and quality control procedures.
- The products are not orally active and often have short plasma half-lives, so special delivery systems may be required, adding further to costs. Like other proteins, biopharmaceutical products do not cross the blood–brain barrier.
- For the above reasons, development generally costs more and takes longer, than it does for synthetic drugs.
- Many biopharmaceuticals are species specific in their effects, making tests of efficacy in animal models difficult or impossible.

is of such low abundance that it cannot be isolated biochemically.

Following the wave of successes by the biotechnology industry in producing biopharmaceuticals such as human insulin, erythropoietin and growth hormone during the 1980s and 1990s, medical biotechnology expanded into many other fields, including the development of therapeutic modalities beyond therapeutic proteins and antibodies. Next we briefly discuss two important developments still in the experimental phase, namely gene-based and cell-based therapies, which are under very active investigation.

GENE THERAPY

Recombinant DNA technology offers the promise of altering the genetic material of cells and thereby correcting the results of genetic defects, whether inherited or acquired. The techniques for manipulating cellular DNA that underpin much of modern molecular biology have great versatility, and can in principle be applied to therapeutic as well as experimental endeavours. Even where the genetic basis of the disease is not well understood, it should be possible to counteract its effects by genetic, as distinct from pharmacological, means. Further technical information about gene therapy is given in Chapter 12, and in reference works such as Meager (1999), Templeton and Lasic (2000), Kresina (2001), Brooks (2002) and Sheridan (2011). Gene therapy has been actively investigated for more than two decades, and many clinical trials have been performed. So far, however, the results have proved disappointing, and there are currently (at the time of publishing) no gene therapy products approved for clinical use, although many clinical trials are still in progress (Sheridan 2011).

The most widely investigated approach involves introducing new genes to replace missing or dysfunctional ones; this is most commonly done by engineering the new gene into a modified virus (the vector), which has the ability to enter the host cell, causing expression of the artificially introduced gene until the cell dies or expels the foreign DNA. Such non-integrated DNA is usually eliminated quite quickly and is not passed on to the cell's progeny, and so this type of transfection is generally only appropriate in situations where transient expression is all that is required. Retroviral vectors are able to incorporate the new DNA into the host cell's chromosomes, where it will remain and be expressed during the lifetime of the cell and will be passed on to any progeny of that cell. More elaborate gene therapy protocols for treating single-gene disorders are designed actually to correct the disease-producing sequence mutation in the host genome, or to alter gene expression so as to silence dysfunctional genes.

At one time gene therapy directed at germline cells was considered a possibility, the advantage being that an inherited gene defect could be prevented from affecting progeny, and effectively eliminated for good. The serious risks and ethical objections to such human genetic engineering, however, have led to a worldwide ban on germ-cell gene-therapy experiments, and efforts are restricted to somatic cell treatments.

How much impact has gene therapy had so far as a therapeutic approach, and what can be expected of it in the future? The first successful trial of gene therapy to be reported was by Anderson and colleagues, who used it in 1990 to replace the dysfunctional gene for the enzyme adenosine deaminase (ADA). ADA deficiency causes *severe combined immunodeficiency syndrome* (SCID), a rare condition which prevents the normal immune response to pathogens, and means that the child can only survive in a germ-free environment. This first gene-therapy trial was successful in partly restoring ADA function, but by no means curative. Hundreds of clinical trials were performed during the 1990s, mainly in three clinical areas, namely cancer, AIDS and single-gene inherited disorders such as cystic fibrosis, haemophilia and SCID. Most of these used viral vectors to deliver the DNA, though some used liposome-packaged DNA or other non-viral vectors for this purpose. The genetic material was delivered systemically in some cases, by intravenous or subcutaneous injection; in other cases it was injected directly into solid tumours. An alternative strategy was to harvest bone marrow cells from the patient, transfect these with the necessary DNA construct ex vivo, and return them to the patient so that the genetically modified cells would recolonize the bone marrow and provide the required protein. These techniques had been extensively worked out in laboratory animals, but the clinical results were uniformly disappointing, mainly because transfection rates were too low and expression was too transient. Repeat administration of viral vectors often elicited an immune response which inactivated the vector. So the very high expectation in the early 1990s that gene therapy would revolutionize treatment in many areas of medicine, from arthritis to mental illness, quickly gave way to much more guarded optimism, and in some cases pessimistic dismissal of the whole concept. There were, however, a few cases in which SCID in children was successfully – and apparently permanently – cured by gene therapy, and there were other trials in haemophilia and certain cancers where results looked promising. Alarm bells sounded, first in 1999 when a teenager, Jesse Gelsinger, who was participating in a gene therapy trial in Philadelphia, developed an intense immunological reaction and suddenly died 4 days after treatment. Official scrutiny uncovered many other cases of adverse reactions that had not been reported as they should have been. Many ongoing trials were halted, and much tighter controls were imposed. Subsequently, in 2000, immune function was successfully restored in 18 SCID children, 17 of whom were alive 5 years later (the first therapeutic success for human gene therapy), but two later developed leukaemia, thought to be because integration of the retroviral transgene occurred in a way that activated a cancer-promoting gene, raising even more serious concerns about the long-term side effects of gene therapy.

In the much more cautious atmosphere now prevailing, some carefully controlled trials are beginning to give positive results, mainly in the treatment of haemophilia, but overall, the general view is that gene therapy, while showing great theoretical potential, has so far proved disappointing in its clinical efficacy, amid concerns about its long-term safety and ongoing problems in designing effective delivery systems (see commentaries by Cavazzana-Calvo et al., 2004; Relph et al., 2004; Sheridan, 2011). Pessimists refer to a decade of failure and note that hundreds of trials have failed so far to produce a single approved therapy. A quick survey of the literature, however, shows a profusion of laboratory studies aimed at improving the technology, and exploring many new ideas for using gene therapy in numerous conditions, ranging from transplant rejection to psychiatric disorders.

The main problems to be overcome are (a) to find delivery vectors that are efficient and selective enough to transfect most or all of the target cells without affecting other cells; (b) to produce long-lasting expression of the therapeutic gene; and (c) to avoid serious adverse effects. Additionally, a method for reversing the effect by turning the foreign gene off if things go wrong would be highly desirable, but has not so far been addressed in trials.

Antisense DNA and small interfering RNA (siRNA) have been investigated as an alternative to the DNA strategies outlined above. Antisense DNA consists of an oligonucleotide sequence complementary to part of a known mRNA sequence. The antisense DNA binds to the mRNA and, by mechanisms that are not fully understood, blocks expression very selectively, though only for as long as the antisense DNA remains in the cell. The practical problems of developing therapeutic antisense reagents are considerable, as unmodified oligonucleotides are quickly degraded in plasma and do not enter cells readily, so either chemical modification or special delivery systems such as liposomal packaging are required (see Kole et al., 2012). So far only one antisense preparation has been approved for clinical use, an oligonucleotide used to treat an ocular virus infection in AIDS patients. *Ribozymes*, specific mRNA sequences that inactivate genes by catalysing DNA cleavage, are being investigated as an alternative to antisense DNA, but so far none has been approved for clinical use. The recent past has seen an explosion of the evaluation of siRNAs following the award of the Nobel Prize for its discovery in 2006 and the demonstration that it can be used to silence important genes in non-human primates (Zimmerman et al., 2006). Most major pharmaceutical companies made large investments in the technology in the hope that it would have broad utility and lend itself to systemic medication against a variety of targets but it now seems that the problems of delivery of the synthetic nucleotide 23mers is a roadblock that is very hard to overcome and most of the early clinical trials currently in progress are using direct injection to the target tissues (Ledford, 2010).

In addition to their chequered clinical trials history, gene therapy products share with other biopharmaceuticals many features that cause major pharmaceutical companies to shy away from investing heavily in such products. The reagents are large molecules, or viruses, that have to be delivered to the appropriate sites in tissues, often to particular cells and with high efficiency. Supplying gene therapy reagents via the bloodstream is only effective for luminal vascular targets, and topical administration is usually needed. Viral vectors do not spread far from the site of injection, nor do they infect all cell types. The vectors have their separate toxicology issues. Commercial production, quality control, formulation and delivery often present problems.

In summary, the theoretical potential of gene therapy is enormous, and the ingenuity being applied to making it work is very impressive. Still, after 30 years of intense research effort no product has been developed, and many of the fundamental problems in delivering genes effectively and controllably still seem far from solution. Most likely, a few effective products for a few specific diseases will be developed and marketed in the next few years, and this trickle will probably grow until gene therapy makes a significant contribution to mainstream therapeutics. Whether it will grow eventually to a flood that supplants much of conventional therapeutics, or whether it will remain hampered by technical problems, nobody can say at this stage. In the foreseeable future, gene therapy is likely to gain acceptance as a useful adjunct to conventional chemotherapy for cancer and viral infections, particularly AIDS. The Holy Grail of a cure for inherited diseases such as cystic fibrosis still seems some way off.

CELL-BASED THERAPIES

Cell-replacement therapies offer the possibility of effective treatment for various kinds of degenerative disease, and much hope currently rests on the potential uses of stem cells, which are undifferentiated progenitor cells that can be maintained in tissue culture and, by the application of appropriate growth factors, be induced to differentiate into functional cells of various kinds. Their ability to divide in culture means that the stock of cells can be expanded as required (see Atala et al., 2011; Lanza et al., 2007).

Autologous cell grafts (i.e. returning treated cells to the same individual) are quite widely used for treating leukaemias and similar malignancies of bone marrow cells. A sample of the patient's bone marrow is taken, cleansed of malignant cells, expanded, and returned to colonize the bone marrow after the patient has been treated with high-dose chemotherapy or radiotherapy to eradicate all resident bone marrow cells. Bone marrow is particularly suitable for this kind of therapy because it is rich in stem cells, and can be recolonized with 'clean' cells injected into the bloodstream.

Apart from this established procedure for treating bone marrow malignancies, only two cell-based therapeutic products have so far gained FDA approval: preparations of autologous chondrocytes used to repair cartilage defects, and autologous keratinocytes, used for treating burns. Other potential applications which have been the focus of much experimental work are reviewed by Fodor (2003). They include:

- Neuronal cells injected into the brain (Isaacson, 2003) to treat neurodegenerative diseases such as Parkinson's disease (loss of dopaminergic neurons), amyotrophic lateral sclerosis (loss of cholinergic neurons) and Huntington's disease (loss of GABA neurons)
- Insulin-secreting cells to treat insulin-dependent diabetes mellitus
- Cardiac muscle cells to restore function after myocardial infarction.

The major obstacle to further development of such cell-based therapies is that the use of embryonic tissues – the preferred source of stem cells – is severely restricted for ethical reasons. Although stem cells can be harvested from adult tissues and organs, they are less satisfactory. Like gene therapy, cell-based therapeutics could in principle have many important applications, and the technical problems that currently stand in the way are the subject of intensive research efforts. Biotechnology companies are active in developing the necessary tools and reagents that are likely to be needed to select and prepare cells for transplantation.

TISSUE AND ORGAN TRANSPLANTATION

Transplantation of human organs, such as heart, liver, kidneys and corneas, is of course a well established procedure, many of the problems of rejection having been largely solved by the use of immunosuppressant drugs such as ciclosporin and fujimycin. Better techniques for preventing rejection, including procedures based on gene therapy, are likely to be developed, but the main obstacle remains the limited supply of healthy human organs, and there is little reason to think that this will change in the foreseeable future. The possibility of xenotransplantation – the use of non-human organs, usually from pigs – has received much attention. Cross-species transplants are normally rejected within minutes by a process known as hyperacute rejection. Transgenic pigs whose organs are rendered resistant to hyperacute rejection have been produced, but trials in humans have so far been ruled out because of the risk of introducing pig retroviruses into humans. Despite much discussion and arguments on both sides, there is no sign of this embargo being lifted. Organ transplantation requires such a high degree of organization to get the correct matched organs to the right patients at the right time, as well as advanced surgical and follow-up resources, that it will remain an option only for the privileged minority.

Building two- (e.g. skin) and three-dimensional (e.g. a heart valve) structures that are intended to function mechanically, either from host cells or from banked, certified primordial or stem cell populations, is at the cutting edge of tissue engineering efforts. The aim is to fashion these tissues and organ parts around artificial scaffold materials, and to do this in culture under the control of appropriate growth and differentiation factors. The development of biocompatible scaffolding materials, and achieving the right growth conditions, are problems where much remains to be done. Artificial skin preparations recently became available and others will probably follow.

Also in an early, albeit encouraging, state of development are bionic devices – the integration of mechanical and electronic prostheses with the human body – which will go beyond what has already been accomplished with devices such as cochlear implants and neurally controlled limb prostheses. The role of the major pharmaceutical companies in this highly technological area is likely to be small. The economic realities of the relatively small patient populations will most likely be the limiting factor governing the full implementation of integrated bionics.

SUMMARY

Small organic molecule drugs of molecular weight <500 Da are the preferred therapeutic modality of the major pharmaceutical companies for most disease applications but the landscape is now changing and it has been predicted that by 2014 the most important therapies for treating human diseases will be biologicals (Reuters Factbox, 2010). The development over the years of large, chemically diverse small-molecule libraries, many already with 'drug-like' properties (see Chapters 8 and 9) built into their structure, reinforces the commitment of the industry to this approach. However, protein and peptide therapeutics also have their place in the pharmaceutical armamentarium, especially with respect to the immune system and hormonal dysregulation. Many pharmaceutical companies began with immune antisera and vaccines, but the first specialized biotechnology companies took advantage of recombinant DNA methods to produce therapeutic proteins. Although the major pharmaceutical companies have almost all adopted protein therapeutics in addition to their traditional small molecule approach, many of the advances in the field have been made by specialist biotechnology companies.

Protein- and DNA- and RNA-based biopharmaceuticals often face difficult pharmacokinetic problems, in particular poor absorption, rapid degradation, and inability to enter cells or cross the blood–brain barrier. Their successful development therefore often depends on developing suitable delivery systems that help to overcome these problems. For this reason (and also to improve the performance of conventional therapeutic drugs) drug delivery technology (see Chapter 16) is currently receiving a great deal of attention, with many new polymer- and liposome-based formulations being invented and tested. The right delivery system is as necessary as the right drug, and for biopharmaceuticals the two will generally need to be developed in tandem, rather than first developing a compound and then optimizing the delivery system (which is the development strategy usually adopted for small-molecule drugs).

Somatic (non-germline) gene therapy initially was thought to have great promise for curing inborn errors that lead to disease. More than 30 years later, although the technology and our understanding have greatly improved, clinical success has proved elusive. Optimizing vectors and delivery systems so as to produce long-lasting gene expression in the tissues where it is needed has proved much more difficult than expected. Nevertheless, there is reason for optimism in the long term. Currently, gene therapy development is being directed mainly at life-threatening disorders such as cancer, AIDs and haemophilia, where the need is greatest and the risks are balanced by the severity of the diseases. It is likely to be another decade or two before gene therapy begins to make a broader clinical impact.

The involvement of pharmaceutical companies in the transplantation field is largely confined to improving the immunosuppressant drugs that are needed to protect transplants from immune rejection. The use of transplants is severely restricted by the availability of human organs, and hopes for improving the situation by the use of xenografts are unlikely to be realized in the foreseeable future. Stem-cell technologies are likely to be used successfully for certain kinds of tissue repair and cell replacement; biotechnology companies, rather than pharmaceutical companies, are likely to make the running in these new fields although some large firms are establishing departments of regenerative medicine. Currently, techniques such as bone marrow transplants are being developed and used successfully by clinical teams without any necessary input from commercial research. Probably their use will become more routine, but it seems unlikely that the market size for commercial products in this area will be enough for a large pharmaceutical company.

REFERENCES

Atala A, Lanza R, Thomson JA, Nerem R, editors. Principles of regenerative medicine. 2nd ed. New York: Academic Press; 2011.

Brooks G, editor. Gene therapy: the use of DNA as a drug. New York: John Wiley and Sons; 2002.

Cavazzana-Calvo M, Thrasher A, Mavilio F. The future of gene therapy. Nature 2004;427:779–81.

Covic A, Kuhlmann MK. Biosimilars: recent developments. International Urology and Nephrology 2007;39:261–6.

Fodor WL. Tissue engineering and cell based therapies, from the bench to the clinic: the potential to replace, repair and regenerate. Reproductive Biology and Endocrinology 2003;1:102–7.

Isaacson O. The production and use of cells as therapeutic agents in neurodegenerative diseases. Lancet Neurology 2003;2:417–24.

Kole R, Krainer AR, Altman S. RNA therapeutics: beyond RNA interference and antisense oligonucleotides. Nature Rev Drug Discov 2012;11:125–40.

Kresina TF, editor. An introduction to molecular medicine and gene therapy. New York: John Wiley and Sons; 2001.

Lanza R, Langer R, Vacanti JP, editors. Principles of tissue engineering. New York: Academic Press; 2007.

Ledford H. Drug giants turn their backs on RNA interference Nature 2010;468:487.

Meager A. Gene therapy technologies: applications and regulations from laboratory to clinic. Chichester: John Wiley and Sons; 1999.

Relph K, Harrington K, Pandha H. Recent developments and current status of gene therapy using viral vectors in the United Kingdom. British Medical Journal 2004;329:839–42.

Reuters Factbox. Apr 13th 2010 Worlds top 2014 vs 2010 www.reuters.com/article/2010/04/13

Scrip Report. (2001) Biopharmaceuticals: a new era of discovery in the biotechnology revolution.

Sheridan C. Gene therapy finds its niche. Nature Biotechnology 2011;29:121–8.

Templeton NS, Lasic DD. Gene therapy: therapeutic mechanisms and strategies. New York: Marcel Dekker; 2000.

Walsh G. Biopharmaceuticals. 2nd ed. Chichester: John Wiley and Sons Ltd; 2003.

Zimmerman TS, Lee ACH, Akinc A, et al. RNAi-mediated gene silencing in non-human primates. Nature 2006;441:111–4.

Section | 2 |

Drug discovery

Chapter 4

The drug discovery process: general principles and some case histories

H P Rang, R G Hill

INTRODUCTION

The creation of a new drug can be broadly divided into three main phases (Figure 4.1):

- Drug discovery – from therapeutic concept to molecule
- Drug development – from molecule to registered product
- Commercialization – from product to therapeutic application to sales.

Traditionally, these functions are performed by Research, Development and Marketing, respectively, reflecting the different professional training and expertise required to do the job. Figure 4.1 greatly oversimplifies what is actually a very complex process. For example, development activities, in the form of additional clinical trials, or testing of new formulations, continue well beyond the point of registration, with the aim of extending the range of applications of the compound or complying with regulatory requirements. The discovery team, having delivered the first candidate drug, will carry on looking for others, to serve as back-ups in case the lead compound should fail in development, or as follow-up compounds intended to have advantages over the lead compound. The three components of the overall process are not independent and consecutive stages, but have to be closely coordinated at all stages of the project. At the outset of any new project, the criteria against which the plan will be judged include not only its scientific strength and originality but, importantly, development and marketing issues. For example, if the therapeutic target is an ill-defined clinical disorder, such as chronic fatigue syndrome, will it be possible to measure clinical efficacy objectively? Does the project face stiff competition from other companies working in the same area, or from drugs already in clinical use? Is it likely that an esoteric drug delivery system will be required, and if so, can this be developed? If the drug is successfully developed, is the expected market sufficient to justify the cost of development? The answers to questions of this kind are likely to change, for better or for worse, during the course of the project, so it is essential to keep such issues constantly under review, and to adapt the project plan if necessary.

To integrate successfully the different interests – and cultures – of research, development and marketing is one of the major challenges for a pharmaceutical company, and the need for such integration is a relatively modern development in the industry. As recently as 25–30 years ago in most companies, the process was much more compartmentalized: scientists produced molecules with interesting pharmacological properties, development functions were responsible for checking their safety and turning them into registrable drugs, and the marketing department generated sales and turned them into revenues. At the time this worked well, and many companies prospered. The drop-out rate was not excessive, because regulatory requirements were less stringent, and the failures that did occur were not unduly expensive in terms of time and resources lost. Since then, biomedical science has advanced dramatically, drug discovery and development have become more technology-driven and, hence, expensive, regulatory requirements are much more stringent, and the competition is more intense. With bigger teams, and more complex multidisciplinary tasks, effective project management has become much more important than it used to be to keep costs and delays to a minimum. An additional complication is that of the increased amount of work being done in partnership with other companies or with academic groups, adding the need for alliance as well as project management (see also Chapter 22).

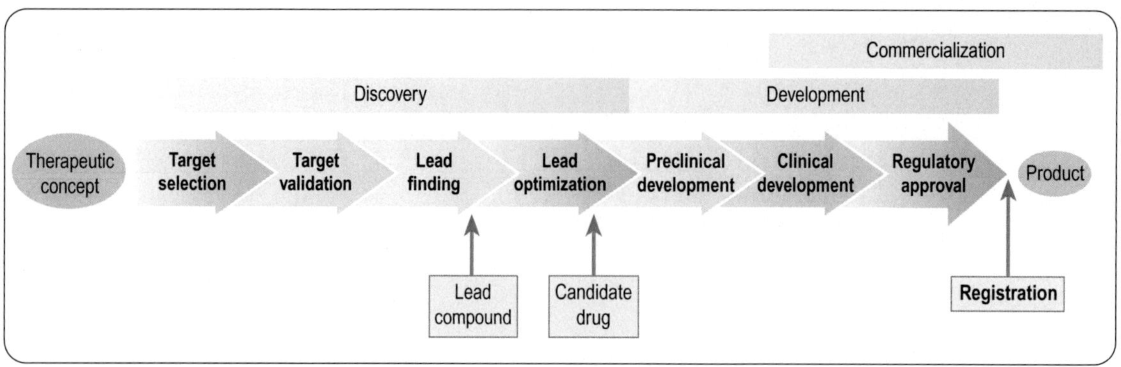

Fig. 4.1 Three main phases of the creation of a new drug: discovery, development and commercialization.

A more detailed overview of the drug discovery phase of a typical project aimed at producing a new synthetic drug is shown in Figure 4.2. It starts with the choice of a disease area and defining the therapeutic need that is to be met. It proceeds to the identification of the biochemical, cellular or pathophysiological mechanism that will be targeted, and, if possible, the identification and validation of a molecular 'drug target'. Next comes the identification of a lead structure, followed by the design, testing and fine-tuning of the drug molecule to the point where it is deemed suitable for development, discussed in more detail in subsequent chapters.

The strong emphasis on defined molecular (normally protein) drug targets as a starting point is too recent to have culminated so far in many actual drugs on the market. Many drugs now being registered have their origins in research going back 20 years or more, in the 'premolecular' drug discovery era, when the selected targets were mainly pathophysiological or biochemical mechanisms, such as blood pressure regulation, inflammation or cholesterol metabolism, of which the molecular components were not yet defined. This earlier period, roughly from 1960 to 1980, was actually highly productive in terms of drug discovery, representing a return on R&D investment considerably greater than what can be achieved today, and the discovery approaches used then remain very much alive despite the increasing emphasis on molecular targets. Nevertheless, we now think increasingly in terms of defined molecular targets as the necessary starting point for drug discovery, and turn automatically to molecular technologies to provide the necessary tools. Until about 1980 this was rarely feasible; even when the 'target' was defined, for example as an enzyme or a receptor, it was seldom available in sufficient quantities in a purified functional form to be used as the basis for screening assays. Instead, the functional activity of the target was measured by indirect means in isolated tissue preparations, or even in whole animals, methods which we nowadays regard as too slow, laborious and error prone to place at the front end of a drug discovery project.

The foregoing remarks apply to the discovery of conventional 'small-molecule' therapeutics, and the strategy for developing biopharmaceuticals – an increasing proportion of new drugs appearing on the market – is generally different. Biopharmaceutical agents (see Chapter 3) are very diverse, including endogenous mediators, monoclonal antibodies and vaccines, and in the future, no doubt, products for siRNA and gene therapy applications. Where endogenous molecules are involved, the concept of targets and lead compounds has much less relevance, as nature has done the discovery part of the work, so once the therapeutic relevance of the substance has been established, the problems mainly revolve around the production, purification and formulation of the material in a form suitable for the market. With other kinds of biopharmaceuticals, such as therapeutic antibodies, the molecular target will generally be chosen in advance, and the main task is to obtain an antibody with the required properties.

A glance at the pharmacopoeia will show that many therapeutic agents, particularly anti-infective and anti-tumour drugs, originate from natural products, rather than synthetic molecules (Table 4.1). Until about 1950, when synthetic chemistry really came into its own as a source of new drugs, most of the pharmacopoeia consisted of natural products, and they continue to be important, as the example of *paclitaxel* described below shows. It is reasonable to suppose that such ready-made, highly evolved biomolecules stand a better chance of interacting with selected drug targets than do random synthetic molecules, and the pool from which they come is huge and largely untapped. Exploiting such a ready-made compound library is seen as an attractive strategy which has led to some important therapeutic breakthroughs, such as the anti-malarial drug *artemesinin*, immunosuppressants such as *ciclosporin fujimycin* (FK506) and *rapamycin*, as well as paclitaxel and other recently introduced anticancer drugs such as *epothilones*. In

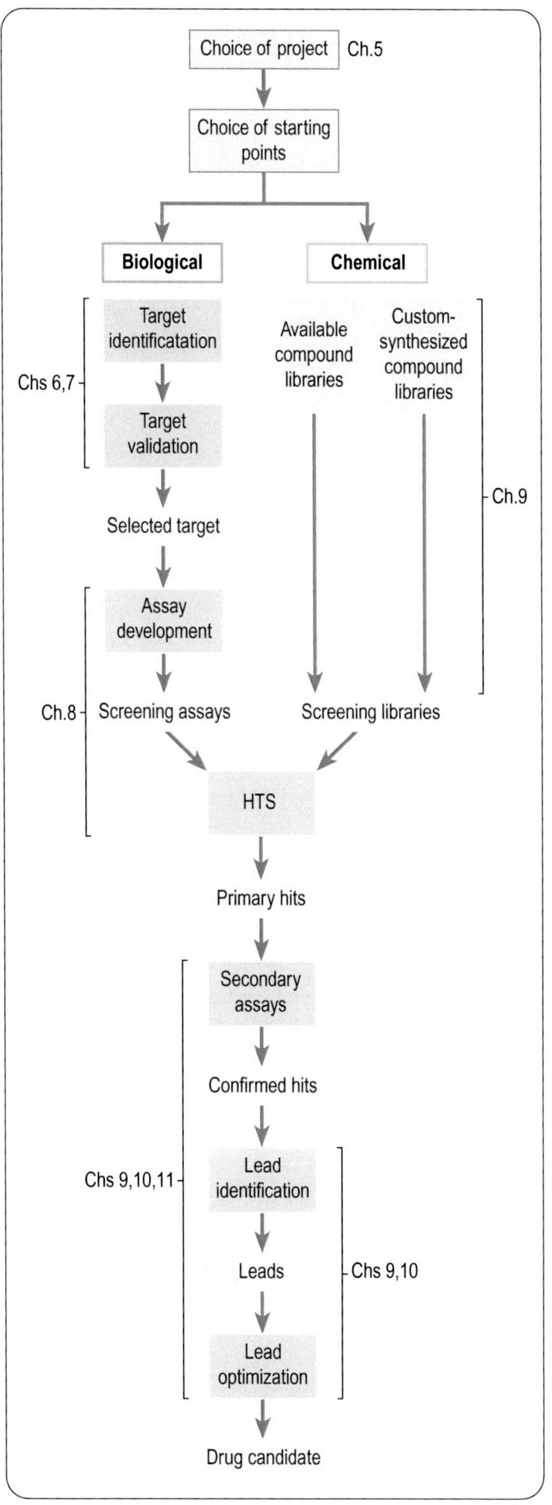

Fig. 4.2 Drug discovery phase of a typical project aimed at producing a new synthetic drug.

Table 4.1 Examples of therapeutic drugs derived from natural products

Warfarin	Anticoagulant. Synthetic compound derived from dicoumarol, found in spoiled sweet clover
Heparin	Anticoagulant, occurring naturally in mammalian tissues
Hirudin	Anticoagulant from leech, now produced by genetic engineering
Opiates	Analgesic compounds from poppies
Methylxanthines (caffeine, theophylline)	Phosphodiesterase inhibitors and adenosine receptor antagonists. Produced by tea, coffee and coca plants
Statins	HMG CoA reductase inhibitors used to reduce plasma cholesterol. Lovastatin is a fungal metabolite. Later compounds (mevastatin, pravastatin) synthesized from lovastatin
Cromoglycate	Asthma prohylaxis. Synthetic compound based on khellin, a plant product used as a herbal medicine
Vinca alkaloids (vincristine, vinblastine)	Anticancer drugs produced by plants of the periwinkle family
Paclitaxel	Anticancer drug from yew tree
Etoposide	Anticancer drug synthesized from podophyllotoxin, produced by mandrake plant; used in folk medicine
Artemether	Antimalarial drug, semisynthetic derivative of artemesin, produced by Chinese herb
Ivermectin	Antihelminthic drug, semisynthetic derivative of avermectin, a fungal metabolite
Antibiotics	Too numerous to list. The majority of current antibiotics are derived from fungal metabolites

In earlier times the pharmacopoeia consisted very largely of plant-derived compounds (e.g. opiates, atropine, ephedrine, ergot alkaloids, strychnine, tubocurarine, digoxin, quinine, veratridine, reserpine, etc.), many of which remain in therapeutic use or provide valuable research tools.

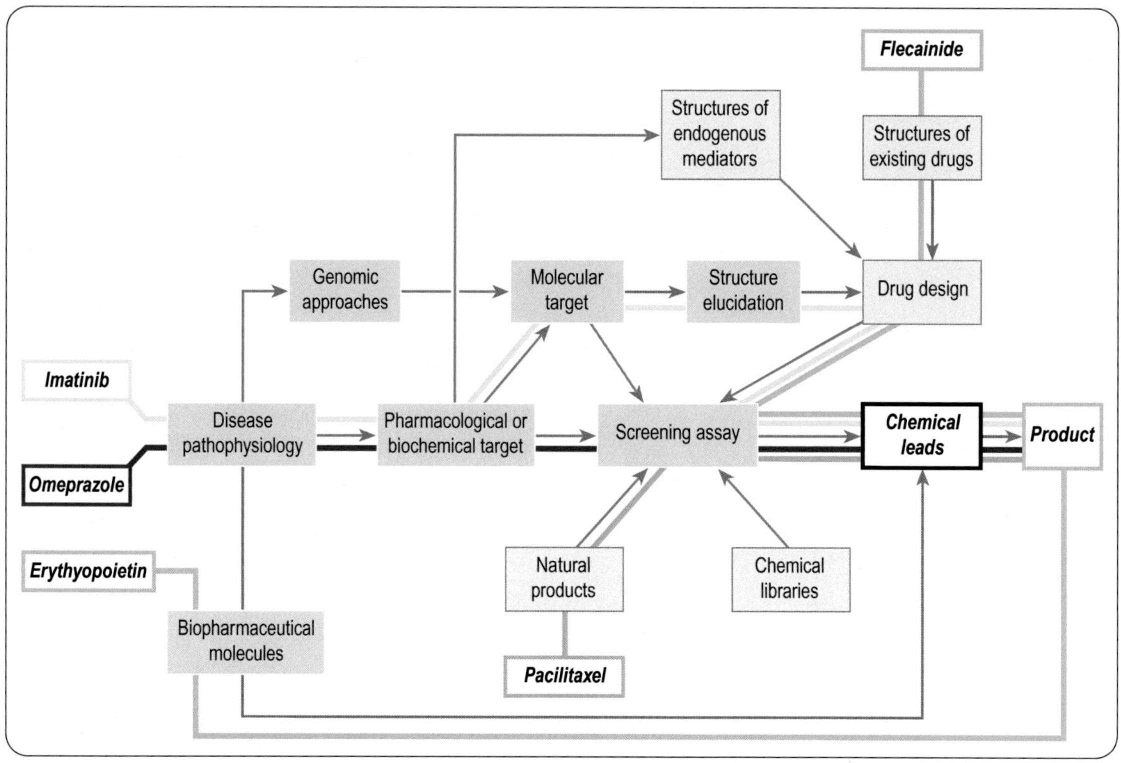

Fig. 4.3 Discovery pathways of some successful projects.

2008–2010, 8 out of 64 novel compounds registered were natural products or derived from natural products. In practice, the theoretical advantages of natural products are balanced by several practical disadvantages. Access to source material in remote places can be troublesome for geographical reasons, as well as being politically sensitive, and the continuing availability of the active compound, if it cannot be synthesized on a commercial basis, may be uncertain. Microorganisms have an advantage over higher species in this regard, but initial positive test data on microbial samples frequently cannot be replicated, presumably because of inconsistencies in the culture conditions. Purification and structure determination of natural products is now fairly routine, but is often difficult and time-consuming. A recent example is the introduction of Sativex, a standardized preparation of cannabinoids, given as intra oral drops for the treatment of spasticity associated with multiple sclerosis.

Some case histories

It is clear that there are many starting points and routes to success in drug discovery projects (Lednicer, 1993; Drews, 2000). The brief case histories of five successful drugs, *paclitaxel (Taxol)*, *flecainide (Tambocor)*, *omeprazol (Losec)*, *imatinib (Gleevec/Glivec)* and *trastuzumab (Herceptin)*, are summarized in Figure 4.3 and Table 4.2, and described in more detail below. Each represents a highly innovative 'breakthrough' project rather than an incremental development based on an existing therapy, and they illustrate the variety of different approaches taken by successful projects over the past 35 years. However, for several reasons we should avoid interpreting these as guidelines for success in the future. For one thing, the approach changes as the underlying technologies advance; furthermore, pharmaceutical companies generally publicize only their successes, and even then the accounts are often somewhat sanitized, and fail to describe the errors that were made, the deadlines missed and the blind alleys that were encountered – the full 'shaggy drug stories' generally remain discreetly hidden. It must be remembered that, of drug discovery projects begun, only about 1 in 50 is successful in terms of bringing a compound to market. Only at the point when official approval for trials in man is granted does the project become visible to the outside world, so data on success rates, timelines, etc., are much

Table 4.2 Timelines for some successful drug discovery projects

Drug	Paclitaxel (Taxol)	Flecainide (Tambocor)	Omeprazol (Losec)	Imatinib (Gleevec/ Glivec)	Trastuzumab (Herceptin)
Mechanism	Natural product inhibitor of tubulin depolymerization	Antidysrhythmic drug. Blocks cardiac Na^+ channels	Inhibitor of gastric acid secretion. Blocks proton pump	Inhibits Abl kinase	Humanized monoclonal antibody. Blocks Her2 oestrogen receptor
Company	US National Cancer Institute/ Bristol Myers Squibb	3M	Astra	Novartis	Genentech/Roche
Indication	Ovarian cancer	Cardiac dysrhythmias	Peptic ulcer	Chronic myeloid leukaemia	Breast cancer
Project start	1964	1965	1966	1983	1988
Compound synthesized or structure determined	1971 (7 years)	1974 (9 years)	1978 (12 years)	1990 (7 years)	1990 (2 years)
Phase I	1983 (19 years)	1976 (11 years)	1981 (15 years)		1991 (3 years)
Registration	1992 (28 years)	1984 (19 years)	1988 (22 years)	2001 (18 years)	1998 (10 years)

more accessible for the minority of projects that progress to Phase I or beyond than for the majority that never get that far. Analysing the success factors for early-stage drug discovery projects is therefore difficult.

Paclitaxel (Taxol)

Paclitaxel is an interesting example of a project based on the development of a natural product (Cragg, 1998). It began in the early 1960s, when the US National Cancer Institute, responding to the Nixon-inspired 'war on cancer', set up one of the first directed screening programmes – still running – to seek new anticancer drugs from plant sources. The sample of bark from the Pacific Yew was collected in 1962 and found to have modest activity against various tumour cell lines. The active substance was isolated in 1969 and joined a collection of moderately active, but not particularly interesting, lead compounds. When this collection was dusted off in 1975 and tested on a new assay, a melanoma cell line, paclitaxel stood out as highly active. Its activity was confirmed in animal models, and it was soon chosen as a development candidate. Interest was further stimulated when its novel mechanism of action, the promotion of microtubule polymerization, was very elegantly demonstrated. Development was difficult, for two main reasons. Paclitaxel is insoluble in water, and the early formulations for injection used in Phase I trials contained a high proportion of the solubilizing agent Cremophor EL, causing frequent severe allergic reactions when given as a bolus intravenous injection. After considerable delay, the problem was overcome by the use of slow infusions and development was resumed. The second problem was the supply of material for clinical trials, and the uncertainty that it could ever be produced on a commercial basis. The Pacific Yew grows slowly and has a restricted habitat, and conservationists were opposed to commercial harvesting. As a result, there was only enough material for limited Phase II studies, on patients with ovarian cancer. The improvement in these patients was dramatic, but continuation of the project, now in collaboration with Bristol Myers Squibb, was seriously hindered by the limited supplies of yew tree bark. The conservation concerns were overcome when a census showed that the tree population was not in fact threatened, and industrial supplies of bark were collected to support the trials programme right through to 1992, when the drug was officially approved.

Commercialization of the material extracted from bark was seen as a major problem, but was solved when it was found that the needles of many yew species contain *baccatin*, from which paclitaxel can be produced. This semisynthetic paclitaxel, made from an abundant and renewable source, was officially approved in 1999 and is a highly successful and clinically valuable form of cancer therapy. The obstacles to progress in this case were (a) the failure of the primary screen to reveal the compound as anything out of the ordinary; (b) the appearance of serious side effects resulting from the properties of the excipient; and (c) the supply problem.

Flecainide (Tambocor)

The story of flecainide (Banitt and Schmid, 1993) represents a completely different route to success, variations of which gave rise to many innovative drugs (e.g. antihypertensive drugs, antidepressants and antipsychotics) during the 1960s. In the early 1960s, the drugs used to treat cardiac dysrhythmias were mainly *quinidine, procainamide, digoxin* (for supraventricular tachycardias) and *lidocaine* (given i.v. for ventricular dysrhythmias). The first three had many troublesome side effects, whereas lidocaine's use was largely confined to intensive care settings. In 1964, the 3M company decided to seek better antidysrhythmic drugs. Their chemists had developed a new synthetic pathway for introducing $-CF_3$ groups, and they started a chemistry programme based on fluorinated derivatives of known local anaesthetic and antidysrythmic drugs. Assays for antidysrhythmic activity at the time involved elaborate studies on anaesthetized dogs, which were quite unsuitable for screening, and so the group developed a simple primary screening assay based on the ability of compounds to prevent ventricular fibrillation induced by chloroform inhalation in mice, which was used to screen hundreds of compounds. Secondary assays on selected compounds were carried out on anaesthetized dogs in the then conventional fashion. Questions of mechanism were not addressed, it being (correctly) assumed that efficacy in these animal models would serve as a good predictor of clinical efficacy irrespective of the cellular mechanisms involved. A potential development compound was synthesized in 1969, but abandoned on account of CNS side effects. After a further 5 years of painstaking chemistry, during which many different structural classes were tested, flecainide was synthesized (1974) and found to have a much improved therapeutic window compared to its predecessors. The first clinical studies were performed in 1976, and development proceeded quite smoothly until the compound was registered in 1984. It was the first deliberate effort to develop an improved antidysrhythmic drug and proved highly successful in the clinic, now accepted as the standard Class 1c antidysrhythmic agent according to the current classification.

With the benefit of hindsight, we can see that the main delaying factor in the flecainide project was simply slow chemistry, guided largely by empiricism. One result of this was that, after encountering side-effect problems with the lead compound, it took 5 years to find the solution (during which, one suspects, the biologists on the team were growing a little bored!). This model of drug discovery research, where chemistry was both the driving force and the rate-limiting factor for the whole project, is typical of many projects conducted in the 1970s (including many that were, like flecainide, ultimately very successful).

Omeprazole (Losec)

Omeprazole, developed by Astra, was the first proton pump inhibitor, and transformed the treatment of peptic ulcers when it was launched in 1988, quickly becoming the company's best-selling drug. The project, however, graphically described by Östholm (1995) had a chequered and death-defying history. In 1966 Astra started a project aimed at developing inhibitors of gastric acid secretion, having previously developed profitable antacid preparations. They started a chemistry programme based on carbamates, and collaborated with an academic group to develop a suitable in vivo screening assay in rats. Compounds with weak activity were quickly identified; initial hepatotoxicity problems were overcome, and a potential development compound was tested in humans in 1968. It had no effect on acid secretion, and the project narrowly escaped termination. In the meantime, good progress was being made by Smith, Kline and French in developing histamine H_2 antagonists for the same indication, thereby adding to the anxiety within Astra. At the same time Searle reported a new class of inhibitory compounds, benzimidazoles, which were active but toxic. Astra began a new chemistry programme based on this series, and in 1973 produced a highly active compound which was proposed for further development. To their dismay, they found that a Hungarian company had a patent on this compound (for a completely different application). However, upon entering licensing negotiations they found that the Hungarian patent had actually lapsed because the company had defaulted on payment of the fees to the patent office! Further studies with this compound revealed problems with thyroid toxicity, however, and more demands to terminate this hapless project were narrowly fought off. The thyroid toxicity was thought to be associated with the thiouracil structure, and further chemistry aimed at eliminating this resulted, in 1976, in the synthesis of *picoprazole*, the forerunner of omeprazole. After yet another toxicological alarm – this time vasculitis in dogs – which turned out to be an artefact, picoprazole was tested in human patients suffering from Zollinger–Ellison syndrome and was found to be highly effective in reducing acid secretion. At around the same time, an academic group showed that acid secretion involved a specific transport mechanism, the proton pump, which was strongly inhibited by the Astra compounds, so their novel mechanism of action was established. Omeprazole, an analogue of picoprazole, was synthesized in 1979, and was chosen for development instead of picoprazole. The chemistry team had by then made over 800 compounds during the 13-year lifetime of the project. The chemical development of omeprazole was complicated by the compound's poor stability and sensitivity to light, requiring special precautions in formulation. Phase II/III clinical trials began in 1981, but were halted for 2 years as a result of yet another toxicology scare – carcinogenicity – which again proved to be a false alarm. Omeprazole was finally registered in 1988.

That omeprazole, one of the most significant new drugs to appear in the early 1990s, should have survived this frightful odyssey is something of a miracle. One setback after another was faced and overcome, a tribute to the sheer determination and persuasive skills of the discovery team. Nowadays, when research managers pride themselves on their decisiveness and courage in terminating projects at the first hint of trouble, omeprazole would surely stand little chance.

Imatinib (Gleevec/Glivec)

Imatinib (Druker and Lydon, 2000; Capdeville et al., 2002), registered in 2001, is the most recent example in these brief histories, and exemplifies the shift towards defined molecular targets that has so altered the approach to drug discovery over the last 20 years. In the mid-1980s, it was discovered that a rare form of cancer, chronic myeloid leukaemia (CML), was almost invariably associated with the expression of a specific oncogene product, Bcr-Abl kinase. The enhanced tyrosine kinase activity of this mutated protein was shown to underlie the malignant transformation of the white blood cells. The proven association between the gene mutation[1], the enhanced kinase activity and the distinct clinical phenotype, provided a particularly clear example of cancer pathogenesis. On this basis, the oncology team of Ciba-Geigy (later Novartis) began a project seeking specific inhibitors of Abl kinase. It is known that there are many different kinases involved in cellular regulatory mechanisms, all using ATP as a phosphate donor and possessing highly conserved ATP-binding domains. Interest in kinase inhibitors as drugs was, and remains, high (Cohen, 2002), but at the time the known inhibitors were all relatively non-specific and distinctly toxic, and the widely held view was that, as the known compounds all acted at the highly conserved ATP-binding site, specific subtype selective kinase inhibitors would be difficult to produce. The commercial potential also appeared weak, as CML is a rare disease. Undaunted, the team started by developing routine biochemical assays for this and other kinases, based on purified enzymes produced in quantity by a genetic engineering technique based on the baculovirus expression system. Screening of synthetic compound libraries revealed that compounds of the 2-phenylaminopyrimidine class showed selectivity in blocking Abl and PDGF-receptor kinases, and systematic chemical derivatization led to the synthesis of imatinib in 1992, roughly 8 years after starting the project. Although crystallographic analysis of the kinase structure played no part in guiding the chemistry that produced imatinib, a later structural study (Schindler et al., 2000) provided an explanation for its selectivity for Abl kinase by showing that its binding site extends beyond the ATP site to other, less conserved domains. Imatinib proved to have no major shortcomings in relation to pharmacokinetics or toxicology, and was highly effective in suppressing the growth of cells engineered to express Bcr-Abl, and of human tumour cells transplanted into mice. Importantly, it also inhibited the growth in culture of peripheral blood or bone marrow cells from CML patients (Druker et al., 1996). The latter result was particularly valuable for the project, as it is rarely possible to carry out such ex vivo tests on material from patients – normally, it is necessary to wait until the compound enters Phase II trials before any evidence relating to clinical efficacy emerges. On that basis the project was given high priority and an accelerated clinical trials programme was devised. The first trials (Druker et al., 2001), beginning in 1998, were performed not on normal subjects, but on 83 CML patients who had failed to respond to treatment with interferon. Different doses were tested in groups of six to eight patients, and the pharmacokinetic parameters, adverse effects and clinical response were measured in parallel. These highly streamlined studies showed an unequivocal clinical effect, with 100% of patients receiving the higher doses showing a good haematological response. As a result, and because the regulatory procedures were dispatched particularly rapidly, the drug was registered in record time, in May 2001, just 3 years after being tested for the first time in humans. Imatinib is the first 'designer' kinase inhibitor to be registered (other drugs, such as *rapamycin*, probably act by kinase inhibition, but this was not known at the time). Imatinib has proved efficacious also in certain gastrointestinal tumours, and is the first of a number of kinase inhibitors now used for treating cancer.

In retrospect, the imatinib project owes its success to several factors, most obviously to the selection of a precisely defined molecular target which was known to be disease relevant, and was amenable to modern assay technologies. Setting up the various kinase assays took 4–5 years, but thereafter screening produced the lead series of compounds rather quickly, and imatinib itself was made within about 4 years of starting the screening programme. Avoiding the pitfalls of pharmacokinetics and toxicology, which so often hinder development, was very fortunate. What was quite exceptional was the speed of clinical development and registration. This was possible partly because CML is resistant to conventional anticancer drugs, and so imatinib did not need to be compared with other treatments. Also, the designation of imatinib as an 'orphan drug' (see Chapter 20), based on the rarity of CML, allowed

[1]Identifiable by a chromosomal staining technique able to detect the translocation of DNA between two chromosomes, producing the characteristic 'Philadelphia chromosome' which gives rise to the abnormal kinase.

the trials programme to be simplified and accelerated. Its action is readily monitored by haematological tests, permitting a rapid clinical readout. The therapeutic effect of the drug on circulating white cells is directly related to its plasma level, which is often not the case for drugs acting on solid tumours. It is an example where the choice of indication, initially made on the basis of a solid biological hypothesis, proved highly advantageous in allowing the clinical development to progress rapidly.

Trastuzumab (Herceptin)

Trastuzumab is a humanized monoclonal antibody which selectively blocks the oestrogen receptor Her2. This project, which took 8 years from compound discovery to registration, shows the speed with which biopharmaceuticals, under the right conditions, can be developed. The Her2 receptor was first cloned in 1985, and 2 years later it was found to be strongly over-expressed in the most aggressive breast cancers. Genentech used its in-house technology to develop a humanized mouse monoclonal antibody that blocked the function of the receptor and suppressed the proliferation of receptor-bearing cells. Compared with conventional lead finding and lead optimization of synthetic molecules, this took very little time – only 2 years from the start of the project. Antibodies generally exhibit much simpler and more predictable pharmacological effects than synthetic compounds, and run into fewer problems with chemical development, formulation and toxicology, so that trastuzumab was able to enter Phase I within 2 years. Clear-cut efficacy was evident in Phase II, and the rest of the clinical development was rapid and straightforward. Trastuzumab represents a significant step forward in the treatment of breast cancer, as well as a commercial success. Given the right circumstances, biopharmaceuticals can be developed more quickly and more cheaply than conventional drugs, a fact reflected in the growing proportion (approximately 35% in 2001 but approaching 50% in 2011) of biopharmaceuticals among new chemical entities being registered.

Comments and conclusions

One common feature that emerges from a survey of the many anecdotal reports of drug discovery projects is that they often have outcomes quite different from what was originally intended. The first tricyclic antidepressant drug, *imipramine*, emerged from a project aimed at developing antihistamines based on the structure of promethazine. *Clonidine* was synthesized in the early 1960s as part of a project intended to develop α-adrenoceptor agonists as vasoconstrictors for use as decongestant nose drops. The physician involved tested the nose drops on his wife, who had a cold, and was surprised by the fact that her blood pressure plummeted. She also slept for 24 hours. It turned out that the dose was about 30 times what was later found effective in humans. The experiment revealed the unexpected hypotensive action of clonidine upon which its subsequent commercial development was based. More recently, it is well known that *sildenafil (Viagra)* was originally intended as a vasodilator for treating angina, and only during clinical testing did its erection-inducing effect become evident and matters have gone full circle with the recent realization that it can be used to treat pulmonary hypertension as well.

It might be supposed that the increasing emphasis now being placed on defined molecular targets as starting points for drug discovery projects would reduce the likelihood of such therapeutic surprises. However, the molecular targets used for screening nowadays lie further, in the functional sense, from the therapeutic response that is being sought than do the physiological responses relied on previously (see Chapter 2, Figure 2.3). Thus compounds aimed with precision at well-defined targets commonly fail to produce the desired therapeutic effect, evidently because we do not sufficiently understand the pathophysiological pathway linking the two. Recent examples of such failures include *ondansetron*, a $5HT_3$-receptor antagonist conceived as an antimigraine drug but ineffective in this indication (developed instead as an antiemetic), and substance P receptor antagonists which were expected to have analgesic properties in humans, but which proved ineffective, although again these agents have found a useful niche as antiemetics. Lack of efficacy in clinical trials – a measure of our inability to predict therapeutic efficacy on the basis of pharmacological properties – remains one of the commonest causes of project failure, accounting for 30% of failures (Kennedy, 1997), second only to pharmacokinetic shortcomings (39%).

THE STAGES OF DRUG DISCOVERY

In this section we are concerned with the initial stages of the overall project outlined in Figure 4.1, up to the point at which a molecule makes its solemn rite of passage from research to development. Figure 4.4 summarizes the main stages that make up a 'typical' drug discovery project, from the identification of a target to the production of a candidate drug[2].

A huge number of 'theoretical' compounds (far too many to be physically accessible) is first 'filtered' in silico to reduce it to a practicable number of compounds that is available, or can be synthesized, in screening libraries. High-throughput screening is then used to identify 'hits',

[2]The process of developing a new biopharmaceutical generally follows a different path, and is described more fully in Chapter 12.

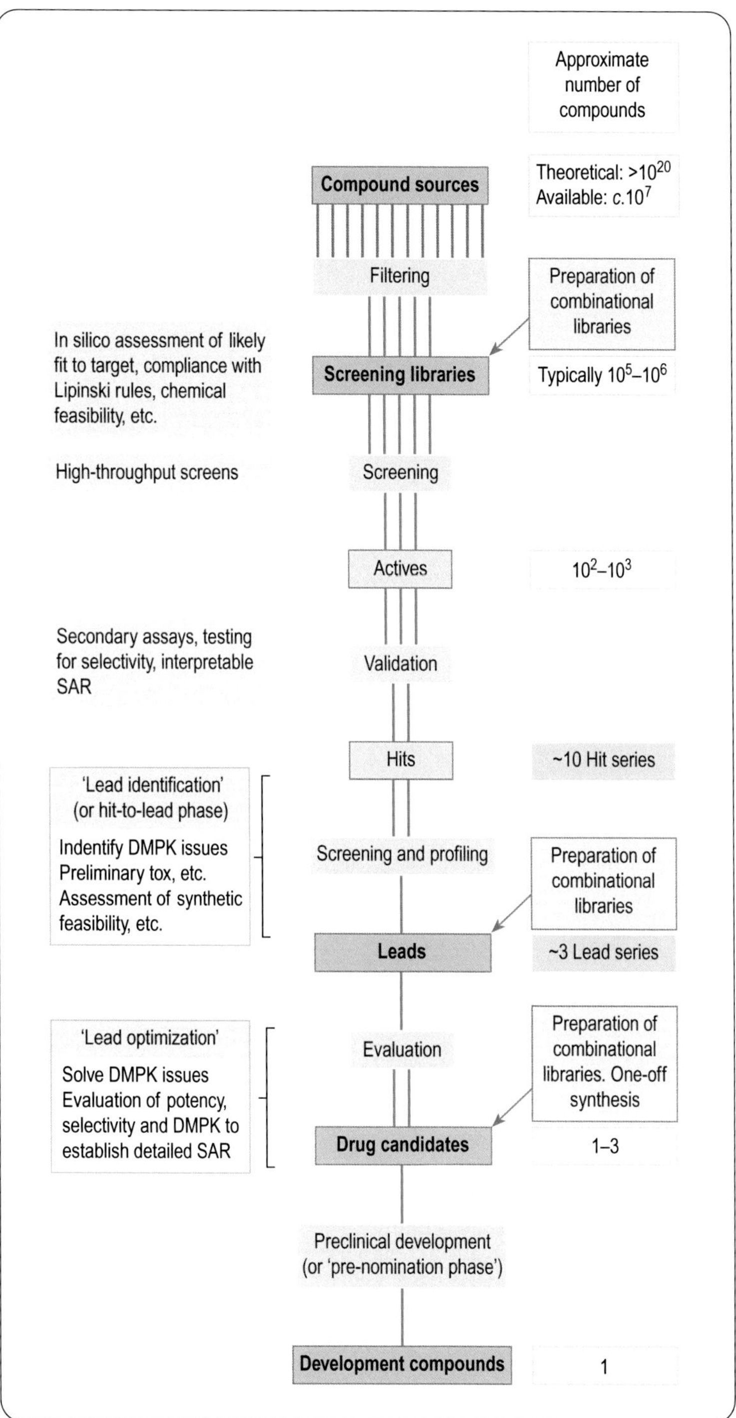

Fig. 4.4 Stages of drug discovery.

which show significant activity in the chosen screen. This may throw up hundreds or thousands of compounds, depending on the nature of the screen and the size and quality of the library. Normally, a significant proportion of these prove to be artefacts of one sort or another, for example results that cannot be repeated when the compound is resynthesized, positives in the assay resulting from non-specific effects, or simply 'noise' in the assay system. 'Validation' of hits is, therefore, necessary to eliminate artefacts, and this may involve repeating the screening of the hits, confirming the result in a different assay designed to measure activity on the chosen target, as well as resynthesis and retesting of the hit compounds. Validation will also entail assessment of the structure–activity relationships within the screening library, and whether the hit belongs to a family of compounds – a 'hit series' – which represents a reasonable starting point for further chemistry.

In the next stage, lead identification, the validated hits are subjected to further scrutiny, particularly in respect of their pharmacokinetic properties and toxicity as well as addressing in more detail the feasibility of building a synthetic chemistry programme. In this process, the handful of 'hit series' is further reduced to one or a few 'lead series'. Up to this point, the aim has been to reduce the number of compounds in contention from millions to a few – 'negative chemistry', if you will.

Synthetic chemistry then begins, in the 'lead optimization' stage. This usually involves parallel synthesis to generate derivatives of the lead series, which are screened and profiled with respect to pharmacology, pharmacokinetics and toxicology, to home in on a small number of 'drug candidates' (often a single compound, or if the project is unlucky, none at all) judged suitable for further development, at which point they are taken into preclinical development.

The flow diagram in Figure 4.4 provides a useful basis for the more detailed accounts of the various activities that contribute to the drug discovery process, described in the chapters that follow. It should be realized, though, that many variations on this basic scheme take place in real life. A project may, for example, work on one lead series and, at the same time, go back to library screening to find new starting points. New biological discoveries, such as the identification of a new receptor subtype, may cause the project to redefine its objectives midstream.

Increasingly, large companies have tended to centralize the early stages of drug discovery, up to the identification of lead series, and to carry out many screens in parallel with very large compound libraries, focusing on putative drug targets often identified on the basis of genomics, rather than on pharmacology and pathophysiology relating to specific disease indications. In this emerging scenario, the work of the drug discovery team effectively begins from the chemical lead. In the last few years there has been a return to a more intuitive approach to drug discovery in some companies as it has been realized that mass screening is not always the best way to generate good-quality chemical leads.

TRENDS IN DRUG DISCOVERY

Increasingly, drug discovery has become focused on cloned molecular targets that can be incorporated into high-throughput screens. Target selection, discussed in Chapter 6, has, therefore, assumed a significance that it rarely had in the past: of the projects described above, three began without any molecular target in mind, which would seldom be the case nowadays.

The examples summarized in Table 4.2 show that it took 7–12 years from the start of the project to identificaton of the compound that was finally developed. That interval has now been substantially reduced, often to 3 years or less once a molecular target has been selected, mainly as a result of (a) high-throughput screening of large compound libraries (including natural product libraries) to identify initial lead compounds; (b) improvements at the lead optimization stage, including the use of automated synthesis to generate large families of related compounds, and increased use of molecular modelling techniques, whereby the results of compound screening are analysed to reveal the molecular configurations that are associated with biological activity.

There is strong motivation to improve not only the speed of lead optimization, but also the 'quality' of the compound selected for development. Quality, in this context, means a low probability that the compound will fail later in development. The main reasons that compounds fail, apart from lack of efficacy or unexpected side effects, are that they show toxicity, or that they have undesirable pharmacokinetic properties (e.g. poor absorption, too long or too short plasma half-life, unpredictable metabolism, accumulation in tissues, etc.). In the past, these aspects of a drug's properties were often not investigated until the discovery/development hurdle had been crossed, as investigating them was traditionally regarded as a responsibility of 'development' rather than 'research'. Frequently a compound would fail after several months in preclinical development – too late for the problem to be addressed by the drug discovery team, which had by then moved on. This highlighted the need to incorporate pharmacokinetic and toxicological studies, as well as pharmacological ones, at an earlier stage of the project, during the lead optimization phase. As described in Chapter 10, studies of this kind are now routinely included in most drug discovery projects. Inevitably this has a cost in terms of time and money, but this will be more than justified by a reduction in the likelihood of compounds failing during clinical development.

Table 4.3 Trends in drug discovery

		c.1800	c.1900	c.2000
Target finding	Sources of targets	Insights from pathophysiology	Known pharmacological targets	Defined human molecular targets based on genomics
		Known pharmacological targets Serendipitous findings	Defined molecular targets	
Hit finding	Compound sources	Available natural products 'one-at-a-time' synthesis	Large compound libraries, selected on basis of availability Natural product libraries	Massive virtual libraries, then focused combinatorial libraries
	Screens	In vitro and in vivo pharmacological screens. Radioligand binding assays	High-throughput screen in vitro Hits validated by secondary functional assays in vitro	Virtual library screened in silico for predicted target affinity 'rule-of-5' compliance, chemical and metabolic stability, toxic groups, etc.
			Selection of leads mainly 'in cerebro'*	Combinatorial libraries screened by HTS, several screens in parallel
Validated hits				
↓ *Lead finding*	Compound sources	Custom synthesis based on medicinal chemistry insights Natural products	Analogues synthesized one at a time or combinatorially	Combinatorial synthesis of analogues
↓	Screens	Low throughput pharmacological assays in vitro and in vivo	Functional assays in vitro and in vivo	Medium throughput in vitro screens for target affinity DMPK characteristics Preliminary measurements of DMPK in vivo
Leads				
↓	Compound sources	Analogues of active compounds synthesized one at a time	Combinatorial or one at a time synthesis of analogues	Combinatorial or one at a time synthesis of analogues
Lead optimization ↓	Screens	Animal models	Efficacy in animal models Simple PK measurements in vivo	Efficacy in animal models Detailed DMPK analysis
Drug candidate			Safety pharmacology In vitro genotoxicity	Safety pharmacology In vitro genotoxicity

*The cerebrum required being that of an experienced medicinal chemist.

The main trends that have occurred over the last two decades are summarized in Table 4.3, the key ones being, as discussed above:

- A massive expansion of the compound collections used as starting points, from large 'white-powder' libraries of 100 000 or more compounds created during the 1990s, to massive virtual libraries of tens of millions
- Use of automated synthesis methods to accelerate lead optimization
- To deal with large, compound libraries, the introduction of high-throughput screens for actual

compounds, and in silico screens for virtual compounds
- Increasing reliance on in silico predictions to generate leads
- Focus on cloned human targets as starting points
- Progressive 'front-loading' of assessment of DMPK (drug metabolism and pharmacokinetic) characteristics, including in silico assessment of virtual libraries.

Project planning

When a project moves from the phase of exploratory research to being an approved drug discovery project to which specific resources are assigned under the direction of a project leader, its objectives, expected timelines and resource requirements need to be agreed by the members of the project team and approved by research management.

The early drug discovery phase of the project will typically begin when a target has been selected and the necessary screening methods established, and its aim will be to identify one or a few 'drug candidates' suitable for progressing to the next stage of preclinical development. The properties required for a drug candidate will vary from project to project, but will invariably include chemical, pharmacological, pharmacokinetic and toxicological aspects of the compound. Table 4.4 summarizes the criteria that might apply to a typical drug acting on a target such as an enzyme or receptor, and intended for oral use. Where appropriate (e.g. potency, oral bioavailability), quantitative limits will normally be set. Such a list of necessary or desirable features, based on results from many independent assessments and experimental tests, provides an essential focus for the project. Some of these, such as potency on target, or oral bioavailability, will be absolute requirements, whereas others, such as water solubility or lack of in vitro genotoxicity, may be highly desirable but not essential. There are, in essence, two balancing components of a typical project:

- Designing and synthesizing novel compounds
- Filtering, to eliminate compounds that fail to satisfy the criteria.

Whereas in an earlier era of drug discovery these two activities took place independently – chemists made compounds and handed over white powders for testing, while pharmacologists tried to find ones that worked – nowadays the process is invariably an iterative and interactive one, whereby the design and synthesis of new compounds continuously takes into account the biological findings and shortcomings that have been revealed to date. Formal project planning, of the kind that would be adopted for the building of a new road, for example, is therefore inappropriate for drug discovery. Experienced managers consequently rely less on detailed advance planning, and more on good communication between the various members of

Table 4.4 Typical selection criteria for drug candidates intended for oral use*

Chemical	Pharmacological	Pharmacokinetic	Toxicological
Patentable structure	Defined potency on target	Cell-permeable in vitro	In vitro genotoxicity tests negative
Water-soluble	Selectivity for specific target relative to other related targets	Adequate oral bioavailability	Preliminary in vivo toxicology tests showing adequate margin between expected 'therapeutic' dose and maximum No Adverse Effect Dose
Chemically stable	Pharmacodynamic activity in vitro and in vivo	For CNS drugs: penetrates blood–brain barrier	
Large-scale synthesis feasible	No adverse effects in standard safety pharmacology tests	Appropriate plasma half-life	
Non-chiral	Active in disease models	Defined metabolism by human liver microsomes	
No known 'toxophoric' groups		No inhibition or induction of cytochrome P450	

*Criteria such as these, which will vary according to the expected therapeutic application of the compound, would normally be applied to compound selection in the drug discovery stage of a project, culminating in lead optimization and the identification of a drug candidate, when preclinical development begins, focusing mainly on pharmacokinetics, toxicology, chemistry and formulation.

the project team, and frequent meetings to review progress and agree on the best way forward.

An important aspect of project planning is deciding what tests to do when, so as to achieve the objectives as quickly and efficiently as possible. The factors that have to be taken into account for each test are:

- Compound throughput
- Cost per compound
- Amount of compound required in relation to amount available
- Time required. Some in vivo pharmacodynamic tests (e.g. bone density changes, tumour growth) are inherently slow. Irrespective of compound throughput, they cannot provide rapid feedback
- 'Salience' of result (i.e. is the criterion an absolute requirement, or desirable but non-essential?)
- Probability that the compound will fail. In a typical high-throughput screen more than 99% of compounds will be eliminated, so it is essential that this is done early. In vitro genotoxicity, in contrast, will be found only occasionally, so it would be wasteful to test for this early in the sequence.

The current emphasis on fast drug discovery, to increase the time window between launch and patent expiry, and on decreasing the rate of failure of compounds during clinical development, is having an important effect on the planning of drug discovery projects. As discussed above, there is increasing emphasis on applying fast-result, high-throughput methods of testing for pharmacokinetic and toxicological properties at an early stage ('front loading'; see Chapter 10), even though the *salience* (i.e. the ability to predict properties needed in the clinic) of such assays may be limited. The growth of high-throughput test methods has had a major impact on the work of chemists in drug discovery (see Chapter 9), where the emphasis has been on preparing 'libraries' of related compounds to feed the hungry assay machines. These changes have undoubtedly improved the performance of the industry in finding new lead compounds of higher quality for new targets. The main bottlenecks now in drug discovery are in lead optimization (see Chapter 9) and animal testing (see Chapter 11), areas so far largely untouched by the high-throughput revolution.

RESEARCH IN THE PHARMACEUTICAL INDUSTRY

Pharmaceutical companies perform research for commercial reasons and seek to ensure that it produces a return on investment. The company owns the data, and is free to publish it or keep it secret as it sees fit. Although most pharmaceutical companies include altruistic as well as commercial aims in their mission statements, the latter necessarily take priority. The company will, therefore, wish to ensure that the research it supports is in some way relevant to its commercial objectives. Clearly, studies aimed directly at drug discovery present no problems. At the other end of the spectrum lies pure curiosity-driven ('blue-skies') research. Although such work may – and often does – lead to progress in drug discovery in the long term, the commercial pay-off is highly uncertain and inevitably long delayed. Generally speaking, only a minimal amount of such long-term research is performed in a commercial setting. Between the two lies a large territory of 'applied' research, more clearly focused on drug discovery, though still medium-term and somewhat uncertain in its applicability. Many technological projects come into this category, such as novel high-throughput screening methods, imaging technologies, etc., as well as research into pathophysiological mechanisms aimed at the identification of new drug targets. The many applications of genomics and molecular biology in drug discovery make up an increasing proportion of work in this applied research category. Small biotechnology companies which started during the 1980s and 1990s moved quickly into this territory, and several large pharmaceutical companies, notably SmithKlineBeecham (now part of GSK), also made major investments. The extent to which pharmaceutical companies invest in medium-term applied research projects varies greatly. A growing tendency seems to be for larger companies to set up what amounts to an in-house biotechnology facility, often incorporating one or more acquired biotech companies. The technological revolution in drug discovery, referred to frequently in this book, has yet to pay dividends in terms of improved performance, so it is uncertain whether this level of commitment to medium-term applied research can be sustained. More recently the view has emerged that much of the information obtained from industry driven genomic studies of disease should be freely available to all and, for example, Merck in the USA has spun out its database to a not-for-profit organization called Sage (see http://www.sagebase.org) for this purpose.

The cultural difference between academic and commercial research is real, but less profound than is often thought. Quality, in the sense of good experimental design, methodology and data interpretation, is equally important to both, as is creativity, the ability to generate new ideas and see them through. Key differences are that, in the industry environment, freedom to choose projects and to publish is undoubtedly more limited, and effective interdisciplinary teamwork is obligatory, rather than a matter of personal choice: there is little room in industry for the lone genius. These differences are, however, becoming narrower as the bodies funding academic research take a more 'corporate' approach to its management. Individual researchers in academia are substantially constrained to work on projects that attract funding support, and are increasingly being required to collaborate in interdisciplinary projects. They are certainly more free to publish, but are also under much more pressure to do so, as, in contrast to the situation in industry, publications are their only measure of research achievement. Pharmaceutical companies also have incentives to publish their work: it gives their scientists visibility in the scientific community and helps them to establish fruitful collaborations, as well as strengthening the company's attractiveness as an employer of good scientists. The main restrictions to publication are the company's need to avoid compromising its future patent position, or giving away information that might help its competitors. Companies vary in their attitude to publication, some being much more liberal than others.

Scientists in industry have to learn to work, and communicate effectively, with the company's management. Managers are likely to ask 'Why do we need this information?' which, to scientists in academia, may seem an irritatingly silly question. To them, the purpose of any research is to add to the edifice of human knowledge, and working towards this aim fully justifies the time, effort and money that support the work. The long-term benefits to humanity are measured in terms of cultural richness and technological progress. In the short term the value of what has been achieved is measured by peer recognition and grant renewal; the long-term judgment is left to history.

Within a pharmaceutical company, research findings are aimed at a more limited audience and their purpose is more focused. The immediate aim is to provide the data needed for prediction of the potential of a new compound to succeed in the clinic. The internal audiences are the research team itself and research management; the external audiences are the external scientific community and, importantly, the regulatory authorities.

We should, however, resist the tendency to think of drug discovery as a commercial undertaking comparable developing a new sports car, where the outcome is assured provided that operatives with the necessary skill and experience fulfil what is asked of them. They are not likely by chance to invent a new kind of aeroplane or vacuum cleaner.

Like all research, drug discovery is more likely than not to come up with unexpected findings, and these can have a major impact on the plan and its objectives. So, frequent review - and, if necessary, amendment - of the plan is essential, and research managers need to understand (as most do, having their own research experiences to draw on) that unexpected results, and the problems that may follow for the project, reflect the complexity of the problem, rather than the failings of the team. Finding by experiment that a hypothesis is wrong is to be seen as a creditable scientific achievement, not at all the same as designing a car with brakes that do not work.

REFERENCES

Banitt EH, Schmid JR. Flecainide. In: Lednicer D, editor. Chronicles of drug discovery. vol. 3. Washington DC: American Chemical Society; 1993.

Capdeville R, Buchdunger E, Zimmermann J, et al. Glivec (STI571, imatinib), a rationally developed, targeted anticancer drug. Nature Reviews Drug Discovery 2002;1: 493–502.

Cohen P. Protein kinases - the major drug targets of the twenty-first century? Nature Reviews Drug Discovery 2002;1:309–16.

Cragg GM. Paclitaxel (Taxol): a success story with valuable lessons for natural product drug discovery and development. Medical Research Review 1998;18:315–31.

Drews J. Drug discovery: a historical perspective. Science 2000;287:1960–4.

Druker BJ, Lydon NB. Lessons learned from the development of an Abl tyrosine kinase inhibitor for chronic myelognous leukemia. Journal of Clinical Investigation 2000;105:3–7.

Druker BJ, Tamura S, Buchdunger E, et al. Effects of a selective inhibitor of the Abl tyrosine kinase on the growth of Bcr-Abl positive cells. Nature Medicine 1996;2:561–6.

Druker BJ, Talpaz M, Resta DJ, et al. Efficacy and safety of a specific inhibitor of the Bcr-Abl tyrosine kinase in chronic myeloid leukemia. New England Journal of Medicine 2001;344:1031–7.

Kennedy T. Managing the drug discovery/development interface. Drug Discovery Today 1997;2: 436–44.

Lednicer D. Chronicles of drug discovery. vol. 3. Washington DC: American Chemical Society; 1993.

Östholm I. Drug discovery: a pharmacist's view. Stockholm: Swedish Pharmaceutical Press; 1995.

Schindler T, Bornmann W, Pellicana P, et al. Structural mechanism for STI-571 inhibition of Abelson tyrosine kinase. Science 2000;289: 1938–42.

Chapter | 5 |

Choosing the project

H P Rang, R G Hill

INTRODUCTION

In this chapter we discuss the various criteria that are applied when making the initial decision of whether or not to embark on a new drug discovery project. The point at which a project becomes formally recognized as a drug discovery project with a clear-cut aim of delivering a candidate molecule for development and the amount of managerial control that is exercised before and after this transition vary considerably from company to company. Some encourage – or at least allow – research scientists to pursue ideas under the general umbrella of 'exploratory research', whereas others control the research portfolio more tightly and discourage their scientists from straying off the straight and narrow path of a specific project. Generally, however, some room is left within the organization for exploratory research in the expectation that it will generate ideas for future drug discovery projects. When successful, this strategy results in research-led project proposals, which generally have the advantage of starting from proprietary knowledge and having a well-motivated and expert in-house team. Historically, such research-led drug discovery projects have produced many successful drugs, including β-blockers, ACE inhibitors, statins, tamoxifen and many others, but also many failures, for example prostanoid receptor ligands, which have found few clinical uses. Facing harder times, managements are now apt to dismiss such projects as 'drugs in search of a disease', so it is incumbent upon research teams to align their work, even in the early exploratory stage, as closely as possible with medical needs and the business objectives of the company, and to frame project proposals accordingly. Increasingly, research is becoming collaborative with large pharmaceutical companies partnering with small biotechnology companies or with academic groups.

MAKING THE DECISION

The first, and perhaps the most important, decision in the life history of a drug discovery project is the decision to start. Imagine a group considering whether or not to climb a mountain. *Strategically*, they decide whether or not they want to get to the top of that particular mountain; *technically*, they decide whether there is a feasible route; and *operationally* they decide whether or not they have the wherewithal to accomplish the climb. In the context of a drug discovery project, the questions are:

- *Should we do it?* (strategic issues)
- *Could we do it?* (scientific and technical issues)
- *Can we do it?* (operational issues).

The main factors that need to be considered are summarized in Figure 5.1.

Strategic issues

Strategic issues relate to the *desirability* of the project from the company's perspective, reflecting its mission (a) to make a significant contribution to healthcare, and (b) to make a profit for its shareholders. These translate into assessments respectively of medical need and market potential.

Unmet medical need

Unmet medical need represents what many would regard as the most fundamental criterion to be satisfied when evaluating any drug discovery project, though defining and evaluating it objectively is far from straightforward. Of course there are common and serious diseases, such as many cancers, viral infections, neurodegenerative diseases,

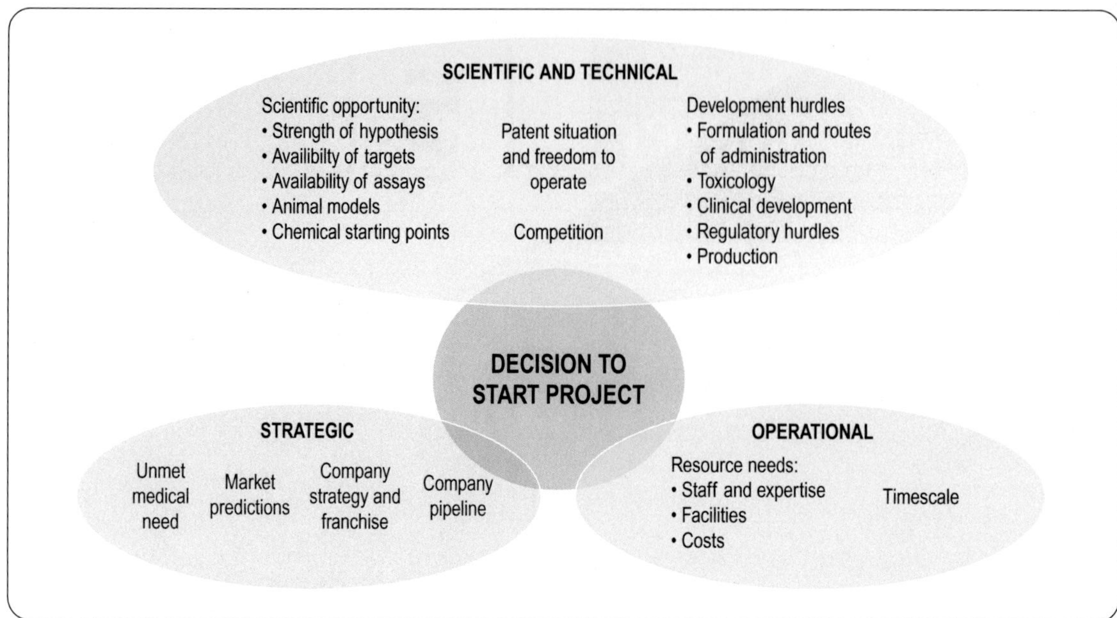

Fig. 5.1 Criteria for project selection.

certain developmental abnormalities, etc., for which current treatments are non-existent or far from ideal, and these would be generally accepted as areas of high unmet need. Nevertheless, trying to rank potential drug discovery projects on this basis is full of difficulties, because it assumes that we can assess disease severity objectively, and somehow balance it against disease prevalence. Does a rare but catastrophic disease represent a greater or a lesser medical need than a common minor one? Is severity best measured in terms of reduced life expectancy, or level of disability and suffering? Does reducing the serious side effects of existing widely used and efficacious drugs (e.g. gastric bleeding with conventional non-steroidal anti-inflammatory drugs) meet a need that is more important than finding a therapy for a condition that was previously untreatable? Does public demand for baldness cures, anti-wrinkle creams and other 'lifestyle' remedies constitute a medical need?

Assessing medical need is not simply a matter of asking customers what they would regard as ideal; this usually results in a product description which falls into the category of 'a free drug, given once orally with no side effects, that cures the condition'. Nevertheless, this trite response can serve a useful purpose when determining the medical need for a new product: how closely do existing and future competitors approach this ideal? How big is the gap between the reality and the ideal, and would it be profitable to try and fill it? Using this type of 'gap analysis' we can ask ourselves the following questions:

- How close do we come to 'free'? In other words, can we be more cost-effective?
- Compliance is important: a drug that is not taken cannot work. Once-daily oral dosing is convenient, but would a long-lasting injection be a better choice for some patients?
- If an oral drug exists, can it be improved, for example by changing the formulation?
- The reduction of side effects is an area where there is often a medical need. Do we have a strategy for improving the side-effect profile of existing drugs?
- Curing a condition or retarding disease progression is preferable to alleviating symptoms. Do we have a strategy for achieving this?

Market considerations

These overlap to some extent with unmet medical need, but focus particularly on assessing the likelihood that the revenue from sales will succeed in recouping the investment. Disease prevalence and severity, as discussed above, obviously affect sales volume and price. Other important factors include the extent to which the proposed compound is likely to be superior to drugs already on the market, and the marketing experience and reputation of the company in the particular disease area. The more innovative the project, the greater is the degree of uncertainty of such assessments. The market for *ciclosporin*, for example, was initially thought to be too small to justify its development – as transplant surgery was regarded as a highly specialized type of intervention that would never become commonplace – but in the end the drug itself gave a large boost to organ transplantation, and proved to be a blockbuster. There are also many examples of innovative and well-researched drugs that fail in development, or perform poorly in the marketplace, so creativity is not an infallible passport to success. Recognizing the uncertainty of market predictions in the early stages of an innovative project, companies generally avoid attaching much weight to these evaluations when judging which projects to support at the research stage. A case in point is the discovery of H_2 receptor blockers for the treatment of peptic ulcer by James Black and his colleagues where throughout the project he was being told by his sales and marketing colleagues that there was no market for this type of product as the medical professional treated ulcers surgically. Fortunately the team persisted in its efforts and again the resulting drug, cimetidine, became a $1 billion per year blockbuster.

Company strategy and franchise

The current and planned franchise of a pharmaceutical company plays a large part in determining the broad disease areas, such as cancer, mental illness, cardiovascular disease, gastroenterology, etc., addressed by new projects, but will not influence the particular scientific approach that is taken. All companies specialize to a greater or lesser extent on particular disease areas, and this is reflected in their research organization and scientific recruitment policies. Biotechnology companies are more commonly focused on particular technologies and scientific approaches, such as drug delivery, genomics, growth factors, monoclonal antibodies, etc., rather than on particular disease areas. They are, therefore, more pragmatic about the potential therapeutic application of their discoveries, which will generally be licensed out at an appropriate stage for development by companies within whose franchise the application falls. In the biotech environment, strategic issues, therefore, tend to be involved more with science and technology than may be the case in larger pharmaceutical companies – a characteristic that is often appealing to research scientists.

The state of a company's development pipeline, and its need to sustain a steady flow of new compounds entering the market, sometimes influences the selection of drug discovery projects. The company may, for example, need a product to replace one that is nearing the end of its patent life, or is losing out to competition, and it may endeavour to direct research to that end. In general, though, in the absence of an innovative scientific strategy such top-down commercially driven priorities often fail. A better, and quicker, solution to the commercial problem will often be to license in a partly developed compound with the required specification.

In general, the management of a pharmaceutical company needs to choose and explain which therapeutic areas it wishes to cover, and to communicate this effectively to the drug discovery research organization, but most will avoid placing too much emphasis on market analysis and commercial factors when it comes to selecting specific projects. This is partly because market analysis is at best a very imprecise business and the commercial environment can change rapidly, but also because success in the past has often come from exploiting unexpected scientific opportunities and building a marketing and commercial strategy on the basis of what is discovered, rather than the other way round. The interface between science and commerce is always somewhat turbulent.

Legislation, government policy, reimbursement and pricing

Unlike the products of many other industries, pharmaceuticals are subject to controls on their pricing, their promotional activities, and their registration as 'safe and effective' products that can be put on the market, and so their commercial environment is significantly altered by government intervention. The socialized medicine that is a feature of European and Canadian healthcare means that the government is not only the major provider of healthcare, but also a monopoly purchaser of drugs for use in the healthcare system. The USA is the only major market where the government does not exert price controls, except as a feature of Medicare, where it acts as a major buyer and expects discounts commensurate with its purchasing power. Governments have great influence on the marketing of drugs, and they have an interest in limiting the prescription of newer, generally more expensive products, and this affects where the industry can sell premium-priced products. Governments and their associated regulatory bodies have gradually extended their power from a position of regulation for public safety to one of guardians of the public purse. Products deemed to be 'clinically essential or life-saving' now may be fast-tracked, whereas those that are thought to be inessential may take twice as long to obtain approval. Many countries, such as Canada, Australia and the UK, have additional reimbursement hurdles, based on the need for cost-efficacy data. As a consequence, the choice of drug development candidate will have to reflect not only the clinical need of the patient, but also government healthcare policies in different countries. The choice of indications for a new drug is thus increasingly affected by the willingness of national healthcare systems to offer accelerated approval and reimbursement for that drug. This is a changing landscape at the time of writing, but the indications are that governments worldwide will exert more rather than less control over drug registration and pricing in the future.

Scientific and technical issues

These issues relate to the *feasibility* of the project, and several aspects need to be considered:

- The scientific and technological basis on which the success of the drug discovery phase of the project will depend
- The nature of the development and regulatory hurdles that will have to be overcome if the development phase of the project is to succeed
- The state of the competition
- The patent situation.

The scientific and technological basis

Evaluation of the *scientific opportunity* should be the main factor on which the decision as to whether or not to embark on a project rests once its general alignment with corporate strategy, as described above, is accepted. Some of the key elements are listed in Figure 5.1. In this context it is important to distinguish between public knowledge and proprietary knowledge, as a secure but well-known scientific hypothesis or technology may provide a less attractive starting point than a shakier scientific platform based on proprietary information. Regardless of the strength of the underlying scientific hypothesis, the other items listed in Figure 5.1 – availability of targets, assays, animal models and chemical starting points – need to be evaluated carefully, as weaknesses in any of these areas are likely to block progress, or at best require significant time and resources to overcome. They are discussed more fully in Chapters 6–9.

Competition

Strictly speaking, competition in drug discovery is unimportant, as the research activities of one company do not impede those of another, except to the limited extent that patents on research tools may restrict a company's 'freedom to operate', as discussed below. What matters greatly is competition in the marketplace. Market success depends in part on being early (not necessarily first) to register a drug of a new type, but more importantly on having a product which is better. Analysis of the external competition faced by a new project therefore involves assessing the chances that it will lead to earlier registration, and/or a better product, than other companies will achieve. Making such an assessment involves long-range predictions based on fragmentary and unreliable information. The earliest solid information comes from patent applications, generally submitted around the time a compound is chosen for preclinical development, and made public soon thereafter (see Chapter 19), and from official clinical trial approvals. Companies are under no obligation to divulge information about their research projects. Information can be gleaned from gossip, publications, scientific meetings and unguarded remarks, and scientists are expected to keep their antennae well tuned to these signals – a process referred to euphemistically as 'competitive intelligence'. There are also professional agencies that specialize in obtaining commercially sensitive information and providing it to subscribers in database form. Such sources may reveal which companies are active in the area, and often which targets they are focusing on, but will rarely indicate how close they are to producing development compounds, and they are often significantly out of date.

At the drug discovery stage of a project overlap with work in other companies is a normal state of affairs and should not, per se, be a deterrent to new initiatives. The fact that 80–90% of compounds entering clinical development are unsuccessful should be borne in mind. So, a single competitor compound in early clinical development theoretically reduces the probability of our new project winning the race to registration by only 10–20%, say from about 2% to 1.7%. In practice, nervousness tends to influence us more than statistical reasoning, and there may be reluctance to start a project if several companies are working along the same lines with drug discovery projects, or if a competitor is well ahead with a compound in development. The incentive to identify novel proprietary drug targets (Chapter 6) stems as much from scientific curiosity and the excitement of breaking new ground as from the potential therapeutic benefits of the new target.

Development and regulatory hurdles

Although many of the problems encountered in developing and registering a new drug relate specifically to the compound and its properties, others are inherent to the therapeutic area and the clinical need being addressed, and can be anticipated at the outset before any candidate compound has been identified. Because development consumes a large proportion of the time and money spent on a project, likely problems need to be assessed at an early stage and taken into account in deciding whether or not to embark on the discovery phase.

The various stages of drug development and registration are described in more detail in Section 3. Here we give some examples of the kinds of issue that need to be considered in the planning phase.

- *Will the drug be given as a short course to relieve an acute illness, or indefinitely to relieve chronic symptoms or prevent recurrence?* Many anti-infective drugs come into the former category, and it is notable that development times for such drugs are much shorter than for, say, drugs used in psychiatry or for lowering plasma cholesterol levels. The need for longer clinical trials and more exhaustive toxicity testing mainly accounts for the difference.
- *Is the intended disease indication rare or common?* Definitive trials of efficacy in rare diseases may be

slow because of problems in recruiting patients. (For recognized 'orphan indications' (see Chapter 20), the clinical trials requirements may be less stringent.)

- *What clinical models and clinical end-points are available for assessing efficacy?* Testing whether a drug relieves an acute symptom, such as pain or nausea, is much simpler and quicker than, for example, testing whether it reduces the incidence of stroke or increases the life expectancy of patients with a rare cancer. Where accepted surrogate markers exist (e.g. lowering of LDL cholesterol as an indicator of cardiovascular risk, or improved bone density on X-ray as a marker of fracture risk in osteoporosis), this enables trials to be carried out more quickly and simply, but there remain many conditions where symptoms and/or life expectancy provide the only available measures of efficacy.
- *How serious is the disease, and what is the status of existing therapies?* Where no effective treatment of a condition exists, comparison of the drug with placebo will generally suffice to provide evidence of efficacy. Where standard therapies exist several comparative trials will be needed, and the new drug will have to show clear evidence of superiority before being accepted by regulatory authorities. For serious disabling or life-threatening conditions the regulatory hurdles are generally lower, and the review process is conducted more quickly.
- *What kind of product is envisaged (synthetic compound, biopharmaceutical, cell or gene-based therapy, etc.), and what route of administration?* The development track and the main obstacles that are likely to be encountered depend very much on the type of product and the route of administration. With protein biopharmaceuticals, for example, toxicology is rarely a major problem, but production may be, whereas the reverse is generally true for synthetic compounds. With proteins, the route of administration is often a difficult issue, whereas with synthetic small molecule compounds the expectation is that they will be developed for oral or topical use. Cell- or gene-based products are likely to face serious safety and ethical questions before clinical trials can be started. The development of a special delivery system, such as a skin patch, nasal spray or slow-release injectable formulation, will add to the time and cost of development.

The patent situation

As described in Chapter 19, patent protection in the pharmaceutical industry relates mainly to specific chemical substances, their manufacture and their uses. Nevertheless, at the start of a project, before the drug substance has been identified, it is important to evaluate the extent to which existing patents on compounds or research tools may limit the company's 'freedom to operate' in the research phase. Existing patents on compounds of a particular class (see Chapter 19) may rule out using such compounds as the starting point for a new project.

By 'research tool' is meant anything that contributes to the discovery or development of a drug, without being part of the final product. Examples include genes, cell lines, reagents, markers, assays, screening methods, animal models, etc.

A company whose business it is to sell drugs is not usually interested in patenting research tools, but it is the business of many biotech companies to develop and commercialize such tools, and these companies will naturally wish to obtain patent protection for them. For pharmaceutical companies, such research tool patents and applications raise issues of freedom to operate, particularly if they contain 'reach-through' claims purporting to cover drugs found by using the patented tools.

Some scientists may believe that research activities, in contrast to manufacture and sale of a product, cannot lead to patent infringement. This is not the case. If I have invented a process that is useful in research and have a valid patent for it, I can enforce that patent against anyone using the process without my permission. I can make money from my patent by granting licenses for a flat fee, or a fee based on the extent to which the process is used; or by selling kits to carry out the process or reagents for use in the process (for example, the enzymes used in the PCR process). What I am not entitled to do is to charge a royalty on the sale of drugs developed with the help of my process. I can patent an electric drill, but I should not expect a royalty on everything it bores a hole in!

Nevertheless, some patents have already been granted containing claims that would be infringed, for example, by the sales of a drug active in a patented assay, and although it is hoped that such claims would be held invalid if challenged in court, the risk that such claims might be enforceable cannot be dismissed.

Should research tool patents be the subject of a freedom to operate search at an early stage of project planning? Probably not. There are simply too many of them, and if no research project could be started without clearance on the basis of such a search, nothing would ever get done. At least for a large company, it is an acceptable business risk to go ahead and assume that if problems arise they can be dealt with at a later stage.

Operational issues

It might seem that it would be a straightforward management task to assess what resources are likely to be needed to carry through a project, and whether they can be made available when required. Almost invariably, however, attempts to analyse the project piece by piece, and to estimate the likely manpower and time required for each phase of the work, end up with a highly over-optimistic prediction, as they start with the assumption that everything will run smoothly according to plan: targets will be established, leads will be found and 'optimized', animal models will work as expected, and the project will most likely be successful in identifying a development compound. In practice, of course, diversionary or delaying events almost invariably occur. The gene that needs to be cloned and expressed proves difficult; obtaining an engineered cell line and devising a workable assay runs into problems; new data are published which necessitate revision of the underlying hypothesis, and possibly a switch to an alternative target; a key member of the team leaves or falls ill; or an essential piece of equipment fails to be delivered on time. However, project champions seeking management support for their ideas do their case no good if they say: 'We plan to set up this animal model and validate it within 3 months, but I have allowed 6 months just in case …'. Happy accidents do occur, of course, but unplanned events are far more likely to slow down a project than to speed it up, so the end result is almost invariably an overrun in terms of time, money and manpower.

Experienced managers understand this and make due allowance for it, but the temptation to approve more projects than the organization can actually cope with is hard for most to resist.

A FINAL WORD

To summarize the key message in a sentence: The drug discovery scientist needs to be aware that many factors other than inherent scientific novelty and quality affect the decision whether or not to embark on a new project. And the subtext: The more the drug discovery scientist understands about the realities of development, patenting, registration and marketing in the pharmaceutical industry, the more effective he or she will be in adapting research plans to the company's needs, and the better at defending them.

Chapter **6**

Choosing the target

H P Rang, R G Hill

INTRODUCTION: THE SCOPE FOR NEW DRUG TARGETS

The word 'target' in the context of drug discovery has several common meanings, including the market niche that the drug is intended to occupy, therapeutic indications for the drug, the biological mechanism that it will modify, the pharmacokinetic properties that it will possess, and – the definition addressed in this chapter – the molecular recognition site to which the drug will bind. For the great majority of existing drugs the target is a protein molecule, most commonly a receptor, an enzyme, a transport molecule or an ion channel, although other proteins such as tubulin and immunophilins are also represented. Some drugs, such as alkylating agents, bind to DNA, and others, such as bisphosphonates, to inorganic bone matrix constituents, but these are exceptions. The search for new drug targets is directed mainly at finding new proteins although approaches aimed at gene-silencing by antisense or siRNA have received much recent attention.

Since the 1950s, when the principle of drug discovery based on identified (then pharmacological or biochemical) targets became established, the pharmaceutical industry has recognized the importance of identifying new targets as the key to successful innovation. As the industry has become more confident in its ability to invent or discover candidate molecules once the target has been defined – a confidence, some would say, based more on hubris than history – the selection of novel targets, preferably exclusive and patentable ones, has assumed increasing importance in the quest for competitive advantage.

In this chapter we look at drug targets in more detail, and discuss old and new strategies for seeking out and validating them.

How many drug targets are there?

Even when we restrict our definition to defined protein targets, counting them is not simple. An obvious starting point is to estimate the number of targets addressed by existing therapeutic drugs, but even this is difficult. For many drugs, we are ignorant of the precise molecular target. For example, several antiepileptic drugs apparently work by blocking voltage-gated sodium channels, but there are many molecular subtypes of these, and we do not know which are relevant to the therapeutic effect. Similarly, antipsychotic drugs block receptors for several amine mediators (dopamine, serotonin, norepinephrine, acetylcholine), for each of which there are several molecular subtypes expressed in the brain. Again, we cannot pinpoint the relevant one or ones that represent the critical targets.

A compendium of therapeutic drugs licensed in the UK and/or US (Dollery, 1999) lists a total of 857 compounds (Figure 6.1), of which 626 are directed at human targets. Of the remainder, 142 are drugs used to treat infectious diseases, and are directed mainly at targets expressed by the infecting organism, and 89 are miscellaneous agents such as vitamins, oxygen, inorganic salts, plasma substitutes, etc., which are not target-directed in the conventional sense.

Drews and Ryser (1997) estimated that these drugs addressed approximately 500 distinct human targets, but this figure includes all of the molecular subtypes of the generic target (e.g. 14 serotonin receptor subtypes and seven opioid receptor subtypes, most of which are not known to be therapeutically relevant, or to be specifically targeted by existing drugs), as well as other putative targets, such as calcineurin, whose therapeutic relevance is unclear. Drews and Ryser estimated that the number of potential targets might be as high as 5000–10 000. Adopting a similar but more restrictive approach, Hopkins and Groom

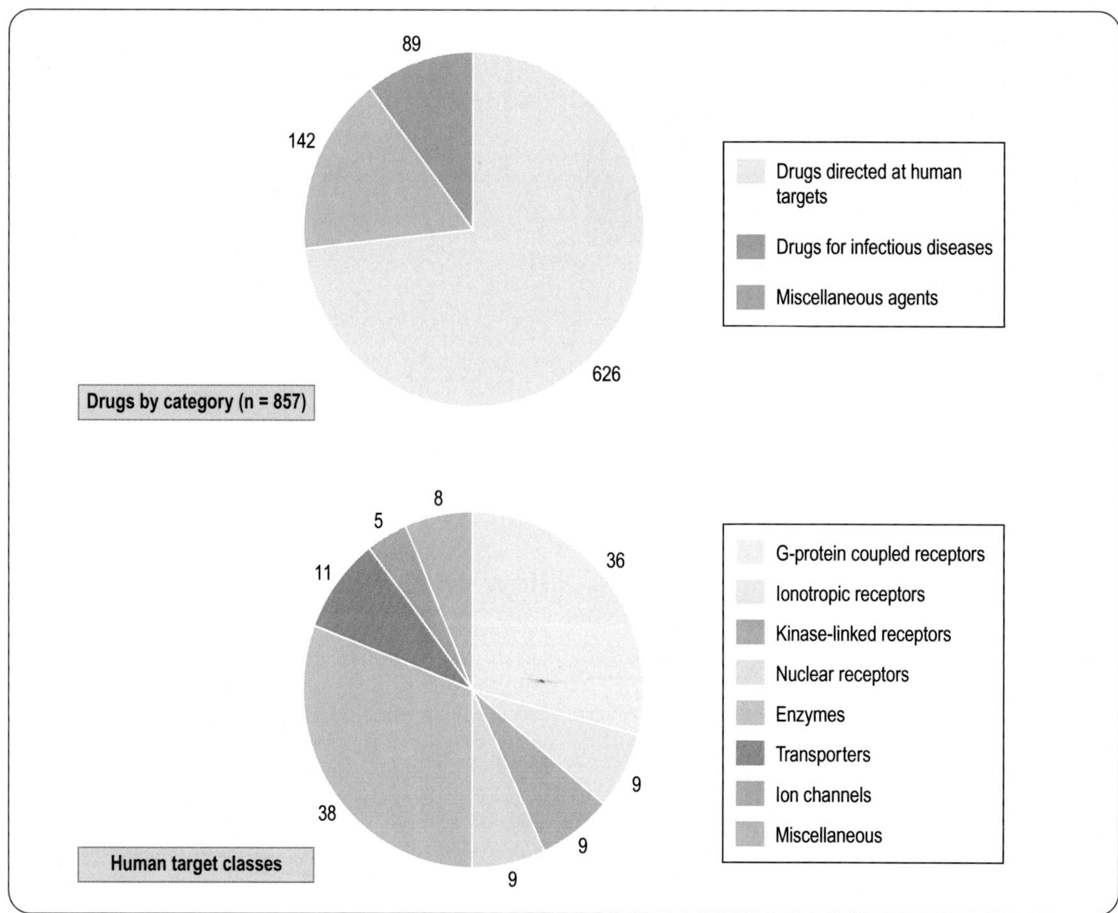

Fig. 6.1 Therapeutic drug targets.

(2002) found that 120 drug targets accounted for the activities of compounds used therapeutically, and estimated that 600–1500 'druggable' targets exist in the human genome. From an analysis of all prescribed drugs produced by the 10 largest pharmaceutical companies, Zambrowicz and Sands (2003) identified fewer than 100 targets; when this analysis was restricted to the 100 best-selling drugs on the market, the number of targets was only 43, reflecting the fact that more than half of the successful targets (i.e. those leading to therapeutically effective and safe drugs) failed to achieve a significant commercial impact. More recently, Imming et al. (2006) identified 218 targets of registered drugs, including those expressed by infectious agents, whereas Overington et al. (2006) found 324 (the difference depending on the exact definition of what constitutes a single identified target). How many targets remain is highly uncertain and Zambrowicz and Sands (2003) suggested that during the 1990s only two or three new targets were exploited by the 30 or so new drugs registered each year, most of which addressed targets that were already well known. The small target base of existing drugs, and the low rate of emergence of new targets, suggests that the number yet to be discovered may be considerably smaller than some optimistic forecasters have predicted. They estimated that 100–150 high-quality targets in the human genome might remain to be discovered. However, a recent analysis of 216 therapeutic drugs registered during the decade 2000–2009 (Rang unpublished) showed that 62 (29%) were first in class compounds directed at novel human targets. This is clearly an increase compared with the previous decade and may give grounds for optimism that many more new targets remain to be found. In the earlier analysis by Drews and Ryser (1997), about one-quarter of the targets identified were associated with drugs used to treat infectious diseases, and belonged to the parasite, rather than the human, genome. Their number is even harder to estimate. Most anti-infective drugs have come from natural products, reflecting the fact that organisms in the natural world have faced strong evolutionary pressure, operating over millions of years, to develop protection against parasites. It is likely, therefore, that the 'druggable genome' of parasitic microorganisms has already been heavily trawled – more so than that of humans, in whom many of the diseases of current concern are too recent for evolutionary counter-measures to have developed.

More recent estimates of the number of possible drug targets (Overington et al., 2006; Imming et al., 2006) are in line with the figure of 600–1500 suggested by Hopkins and Groom (2002). The increased use of gene deletion mutant mice and si RNA for gene knock down coupled with a bioinformatic approach to protein characterization is starting to increase the reliability of target identification (Imming et al., 2006; Wishart et al., 2008; Bakheet and Doig, 2009). New approaches, in which networks of genes are associated with particular disease states, are likely to throw up additional targets that may not have been discovered otherwise (e.g. see Emilsson et al., 2008).

The nature of existing drug targets

The human targets of the 626 drugs, where they are known, are summarized in Figure 6.1. Of the 125 known targets, the largest groups are enzymes and G-protein-coupled receptors, each accounting for about 30%, the remainder being transporters, other receptor classes, and ion channels. This analysis gives only a crude idea of present-day therapeutics, and underestimates the number of molecular targets currently addressed, since it fails to take into account the many subtypes of these targets that have been identified by molecular cloning. In most cases we do not know which particular subtypes are responsible for the therapeutic effect, and the number of distinct targets will certainly increase as these details become known. Also there are many drugs whose targets we do not yet know. There are a growing number of examples where drug targets consist, not of a single protein, but of an oligomeric assembly of different proteins. This is well established for ion channels, most of which are hetero-oligomers, and recent studies show that G-protein-coupled receptors (GPCRs) may form functional dimers (Bouvier, 2001) or may associate with accessory proteins known as RAMPs (McLatchie et al., 1998; Morphis et al., 2003), which strongly influence their pharmacological characteristics. The human genome is thought to contain about 1000 genes in the GPCR family, of which about one-third could be odorant receptors. Excluding the latter, and without taking into account the possible diversity factors mentioned, the 40 or so GPCR targets for existing drugs represent only about 7–10% of the total. Roughly one-third of cloned GPCRs are classed as 'orphan' receptors, for which no endogenous ligand has yet been identified, and these could certainly emerge as attractive drug targets when more is known about their physiological role. Broadly similar conclusions apply to other major classes of drug target, such as nuclear receptors, ion channels and kinases.

The above discussion relates to drug targets expressed by human cells, and similar arguments apply to those of infective organisms. The therapy of infectious diseases, ranging from viruses to multicellular parasites, is one of medicine's greatest challenges. Current antibacterial drugs – the largest class – originate mainly from natural products (with a few, e.g. sulfonamides and oxazolidinediones, coming from synthetic compounds) first identified through screening on bacterial cultures, and analysis of their biochemical mechanism and site of action came later. In many cases this knowledge remains incomplete, and the molecular targets are still unclear. Since the pioneering work of Hitchings and Elion (see Chapter 1), the strategy of target-directed drug discovery has rarely been applied in this field[1]; instead, the 'antibiotic' approach, originating with the discovery of penicillin, has held sway. For the 142 current anti-infective drugs (Figure 6.1), which include antiviral and antiparasitic as well as antibacterial drugs, we can identify approximately 40 targets (mainly enzymes and structural proteins) at the biochemical level, only about half of which have been cloned. The urgent need for drugs that act on new targets arises because of the major problem of drug resistance, with which the traditional chemistry-led strategies are failing to keep up. Consequently, as with other therapeutic classes, genomic technologies are being increasingly applied to the problem of finding new antimicrobial drug targets (Rosamond and Allsop, 2000; Buysse, 2001). In some ways the problem appears simpler than finding human drug targets. Microbial genomes are being sequenced at a high rate, and identifying prokaryotic genes that are essential for survival, replication or pathogenicity is generally easier than identifying genes that are involved in specific regulatory mechanisms in eukaryotes.

CONVENTIONAL STRATEGIES FOR FINDING NEW DRUG TARGETS

Two main routes have been followed so far:

- Analysis of pathophysiology
- Analysis of mechanism of action of existing therapeutic drugs.

There are numerous examples where the elucidation of pathophysiological pathways has pointed to the existence of novel targets that have subsequently resulted in successful drugs, and this strategy is still adopted by most pharmaceutical companies. To many scientists it seems the safe and logical way to proceed – first understand the pathway leading from the primary disturbance to the

[1]A notable exception is the discovery (Wengelnik et al., 2002) of a new class of antimalarial drug designed on biochemical principles to interfere with choline metabolism, which is essential for membrane synthesis during the multiplicatory phase of the malaria organism within the host's red blood cells. Hitchings and Elion would have approved.

appearance of the disease phenotype, then identify particular biochemical steps amenable to therapeutic intervention, then select key molecules as targets. The pioneers in developing this approach were undoubtedly Hitchings and Elion (see Chapter 1), who unravelled the steps in purine and pyrimidine biosynthesis and selected the enzyme dihydrofolate reductase as a suitable target. This biochemical approach led to a remarkable series of therapeutic breakthroughs in antibacterial, anticancer and immunosuppressant drugs. The work of Black and his colleagues, based on mediators and receptors, also described in Chapter 1, was another early and highly successful example of this approach, and there have been many others (Table 6.1a). In some cases the target has emerged

Table 6.1 Examples of drug targets identified, (a) by analysis of pathophysiology, and (b) by analysis of existing drugs

(a) Targets identified via pathophysiology

Disease indication	Target identified	Drugs developed
AIDS	Reverse transcriptase HIV protease	Zidovudine Saquinavir
Asthma	Cysteinyl leukotriene receptor	Zafirlukast
Bacterial infections	Dihydrofolate reductase	Trimethoprim
Malignant disease	Dihydrofolate reductase	6-mercaptopurine Methotrexate
Depression	5HT transporter	Fluoxetine
Hypertension	Angiotensin-converting enzyme Type 5 phosphodiesterase Angiotensin-2 receptor	Captopril Sildenafil Losartan
Inflammatory disease	COX-2	Celecoxib Rofecoxib
Alzheimer's disease	Acetylcholinesterase	Donepezil
Breast cancer	Oestrogen receptor	Tamoxifen Herceptin
Chronic myeloid leukemia	Abl kinase	Imatinib
Parkinson's disease	Dopamine synthesis MAO-B	Levodopa Selegiline
Depression	MAO-A	Moclobemide

(b) Targets identified via drug effects

Drug	Disease	Target
Benzodiazepines	Anxiety, sleep disorders	BDZ binding site on $GABA_A$ receptor
Aspirin-like drugs	Inflammation, pain	COX enzymes
Ciclosporin, FK506	Transplant rejection	Immunophilins
Vinca alkaloids	Cancers	Tubulin
Dihydropyridines	Cardiovascular disease	L-type calcium channels
Sulfonylureas	Diabetes	K_{ATP} channels
Classic antipsychotic drugs	Schizophrenia	Dopamine D_2 receptor
Tricyclic antidepressants	Depression	Monoamine transporters
Fibrates	Raised blood cholesterol	PPARα

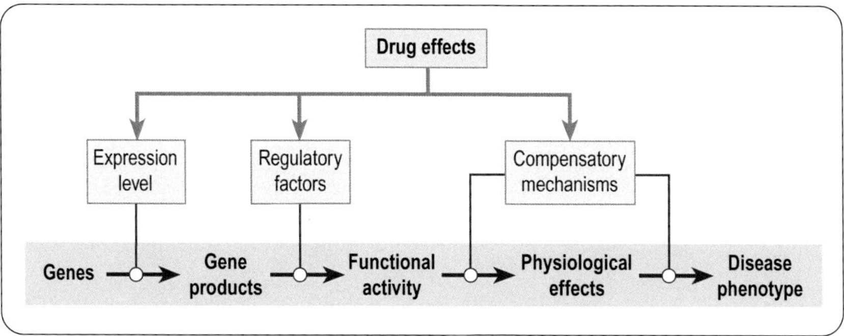

Fig. 6.2 Drug effects in relation to disease aetiology.

from pharmacological rather than pathophysiological studies. The $5HT_3$ receptor was identified from pharmacological studies and chosen as a potential drug target for the development of antagonists, but its role in pathophysiology was at the time far from clear. Eventually animal and clinical studies revealed the antiemetic effect of drugs such as *ondansetron*, and such drugs were developed mainly to control the nausea and vomiting associated with cancer chemotherapy. Similarly, the $GABA_B$ receptor (target for relaxant drugs such as *baclofen)* was discovered by analysis of the pharmacological effects of GABA, and only later exploited therapeutically to treat muscle spasm.

The identification of drug targets by the 'backwards' approach – involving analysis of the mechanism of action of empirically discovered therapeutic agents – has produced some major breakthroughs in the past (see examples in Table 6.1b). Its relevance is likely to decline as drug discovery becomes more target focused, though natural product pharmacology will probably continue to reveal novel drug targets.

It is worth reminding ourselves that there remain several important drug classes whose mechanism of action we still do not fully understand (e.g. acetaminophen (paracetamol)[2], valproate). Whether their targets remain elusive because their effects depend on a cocktail of interactions at several different sites, or whether novel targets will emerge for such drugs, remains uncertain.

New strategies for identifying drug targets

Figure 6.2 summarizes the main points at which drugs may intervene along the pathway from genotype to phenotype, namely by altering gene expression, by altering the functional activity of gene products, or by activating compensatory mechanisms. This is of course an oversimplification, as changes in gene expression or the activation of compensatory mechanisms are themselves indirect effects, following pathways similar to that represented by the primary track in Figure 6.2. Nevertheless, it provides a useful framework for discussing some of the newer genomics-based approaches. A useful account of the various genetic models that have been developed in different organisms for the identification of new drug targets, and elucidating the mechanisms of action of existing drugs, is given by Carroll and Fitzgerald (2003).

Trawling the genome

The conventional route to new drug targets, starting from pathophysiology, will undoubtedly remain as a standard approach. Understanding of the disease mechanisms in the major areas of therapeutic challenge, such as Alzheimer's disease, atherosclerosis, cancer, stroke, obesity, etc., is advancing rapidly, and new targets are continually emerging. But this is generally slow, painstaking, hypothesis-driven work, and there is a strong incentive to seek shortcuts based on the use of new technologies to select and validate novel targets, starting from the genome. In principle, it is argued, nearly all drug targets are proteins, and are, therefore, represented in the proteome, and also as corresponding genes in the genome. There are, however, some significant caveats, the main ones being the following:

- Splice variants may result in more than one pharmacologically distinct type of receptor being encoded in a single gene. These are generally predictable from the genome, and represented as distinct species in the transcriptome and proteome.
- There are many examples of multimeric receptors, made up of non-identical subunits encoded by different genes. This is true of the majority of ligand-gated ion channels, whose pharmacological characteristics depend critically on the subunit

[2]COX-3, a novel splice variant of cyclooxygenase-1, was suggested as apossible target underlying the analgesic action of acetaminophen (Chandrasekharan et al., 2002), spurring several companies to set up screens for new acetaminophen-like drugs. This now seems to have been a dry well and recent suggestions on mechanism have included activation of TRPV1 and cannabinoid receptors by a metabolite (Mallet et al., 2010) and the inhibition of prostaglandin H synthase (Aronoff et al., 2006).

composition (Hille, 2001). Recent work also shows that G-protein-coupled receptors often exist as heteromeric dimers, with pharmacological properties distinct from those of the individual units (Bouvier, 2001). Moreover, association between receptors and non-receptor proteins can determine the pharmacological characteristics of certain G-protein-coupled receptors (McLatchie et al., 1998).

Despite these complications, studies based on the appealingly simple dogma:

one gene → one protein → one drug target

have been extremely productive in advancing our knowledge of receptors and other drug targets in recent years, and it is expected that genome trawling will reveal more 'single-protein' targets, even though multiunit complexes are likely to escape detection by this approach.

How might potential drug targets be recognized among the 25 000 or so genes in the human genome?

Several approaches have been described for homing in on genes that may encode novel drug targets, starting with the identification of certain gene categories:

- 'Disease genes', i.e. genes, mutations of which cause or predispose to the development of human disease.
- 'Disease-modifying' genes. These comprise (a) genes whose altered expression is thought to be involved in the development of the disease state; and (b) genes that encode functional proteins, whose activity is altered (even if their expression level is not) in the disease state, and which play a part in inducing the disease state.
- 'Druggable genes', i.e. genes encoding proteins likely to possess binding domains that recognize drug-like small molecules. Included in this group are genes encoding targets for existing therapeutic and experimental drugs. These genes and their paralogues (i.e. closely related but non-identical genes occurring elsewhere in the genome) comprise the group of druggable genes.

On this basis (Hopkins and Groom, 2002), novel targets are represented by the intersection of disease-modifying and druggable gene classes, excluding those already targeted by therapeutic drugs. Next, we consider these categories in more detail.

Disease genes

The identification of genes in which mutations are associated with particular diseases has a long history in medicine (Weatherall, 1991), starting with the concept of 'inborn errors of metabolism' such as phenylketonuria. The strategies used to identify disease-associated genes, described in Chapter 7, have been very successful. Examples of common diseases associated with mutations of a single gene are summarized in Table 7.3. There are many more examples of rare inherited disorders of this type. Information of this kind, important though it is for the diagnosis, management and counselling of these patients, has so far had little impact on the selection of drug targets. None of the gene products identified appears to be directly 'targetable'. Much more common than single-gene disorders are conditions such as diabetes, hypertension, schizophrenia, bipolar depressive illness and many cancers in which there is a clear genetic component, but, together with environmental factors, several different genes contribute as risk factors for the appearance of the disease phenotype. The methods for identifying the particular genes involved (see Chapter 7) were until recently difficult and laborious, but are becoming much easier as the sequencing and annotation of the human genome progresses. The Human Genome Consortium (2001) found 971 'disease genes' already listed in public databases, and identified 286 paralogues of these in the sequenced genome. Progress has been rapid and Lander (2011) contrasts the situation in 2000, when only about a dozen genetic variations outside the HLA locus had been associated with common diseases, with today, when more than 1100 loci associated with 165 diseases have been identified. Notably most of these have been discovered since 2007. The challenge of obtaining useful drug targets from genome-wide association studies remains considerable (Donnelly, 2008).

The value of information about disease genes in better understanding the pathophysiology is unquestionable, but just how useful is it as a pointer to novel drug targets? Many years after being identified, the genes involved in several important single-gene disorders, such as thalassaemia, muscular dystrophy and cystic fibrosis, have not so far proved useful as drug targets, although progress is at last being made. On the other hand, the example of Abl-kinase, the molecular target for the recently introduced anticancer drug *imatinib (Gleevec;* see Chapter 4), shows that the proteins encoded by mutated genes can themselves constitute drug targets, but so far there are few instances where this has proved successful. The findings that rare forms of familial Alzheimer's disease were associated with mutations in the gene encoding the amyloid precursor protein (APP) or the secretase enzyme responsible for formation of the β-amyloid fragment present in amyloid plaques were strong pointers that confirmed the validity of secretase as a drug target (although it had already been singled out on the basis of biochemical studies). Secretase inhibitors reached late-stage clinical development as potential anti-Alzheimer's drugs in 2001, but none at the time of writing have emerged from the development pipeline as useful drugs. Similar approaches have been successful in identifying disease-associated genes in defined subgroups of patients with conditions such as diabetes, hypertension and hypercholesterolaemia, and there is reason to hope that novel drug targets will emerge in these areas. However, in other fields, such as schizophrenia and asthma, progress in pinning down disease-related genes has been very limited. The most promising field for identifying novel drug targets among disease-associated mutations is likely to be in cancer therapies, as mutations are the basic cause of malignant transformation and real progress is being made in exploiting our knowledge of the cancer genome (Roukos, 2011). In general, one can say that identifying disease genes may provide valuable pointers to possible drug targets further down the pathophysiological pathway, even though their immediate gene products may not always be targetable. The identification of a new disease gene often hits the popular headlines on the basis that an effective therapy will quickly follow, though this rarely happens, and never quickly.

In summary, the class of disease genes does not seem to include many obvious drug targets.

Disease-modifying genes

In this class lie many non-mutated genes that are directly involved in the pathophysiological pathway leading to the disease phenotype. The phenotype may be associated with over- or underexpression of the genes, detectable by expression profiling (see below), or by the over- or underactivity of the gene product – for example, an enzyme – independently of changes in its expression level.

This is the most important category in relation to drug targets, as therapeutic drug action generally occurs by changing the activity of functional proteins, whether or not the disease alters their expression level. Finding new ones, however, is not easy, and there is as yet no shortcut screening strategy for locating them in the genome.

Two main approaches are currently being used, namely gene expression profiling and comprehensive gene knockout studies.

Gene expression profiling

The principle underlying gene expression profiling as a guide to new drug targets is that the development of any disease phenotype necessarily involves changes in gene expression in the cells and tissues involved. Long-term changes in the structure or function of cells cannot occur without altered gene expression, and so a catalogue of all the genes whose expression is up- or down-regulated in the disease state will include genes where such regulation is actually required for the development of the disease phenotype. As well as these 'critical path genes', which may represent potential drug targets, others are likely to be affected as genes involved in secondary reinforcing of compensatory mechanisms following the development of the disease phenotype (which may also represent potential drug targets), but many will be irrelevant 'bystander genes' (Figure 6.3). The important problem, to which there is no simple answer, is how to eliminate the bystanders, and how to identify potential drug targets among the rest. Zanders (2000), in a thoughtful review, emphasizes the importance of focusing on signal transduction pathways as the most likely source of novel targets identifiable by gene expression profiling.

The methods available for gene expression profiling are described in Chapter 7. DNA microarrays ('gene chips') are most commonly used, their advantage being that they are quick and easy to use. They have the disadvantage that the DNA sequences screened are selected in advance, but this is becoming less of a limitation as more genomic information accumulates. They also have limited sensitivity, which (see Chapter 7) means that genes expressed at low levels – including, possibly, a significant proportion of potential drug targets – can be missed. Methods based on the polymerase chain reaction (PCR), such as serial

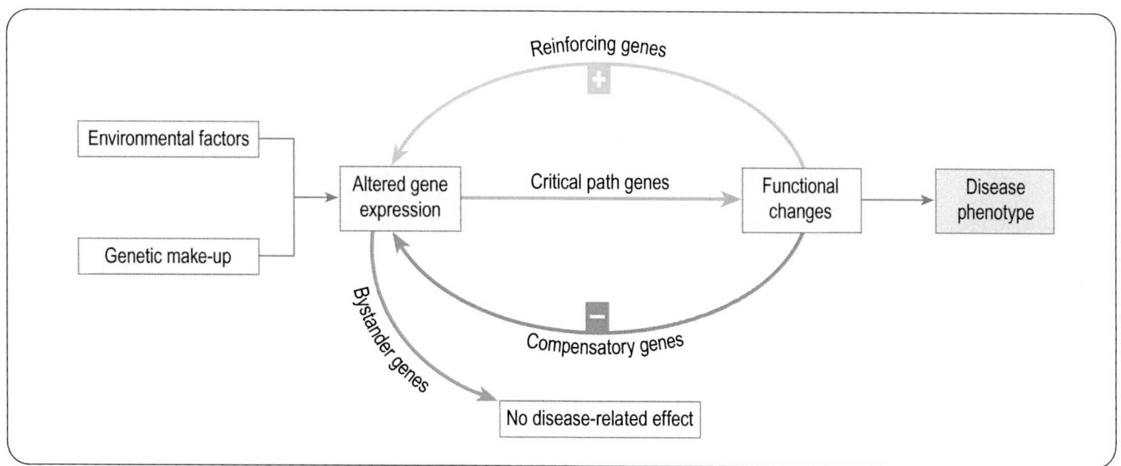

Fig. 6.3 Gene expression in disease.

analysis of gene expression (SAGE; Velculescu et al., 1995), are, in principle, capable of detecting all transcribed RNAs without preselection, with higher sensitivity than microarrays, but are more laborious and technically demanding. Both technologies produce the same kind of data, namely a list of genes whose expression is significantly altered as a result of a defined experimental intervention. A large body of gene expression data has been collected over the last few years, showing the effects of many kinds of disturbance, including human disease, animal models of disease and drug effects; some examples are listed in Table 6.2. In most cases, several thousand genes have been probed with microarrays, covering perhaps 20% of the entire genome, so the coverage is by no means complete. Commonly, it is found that some 2–10% of the genes studied show significant changes in response to such disturbances. Thus, given a total of about 25 000 genes in man, with perhaps 20% expressed in a given tissue, we can expect several hundred to be affected in a typical disease state. Much effort has gone into (a) methods of analysis and pattern recognition within these large data sets, and (b) defining the principles for identifying possible drug targets within such a group of regulated genes. Techniques for analysis and pattern recognition fall within the field of bioinformatics (Chapter 7), and the specific problem of analysing transcription data is discussed by Quackenbush (2001) and Butte (2002), and also Lander (2011). Because altered mRNA levels do not always correlate with changes in protein expression, protein changes should be confirmed independently where possible. This normally entails the production and validation of an antibody-based assay or staining procedure.

Identifying potential drug targets among the array of differentially expressed genes that are revealed by expression profiling is neither straightforward nor exact. Possible approaches are:

- On the basis of prior biological knowledge, genes that might plausibly be critical in the pathogenesis of the disease can be distinguished from those (e.g. housekeeping genes, or genes involved in intermediary metabolism) that are unlikely to be critical. This, the plausibility criterion, is in practice the most important factor in identifying likely drug targets. As genomic analysis proceeds, it is becoming possible to group genes into functional classes, e.g. tissue growth and repair, inflammation, myelin formation, neurotransmission, etc., and changes in expression are often concentrated in one or more of these functional groups, giving a useful pointer to the biological pathways involved in pathogenesis.
- Anatomical studies can be used to identify whether candidate genes are regulated in the cells and tissues affected by the disease.
- Timecourse measurements reveal the relationship between gene expression changes and the development of the disease phenotype. With many acute interventions, several distinct temporal patterns are detectable in the expression of different genes. 'Clustering' algorithms (see Chapter 7; Quackenbush, 2001) are useful to identify genes which are co-regulated and whose function might point to a particular biochemical or signalling pathway relevant to the pathogenesis.
- The study of several different clinical and animal models with similar disease phenotypes can reveal networks of genes whose expression is consistently affected and hence representative of the phenotype (see Emilsson et al. 2008; Schadt 2009).
- The effects of drug or other treatments can be studied in order to reveal genes whose expression is normalized in parallel with the 'therapeutic' effect.

Gene knockout screening

Another screening approach for identifying potential drug target genes, based on generating transgenic 'gene knockout' strains of mice, as performed by biotechnology company Lexicon Pharmaceuticals (Walke et al., 2001; Zambrowicz and Sands, 2003), aimed to study 5000 genes within 5 years. The 5000 genes were selected on several criteria, including existing evidence of association with disease and membership of families of known drug targets (GPCRs, transporters, kinases, etc.). The group has developed an efficient procedure for generating transgenic knockout mice, and a standardized set of tests to detect phenotypic effects relevant to a range of disease states. In a recent review, Zambrowicz and Sands (2003) present many examples where the effects of gene knockouts in mice produce effects consistent with the known actions and side effects of therapeutic drugs. For example, inactivation of the genes for angiotensin converting enzyme (ACE) or the angiotensin receptor results in lowering of blood pressure, reflecting the clinical effect of drugs acting on these targets. Similarly, elimination of the gene encoding one of the subunits of the $GABA_A$ receptor produces a state of irritability and hyperactivity in mice, the opposite of the effect of benzodiazepine tranquillizers, which enhance $GABA_A$ receptor function. However, using transgenic gene knockout technology (sometimes dubbed 'reverse genetics') to confirm the validity of previously well-established drug targets is not the same as using it to discover new targets. Success in the latter context will depend greatly on the ability of the phenotypic tests that are applied to detect therapeutically relevant changes in the knockout strains. Some new targets have already been identified in this way, and deployed in drug discovery programmes; they include *cathepsin K*, a protease involved in the genesis of osteoporosis, and *melanocortin receptors*, which may play a role in obesity. The Lexicon group has developed a systems-based panel of primary screens to look for relevant effects on the main physiological systems (cardiovascular, CNS, immune

Table 6.2 Examples of gene expression profiling studies, showing numbers of mRNAs affected under various conditions

Test system	Method	Number of genes analysed	Number of genes affected (threshold)	Number up	Number down	Ref
Activated vs quiescent human fibroblasts	Microarray	8600	517 (2.2-fold)) (Some genes showed both up- and down-regulation at different times)	148	242	Iyer et al (1999)
Differentiated vs undifferentiated mouse neural stem cells	Microarray	8700	156 (twofold)	94	62	Somogyi (1999)
Small diameter vs large diameter rat sensory neurons	Microarray	477	40 (1.5-fold)	26	14	Luo et al. (1999)
Ischaemic vs control rat brain	Microarray	1179	20 (1.8-fold)	6	14	Keyvani et al. (2002)
Inflamed vs normal mouse lung	Microarray	6000	470 (twofold) (Many genes showed both up- and down-regulation at different times)			Kaminski et al. (2000)
Old vs young mouse brain (cortex)	Microarray	6347	110 (1.7-fold)	63	47	Lee et al. (2000)
Old vs young mouse skeletal muscle	Microarray	6300	113 (twofold)	58	55	Lee et al. (1999)
Human colorectal cancer vs normal tissue	SAGE	~49 000	289 (difference significant at $p < 0.01$)	108	181	Zhang et al. (1997)
Human MS plaques vs normal brain	Microarray	>5000	(~twofold)	29	ND	Whitney et al. (1999)
Human ovarian cancer vs normal ovary	Microarray	5766	726 (threefold)	295	431	Wang et al. (1999)
Human Alzheimer's disease plaques vs non-plaque regions	Microarray	6800	18 (1.8-fold)	–	18	Ho et al. (2001)
Mouse liver, thyroid treated vs hypothyroid	Microarray	2225	55 (twofold)	14	41	Feng et al. (2000)
Mouse, hypertophied vs normal heart muscle	Microarray	>4000	47 (~1.8-fold)	21	26	Friddle et al. (2000)
Human postmortem prefrontal cortex, schizophrenia vs control	Microarray	~7000	179 (1.9-fold)	97	82	Mirnics et al. (2000)

Continued

Table 6.2 *Continued*

Test system	Method	Number of genes analysed	Number of genes affected (threshold)	Number up	Number down	Ref
Human postmortem prefrontal cortex, schizophrenia vs control	Microarray	~6000	88 (1.4-fold)	71	17	Hakak et al. (2001)
Single neurons from human postmortem entorhinal cortex, schizophrenia vs control	Microarray	>18000	4139 (2-fold)	2574	1565	Hemby et al. (2002)

system, etc.). On the basis of their experience with the first 750 of the planned 5000 gene knockouts, they predicted that about 100 new high-quality targets could be revealed in this way. Programmes such as this, based on mouse models, are time-consuming and costly, but have the great advantage that mouse physiology is fairly similar to human. The use of species such as flatworm (*Caenorhabditis elegans*) and zebra-fish *(Danio rerio)* is being explored as a means of speeding up the process (Shin and Fishman, 2002) and more recently studies in yeast have successfully facilitated the discovery of molecules that interact with mammalian drug targets (Brown et al., 2011).

'Druggable' genes

For a gene product to serve as a drug target, it must possess a recognition site capable of binding small molecules. Hopkins and Groom (2002) found a total of 399 protein targets for registered and experimental drug molecules. The 399 targets belong to 130 distinct protein families, and the authors suggest that other members of these families – a total of 3051 proteins – are also likely to possess similar binding domains, even though specific ligands have not yet been described, and propose that this total represents the current limit of the druggable genome. Of course, it is likely that new targets, belonging to different protein families, will emerge in the future, so this number may well expand. 'Druggable' in this context implies only that the protein is likely to possess a binding site for a small molecule, irrespective of whether such an interaction is likely be of any therapeutic value. To be useful as a starting point for drug discovery, a potential target needs to combine 'druggability' with disease-modifying properties. One new approach is to look at the characteristics of a typical human protein drug target (e.g. hydrophobic, high length, signal motif present) and to then look for these characteristics in a non-target set of proteins so as to identify new potential targets (Bakheet and Doig, 2009).

TARGET VALIDATION

The techniques discussed so far are aimed at identifying potential drug targets within the diversity warehouse represented by the genome, the key word being 'potential'.

Few companies will be willing to invest the considerable resources needed to mount a target-directed drug discovery project without more direct evidence that the target is an appropriate one for the disease indication. Target validation refers to the experimental approaches by which a potential drug target can be tested and given further credibility. It is an open-ended term, which can be taken to embrace virtually the whole of biology, but for practical purposes the main approaches are *pharmacological* and *genetic*.

Although these experimental approaches can go a long way towards supporting the validity of a chosen target, the ultimate test is in the clinic, where efficacy is or is not confirmed. Lack of clinical efficacy causes the abandonment of roughly one-third of drugs in Phase II, reflecting the unreliability of the earlier surrogate evidence for target validity.

Pharmacological approaches

The underlying question to be addressed is whether drugs that influence the potential drug target actually produce the expected effects on cells, tissues or whole animals. Where a known receptor, for example the metabotropic glutamate receptor (mGluR), was identified as a potential target for a new indication (e.g. pain) its validity could be tested by measuring the analgesic effect of known mGluR antagonists in relevant animal models. For novel targets, of course, no panel of active compounds will normally be available, and so it will be necessary to set up a screening assay to identify them. Where a company is already active in a particular line of research – as was the case with Ciba

Geigy in the kinase field – it may be straightforward to refine its assay methods in order to identify selective inhibitors. Ciba Geigy was able to identify active Abl kinase inhibitors within its existing compound collection, and hence to show that these were effective in cell proliferation assays.

A variant of the pharmacological approach is to use antibodies raised against the putative target protein, rather than small-molecule inhibitors.

Many experts predict that, as high-throughput screening and automated chemistry develop (see Chapters 8 and 9), allowing the rapid identification of families of selective compounds, these technologies will be increasingly used as tools for target validation, in parallel with lead finding. 'Hits' from screening that show a reasonable degree of target selectivity, whether or not they represent viable lead compounds, can be used in pharmacological studies designed to test their efficacy in a selection of in vitro and in vivo models. Showing that such prototype compounds, regardless of their suitability as leads, do in fact produce the desired effect greatly strengthens the argument for target validity. Although contemporary examples are generally shrouded in confidentiality, it is clear that this approach is becoming more common, so that target validation and lead finding are carried out simultaneously. More recently the move has been towards screening enriched libraries containing compounds of a particular chemical phenotype known to, for example, be disposed towards kinase inhibition rather than screening entire compound collections in a random fashion.

Genetic approaches

These approaches involve various techniques for suppressing the expression of specific genes to determine whether they are critical to the disease process. This can be done acutely in genetically normal cells or animals by the use of antisense oligonucleotides or RNA interference, or constitutively by generating transgenic animals in which the genes of interest are either overactive or suppressed.

Antisense oligonucleotides

Antisense oligonucleotides (Phillips, 2000; Dean, 2001) are stretches of RNA complementary to the gene of interest, which bind to cellular mRNA and prevent its translation. In principle this allows the expression of specific genes to be inhibited, so that their role in the development of a disease phenotype can be determined. Although simple in principle, the technology is subject to many pitfalls and artefacts in practice, and attempts to use it, without very careful controls, to assess genes as potential drug targets are likely to give misleading results. As an alternative to using synthetic oligonucleotides, antisense sequences can be introduced into cells by genetic engineering. Examples where this approach has been used to validate putative drug targets include a range of recent studies on the novel cell surface receptor uPAR (urokinase plasminogen-activator receptor; see review by Wang, 2001). This receptor is expressed by certain malignant tumour cells, particularly gliomas, and antisense studies have shown it to be important in controlling the tendency of these tumours to metastasize, and therefore to be a potential drug target. In a different field, antisense studies have supported the role of a recently cloned sodium channel subtype, PN3 (now known to be Nav 1.87) (Porreca et al., 1999) and of the metabotropic glutamate receptor mGluR1 (Fundytus et al., 2001) in the pathogenesis of neuropathic pain in animal models. Antisense oligonucleotides have the advantage that their effects on gene expression are acute and reversible, and so mimic drug effects more closely than, for example, the changes seen in transgenic animals (see below), where in most cases the genetic disturbance is present throughout life. It is likely that, as more experience is gained, antisense methods based on synthetic oligonucleotides will play an increasingly important role in drug target validation.

RNA interference (RNAi)

This technique depends on the fact that short lengths of double-stranded RNA *(short interfering RNAs, or siRNAs)* activate a sequence-specific *RNA-induced silencing complex (RISC)*, which destroys by cleavage the corresponding functional mRNA within the cell (Hannon, 2000; Kim, 2003). Thus specific mRNAs or whole gene families can be inactivated by choosing appropriate siRNA sequences. Gene silencing by this method is highly efficient, particularly in invertebrates such as *Caenorhabditis elegans* and *Drosophila*, and can also be used in mammalian cells and whole animals. Its use for studying gene function and validating potential drug targets is increasing rapidly, and it also has potential for therapeutic applications. It has proved to be a rapid and effective tool for discovering new targets and automated cell assays have allowed the rapid screening of large groups of genes.

Transgenic animals

The use of the gene knockout principle as a screening approach to identify new targets is described above. The same technology is also valuable, and increasingly being used, as a means of validating putative targets. In principle, deletion or overexpression of a specific gene in vivo can provide a direct test of whether or not it plays a role in the sequence of events that gives rise to a disease phenotype. The generation of transgenic animal – mainly mouse – strains is, however, a demanding and time-consuming process (Houdebine, 1997; Jackson and Abbott, 2000). Therefore, although this technology has an increasingly important role to play in the later stages of drug discovery and development, some have claimed it is too cumbersome to be used routinely at the stage of target selection, though Harris and Foord (2000) predicted that high-throughput 'transgenic factories' may be used in this way. One problem relates to the genetic background of the transgenic colony. It is well known that different mouse strains differ in many significant ways, for example in their behaviour, susceptibility to tumour development, body weight, etc. For technical reasons, the strain into which the transgene is introduced is normally different from that used to establish the breeding colony, so a protocol of back-crossing the transgenic 'founders' into the breeding strain has to proceed for several generations before a genetically homogeneous transgenic colony is obtained. Limited by the breeding cycle of mice, this normally takes about 2 years. It is mainly for this reason that the generation of transgenic animals for the purposes of target validation is not usually included as a stage on the critical path of the project. Sometimes, studies on transgenic animals tip the balance of opinion in such a way as to encourage work on a novel drug target. For example, the vanilloid receptor, TRPV1, which is expressed by nociceptive sensory neurons, was confirmed as a potential drug target when the knockout mouse proved to have a marked deficit in the development of inflammatory hyperalgesia (Davis et al., 2000), thereby confirming the likely involvement of this receptor in a significant clinical condition. Most target-directed projects, however, start on the basis of other evidence for (or simply faith in) the relevance of the target, and work on developing transgenic animals begins at the same time, in anticipation of a need for them later in the project. In many cases, transgenic animals have provided the most useful (sometimes the only available) disease models for drug testing in vivo. Thus, cancer models based on deletion of the p53 tumour suppressor gene are widely used, as are atherosclerosis models based on deletion of the ApoE or LDL-receptor genes. Alzheimer's disease models involving mutation of the gene for amyloid precursor protein, or the presenilin genes, have also proved extremely valuable, as there was hitherto no model that replicated the amyloid deposits typical of this disease. In summary, transgenic animal models are often helpful for post hoc target validation, but their main – and increasing – use in drug discovery comes at later stages of the project (see Chapter 11).

SUMMARY AND CONCLUSIONS

In the present drug discovery environment most projects begin with the identification of a molecular target, usually one that can be incorporated into a high-throughput screening assay. Drugs currently in therapeutic use cover about 200–250 distinct human molecular targets, and the great majority of new compounds registered in the last decade are directed at targets that were already well known; on average, about three novel targets are covered by drugs registered each year. The discovery and exploitation of new targets is considered essential for therapeutic progress and commercial success in the long term. Estimates from genome sequence data of the number of potential drug targets, defined by disease relevance and 'druggability', suggest that from about 100 to several thousand 'druggable' new targets remain to be discovered. The uncertainty reflects two main problems: the difficulty of recognizing 'druggability' in gene sequence data, and the difficulty of determining the relevance of a particular gene product in the development of a disease phenotype. Much effort is currently being applied to these problems, often taking the form of new 'omic' disciplines whose role and status are not yet defined. Proteomics and structural genomics are expected to improve our ability to distinguish druggable proteins from the rest, and 'transcriptomics' (another name for gene expression profiling) and the study of transgenic animals will throw light on gene function, thus improving our ability to recognize the disease-modifying mechanisms wherein novel drug targets are expected to reside.

REFERENCES

Aronoff DM, Oates JA, Boutaud O. New insights into the mechanism of action of acetaminophen: its clinical pharmacologic characteristics reflect its inhibition of the two prostaglandin H2 synthases. Clinical Pharmacology and Therapeutics 2006;79:9–19.

Bakheet TM, Doig AJ. Properties and identification of human protein drug targets. Bioinformatics 2009; 25:451–7.

Bouvier M. Oligomerization of G-protein-coupled transmitter receptors. Nature Reviews Neuroscience 2001;2:274–86.

Brown AJ, Daniels DA, Kassim M, et al. Pharmacology of GPR-55 in yeast and identification of GSK494581A as a mixed-activity glycine transporter subtype 1 imhibitor and GPR55 agonist. Journal of Pharmacology and Experimental Therapeutics 2011;337:236–46.

Butte A. The use and analysis of microarray data. Nature Reviews Drug Discovery 2002;1:951–60.

Buysse JM. The role of genomics in antibacterial drug discovery. Current Medicinal Chemistry 2001;8:1713–26.

Carroll PM, Fitzgerald K, editors. Model organisms in drug discovery. Chichester: John Wiley; 2003.

Chandrasekharan NV, Dai H, Roos KL, et al. COX-3, a cyclooxygenase-1 variant inhibited by acetaminophen and other analgesic/antipyretic drugs: cloning, structure, and expression. Proceedings of the National Academy of Sciences of the USA 2002;99:13926–31.

Davis JB, Gray J, Gunthorpe MJ, et al. Vanilloid receptor-1 is essential for inflammatory thermal hyperalgesia. Nature 2000;405:183–7.

Dean NM. Functional genomics and target validation approaches using antisense oligonucleotide technology. Current Opinion in Biotechnology 2001;12:622–5.

Dollery CT, editor. Therapeutic drugs. Edinburgh: Churchill Livingstone; 1999.

Donnelly P. Progress and challenges in genome-wide association studies. Nature 2008;456:728–31.

Drews J, Ryser S. Classic drug targets. Nature Biotechnology 1997;15:1318–9.

Emilsson V, Thorleifsson G, Zhang B, et al. Genetics of gene expression and its effect on disease. Nature 2008;452:423–8.

Feng X, Jiang Y, Meltzer P, et al. Thyroid hormone regulation of hepatic genes in vivo detected by complementary DNA microarray. Molecular Endocrinology 2000;14:947–55.

Friddle CJ, Koga T, Rubin EM, et al. Expression profiling reveals distinct sets of genes altered during induction and regression of cardiac hypertrophy. Proceedings of the National Academy of Sciences of the USA 2000;97:6745–50.

Fundytus ME, Yashpal K, Chabot JG, et al. Knockdown of spinal metabotropic receptor 1 (mGluR1) alleviates pain and restores opioid efficacy after nerve injury in rats. British Journal of Pharmacology 2001;132:354–67.

Hakak Y, Walker JR, Li C, et al. Genome-wide expression analysis reveals dysregulation of myelination-related genes in chronic schizophrenia. Proceedings of the National Academy of Sciences of the USA 2001;98:4746–51.

Hannon GJ. RNA interference. Nature 2000;418:244–51.

Harris S, Foord SM. Transgenic gene knock-outs: functional genomics and therapeutic target selection. Pharmacogenomics 2000;1:433–43.

Hemby SE, Ginsberg SD, Brunk B, et al. Gene expression profile for schizophrenia: discrete neuron transcription patterns in the entorhinal cortex. Archives of General Psychiatry 2002;59:631–40.

Hille B. Ion channels of excitable membranes. 3rd ed. Sunderland, MA: Sinauer; 2001.

Ho L, Guo Y, Spielman L et al. Altered expression of a-type but not b-type synapsin isoform in the brain of patients at high risk for Alzheimer's disease assessed by DNA microarray technique. Neuroscience Letters 2001;298:191–4.

Hopkins AL, Groom CR. The druggable genome. Nature Reviews Drug Discovery 2002;1:727–30.

Houdebine LM. Transgenic animals – generation and use. Amsterdam: Harwood Academic; 1997.

Imming P, Sinning C, Meyer A. Drugs, their targets and the nature and number of drug targets. Nature Reviews. Drug Discovery 2006; 5:821–34.

Iyer VR, Eisen MB, Ross DT, et al. The transcriptional program in the response of human fibroblasts to serum. Science 1999;283:83–7.

Jackson IJ, Abbott CM. Mouse genetics and transgenics. Oxford: Oxford University Press; 2000.

Kaminski N, Allard JD, Pittet JF, et al. Global analysis of gene expression in pulmonary fibrosis reveals distinct programs regulating lung inflammation and fibrosis. Proceedings of the National Academy of Sciences of the USA 2000;97:1778–83.

Keyvani K, Witte OW, Paulus W. Gene expression profiling in perilesional and contralateral areas after ischemia in rat brain. Journal of Cerebral Blood Flow and Metabolism 2002;22:153–60.

Kim VN. RNA interference in functional genomics and medicine. Journal of Korean Medical Science 2003;18: 309–18.

Lander ES. Initial impact of the sequencing of the human genome. Nature 2011;470:187–97.

Lee CK, Klopp RG, Weindruch R, et al. Gene expression profile of aging and its retardation by caloric restriction. Science 1999;285:1390–3.

Lee CK, Weindruch R, Prolla TA. Gene-expression profile of the ageing brain in mice. Nature Genetics 2000;25:294–7.

Luo L, Salunga RC, Guo H, et al. Gene expression profiles of laser-captured adjacent neuronal subtypes. Nature Medicine 1999;5:117–22.

McLatchie LM, Fraser NJ, Main MJ, et al. RAMPs regulate the transport and ligand specificity of the calcitonin-receptor-like receptor. Nature 1998;393:333–9.

Mallet C, Barriere DA, Ermund A, et al. TRPV1 in brain is involved in acetaminophen-induced antinociception. PLoS ONE 2010;5:1–11.

Mirnics K, Middleton FA, Marquez A, et al. Molecular characterization of schizophrenia viewed by microarray analysis of gene expression in prefrontal cortex. Neuron 2000; 28:53–67.

Morphis M, Christopoulos A, Sexton PM. RAMPs: 5 years on, where to now? Trends in Pharmacological Sciences 2003;24:596–601.

Overington JP, Bissan A-L, Hopkins AL. How many drug targets are there? Nature Reviews. Drug Discovery 2006;5:993–6.

Phillips MI. Antisense technology, Parts A and B. San Diego: Academic Press; 2000.

Porreca F, Lai J, Bian D, et al. A comparison of the potential role of the tetrodotoxin-insensitive sodium channels, PN3/SNS and NaN/SNS2, in rat models of chronic pain. Proceedings of the National Academy of Sciences of the USA 1999;96:7640–4.

Quackenbush J. Computational analysis of microarray data. Nature Reviews Genetics 2001;2:418–27.

Rosamond J, Allsop A. Harnessing the power of the genome in the search for new antibiotics. Science 2000; 287:1973–6.

Roukos DH. Trastuzumab and beyond: sequencing cancer genomes and predicting molecular networks. Pharmacogenomics Journal 2011;11: 81–92.

Schadt EE. Molecular networks as sensors and drivers of common human diseases. Nature 2009;461: 218–23.

Shin JT, Fishman MC. From zebrafish to human: molecular medical models. Annual Review of Genomics and Human Genetics 2002;3:311–40.

Somogyi R. Making sense of gene-expression data. In: Pharma Informatics, A Trends Guide. Elsevier Trends in Biotechnology 1999;17 (Suppl. 1):17–24.

Velculescu VE, Zhang L, Vogelstein B, et al. Serial analysis of gene expression. Science 1995;270:484–7.

Walke DW, Han C, Shaw J, et al. In vivo drug target discovery: identifying the best targets from the genome. Current Opinion in Biotechnology 2001;12:626–31.

Wang Y. The role and regulation of urokinase-type plasminogen activator receptor gene expression in cancer invasion and metastasis. Medicinal Research Reviews 2001;21: 146–70.

Wang K, Gan L, Jeffery E, et al. Monitoring gene expression profile changes in ovarian carcinomas using cDNA microarray. Gene 1999;229:101–8.

Weatherall DJ. The new genetica and clinical practice. 3rd ed. Oxford: Oxford University Press; 1991.

Wengelnik K, Vidal V, Ancelin ML, et al. A class of potent antimalarials and their specific accumulation in infected erythrocytes. Science 2002;295:1311–4.

Whitney LW, Becker KG, Tresser NJ, et al. Analysis of gene expression in mutiple sclerosis lesions using cDNA microarrays. Annals of Neurology 1999;46:425–8.

Wishart DS, Knox, C, Guo AC, et al. DrugBank: a knowledgebase for drugs, drug actions and drug targets. Nucleic Acids Research 2008;36: D901–D906.

Zambrowicz BP, Sands AT. Knockouts model the 100 best-selling drugs – will they model the next 100? Nature Reviews. Drug Discovery 2003;2:38–51.

Zanders ED. Gene expression profiling as an aid to the identification of drug targets. Pharmacogenomics 2000;1:375–84.

Zhang L, Zhou W, Velculescu VE, et al. Gene expression profiles in normal and cancer cells. Science 1997;276: 1268–72.

Chapter | 7 |

The role of information, bioinformatics and genomics

B Robson, R McBurney

THE PHARMACEUTICAL INDUSTRY AS AN INFORMATION INDUSTRY

As outlined in earlier chapters, making drugs that can affect the symptoms or causes of diseases in safe and beneficial ways has been a substantial challenge for the pharmaceutical industry (Munos, 2009). However, there are countless examples where safe and effective biologically active molecules have been generated. The bad news is that the vast majority of these are works of nature, and to produce the examples we see today across all biological organisms, nature has run a 'trial-and-error' genetic algorithm for some 4 billion years. By contrast, during the last 100 years or so, the pharmaceutical industry has been heroically developing handfuls of successful new drugs in 10–15 year timeframes. Even then, the overwhelming majority of drug discovery and development projects fail and, recently, the productivity of the pharmaceutical industry has been conjectured to be too low to sustain its current business model (Cockburn, 2007; Garnier, 2008).

A great deal of analysis and thought is now focused on ways to improve the productivity of the drug discovery and development process (see, for example, Paul et al., 2010). While streamlining the process and rebalancing the effort and expenditures across the various phases of drug discovery and development will likely increase productivity to some extent, the fact remains that *what we need to know to optimize productivity in drug discovery and development far exceeds what we do know right now*. To improve productivity substantially, the pharmaceutical industry must increasingly become what in a looser sense it always was, an *information industry* (Robson and Baek, 2009).

Initially, the present authors leaned towards extending this idea by highlighting the pharmaceutical process as an information flow, a flow seen as a probabilistic and information theoretic network, from the computations of probabilities from genetics and other sources, to the probability that a drug will play a useful role in the marketplace. As may easily be imagined, such a description is rich, complex, and evolving (and rather formal), and the chapter was rapidly reaching the size of a book while barely scratching the surface of such a description. It must suffice to concentrate on the nodes (old and new) of that network, and largely on those nodes that represent the sources and pools of data and information that are brought together in multiple ways.

This chapter begins with general concepts about information then focuses on information about biological molecules and on its relationship to drug discovery and development. Since most drugs act by binding to and modulating the function of proteins, it is reasonable for pharmaceutical industry scientists to want to have as much information as possible about the nature and behaviour of proteins in health and disease. Proteins are vast in numbers (compared to genes), have an enormous dynamic range of abundances in tissues and body fluids, and have complex variations that underlie specific functions. At present, the available information about proteins is limited by lack of technologies capable of cost-efficiently identifying, characterizing and quantifying the protein content of body fluids and tissues. So, this chapter deals primarily with information about genes and its role in drug discovery and development.

INNOVATION DEPENDS ON INFORMATION FROM MULTIPLE SOURCES

Information from three diverse domains sparks *innovation* in drug discovery and development (http://dschool.

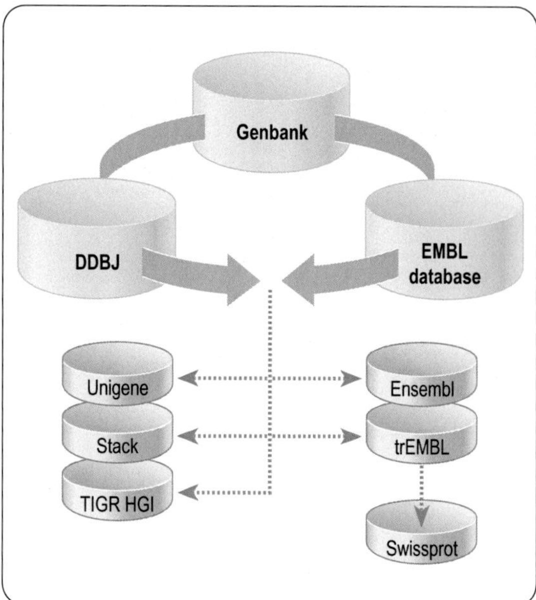

Fig. 7.1 Flow of public sequence data between major sequence repositories. Shown in blue are the components of the International Nucleotide Sequence Database Collaboration (INSDC) comprising Genbank (USA), the European Molecular Biology Laboratory (EMBL) Database (Europe) and the DNA Data Bank of Japan (DDBJ).

stanford.edu/big_picture/multidisciplinary_approach.php):

- Feasibility (Is the product technically/scientifically possible?)
- Viability (Can such a product be brought cost-effectively to the marketplace?)
- Desirability (Is there a real need for such a product?).

The viability and desirability domains include information concerning public health and medical need, physician judgment, patient viewpoints, market research, healthcare strategies, healthcare economics and intellectual property. The feasibility domain includes information about biology, chemistry, physics, statistics and mathematics. Currently, the totality of available information can be obtained from diverse, unconnected ('siloed') public or private sources, such as the brains of human beings, books, journals, patents, general literature, databases available via the Internet (see, for example, Fig. 7.1) and results (proprietary or otherwise) of studies undertaken as part of drug discovery and development. However, due to its siloed nature, discreet sets of information from only one domain are often applied, suboptimally, in isolation to particular aspects of drug discovery and development. One promising approach for optimizing the utility of available, but diverse, information across all aspects of drug discovery and development is to connect apparently disparate information sets using a common format and a collection of rules (a language) that relate elements of the content to each other. Such connections make it possible for users to access the information in any domain or set then traverse across information in multiple sets or domains in a fashion that sparks innovation. This promising approach is embodied in the Semantic Web, a vision for the connection of not just web pages but of data and information (see http://en.wikipedia.org/wiki/Semantic_Web and http://www.w3.org/2001/sw/), which is already beginning to impact the life sciences, generally, and drug discovery and development, in particular (Neumann and Quan, 2006; Stephens et al., 2006; Ruttenberg et al., 2009).

BIOINFORMATICS

The term *bioinformatics* for the creation, analysis and management of information about living organisms, and particularly nucleotide and protein sequences, was probably first coined in 1984, in the announcement of a funding programme by the European Economic Community (EC COM84 Final). The programme was in response to a memo from the White House that Europe was falling behind America and Japan in biotechnology.

The overall task of bioinformatics as it was defined in that announcement is to generate information from biological data (*bioinformation*) and to make that information accessible to humans and machines that are in need of information to advance toward the achievement of an objective. Handling all the data and information about life forms, even the currently available information on nucleotide and protein sequences, is not trivial. Overviews of established basic procedures and databases in bioinformatics, and the ability to try one's hand at them, are provided by a number of high-quality sources many of which have links to other sources, for example:

- The European Bioinformatics Institute (EMBL-EBI), which is part of the European Molecular Biology Laboratory (EMBL) (http://www.ebi.ac.uk/2can/home.html)
- The National Center for Biotechnology Information of the National Institutes of Health (http://www.ncbi.nlm.nih.gov/Tools/)
- The Biology Workbench at the University of San Diego (http://workbench.sdsc.edu/).

Rather than give a detailed account of specific tools for bioinformatics, our focus will be on the general ways by which bioinformation is generated by bioinformatics, and the principles used to analyse and interpret information.

Bioinformatics is the management and *data analytics* of bioinformation. In genetics and molecular biology applications, that includes everything from classical statistics and specialized applications of statistics or probability theory, such as the Hardy–Weinberg equilibrium law and linkage analysis, to modelling interactions between the products of gene expression and subsequent biological interpretation (for interpretation tool examples see www.ingenuity.com and www.genego.com). According to taste, one may either say that a new part of data analytics is bioinformatics, or that bioinformatics embraces most if not all of data analytics as applied to genes and proteins and the consequences of them. Here, we embrace much as bioinformatics, but also refer to the more general field of data analytics for techniques on which bioinformatics draws and will continue to borrow.

The term bioinformatics does have the merit of addressing not only the analysis but also the management of data using information technology. Interestingly, it is not always easy to distinguish data management from the processing and analysis of data. This is not least because computers often handle both. Sometimes, efficiency and insight can be gained by not segregating the two aspects of bioinformatics.

Bioinformatics as data mining and inference

Data mining includes also analysis of market, business, communications, medical, meteorological, ecological, astronomical, military and security data, but its tools have been implicit and ubiquitous in bioinformatics from the outset, even if the term 'data mining' has only fairly recently been used in that context. All the principles described below are relevant to a major portion of traditional bioinformatics. The same data mining programme used by one of the authors has been applied to both joint market trends in South America and the relationship of protein sequences to their secondary structure and immunological properties. In the broader language of data analytics, bioinformatics can be seen as having two major modes of application in the way it obtains information from data – *query* or *data mining*. In the *query* mode (directed analysis), for example, a nucleotide sequence might be used to find its occurrence in other gene sequences, thus 'pulling them from the file'. That is similar to a Google search and also somewhat analogous to testing a hypothesis in classical statistics, in that one specific question is asked and tested as to the hypothesis that it exists in the data.

In the *data mining* mode (undirected or unsupervised analysis), one is seeking to discover anything interesting in the data, such as a hidden pattern. Ultimately, finding likely (and effectively testing) hypotheses for combinations of N symbols or factors (states, events, measurements, etc.) is equivalent to making 2^N-1 queries or classical statistical tests of hypotheses. For $N = 100$, this is 10^{30}. If such an activity involves continuous variables of interest to an error of e percent (and e is usually much less than 50%) then this escalates to $(100/e)^N$. Clearly, therefore, data mining is a strategy, not a guaranteed solution, but, equally clearly, delivers a lot more than one query. Insomuch as issuing one query is simply a limiting case of the ultimate in highly constrained data mining, both modes can be referred to as data mining.

Both querying and data mining seem a far cry from *predicting* what regions of DNA are likely to be a gene, or the role a pattern of gene variants might play in disease or drug response, or the structure of a protein, and so on. As it happens, however, prediction of what regions of DNA are genes or control points, what a gene's function is, of protein secondary and tertiary structure, of segments in protein primary structure that will serve as a basis for a synthetic diagnostic or vaccine, are all longstanding examples of what we might today call data mining followed by its application to prediction. In those activities, the mining of data, as a *training set*, is used to generate probabilistic parameters often called 'rules'. These rules are preferably validated in an independent *test set*. The further step required is some process for using the validated rules to draw a conclusion based on new data or data sets, i.e. formally the process of *inference*, as a *prediction*.

An *Expert System* also uses rules and inference except the rules and their probabilities are drawn from human experts at the rate of 2–5 a day (and, by definition, are essentially anecdotal and likely biased). Computer-based data mining can generate hundreds of thousands of unbiased probabilistic rules in the order of minutes to hours (which is essentially in the spirit of evidence based medicine's *best evidence*). In the early days of bioinformatics, pursuits like predicting protein sequence, signal polypeptide sequences, immunological epitopes, DNA consensus sequences with special meaning, and so forth, were often basically like Expert Systems using rules and recipes devised by experts in the field. Most of those pursuits have now succumbed to use rules provided from computer-based mining of increasingly larger amounts of data, and those rules bear little resemblance to the original expert rules.

General principles for data mining

Data mining is usually undertaken on a *sample dataset*. Several difficulties have dogged the field. At one end of the spectrum is the counterintuitive concern of 'too much (relevant) information'. Ideally, to make use of maximum data available for testing a method and quality of the rules, it quickly became clear that one should use the *jackknife method*. For example, in predicting something about each and every accessible gene or protein in order to test a method, that gene or protein is removed from the sample data set used to generate the rules for its prediction. So for a comprehensive test of predictive power, the rules are regenerated afresh for every gene or protein in the database, or more correctly put, for the absence of each in the database. The reason is that probabilistic rules are really terms in a probabilistic or information theoretic expansion that, when brought together correctly, can predict something with close to 100% accuracy, if the gene or protein was in the set used to derive the rules. That has practical applications, but for most purposes would be 'cheating' and certainly misleading. Once the accuracy is established as acceptable, the rules are generated from all genes or proteins available, because they will typically be applied to new genes or proteins that emerge and which were not present in the data. On the other hand, once these become 'old news', they are added to the source data, and at intervals the rules are updated from it.

At the other end of the scale are the concerns of too little relevant information. For example, data may be too sparse for rules with many parameters or factors (the so-called 'curse of high dimensionality'), and this includes the case where no observations are available at all. Insight or predictions may then be incorrect because many relevant rules may need to come together to make a final pronouncement. It is rare that a single probabilistic rule will say all that needs to be said. Perhaps the greatest current concern, related to the above, is that the information obtained will only be of general utility if the sample dataset is a sufficient representation of the *entire population*. This is a key consideration in any data mining activity and likely underlies many disputes in the literature and elsewhere about the validity of the results of various studies involving data mining. To generate useful information from any such study, it is essential to pay particular attention to the design of the study and to replicate and validate the results using other sample datasets from the entire population. The term *data dredging* is often used in reference to preliminary data mining activities on sample datasets that are too small to generate results of sufficient statistical power to likely be valid but can generate hypotheses for exploration using large sample datasets.

A further concern is that sparse events in data can be particularly important precisely because they *are* sparse. What matters is not the support for a rule in terms of the amount and quality of data concerning it, but (in many approaches at least) whether the event occurred with an abundance much more, or *much less*, than expected, say on a chance basis. Negative associations are of great importance in medicine when we want to prevent something, and we want a negative relationship between a therapy and disease. The so-called *unicorn events* about observations never seen at all are hard to handle. A simple pedagogic example is the absence of pregnant males in a medical database. Whilst this particular example may only be of interest to a Martian, most complex rules that are not deducible from simpler ones (that are a kind of subset to them) might be of this type. Of particular concern is that drugs A, B, and C might work 100% used alone, and so might AB, BC, and AC, but ABC might be a useless (or, perhaps, lethal) combination. Yet, traditionally, unicorn events are not even seen to justify consideration, and in computing terms they are not even 'existentially qualified', no variables may even be created to consider them. If we do force creation of them, then the number of things to allow for because they just might be, in principle, can be astronomical.

Data mining algorithms can yield information about:

- the presence of subgroups of samples within a sample dataset that are similar on the basis of patterns of characteristics in the variables for each sample (*clustering* samples into *classes*)
- the variables that can be used (with *weightings* reflecting the importance of each variable) to classify a new sample into a specified class (*classification*)
- mathematical or logical functions that model the data (for example, *regression analysis*) or
- relationships between variables that can be used to explore the behaviour of the system of variables as a whole and to reveal which variables provide either novel (unique) or redundant information (*association* or *correlation*).

Some general principles for data mining in medical applications are exemplified in the mining of 667 000 patient records in Virginia by Mullins et al. (2006). In that study, which did not include any genomic data, three main types of data mining were used (pattern discovery, predictive analysis and association analysis). A brief description of each method follows.

Pattern discovery

Pattern discovery is a data mining technique which seeks to find a pattern, not necessarily an exact match, that occurs in a dataset more than a specified number of times k. It is itself a 'number of times', say n(A & B & C &...). Pattern discovery is not *pattern recognition*, which is the use of these results. In the pure form of the method, there is no normalization to a probability or to an association measure as for the other two data mining types discussed below. Pattern discovery is excellent at picking up complex patterns with multiple factors A, B, C, etc., that tax the next two methods. The A, B, C, etc. may be nucleotides (A, T, G, C) or amino acid residues (in IUPAC one letter code), but not necessarily contiguous, or any other variables. In practice, due to the problems typically addressed and the nature of natural gene sequences, pattern discovery for nucleotides tends to focus on runs of, say, 5–20 symbols. Moreover, the patterns found can be quantified in the same terms as either of the other two methods below. However, if one takes this route alone, important relationships are missed. It is easy to see that this technique cannot pick up a pattern occurring less than k times, and $k = 1$ makes no sense (everything is a pattern). It must also miss alerting to patterns that statistically ought to occur but do not, i.e. the so-called unicorn events. Pattern discovery is an excellent example of an application that does have an analogue at operating system level, the use of the *regular expression* for partial pattern matching (http://en.wikipedia.org/wiki/Regular_expression), but it is most efficiently done by an algorithm in a domain-specific application (the domain in this case is fairly broad, however, since it has many other applications, not just in bioinformatics, proteomics, and biology generally). An efficient pattern discovery algorithm developed by IBM is available as Teireisis (http://www.ncbi.nlm.nih.gov/pmc/articles/PMC169027/).

Predictive analysis

Predictive analysis encompasses a variety of techniques from statistics and game theory that analyse current and historical facts to predict future events (http://en.wikipedia.org/wiki/Predictive_analytics). 'Predictive analysis' appears to be the term most frequently used for the part of data mining that involves normalizing n(A & B & C) to conditional probabilities, e.g.

$$P(A \mid B \& C) = n(A \& B \& C) / n(B \& C) \quad (1)$$

In usual practice, predictive analysis tends to focus on 2–3 symbols or factors. This approach is an excellent form for inference of the type that uses 'If B & C then A', but takes no account of the fact that A could occur by chance anyway. In practice, predictive analysis usually rests heavily on the commonest idea of *support*, i.e. if the pattern is not seen a significant number of times, the conditional probability of it is not a good estimate. So again, it will not detect important negative associations and unicorn events. Recently, this approach has probably been the most popular kind of data mining for the general business domain.

Association analysis

Association analysis is often formulated in log form as Fano's mutual information, e.g.

$$I(A; B \& C) = \log_e\{P(A \& B \& C)/[P(A)P(B \& C)]\} \quad (2)$$

(Robson, 2003, 2004, 2005, 2008; Robson and Mushlin, 2004; Robson and Vaithiligam, 2010). Clearly it does take account of the occurrence of A. This opens up the full power of information theory, of instinctive interest to the pharmaceutical industry as an information industry, and of course to other mutual information measures such as:

$$I(A; B \mid C) = \log_e\{P(A \& B \& C)/[P(A \& C)P(B \& C)]\} \quad (3)$$

and

$$I(A; B; C) = \log_e\{P(A \& B \& C)/[P(A)P(B)P(C)]\} \quad (4)$$

The last *atomic form* is of interest since other measures can be calculated from it (see below). Clearly it can also be calculated from the conditional probabilities of predictive analysis. To show relationship with other fields such as evidence based medicine and epidemiology,

$$I(A:\sim A; B) = I(A; B) - I(\sim A; B) \quad (5)$$

where ~A is a negative of complementary state or event such that

$$P(\sim A) = 1 - P(A) \quad (6)$$

is familiar as log *predictive odds*, while

$$I(A:\sim A; B) - I(A:\sim A; \sim B) \quad (7)$$

is the log *odds ratio*.

The association analysis approach handles positive, zero, and negative associations including treatment sparse joint events. To that end, it may use the more general definition of information in terms of *zeta functions*, ζ. Unlike predictive analysis, the approach used in this way returns *expected information*, basically building into the final value the idea of support. In the Virginia study, using the above 'zeta approach', one could detect patterns of 2–7 symbols or factors, the limit being the sparseness of data for many such. As data increase, I(males; tall) = ζ(1, observed[males, tall]) − ζ(1, expected[males, tall]) will rapidly approach $\log_e$ (observed[males, tall]) − $\log_e$ (expected[males, tall]), but unlike log ratios, ζ(1, observed[males, pregnant]) − ζ(1, expected[males, pregnant]) works appropriately with the data for the terms that are very small or zero. To handle unicorn events still requires variables to be created in the programme, but the overall approach is more natural.

The above seem to miss out various forms of data mining such as *time series analysis* and *clustering analysis*, although ultimately these can be expressed in the above terms. What seems to require an additional comment is *correlation*. While biostatistics courses often use *association* and *correlation* synonymously, data miners do not. Association relates to the extent to the number of times things are observed together more, or less, than on a chance basis in a 'presence or absence' fashion (such as the association between a categorical SNP genotype and a categorical phenotype). This is reminiscent of the classical chi square test, but revealing the individual contributions to non-randomness within the data grid (as well as the positive or negative nature of the association). In contrast, correlation relates to trends in values of potentially continuous variables (independence between the variances), classically exemplified by use of Pearson's correlation. Correlation is important in gene expression analysis, in proteomics and in metabolomics, since a gene transcript (mRNA) or a protein or a small molecule metabolite, in general, has a level of abundance in any sample rather than a quantized presence/absence. Despite the apparent differences, however, the implied comparison of covariance with what is expected on independent, i.e. chance, basis is essentially the same general idea as for association. Hence results can be expressed in mutual information format, based on a kind of fuzzy logic reasoning (Robson and Mushlin, 2004).

Much of the above may not seem like bioinformatics, but only because the jargon is different. That this 'barrier' is progressively coming down is important, as each discipline has valuable techniques less well known in the other. Where they do seem to be bioinformatics it is essentially due to the fact that they come packaged in distinct suites of applications targeted at bioinformatics users, and where they do not seem to be bioinformatics, they do not come simply packaged for bioinformatics users.

GENOMICS

The genome and its offspring '-omes'

In contrast to *bioinformatics*, the term *genome* is much older, first believed to be used in 1920 by Professor Hans Winkler at the University of Hamburg, as describing the world or system within the discipline of biology and within each cell of an organism that addresses the inherited executable information. The word *genome* (Gk: γίνομαι) means *I become, I am born, to come into being*, and the Oxford English Dictionary gives its aetiology as being from ***gene*** and *chromo**some***. This aetiology may not be entirely correct.

In this chapter, *genomes* of organisms are in computer science jargon the 'primary objects' on which bioinformatics 'acts'. Their daughter molecular objects, such as the corresponding *transcriptomes, proteomes* and *metabolomes*, should indeed be considered in their own right but may also be seen as subsets or derivatives of the genome concept. The remainder of this chapter is largely devoted to genomic information and its use in drug discovery and development.

While the term genome has recently spawned many offspring '-omes' relating to the disciplines that address various matters downstream from inherited information in DNA, e.g. the *proteome*, these popular *-ome* words have an even earlier origin in the 20th century (e.g. *biome* and *rhizome*). Adding the plural '-ics' suffix seems recent. The use of 'omics' as a suffix is more like an analogue of the earlier '-netics' and '-onics' in engineering. The current rising hierarchy of '-omes' is shown in Table 7.1, and these and others are discussed by Robson and Baek (2009). There are constant additions to the '-omes'.

The new '-omes' are not as simple as a genome. For one thing, there is typically no convenient common file format or coding scheme for them comparable with the linear DNA and protein sequence format provided by nature. Whereas the genome contains a static compilation of the sequence of the four DNA bases, the subject matters of the other '-omes' are dynamic and much more complex, including the interactions with each other and the surrounding ecosystem. It is these shifting, adapting pools of cellular components that determine health and pathology. Each of them as a discipline is currently a 'mini' (or, perhaps more correctly, 'maxi') genome project, albeit

Table 7.1 Gene to function is paved with '-omes'

Commonly used terms		
Genome	Full complement of genetic information (i.e. DNA sequence, including coding and non-coding regions)	Static
Transcriptome	Population of mRNA molecules in a cell under defined conditions at a given time	Dynamic
Proteome	Either: the complement of proteins (including post-translational modifications) encoded by the genome	Static
	or: the set of proteins and their post-translational modifications expressed in a cell or tissue under defined conditions at a specific time (also sometimes referred to as the translatome)	Dynamic
Terms occasionally encountered (to be interpreted with caution)		
Secretome	Population of secreted proteins produced by a cell	Dynamic
Metabolome	Small molecule content of a cell	Dynamic
Interactome	Grouping of interactions between proteins in a cell	Dynamic
Glycome	Population of carbohydrate molecules in a cell	Dynamic
Foldome	Population of gene products classified by tertiary structure	Dynamic
Phenome	Population of observable phenotypes describing variations of form and function in a given species	Dynamic

with ground rules that are much less well defined. Some people have worried that '-omics' will prove to be a spiral of knowing less and less about more and more. *Systems biology* seeks to integrate the '-omics' and simulate the detailed molecular and macroscopic processes under the constraint of as much real-world data as possible (van der Greef and McBurney, 2005; van der Greef et al., 2007).

For the purposes of this chapter, we follow the United States Food and Drug Administration (FDA) and European Medicines Evaluation Agency (EMEA) agreed definition of 'genomics' as captured in the definition of a 'genomic biomarker', which is defined as: *A measurable DNA and/or RNA characteristic that is an indicator of normal biologic processes, pathogenic processes, and/or response to therapeutic or other interventions* (see http://www.fda.gov/downloads/Drugs/GuidanceComplianceRegulatoryInformation/Guidances/ucm073162.pdf). A genomic biomarker can consist of one or more deoxyribonucleic acid (DNA) and/or ribonucleic acid (RNA) characteristics.

DNA characteristics include, but are not limited to:

- Single nucleotide polymorphisms (SNPs);
- Variability of short sequence repeats
- Haplotypes
- DNA modifications
- Deletions or insertions of (a) single nucleotide(s)
- Copy number variations
- Cytogenetic rearrangements, e.g., translocations, duplications, deletions, or inversions.

RNA characteristics include, but are not limited to:

- RNA sequences
- RNA expression levels
- RNA processing, e.g. splicing and editing
- MicroRNA levels.

The definition of a genomic biomarker does not include the measurement and characterization of proteins or small molecule metabolites and, therefore, to limit the scope of this chapter, the roles of proteomics and metabolomics in drug discovery and development will not be discussed.

It remains that the genome currently rules in the sense of being the basic instruction set from which various subsets of gene products are derived (Greenbaum et al., 2001), and hence largely responsible for the manifestation of all the '-omes', albeit the details of that manifestation are contingent upon the environment of the cell and organism (see below). The coded information is a strength in terms of simplicity, and as an essentially invariant feature of a patient, while all else on the lifelong 'health record' may change. And whereas the downstream '-omes' seen can have a huge role in interpreting the genome, inspection of features in the genome alone will often inform what is not possible, or likely to be a malfunction. Although it will ultimately be important to know all of the possible gene products that a species is capable of producing and to understand all the mechanistic details concerning the behaviour of an organism, understanding which ones are altered in disease or play a role in drug responses is most relevant to drug discovery and development. Furthermore, while detailed mechanisms may never be fully understood, physicians can certainly make use of validated relationships between genome features and the efficacy or safety outcomes of various treatments to tailor treatment strategies for individual patients, often referred to as *personalized medicine*.

A few genome details

A great deal of technology had to be invented to accomplish the sequencing of genomes (Cantor and Smith, 1999). Recent years have seen dramatic progress. By the middle of 2010, the sequences of the genomes of more than 2400 organisms were either complete (770 prokaryotes; 37 eukaryotes), in draft assembly (568 prokaryotes; 240 eukaryotes) or in progress (551 prokaryotes; 266 eukaryotes) (http://www.ncbi.nlm.nih.gov/sites/genome). Most sequenced genomes are for bacteria, but the eukaryote genomes sequenced include *Homo sapiens* (Lander et al., 2001; Venter et al., 2001) and a wide variety of animals that play a role in the discovery of disease mechanisms or in drug discovery and development, such as the fruit fly (*Drosophila simulans* (*melanogaster*)), flatworm (*Caenorhabditis elegans*), guinea pig (*Cavia porcellus*), mouse (*Mus musculus*), rat (*Rattus norvegicus*), dog (*Canis lupus*) and monkey (*Macaca mulatta*). The massive amount of information generated in the various genome projects and gene mapping studies has to be stored, disseminated and analysed electronically, relying heavily on bioinformatics software systems and the Internet (see, for example, Fig. 7.2). Here we may note that defining the nucleotide sequence is only the starting point of the genomic approach.

While the percentage of human DNA spanned by genes is 25.5–37.8%, only about 2% of the human genome is nucleotide sequence that actually codes for protein, or indeed for structural or catalytic RNA. The other 98%, initially considered to be 'junk' DNA, may indeed include evolution's junk, i.e. fossil relics of evolution or, more kindly put, non-functional genes that might serve as the basis of evolution in the longer term. However, information about this 'junk' DNA is not uninteresting or useless. Even truly non-functional DNA may have significant medical and forensic value. Significant human individual differences represented by *genomic biomarkers* are an exploding opportunity for improving healthcare and transforming the activities of the pharmaceutical industry (Svinte et al., 2007), but these genomic biomarkers frequently are found not to lie in protein coding regions. They have often travelled with the genes about which they carry information, in the course of the migrations of human prehistory and history. The so-called 'junk', including the introns discussed below and *control segments*, is involved in chromatin structure, recombination templating, and is

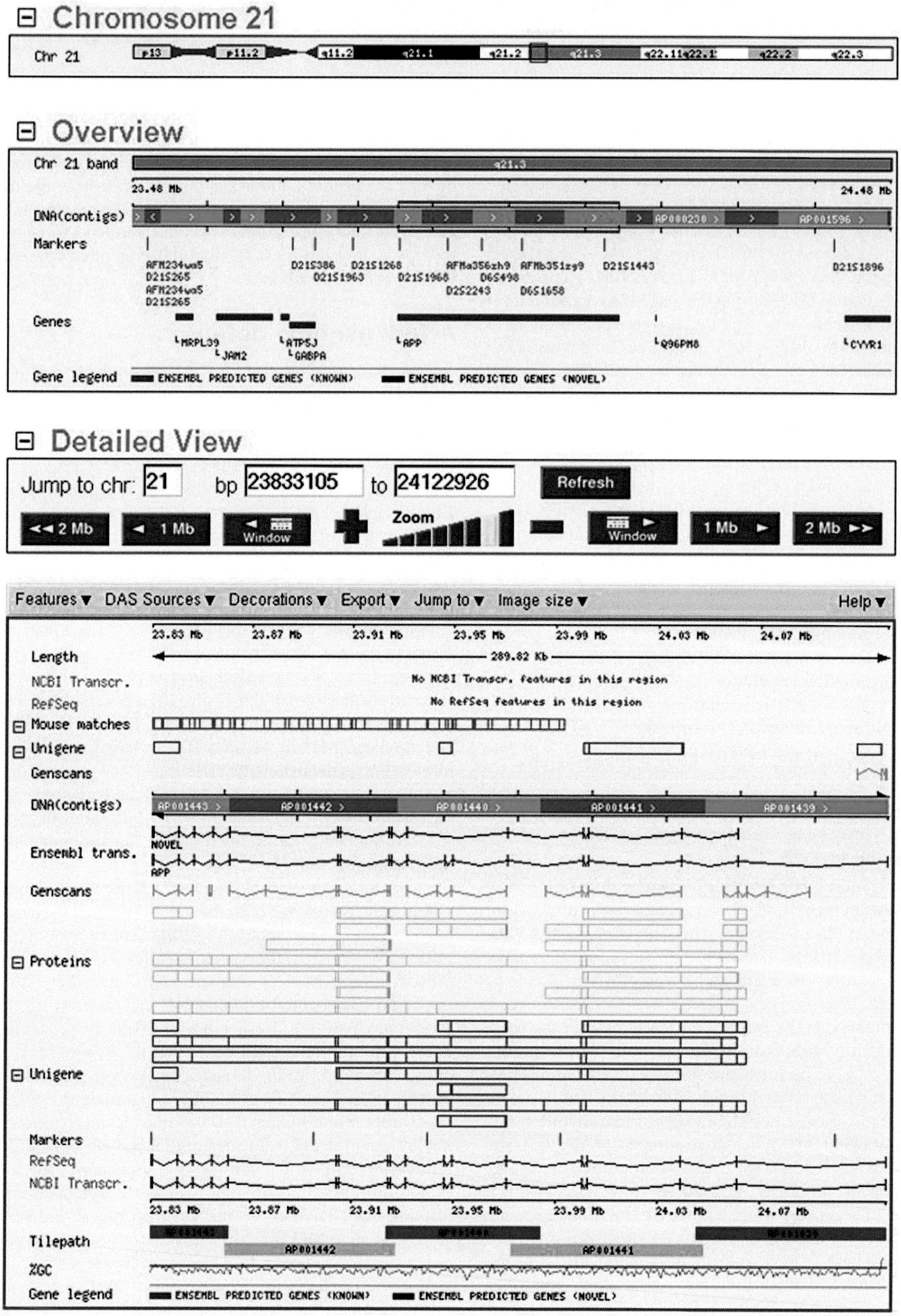

Chromosome 21

Overview

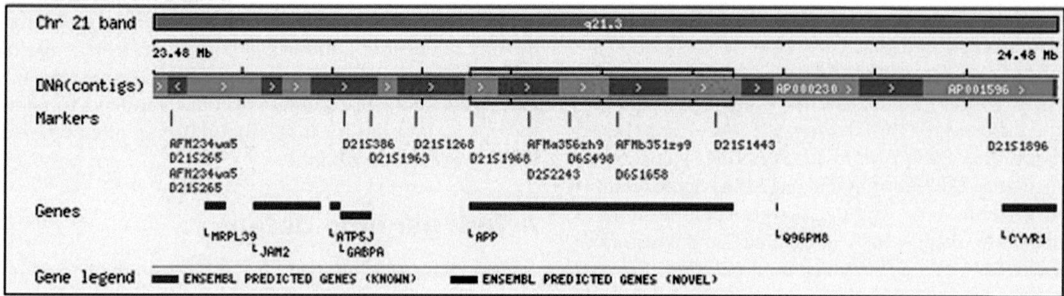

Detailed View

Fig. 7.2 Screenshot from the Ensembl website. Shown is a chromosomal overview and a regional view of chromosome 21 surrounding the gene APP, the Alzheimer's disease amyloid A4 protein precursor. In the detailed view the precise exon–intron structure of the gene is shown, including sequence homology matches to a variety of databases or de novo gene predictions. The viewer is highly customizable and users can easily navigate along the genomic axis.

Reproduced with kind permission of European Bioinformatics Institute and Wellcome Trust Sanger Institute.

now seen as representing hotspots for sponsoring heterogeneity (see comment on epigenetics below).

There was, for a time, a surprising reduction in the promised amount of what constitutes really interesting genomic information in humans. Although identifying genes within the genome sequence is not straightforward, earlier estimates of about 100 000 genes in the human genome based on the variety of proteins produced came down, rather startlingly, to about 35 000 when the genome was determined, and later (International Human Genome Sequencing Consortium, 2004) to about 25 000. A clue as to how this can be so was already well known in the late 1970s and 1980s – that genes in complex organisms are suspiciously much larger than would be expected from the number of amino acid residues in the proteins for which they code. It was found that only the regions of a gene called exons actually code for proteins, and the intervening introns are removed by RNA splicing at the messenger RNA (mRNA) level. The average human gene has some 30 000 nucleotides and 7 exons. The largest known human gene, for titin, has 363 introns.

Genome variability and individual differences

Personalized medicine in the clinical setting is an emerging field. Human individuality underpins susceptibility to disease and response to treatment. Fundamental to human individuality is the content of each individual's genome. All humans have 99.5–99.9% of nucleotide sequence identity in their genomes, depending upon whether one takes into account just SNPs or all forms of genetic variation (see http://www.genome.gov/19016904 and also Freeman et al., 2006). However, the 0.1% difference in SNPs represents 6 million bases in a genome of 6 billion bases – plenty of scope for individuality. Even monozygotic twins can develop individuality at the genome (epigenome) level in individual body cells or tissues through 'life experience'. Understanding human individuality at the genomic level has the potential to enable great advances in drug discovery and development. *Pharmacogenomics* addresses the matter of whether the same drug will cure, do little, or harm according to the unique genomics of the patient.

The epigenome

In addition to the linear sequence code of DNA that contains the information necessary to generate RNA and, ultimately, the amino acid sequences of proteins, there is an additional level of information in the DNA structure in the form of the complex nucleoprotein entity *chromatin*. Genetic information is encoded not only by the linear sequence of DNA nucleotides but by modifications of chromatin structure which influence gene expression. *Epigenetics* as a field of study is defined as '... the study of changes in gene function ... that do not entail a change in DNA sequence' (Wu and Morris, 2001). The word was coined by Conrad Waddington in 1939 (Waddington, 1939) in recognition of relationship between genetics and developmental biology and of the sum of all mechanisms necessary for the unfolding of the programme for development of an organism.

The modifications of chromatin structure that can influence gene expression comprise histone variants, post-translational modifications of amino acids on the amino-terminal tail of histones, and covalent modifications of DNA bases – most notably methylation of cytosine bases at CpG sequences. CpG-rich regions are not evenly distributed in the genome, but are concentrated in the promoter regions and first exons of certain genes (Larsen et al., 1992). If DNA is methylated, the methyl groups protrude from the cytosine nucleotides into the major groove of the DNA and inhibit the binding of transcription factors that promote gene expression (Hark et al., 2000). Changes in DNA methylation can explain the fact that genes switch on or off during development and the pattern of methylation is heritable (first proposed by Holliday and Pugh, 1975). It has been shown that DNA methylation can be influenced by external stressors, environmental toxins, and aging (Dolinoy et al., 2007; Hanson and Gluckman, 2008), providing a key link between the environment and life experience and the regulation of gene expression in specific cell types.

A key finding in epigenetics was reported by Fraga et al. in 2005. In a large cohort of monozygotic twins, DNA methylation was found to increase over time within different tissues and cell types. Importantly, monozygotic twins were found to be indistinguishable in terms of DNA methylation early in life but were found to exhibit substantial differences in DNA methylation with advancing age. The authors of the landmark paper stated that 'distinct profiles of DNA methylation and histone acetylation patterns that among different tissues arise during the lifetime of monozygotic twins may contribute to the explanation of some of their phenotypic discordances and underlie their differential frequency/onset of common disease.'

The transcriptome

The fact that the cell must cut out the introns from mRNA and splice together the ends of the remaining exons is the 'loophole' that allows somatic diversity of proteins, because the RNA coding for exons can be spliced back together in different ways. Alternative splicing might therefore reasonably be called recombinant splicing, though that term offers some confusion with the term 'recombinant' as used in classical genetics. That some 100 000 genes were expected on the basis of protein diversity and about 25 000 are found does not mean that the diversity so generated is simply a matter of about four proteins made from each gene on average. Recent work has shown

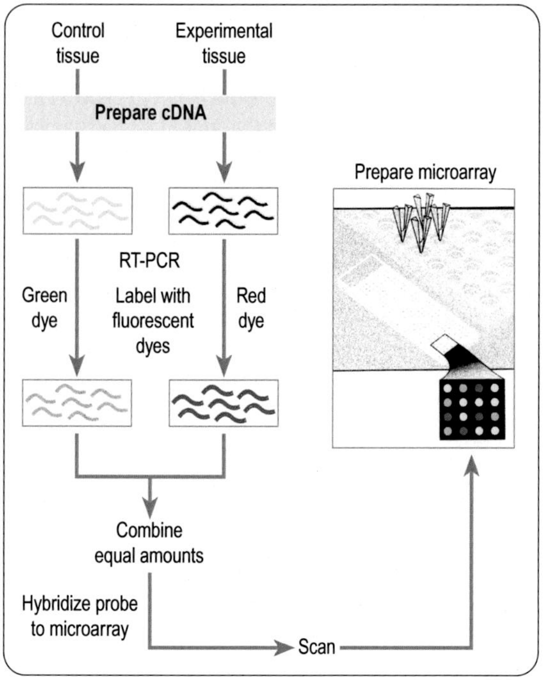

Fig. 7.3 Microarray experiment: technology for analysing mRNA expression.

that alternative splicing can be associated with thousands of important signals.

The above is one aspect of the transcriptome, i.e. the world of RNA produced from DNA. Whereas one may defer discussion of other 'omes' (e.g. of proteins, except as the 'ultimate' purpose of many genes), the above exemplifies that one makes little further progress at this stage by ignoring the *transcriptome*. A primary technology for measuring differences in mRNA levels between tissue samples is the microarray, illustrated in Figs. 7.3 & 7.4.

The RNA world now intermediates between the genome and the proteome, including carrying transcripts of DNA in order to determine the amino acid sequences of proteins, but is believed to be the more ancient genomic world before DNA developed as a sophisticated central archive. Not least, since unlike a protein any RNA is a direct copy of regions of DNA (except for U replacing T), much of an account of the transcriptome looks like and involves an account of the genome, and *vice versa*.

To be certain, the transcriptome does go beyond that. The RNA produced by DNA can perform many complex roles, of which mRNA and its alternative splicing provide just one example. Many of the sites for producing these RNAs lie not in introns but outside the span of a gene, i.e. in the intergenic regions. Like elucidation of the exon/intron structure within genes, intergenic regions are similarly yielding to more detailed analysis. The longest known intergenic length is about 3 million nucleotides. While 3% of DNA is short repeats and 5% is duplicated large pieces, 45% of intergenic DNA comprises four classes of 'parasitic elements' arising from reverse transcription. In fact it may be that this DNA is 'a boiling foam' of RNA transcription and reverse transcription. It now appears that both repeats and boiling foam alike appear to harbour many control features.

At first, the fact that organisms such as most bacteria have 75–85% of coding sequences, and that even the puffer fish has little intergenic DNA and few repeats, may bring into question the idea that the intergenic DNA and its transcriptome can be important. However, there is evidently a significant difference in sophistication between humans and such organisms. This thinking has now altered somewhat the original use of the term genome. The *human genome* now refers to all nuclear DNA (and ideally mitochondrial DNA as well). That is, the word has been increasingly interpreted as 'the full complement of genetic information' coding for proteins or not. The implication is that 'genome' is all DNA, including that which does *not appear* to carry biological information, on the basis of the growing suspicion that it does. As it happens, the term 'coding' even traditionally sometimes included genes that code for tRNA and rRNA to provide the RNA-based protein-synthesizing machinery, since these are long known. The key difference may therefore mainly lie in departure from the older idea that RNA serves universal *housekeeping features* of the cell as 'a given' that do not reflect the *variety* of cell structure and function, and *differentiation*. That, in contrast, much RNA serves *contingency* functions relating to the embryonic development of organisms is discussed below.

There are still many unidentified functionalities of RNA coding regions in the 'junk DNA', but one that is very topical and beginning to be understood is microRNA (or miRNA). miRNAs are short lengths of RNA, just some 20–25 nucleotides, which may base pair with RNA and in some cases DNA – possibly to stop it binding and competing with its own production, but certainly to enable control process that hold the miRNAs in check.

The maturation of miRNAs is quite complicated. Two complementary regions in the immature and much larger miRNA associate to form a hairpin, and a nuclear enzyme *Drosha* cleaves at the base of the hairpin. The enzyme *Dicer* then extracts the mature miRNA from its larger parent. A typical known function of a mature miRNA is as an antisense inhibitor, i.e. binding messenger mRNA, and then initiating its degradation, so that no protein molecule can be made from the mRNA. Note that in the above, one could think largely of recognition regions in the proto-miRNA transcript as simply mapping to patterns of nucleotides in DNA. But it would be impossible to meaningfully discuss, or at least not be insightful, without consideration of the biochemical processes downstream of the first transcription step.

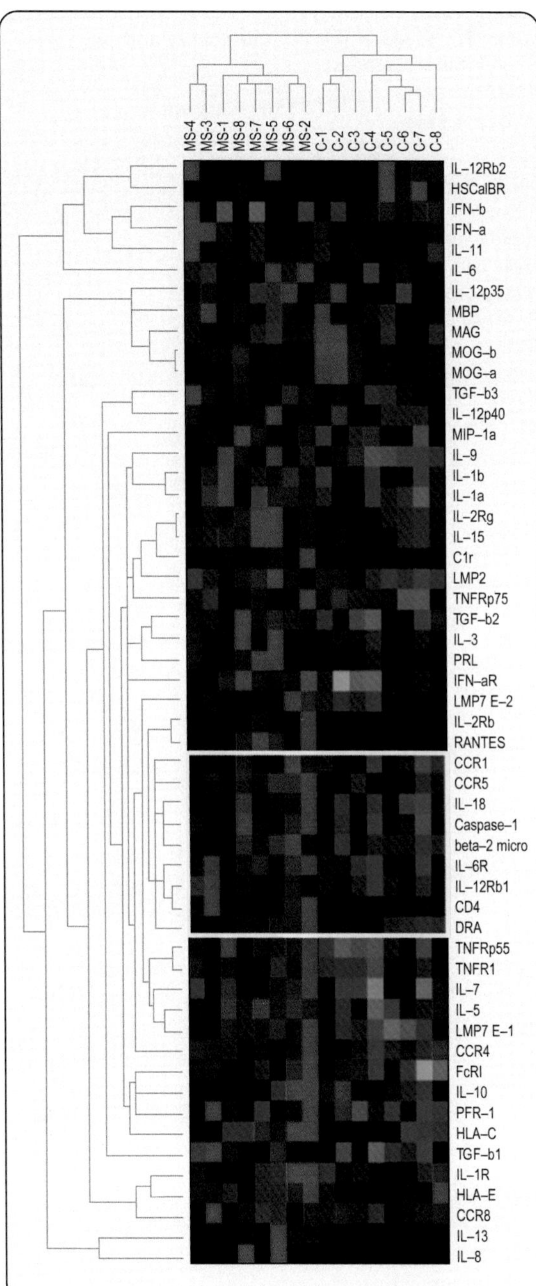

Fig. 7.4 Cluster analysis of gene expression experiment. Expression levels of 54 genes (listed on right) in eight control and eight multiple sclerosis brain samples (listed above). Relative expression levels are indicated in shades of red for high values and green for low values. A computer algorithm was used to calculate similarity between the expression pattern of each gene for all subjects, and the expression pattern for each subject for all genes, and to display the results as a dendrogram. The top dendrogram shows that MS and control samples are clearly distinguishable, the intragroup distance being much greater than the intersample difference within each group. The left-hand dendrogram shows the grouping of genes into clusters that behave similarly. A group of genes with highly similar expression patterns is outlined in yellow.

Adapted, with permission, from Baranzini et al., 2000.

In defence of the genome

The complexities contained in the discussion above challenge the authority of the genome as 'king'. At present, the genome rules much because of our ignorance. DNA is potentially no more, and no less, important than the magnetic tapes, floppy disks, CDs, and Internet downloads that we feed into our computers, indispensible and primary, but cold and lifeless without all the rest. While genomic data now represent a huge amount of information that is relevant to the pharmaceutical industry, it cannot be denied that complete pharmaceutical utility lies in understanding how the information in DNA, including interaction between many genes and gene products, translates into function at the organism level. Not least, drugs influence that translation process. The rise of systems biology reflects this awareness of the organism as a dynamic system dwelling in three dimensions of space and one of time.

The problem is that the child '-omes' are still immature and rather weak. We are assembling a very rich lexicon from the genomes, but are left with the questions of when, how, and why, the patterns of life, molecular and macroscopic, unfold. And one may say *fold* too, since the folding of proteins, the key step at which linear information in DNA becomes three-dimensional biology, remains largely unsolved. Perhaps for all such reasons, the earlier pharmaceutical industry hopes for genomics and bioinformatics (Li and Robson, 2000) have not yet been realized (Drews, 2003).

But low-hanging fruits have been picked to keep the pharmaceutical industry buoyant. Biotechnology companies drink of biological knowledge much closer to the genome than pharmaceutical companies usually do, and they largely enabled the methodologies that made the Human Genome Project a reality. Thus, they currently position themselves as leaders in managing and tapping this vast new information resource. Companies specializing in genomic technology, bioinformatics, and related fields were the fastest expanding sector of the biotechnology industry during the 1990s, aspiring to lead the pharmaceutical industry into an era of rapid identification and exploitation of novel targets (Chandra and Caldwell, 2003).

Not the least because the biotechnology industry has provided proof of concept, there is still consensus that the Human Genome Project will be worth *to the pharmaceutical industry* the billions of dollars and millions of man-hours that nations have invested. But it still remains unclear as to exactly how all the available and future information can be used cost-effectively to optimize drug discovery and development.

So just how prominent should genome-based strategies be, right now, in the research portfolio of pharmaceutical companies, and what should those strategies be? The principle of using genomic information as the starting point for identifying novel drug targets was described in Chapter 6. Following is an overview of the ways in which genomic information can, or might, impact almost every aspect of the drug discovery and development process.

Genomic information in drug discovery and development

Drug discovery and development is mankind's most complicated engineering process, integrating a wide variety of scientific and business activities, some of which are presented in Table 7.2.

Table 7.2 Steps in the drug discovery and development process

Process step
Understanding human disease intrinsic mechanisms
Understanding the biology of infectious agents
Identifying potential drug targets
Validating drug targets
Selecting targets for assay development
Assay development
Discovering hits
Hits to leads
Preclinical pharmacokinetics
Preclinical efficacy pharmacology
Preclinical safety pharmacology
Preclinical toxicology
Phase 0 clinical studies for low dose agents (e.g. molecular imaging)
Phase I clinical studies – pharmacokinetics
Phase I clinical studies – safety
Phase II clinical studies – pharmacokinetics
Phase II clinical studies – efficacy
Phase II clinical studies – safety
Phase III clinical studies – efficacy
Phase III clinical studies – safety
Phase IV clinical studies – efficacy
Phase IV clinical studies – safety
Drug repurposing – additional/alternate uses
Drug rescue

With regard to the relevance of genomic information in the drug discovery and development process, a key consideration is how best (cost-effectively) to use the information that underpins human individuality to improve the process such that:

- Diseases are characterized, or defined, by molecular means rather than by symptoms – a key advance since pharmaceutical scientists make drug candidate molecules which interact with other molecules not with symptoms
- Diseases are detected by molecular means earlier than currently possible, at a time when the underlying pathologies are reversible
- Subgroups of patients with similar molecular characteristics can be identified within the larger group of patients with similar symptoms, enabling clinical trials to be focused on those subgroups of patients most likely to benefit from a particular pharmacological approach
- The best drug targets are selected for specific diseases or subgroups of patients
- Individual human variation in drug exposure or drug response in terms of efficacy or side effects can be anticipated or explained in the drug discovery

and development process, with the resulting reduction in the frequency of clinical trials that fail because of unanticipated 'responder versus non-responder' treatment outcomes and overall increase in productivity of drug discovery and development.

Following are comments on the impact that genomics and genomic information can, or will, have on some of the steps in Table 7.2.

Understanding human disease intrinsic mechanisms

Many common human diseases are thought to result from the interaction of genetic risk profiles with life style and environmental risk factors. Over the past few decades, large scale studies of healthy humans and human suffering from diseases have associated specific gene variants with diseases. In many cases, these studies have revealed only relatively weak associations between many individual gene variants and diseases (Robinson, 2010). To date, this area of investigation has not returned the immediate benefit hoped for, and perhaps 'hyped for', by the genomic community. Nevertheless, insights have been gained into intrinsic biochemical mechanisms underlying certain diseases.

Insight into the biochemical mechanisms of common diseases has definitely been gained from the study of inherited monogenic diseases in special families (Peltonen et al., 2006). In these cases, the association between the gene variant and disease phenotype is very strong, although the application of the information to common diseases must be undertaken with caution.

Understanding the biology of infectious agents

The availability of complete genome sequences for many infectious agents has provided a great deal of insight into their biology (Pucci, 2007). Furthermore, such genetic information has also revealed the mutations in the genetic material of these organisms that are responsible for drug resistance (Kidgell and Winzeler, 2006) – of great interest to those involved in the discovery of new drugs to treat major infections. There is a strong interplay with the human genome, especially the HLA genes, which determine whether the T cell system will recognize certain features of proteins expressed by pathogens.

Identifying potential drug targets

Studies of the association of gene variants with the phenotypes of common diseases have revealed, in some cases, hundreds of gene variants that can predispose humans to certain diseases. When the proteins coded for by the genes associated with a specific disease are mapped onto known biochemical pathways (see, for example, www.ingenuity.com or www.genego.com), it is sometimes possible to gain an overall picture of likely disease mechanisms and to identify and prioritize potential drug targets for the disease (see Chapter 6).

Validating drug targets

Transgenic animals, in which the gene coding for the drug target protein can be knocked out or its expression down-regulated, can provide validation for the pharmacological effect of an inhibitor drug prior to availability of any candidate drug molecules (Sacca et al., 2010).

Assay development for selected drug targets

An analysis of variation in the gene coding for the drug target across a diverse human population can identify potential drug response variability in patients (Sadee et al., 2001; Niu et al., 2010; Zhang et al., 2010). For example, at SNP locations, the relative frequencies of occurrence of each of the genotypes (for example, AA, AG or GG) can provide information on likely differences in the abundance or structure of the drug target across the human population. Different protein isoforms with even slightly different structures could be associated with altered drug binding or activation/inhibition of downstream biochemical mechanisms. To avoid the discovery of drug candidates which interact effectively with only one isoform of the protein drug target or, alternatively, to focus on discovering such drug candidates, multiple assays based on different protein isoforms expressed from variants of each drug target gene could be established. These parallel assays could be used for screening chemical libraries to select hits which were selective for one isoform of the drug target protein, for enabling *personalized medicine*, or were able to interact effectively with more than one isoform, for enabling *population-focused medicine*.

Phase 0 clinical studies – understanding from compounds in low concentration

This relatively recent term relates to trials which are safe because they need such low doses of a new chemical entity being tested. Usually this applies to testing the very low concentrations of radioactively labelled compounds for molecular imaging; concentrations still are sufficient to see how they travel, where they go, where they accumulate, and how they are metabolized. A compound can be labelled at several points to track its components and derivatives formed in metabolism. It is inevitable that many differences in transport and metabolism will occur in individuals, so genomics will play a strong supporting role. It is likely that these kinds of trial will increasingly frequently be applied not just to develop a research agent, but to gather data for the compound to be used in the following trials.

Phase I clinical studies – pharmacokinetics and safety

Preclinical drug metabolism studies conducted on drug candidates in line with the guidance provided by the US FDA (see http://www.fda.gov/downloads/Drugs/GuidanceComplianceRegulatoryInformation/Guidances/ucm072101.pdf) can provide a wealth of information on the likely routes of metabolism of the drug, the enzymes and transporters involved in the metabolism, and the drug metabolites generated. Enzymes of particular interest are the cytochromes P450 (CYPs) which introduce a polar functional group into the parent molecule in the first phase of biotransformation of a drug.

An analysis of the genotypes of Phase I human subjects with respect to drug metabolizing enzymes can provide explanations for unusual pharmacokinetics and even adverse drug effects in certain subjects (Crettol et al., 2010). In particular, subjects with a CYP2D6 gene variant associated with lower than normal enzyme expression or activity (referred to as 'poor metabolizers') might have an exaggerated response to a standard dose of the drug. In those subjects, drug exposure might reach toxic levels and trigger adverse effects. On the other hand, subjects with a different CYP2D6 variant, associated with higher than normal enzyme expression or activity (referred to as 'rapid metabolizers' or 'ultra rapid metabolizers') might not exhibit any drug effects whatsoever. Clearly, information concerning each individual's genotype, with respect to drug metabolizing enzymes, in concert with information about the routes of metabolism of a drug candidate, can be used to interpret the response to drug dosing in Phase I studies but, more comprehensively, can potentially be used to optimize the probability of success for the development of the drug and even the strategies for using an approved drug in medical practice.

Phase II and III clinical studies – efficacy and safety

In clinical studies to determine the efficacy and safety of drug candidates in patients, it is important to recognize and take steps to deal with the likelihood that the different genotypes across the clinical trial population could influence overall trial outcome. A not uncommon feature of clinical trials is that, with respect to treatment outcome (efficacy or safety), patients fall into two broad groups – 'responders' and 'non-responders'. The balance between these two groups of patients can have a profound effect on the overall results of a trial. While variants in the genes encoding drug metabolizing enzymes might explain some such results, as mentioned above, other genetic variations across the population could also play a role in diverse responses to drug treatment in a clinical trial population. For example, drug treatment response could be altered in patients with variants in individual genes encoding the drug receptors or with variants in individual genes encoding associated signalling proteins or with patterns of variants in the genes encoding multiple proteins in relevant biochemical signalling pathways.

At present there are relatively few clear examples of the influence of genomic variation on clinical trial outcome (see http://www.fda.gov/Drugs/ScienceResearch/ResearchAreas/Pharmacogenetics/ucm083378.htm). Nevertheless, this area of investigation has a substantial place in drug discovery and development strategies in the future. All clinical studies should now incorporate DNA collection from every subject and patient. The costs of whole genome analysis are constantly diminishing and bioinformatic methods for data mining to discover associations between genomic variables and treatment–response variables are continually improving.

A research effort undertaken in Phase I and Phase II clinical studies to discover information about genetic variants which influence the response to a drug candidate can contribute substantially to the planning for pivotal Phase III trials and the interpretation of the results of those trials, enhancing the overall prospects for successful completion of the development programme for a drug candidate. More information on clinical trials can be found later in the book.

Genomic information and drug regulatory authorities

Successful drug discovery and development culminates in the approval for marketing of a product containing the drug. Approval for marketing in a specific country or region is based on a review by the appropriate drug regulatory authority of a substantial amount of information submitted to the regulatory authority by the sponsor (e.g. pharmaceutical company) – on manufacturing, efficacy and safety of the product.

How has the growing availability of vast amounts of genomic information affected the drug approval process? What changes are taking place at the regulatory authorities? What new types of information do pharmaceutical and biotechnology companies need to provide in the regulatory submissions associated with the drug discovery and development process?

Over the past 10 years, in response to the changing landscape of genomics information and its potential to improve the drug discovery and development process and the cost-effectiveness of new medicines, there has been a steep learning curve around the world within regulatory authorities and pharmaceutical/biotechnology companies. Fortunately, representatives of the regulatory authorities and the companies have joined together to explore and define the role of genomic information in drug discovery and development, and marketing approval.

Critical Path Initiative and the EMEA's equivalent programme

In the early 2000s, the US Food and Drug Administration (FDA) and the European Medicines Evaluation Agency (EMEA) separately initiated efforts to improve the drug discovery and development process. In part, these efforts were stimulated by a trend in the preceding years of fewer and fewer drug approvals each year. Additionally, there was an understanding at these regulatory agencies that new developments in scientific and medical research, such as the explosion of genomic information, were not being incorporated into the drug evaluation processes. The FDA kicked-off its initiative in March 2004 with an insightful white paper entitled 'Innovation/Stagnation: Challenge and Opportunity on the Critical Path to New Medical Products' (http://www.fda.gov/downloads/ScienceResearch/SpecialTopics/CriticalPathInitiative/CriticalPathOpportunitiesReports/ucm113411.pdf) and the initiative became known as the Critical Path Initiative. Also in 2004, the EMEA set up the EMA/CHMP Think-Tank Group on Innovative Drug Development (http://www.ema.europa.eu/ema/index.jsp?curl=pages/special_topics/general/general_content_000339.jsp&murl=menus/special_topics/special_topics.jsp&mid=WC0b01ac05800baed8&jsenabled=true).

Voluntary exploratory data submissions and guidance documents

In November 2003, the FDA published a draft guidance document on Pharmacogenomic Data Submissions (final guidance published in March 2005, http://www.fda.gov/downloads/RegulatoryInformation/Guidances/ucm126957.pdf) and introduced a programme to encourage pharmaceutical/biotechnology companies to make Voluntary Genomic Data Submissions (VGDS) concerning aspects of their drug discovery or development projects, under 'safe harbour' conditions without immediate regulatory impact. The goal of the VGDS programme was to provide 'real-world' examples around which to create dialogue between the FDA and pharmaceutical/biotechnology companies about the potential roles of genomic information in the drug development process and to educate both regulators and drug developers. Within a short time of its initiation, the programme was expanded to include other molecular data types and is now known as the Voluntary Exploratory Data Submissions (VXDS) programme and also involves collaboration with the EMEA. A recent article (Goodsaid et al., 2010) provides an overview of the first 5 years of operation of the programme and presents a number of selected case studies.

Overall the VXDS programme has been of mutual benefit to regulators, pharmaceutical companies, technology providers and academic researchers. As envisioned by the FDA's Critical Path Initiative, the VXDS programme will continue to shape the ways that pharmaceutical companies incorporate, and regulators review, genomic information in the drug discovery, development and approval process.

The FDA and EMEA guidance documents and meeting reports are presented in Table 7.3.

CONCLUSION

The biopharmaceutical industry depends upon vast amounts of information from diverse sources to support the discovery, development and marketing approval of its products. In recent years, the sustainability of the industry's business model has been questioned because the frequency of successful drug discovery and development projects, in terms of approved products, is considered too low in light of the associated costs – particularly in a social context where healthcare costs are spiralling upwards and 'out of control'.

The lack of successful outcome for the overwhelming majority of drug discovery and development projects results from the fact that we simply do not know enough about biology in general, and human biology in particular, to avoid unanticipated 'roadblocks' or 'minefields' in the path to drug approval. In short, we do not have enough bioinformation.

Most drugs interact with protein targets, so it would be natural for pharmaceutical scientists to want comprehensive information about the nature and behaviour of proteins in health and disease. Unfortunately, because of the complexity of protein species, availability proteomic technologies have not yet been able to reveal such comprehensive information about proteins – although substantial advances have been made over the past few decades.

However, as a result of tremendous advances in genomic and bioinformatic technologies during the second half of the 20th century and over the past decade, comprehensive information about the genomes of many organisms is becoming available to the biomedical research community, including pharmaceutical scientists. Genomic information is the primary type of bioinformation and the nature and behaviour of the genome of an organism underpins all of its activities. It is also 'relatively' simple in structure compared to proteomic or metabolomic information.

Genomic information, by itself, has the potential to transform the drug discovery and development process, to enhance the probability of success of any project and to reduce overall costs. Such a transformation will be brought about through new drug discovery and development strategies focused on understanding molecular subtypes underpinning disease symptoms, discovering drug targets relevant to particular disease molecular subtypes and undertaking clinical studies informed by the knowledge of how human genetic individuality can influence treatment outcome. Onward!

Table 7.3 EMEA and FDA Genomics guidance documents, concept papers and policies

EMEA guidance documents and concept papers	
Reflection paper on co-development of pharmacogenomic biomarkers and assays in the context of drug development	http://www.ema.europa.eu/docs/en_GB/document_library/Scientific_guideline/2010/07/WC500094445.pdf
Use of pharmacogenetic methodologies in the pharmacokinetic evaluation of medicinal products	http://www.ema.europa.eu/docs/en_GB/document_library/Scientific_guideline/2010/05/WC500090323.pdf
ICH concept paper on pharmacogenomic (PG) biomarker qualification: Format and data standards	http://www.ema.europa.eu/docs/en_GB/document_library/Scientific_guideline/2009/09/WC500003863.pdf
Reflection paper on pharmacogenomics in oncology	http://www.ema.europa.eu/docs/en_GB/document_library/Scientific_guideline/2009/09/WC500003866.pdf
ICH Topic E15: Definitions for genomic biomarkers, pharmacogenomics, pharmacogenetics, genomic data and sample coding categories	http://www.ema.europa.eu/docs/en_GB/document_library/Scientific_guideline/2009/09/WC500003888.pdf
Reflection paper on pharmacogenomic samples, testing and data handling	http://www.ema.europa.eu/docs/en_GB/document_library/Scientific_guideline/2009/09/WC500003864.pdf
Guiding principles: Processing joint FDA EMEA voluntary genomic data submissions (VGDSs) within the framework of the confidentiality arrangement	http://www.ema.europa.eu/docs/en_GB/document_library/Scientific_guideline/2009/09/WC500003887.pdf
Reflection paper on the use of genomics in cardiovascular clinical trials	http://www.ema.europa.eu/docs/en_GB/document_library/Scientific_guideline/2009/09/WC500003865.pdf
Reflection paper on the use of pharmacogenetics in the pharmacokinetic evaluation of medicinal products	http://www.ema.europa.eu/docs/en_GB/document_library/Scientific_guideline/2009/09/WC500003890.pdf
Pharmacogenetics briefing meeting	http://www.ema.europa.eu/docs/en_GB/document_library/Scientific_guideline/2009/09/WC500003886.pdf
Position paper on terminology in pharmacogenetics	http://www.ema.europa.eu/docs/en_GB/document_library/Scientific_guideline/2009/09/WC500003889.pdf
FDA guidance documents, concept papers and policy documents	
Guiding Principles for Joint FDA EMEA Voluntary Genomic Data Submission Briefing Meetings	http://www.fda.gov/downloads/Drugs/ScienceResearch/ResearchAreas/Pharmacogenetics/UCM085378.pdf
Pharmacogenetic Tests and Genetic Tests for Heritable Markers	http://www.fda.gov/MedicalDevices/DeviceRegulationandGuidance/GuidanceDocuments/ucm077862.htm
Guidance for Industry: Pharmacogenomic Data Submissions	http://www.fda.gov/downloads/Drugs/GuidanceComplianceRegulatoryInformation/Guidances/ucm079849.pdf
Pharmacogenomic Data Submissions – Companion Guidance	http://www.fda.gov/downloads/Drugs/GuidanceComplianceRegulatoryInformation/Guidances/ucm079855.pdf
E15 Definitions for Genomic Biomarkers, Pharmacogenomics, Pharmacogenetics, Genomic Data and Sample Coding Categories	http://www.fda.gov/downloads/RegulatoryInformation/Guidances/ucm129296.pdf
Class II Special Controls Guidance Document: Drug Metabolizing Enzyme Genotyping System – Guidance for Industry and FDA Staff	http://www.fda.gov/MedicalDevices/DeviceRegulationandGuidance/GuidanceDocuments/ucm077933.htm
Drug-Diagnostic Co-Development Concept Paper	http://www.fda.gov/downloads/Drugs/ScienceResearch/ResearchAreas/Pharmacogenetics/UCM116689.pdf

Table 7.3 ***Continued***

Guiding principles Processing Joint FDA EMEA Voluntary Genomic Data Submissions (VGDSs) within the framework of the Confidentiality Arrangement	http://www.fda.gov/downloads/Drugs/ScienceResearch/ResearchAreas/Pharmacogenetics/UCM085378.pdf
Management of the Interdisciplinary Pharmacogenomics Review Group (IPRG)	http://www.fda.gov/downloads/AboutFDA/CentersOffices/CDER/ManualofPoliciesProcedures/UCM073574.pdf
Processing and Reviewing Voluntary Genomic Data Submissions (VGDSs)	http://www.fda.gov/downloads/AboutFDA/CentersOffices/CDER/ManualofPoliciesProcedures/UCM073575.pdf
Examples of Voluntary Submissions or Submissions Required Under 21 CFR 312, 314, or 601	http://www.fda.gov/downloads/Drugs/GuidanceComplianceRegulatoryInformation/Guidances/UCM079851.pdf

REFERENCES

Baranzini SL, Elfstrom C, Chang SY, et al. Transcriptional analysis of multiple sclerosis brain lesions reveals a complex pattern of cytokine expression. Journal of Immunology 2000;165:6576–82.

Cantor CR, Smith CL. Genomics. The science and technology behind the Human Genome Project. New York: John Wiley and Sons; 1999.

Chandra SK, Caldwell JS. Fulfilling the promise: drug discovery in the post-genomic era. Drug Discovery Today 2003;8:168–74.

Cockburn IM. Is the pharmaceutical industry in a productivity crisis? Innovation Policy and the Economy 2007;7:1–32.

Crettol S, Petrovic N, Murray M. Pharmacogenetics of Phase I and Phase II drug metabolism. Current Pharmaceutical Design 2010;16:204–19.

Dolinoy DC, Huang D, Jirtle RL. Maternal nutrient supplementation counteracts bisphenol A-induced DNA hypomethylation in early development. Proceedings of the National Academy of Sciences of the USA 2007;104:13056–61.

Drews J. Strategic trends in the drug industry. Drug Discovery Today 2003;8:411–20.

Fraga MF, Ballestar E, Paz MF, et al. Epigenetic differences arise during the lifetime of monozygotic twins. Proceedings of the National Academy of Sciences of the USA 2005;102:10604–9.

Freeman JL, Perry GH, Feuk L, et al. Copy number variation: new insights in genome diversity. Genome Research 2006;16:949–61.

Garnier JP. Rebuilding the R&D engine in big pharma. Harvard Business Review 2008;86:68–70, 72–6, 128.

Goodsaid FM, Amur S, Aubrecht J, et al. Voluntary exploratory data submissions to the US FDA and the EMA: experience and impact. Nature Reviews Drug Discovery 2010;9:435–45.

Greenbaum D, Luscombe NM, Jansen R, et al. Interrelating different types of genomic data, from proteome to secretome: 'oming in on function. Genome Research 2001;11:1463–8.

Hanson, MA, Gluckman, PD. Developmental origins of health and disease: new insights. Basic and Clinical Pharmacology and Toxicology 2008;102:90–3.

Hark AT, Schoenherr CJ, Katz DJ, et al. CTCF mediates methylation-sensitive enhancer-blocking activity at the H19/Igf2 locus. Nature 2000;405:486–9.

Holliday R, Pugh JE. DNA modification mechanisms and gene activity during development. Science 1975;187:226–32.

International Genome Sequencing Consortium. Finishing the euchromatic sequence of the human genome. Nature 2004; 431:915–6.

Kidgell C, Winzeler EA. Using the genome to dissect the molecular basis of drug resistance. Future Microbiology 2006;1:185–99.

Lander ES, Linton LM, Birren B, et al. Initial sequencing and analysis of the human genome. Nature 2001;409:860–921.

Larsen F, Gundersen G, Lopez R, et al. CpG islands as gene markers in the human genome. Genomics 1992;13:1095–107.

Li J, Robson B. Bioinformatics and computational chemistry in molecular design. Recent advances and their application. In: Peptide and protein drug analysis. NY: Marcel Dekker; 2000. p. 285–307.

Mullins IM, Siadaty MS, Lyman J, et al. Data mining and clinical data repositories: insights from a 667,000 patient data set. Computers in Biology and Medicine 2006;36: 1351–77.

Munos BH. Lessons from 60 years of pharmaceutical innovation. Nature Reviews Drug Discovery 2009;8: 959–68.

Neumann EK, Quan D. Biodash: a semantic web dashboard for drug development. Pacific Symposium on Biocomputing 2006;11:176–87.

Niu Y, Gong Y, Langaee TY, et al. Genetic variation in the β2 subunit of the voltage-gated calcium channel and pharmacogenetic association with adverse cardiovascular outcomes in the International VErapamil SR-Trandolapril STudy GENEtic Substudy (INVEST-GENES).

Circulation. Cardiovascular Genetics 2010;3:548–55.

Paul SM, Mytelka DS, Dunwiddie CT, et al. How to improve R&D productivity: the pharmaceutical industry's grand challenge. Nature Reviews Drug Discovery 2010;9:203–14.

Peltonen L, Perola M, Naukkarinen J, et al. Lessons from studying monogenic disease for common disease. Human Molecular Genetics 2006;15:R67–R74.

Pucci MJ. Novel genetic techniques and approaches in the microbial genomics era: identification and/or validation of targets for the discovery of new antibacterial agents. Drugs R&D 2007;8:201–12.

Robinson R. Common disease, multiple rare (and distant) variants. PLoS Biology 2010;8(1): e1000293.

Robson B. Clinical and pharmacogenomic data mining. 1. The generalized theory of expected information and application to the development of tools. Journal of Proteome Research 2003;2:283–301.

Robson B. The dragon on the gold: Myths and realities for data mining in biotechnology using digital and molecular libraries. Journal of Proteome Research 2004;3:1113–9.

Robson B. Clinical and pharmacogenomics data mining. 3 Zeta theory as a general tactic for clinical bioinformatics. Journal of Proteome Research 2005;4;445–55.

Robson B. Clinical and phamacogenomic data mining. 4. The FANO program and command set as an example of tools for biomedical discovery and evidence based medicine. Journal of Proteome Research 2008;7:3922–47.

Robson B, Baek OK. The engines of Hippocrates: from medicine's early dawn to medical and pharmaceutical informatics. New York: John Wiley & Sons; 2009.

Robson B, Mushlin R. Clinical and pharmacogenomic data mining. 2. A simple method for the combination of information from associations and multivariances to facilitate analysis, decision and design in clinical research and practice. Journal of Proteome Research 2004;3:697–711.

Robson B, Vaithiligam A. Drug gold and data dragons: Myths and realities of data mining in the pharmaceutical industry. In: Balakin KV, editor. Pharmaceutical Data Mining. John Wiley & Sons; 2010. p. 25–85.

Ruttenberg A, Rees JA, Samwald M, et al. Life sciences on the semantic web: the neurocommons and beyond. Briefings in Bioinformatics 2009;10:193–204.

Sacca R, Engle SJ, Qin W, et al. Genetically engineered mouse models in drug discovery research. Methods in Molecular Biology 2010;602:37–54.

Sadee W, Hoeg E, Lucas J, et al. Genetic variations in human g protein-coupled receptors: implications for drug therapy. AAPS PharmSci 2001;3:E22.

Stephens S, Morales A, Quinlan M. Applying semantic web technologies to drug safety determination. IEEE Intelligent Systems 2006;21:82–6.

Svinte M, Robson B, Hehenberger M. Biomarkers in drug development and patient care. Burrill 2007 Person. Medical Report 2007;6:3114–26.

van der Greef J, McBurney RN. Rescuing drug discovery: in vivo systems pathology and systems pharmacology. Nature Reviews Drug Discovery 2005;4:961–7.

van der Greef J, Martin S, Juhasz P, et al. The art and practice of systems biology in medicine: mapping patterns of relationships. Journal of Proteome Research 2007;4:1540–59.

Venter JC, Adams MD, Myers EW, et al. The sequence of the human genome. Science 2001;291:1304–51.

Waddington CH. Introduction to modern genetics. London: Allen and Unwin; 1939.

Wu CT, Morris JR. Genes, genetics, and epigenetics: a correspondence. Science 2001;293:1103–5.

Zhang JP, Lencz T, Malhotra AK. D2 receptor genetic variation and clinical response to antipsychotic drug treatment: a meta-analysis. American Journal of Psychiatry 2010;167:763–72.

Chapter | 8 |

High-throughput screening

D Cronk

INTRODUCTION: A HISTORICAL AND FUTURE PERSPECTIVE

Systematic drug research began about 100 years ago, when chemistry had reached a degree of maturity that allowed its principles and methods to be applied to problems outside the field, and when pharmacology had in turn become a well-defined scientific discipline. A key step was the introduction of the concept of selective affinity through the postulation of 'chemoreceptors' by Paul Ehrlich. He was the first to argue that differences in chemoreceptors between species may be exploited therapeutically. This was also the birth of chemotherapy. In 1907, Ehrlich identified compound number 606, Salvarsan (diaminodioxy-arsenobenzene) (Ehrlich and Bertheim, 1912), which was brought to the market in 1910 by Hoechst for the treatment of syphilis, and hailed as a miracle drug (Figure 8.1).

This was the first time extensive pharmaceutical screening had been used to find drugs. At that time screening was based on phenotypic readouts e.g. antimicrobial effect, a concept which has since led to unprecedented therapeutic triumphs in anti-infective and anticancer therapies, based particularly on natural products. In contrast, today's screening is largely driven by distinct molecular targets and relies on biochemical readout.

In the further course of the 20th century drug research became influenced primarily by biochemistry. The dominant concepts introduced by biochemistry were those of enzymes and receptors, which were empirically found to be drug targets. In 1948 Ahlquist made a crucial, further step by proposing the existence of two types of adrenoceptor (α and β) in most organs. The principle of receptor classification has been the basis for a large number of diverse drugs, including β-adrenoceptor agonists and antagonists, benzodiazepines, angiotensin receptor antagonists and ultimately monoclonal antibodies.

Today's marketed drugs are believed to target a range of human biomolecules (see Chapters 6 and 7), ranging from various enzymes and transporters to G-protein-coupled receptors (GPCRs) and ion channels. At present the GPCRs are the predominant target family, and more than 800 of these biomolecules have been identified in the human genome (Kroeze et al., 2003). However, it is predicted that less than half are druggable and in reality proteases and kinases may offer greater potential as targets for pharmaceutical products (Russ and Lampel, 2005). Although the target portfolio of a pharmaceutical company can change from time to time, the newly chosen targets are still likely to belong to one of the main therapeutic target classes. The selection of targets and target families (see Chapter 6) plays a pivotal role in determining the success of today's lead molecule discovery.

Over the last 15 years significant technological progress has been achieved in genomic sciences (Chapter 7), high-throughput medicinal chemistry (Chapter 9), cell-based assays and high-throughput screening. These have led to a 'new' concept in drug discovery whereby targets with therapeutic potential are incorporated into biochemical or cell-based assays which are exposed to large numbers of compounds, each representing a given chemical structure space. Massively parallel screening, called high-throughput screening (HTS), was first introduced by pharmaceutical companies in the early 1990s and is now employed routinely as the most widely applicable technology for identifying chemistry starting points for drug discovery programmes.

Nevertheless, HTS remains just one of a number of possible lead discovery strategies (see Chapters 6 and 9). In the best case it can provide an efficient way to obtain

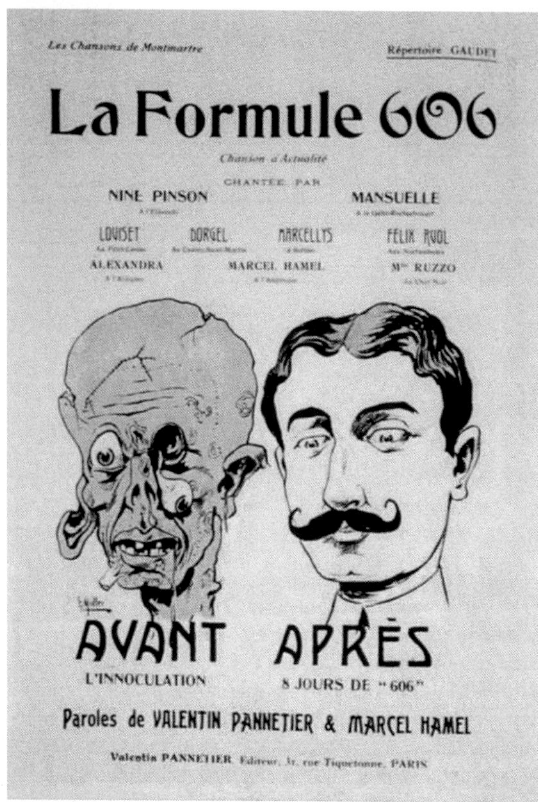

Fig. 8.1 In France, where Salvarsan was called 'Formule 606', true miracles were expected from the new therapy.

useful data on the biological activity of large numbers of test samples by using high-quality assays and high-quality chemical compounds. Today's lead discovery departments are typically composed of the following units: (1) compound logistics; (2) assay development and screening (which may utilize automation); (3) tool (reagent) production; and (4) profiling. Whilst most HTS projects focus on the use of synthetic molecules typically within a molecular weight range of 250–600 Da, some companies are interested in exploring natural products and have dedicated research departments for this purpose. These groups work closely with the HTS groups to curate the natural products, which are typically stored as complex mixtures, and provide the necessary analytical skills to isolate the single active molecule.

Compared with initial volume driven HTS in the 1990s there is now much more focus on quality-oriented output. At first, screening throughput was the main emphasis, but it is now only one of many performance indicators. In the 1990s the primary concern of a company's compound logistics group was to collect all its historic compound collections in sufficient quantities and of sufficient quality to file them by electronic systems, and store them in the most appropriate way in compound archives. This resulted in huge collections that range from several hundred thousand to a few million compounds. Today's focus has shifted to the application of defined electronic or physical filters for compound selection before they are assembled into a library for testing. The result is a customized ensemble of either newly designed or historic compounds for use in screening, otherwise known as 'cherry picking'. However, it is often the case that the HTS departments have sufficient infrastructure to enable routine screening of the entire compound collection and it is only where the assay is complex or relatively expensive that the time to create 'cherry picked', focused, compound sets is invested (Valler and Green, 2000).

In assay development there is a clear trend towards mechanistically driven high-quality assays that capture the relevant biochemistry (e.g. stochiometry, kinetics) or cell biology. Homogeneous assay principles, along with sensitive detection technologies, have enabled the miniaturization of assay formats producing a concomitant reduction of reagent usage and cost per data point. With this evolution of HTS formats it is becoming increasingly common to gain more than one set of information from the same assay well either through multiparametric analysis or multiplexing, e.g. cellular function response and toxicity (Beske and Goldbard, 2002; Hanson, 2006; Hallis et al., 2007). The drive for information rich data from HTS campaigns is no more evident than through the use of imaging technology to enable subcellular resolution, a methodology broadly termed high content screening (HCS). HCS assay platforms facilitate the study of intracellular pharmacology through spatiotemporal resolution, and the quantification of signalling and regulatory pathways. Such techniques increasingly use cells that are more phenotypically representative of disease states, so called disease-relevant cell lines (Clemons, 2004), in an effort to add further value to the information provided.

Screening departments in large pharmaceutical companies utilize automated screening platforms, which in the early days of HTS were large linear track systems, typically five metres or more in length. The more recent trends have been towards integrated networks of workstation-based instrumentation, typically arranged around the circumference of a static, rotating robotic arm, which offers greater flexibility and increased efficiency in throughput due to reduced plate transit times within the automated workcell. Typically, the screening unit of a large pharmaceutical company will generate tens of millions of single point determinations per year, with fully automated data acquisition and processing. Following primary screening, there has been an increased need for secondary/complementary screening to confirm the primary results, provide information on test compound specificity and selectivity and to refine these compounds further. Typical data formats include half-maximal concentrations at which a compound causes a defined modulatory effect in functional assays, or binding/inhibitory constants. Post-HTS, broader selectivity profiling may be required, for active compounds against panels of related target families. As HTS technologies are adopted into other related disciplines compound potency and selectivity are no longer the only parameters to be optimized during hit-finding. With this broader acceptance of key technologies, harmonization and standardization of data across disciplines are crucial to facilitate analysis and mining of the data. Important information such as compound purity and its associated physicochemical properties such as solubility can be derived very quickly on relatively large numbers of compounds and thus help prioritize compounds for progression based on overall suitability, not just potency (Fligge and Schuler, 2006). These quality criteria, and quality assessment at all key points in the discovery process, are crucial. Late-stage attrition of drug candidates, particularly in development and beyond, is extremely expensive and such failures must be kept to a minimum. This is typically done by an extensive assessment of chemical integrity, synthetic accessibility, functional properties, structure–activity relationship (SAR) and biophysicochemical properties, and related absorption, distribution, metabolism and excretion (ADME) characteristics, as discussed further in Chapters 9 and 10.

In summary, significant technological progress has been made over the last 15 years in HTS. Major concepts such as miniaturization and parallelization have been introduced in almost all areas and steps of the lead discovery process. This, in turn, has led to a great increase in screening capacity, significant savings in compound or reagent consumption, and, ultimately, improved cost-effectiveness. More recently, stringent quality assessment in library management and assay development, along with consistent data formats in automated screening, has led to much higher-quality screening outcomes. The perception of HTS has also changed significantly in the past decade and is now recognized as a multidisciplinary science, encompassing biological sciences, engineering and information technology. HTS departments generate huge amounts of data that can be used together with computational chemistry tools to drive compound structure–activity relationships and aid selection of focused compound sets for further testing from larger compound libraries. Where information rich assays are used complex analysis algorithms may be required to ensure the relevant data are extracted. Various statistical, informatics and filtering methods have recently been introduced to foster the integration of experimental and *in silico* screening, and so maximize the output in lead discovery. As a result, lead-finding activities continue to benefit greatly from a more unified and knowledge-based approach to biological screening, in addition to the many technical advances towards even higher-throughput screening.

LEAD DISCOVERY AND HIGH-THROUGHPUT SCREENING

A lead compound is generally defined as a new chemical entity that could potentially be developed into a new drug by optimizing its beneficial effects and minimizing its side effects (see Chapter 9 for a more detailed discussion of the criteria). HTS is currently the main approach for the identification of lead compounds, i.e. large numbers of compounds (the 'compound library') are usually tested in a random approach for their biological activity against a disease-relevant target. However, there are other techniques in place for lead discovery that are complementary to HTS.

Besides the conventional literature search (identification of compounds already described for the desired activity), structure-based virtual screening is a frequently applied technique (Ghosh et al., 2006; Waszkowycz, 2008). Molecular recognition events are simulated by computational techniques based on knowledge of the molecular target, thereby allowing very large 'virtual' compound libraries (greater than 4 million compounds) to be screened in silico and, by applying this information, pharmacophore models can be developed. These allow the identification of potential leads *in silico*, without experimental screening and the subsequent construction of smaller sets of compounds ('focused libraries') for testing against a specific target or family of targets (Stahura et al., 2002; Muegge and Oloff, 2006). Similarly, X-ray analysis of the target can be applied to guide the *de novo* synthesis and design of bioactive molecules. In the absence of computational models, very low-molecular-weight compounds (typically 150–300 Da, so-called fragments), may be screened using biophysical methods to detect low-affinity interactions. The use of protein crystallography and X-ray diffraction techniques allows elucidation of the binding mode of these fragments and these can be used as a starting point for developing higher affinity leads by assemblies of the functional components of the fragments (Rees et al., 2004; Hartshorn et al., 2005; Congreve et al., 2008).

Typically, in HTS, large compound libraries are screened ('primary' screen) and numerous bioactive compounds ('primary hits' or 'positives') are identified. These compounds are taken through successive rounds of further screening ('secondary' screens) to confirm their activity, potency and where possible gain an early measure of specificity for the target of interest. A typical HTS activity cascade is shown in Figure 8.2 resulting in the identification of hits, usually with multiple members of a similar chemical core or chemical series. These hits then enter into the 'hit-to-lead' process during which medicinal chemistry teams synthesize specific compounds or small arrays of compounds for testing to develop an understanding of the

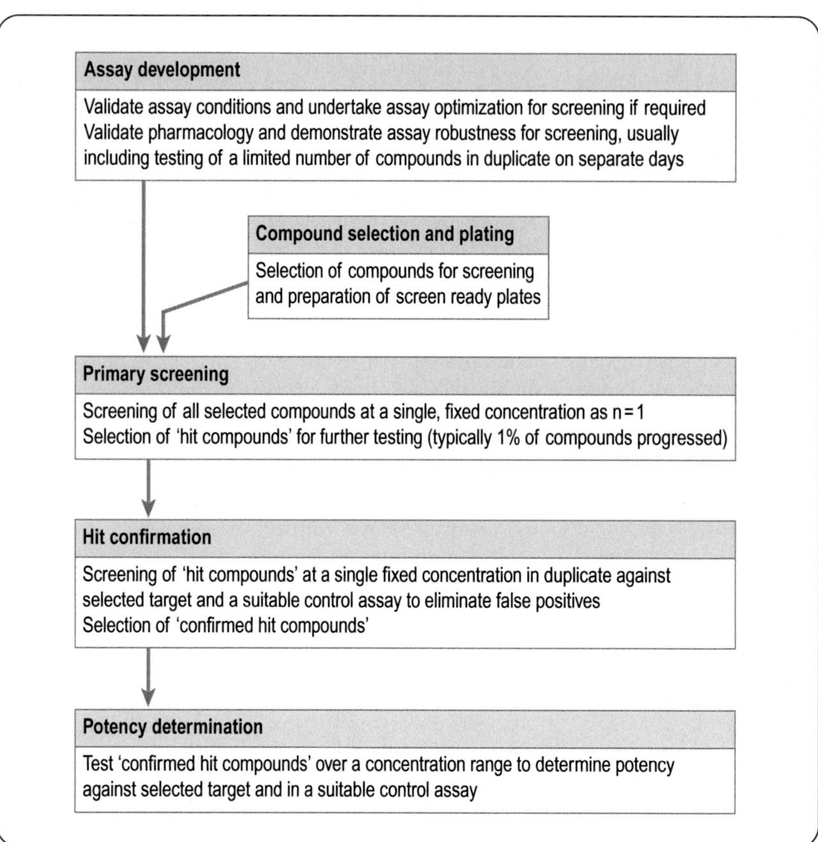

Fig. 8.2 The typical high throughput screening process.

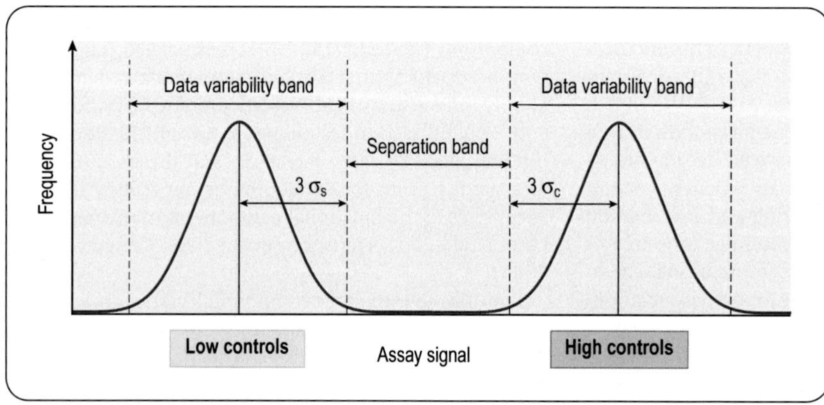

Fig. 8.3 Illustration of data variability and the signal window, given by the separation band between high and low controls. *Adapted, with permission, from Zhang et al., 1999.*

structure–activity relationship (SAR) of the underlying chemical series. The result of the hit-to-lead phase is a group of compounds (the lead series) which has appropriate drug-like properties such as specificity, pharmacokinetics or bioavailability. These properties can then be further improved by medicinal chemistry in a 'lead optimization' process (Figure 8.3). Often the HTS group will provide support for these hit-to-lead and lead optimization stages through ongoing provision of reagents, provision of assay expertise or execution of the assays themselves.

Assay development and validation

The target validation process (see Chapters 6 and 7) establishes the relevance of a target in a certain disease pathway. In the next step an assay has to be developed, allowing the quantification of the interaction of molecules with the chosen target. This interaction can be inhibition, stimulation, or simply binding. There are numerous different assay technologies available, and the choice for a specific assay type will always be determined by factors such as type of target, the required sensitivity, robustness, ease of automation and cost. Assays can be carried out in different formats based on 96-, 384-, or 1536-well microtitre plates. The format to be applied depends on various parameters, e.g. readout, desired throughput, or existing hardware in liquid handling and signal detection with 384- (either standard volume or low volume) and 1536-well formats being the most commonly applied. In all cases the homogeneous type of assay is preferred, as it is quicker, easier to handle and cost-effective, allowing 'mix and measure' operation without any need for further separation steps.

Next to scientific criteria, cost is a key factor in assay development. The choice of format has a significant effect on the total cost per data point: the use of 384-well low-volume microtitre plates instead of a 96-well plate format results in a significant reduction of the reaction volume (see Table 8.1). This reduction correlates directly with reagent costs per well. The size of a typical screening library is between 500 000 and 1 million compounds. Detection reagent costs per well can easily vary between US$0.05 and more than U$0.5 per data point, depending on the type and format of the assay. Therefore, screening an assay with a 500 000 compound library may cost either US$25 000 or US$250 000, depending on the selected assay design – a significant difference! It should also be borne in mind that these costs are representative for reagents only and the cost of consumables (assay plates and disposable liquid handling tips) may be an additional consideration. Whilst the consumables costs are higher for the higher density formats, the saving in reagent costs and increased throughput associated with miniaturization usually result in assays being run in the highest density format the HTS department has available.

Table 8.1 Reaction volumes in microtitre plates

Plate format	Typical assay volume
96	100–200 µL
384	25–50 µL
384 low volume	5–20 µL
1536	2–10 µL

Once a decision on the principal format and readout technology is taken, the assay has to be validated for its sensitivity and robustness. Biochemical parameters, reagents and screening hardware (e.g. detectors, microtitre plates) must be optimized. To give a practical example, in a typical screen designed for inhibitors of protease activity, test compounds are mixed together with the enzyme and finally substrate is added. The substrate consists of a cleavable peptide linked to a fluorescent label, and the reaction is quantified by measuring the change in fluoresecence intensity that accompanies the enzymic cleavage. In the process of validation, the best available labelled substrate (natural or synthetic) must be selected, the reaction conditions optimized (for example reaction time, buffers and temperature), enzyme kinetic measurements performed to identify the linear range, and the response of the assay to known inhibitors (if available) tested. Certain types of compound or solvent (which in most cases will be dimethylsulfoxide, DMSO) may interfere with the assay readout and this has to be checked. The stability of assay reagents is a further important parameter to be determined during assay validation, as some assay formats require a long incubation time.

At this point other aspects of screening logistics have to be considered. If the enzyme is not available commercially it has to be produced in-house by process development, and batch-to-batch reproducibility and timely delivery have to be ensured. With cell-based screens it must be guaranteed that the cell production facility is able to deliver sufficient quantities of consistently functioning, physiologically intact cells during the whole screening campaign and that there is no degradation of signal or loss of protein expression from the cells with extended periods of subculture.

The principal goal of developing HTS assays is the fast and reliable identification of active compounds ('positives' or 'hits') from chemical libraries. Most HTS programmes test compounds at only one concentration. In most instances this approximates to a final test concentration in the assay of 10 micromolar. This may be adjusted depending on the nature of the target but in all cases must be within the bounds of the solvent tolerance of the assay determined earlier in the development process. In order to identify hits with confidence, only small variations in signal measurements can be tolerated. The statistical parameters used to determine the suitability of assays for HTS are the calculation of standard deviations, the coefficient of variation (CV), signal-to-noise (S/N) ratio or signal-to-background (S/B) ratio. The inherent problem with using these last two is that neither takes into account the dynamic range of the signal (i.e. the difference between the background (low control) and the maximum (high control) signal), or the variability in the sample and reference control measurements. A more reliable assessment of assay quality is achieved by the Z′-factor equation (Zhang et al., 1999):

$$Z' = 1 - \frac{(3(\text{SD of High Control}) + 3(\text{SD of Low Control}))}{[\text{Mean of High Control} - \text{Mean of Low Control}]}$$

where SD = standard deviation and the maximum possible value of Z is 1. For biochemical assays a value greater than 0.5 represents a good assay whereas a value less than 0.5 is generally unsatisfactory for HTS. A lower Z′ threshold of 0.4 is usually considered acceptable for cell-based assays.

This equation takes into account that the quality of an assay is reflected in the variability of the high and low controls, and the separation band between them (Figure 8.3). Z′-factors are obtained by measuring plates containing 50% low controls (in the protease example: assay plus reference inhibitor, minimum signal to be measured) and 50% high controls (assay without inhibitor; maximum signal to be measured). In addition, inter- and intra-plate coefficients of variation (CV) are determined to check for systematic sources of variation. All measurements are normally made in triplicate. Once an assay has passed these quality criteria it can be transferred to the robotic screening laboratory. A reduced number of control wells can be employed to monitor Z′-values when the assay is progressed to HTS mode, usually 16 high- and 16 low-controls on a 384-well plate, with the removal of no more than two outlying controls to achieve an acceptable Z′-value. The parameter can be further modified to calculate the Z-value, whereby the average signal and standard deviation of test compound wells are compared to the high-control wells (Zhang et al., 1999). Due to the variability that will be present in the compound wells, and assuming a low number of active compounds, the Z-value is usually lower than the Z′-value.

Whilst there are been several alternatives of Zhang's proposal for assessing assay robustness, such as power analysis (Sui and Wu, 2007), the simplicity of the equation still make the Z′-value the primary assessment of assay suitability for HTS.

The Assay Guidance Website hosted by the National Institutes of Health Center for Translational Therapeutics (NCTT) (http://assay.nih.gov/assay/index.php/Table_of_Contents) provides comprehensive guidance of factors to consider for a wide range of assay formats.

Biochemical and cell-based assays

There is a wide range of assays formats that can be deployed in the drug discovery arena (Hemmilä and Hurskainen, 2002), although they broadly fall into two categories: **biochemical** and **cell-based**.

Biochemical assays (Figure 8.4) involve the use of cell-free *in-vitro* systems to model the biochemistry of a subset of cellular processes. The assay systems vary from simple interactions, such as enzyme/substrate reactions, receptor binding or protein–protein interactions, to more complex models such as *in-vitro* transcription systems. In contrast to cell-based assays, biochemical assays give direct information regarding the nature of the molecular interaction (e.g. kinetic data) and tend to have increased solvent

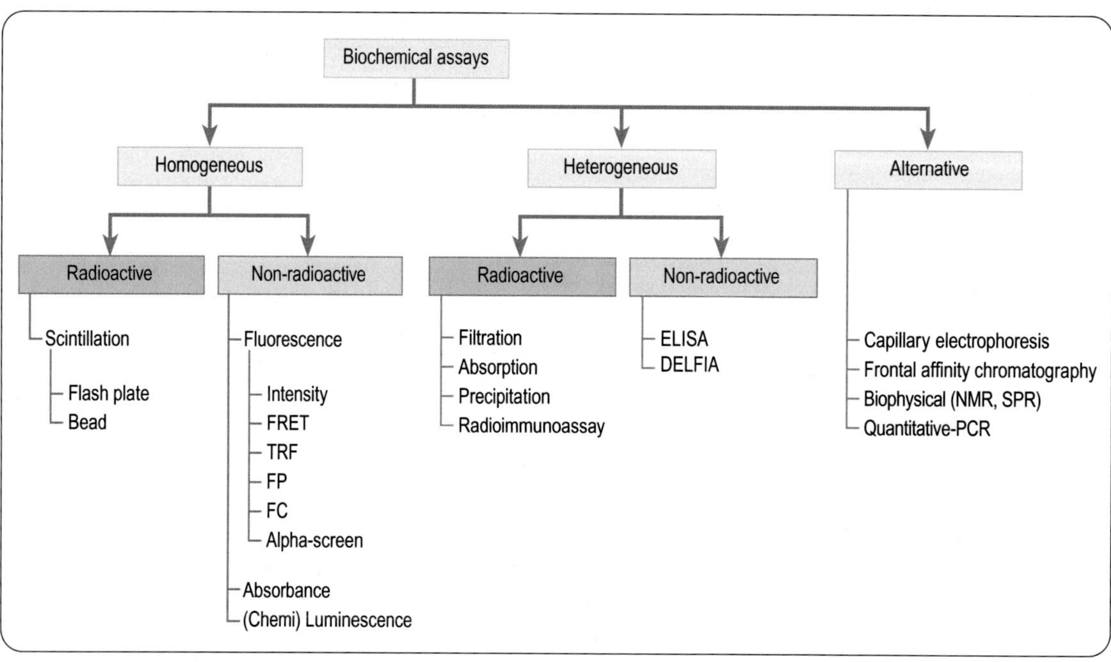

Fig. 8.4 Types of biochemical assay.

tolerance compared to cellular assays, thereby permitting the use of higher compound screening concentration if required. However, biochemical assays lack the cellular context, and are insensitive to properties such as membrane permeability, which determine the effects of compounds on intact cells.

Unlike biochemical assays, cell-based assays (Figure 8.5) mimic more closely the *in-vivo* situation and can be adapted for targets that are unsuitable for screening in biochemical assays, such as those involving signal transduction pathways, membrane transport, cell division, cytotoxicity or antibacterial actions. Parameters measured in cell-based assays range from growth, transcriptional activity, changes in cell metabolism or morphology, to changes in the level of an intracellular messenger such as cAMP, intracellular calcium concentration and changes in membrane potential for ion channels (Moore and Rees, 2001). Importantly, cell-based assays are able to distinguish between receptor antagonists, agonists, inverse agonists and allosteric modulators which cannot be done by measuring binding affinity in a biochemical assay.

Many cell-based assays have quite complex protocols, for example removing cell culture media, washing cells, adding compounds to be tested, prolonged incubation at 37°C, and, finally, reading the cellular response. Therefore, screening with cell-based assays requires a sophisticated infrastructure in the screening laboratory (including cell cultivation facilities, and robotic systems equipped to maintain physiological conditions during the assay procedure) and the throughput is generally lower.

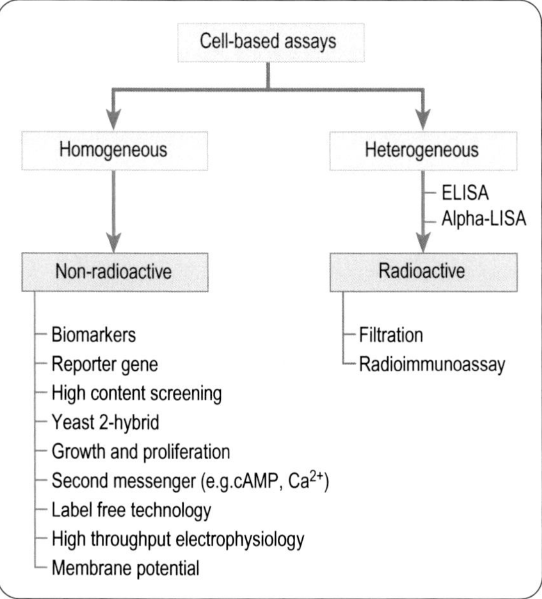

Fig. 8.5 Types of cell-based assay.

Cell-based assays frequently lead to higher hit rates, because of non-specific and 'off-target' effects of test compounds that affect the readout. Primary hits therefore need to be assessed by means of secondary assays such as non- or control-transfected cells in order to determine the mechanism of the effect (Moore and Rees, 2001).

Although cell-based assays are generally more time-consuming than cell-free assays to set up and run in high-throughput mode, there are many situations in which they are needed. For example, assays involving G-protein coupled receptors (GPCRs), membrane transporters and ion channels generally require intact cells if the functionality of the test compound is to be understood, or at least membranes prepared from intact cells for determining compound binding. In other cases, the production of biochemical targets such as enzymes in sufficient quantities for screening may be difficult or costly compared to cell-based assays directed at the same targets. The main pros and cons of cell-based assays are summarized in Table 8.2.

Table 8.2 Advantages and disadvantages of cell-based assays

Advantages	Disadvantages
Cytotoxic compounds can be detected and eliminated at the outset	Require high-capacity cell culture facilities and more challenging to fully automate
In receptor studies, agonists can be distinguished from antagonists	Often require specially engineered cell lines and/or careful selection of control cells
Detection of allosteric modulators	Reagent provision and control of variability of reagent batches
Binding and different functional readouts can be used in parallel – high information content	Cells liable to become detached from support
Phenotypic readouts are enabling when the molecular target is unknown (e.g. to detect compounds that affect cell division, growth, differentiation or metabolism)	High rate of false positives due to non-specific effects of test compounds on cell function
More disease relevant than biochemical asays	Assay variability can make assays more difficult to miniaturize
No requirement for protein production/scale up	Assay conditions (e.g. use of solvents, pH) limited by cell viability

Assay readout and detection

Ligand binding assays

Assays to determine direct interaction of the test compound with the target of interest through the use of radiolabelled compounds are sensitive and robust and are widely used for ligand-binding assays. The assay is based on measuring the ability of the test compound to inhibit the binding of a radiolabelled ligand to the target, and requires that the assay can distinguish between bound and free forms of the radioligand. This can be done by physical separation of bound from unbound ligand (*heterogeneous* format) by filtration, adsorption or centrifugation. The need for several washing steps makes it unsuitable for fully automated HTS, and generates large volumes of radioactive waste, raising safety and cost concerns over storage and disposal. Such assays are mainly restricted to 96-well format due to limitations of available multiwell filter plates and achieving consistent filtration when using higher density formats. Filtration systems do provide the advantage that they allow accurate determination of maximal binding levels and ligand affinities at sufficient throughput for support of hit-to-lead and lead optimization activities.

In the HTS arena, filtration assays have been superseded by *homogeneous* formats for radioactive assays. These have reduced overall reaction volume and eliminate the need for separation steps, largely eliminating the problem of waste disposal and provide increased throughput.

The majority of homogenous radioactive assay types are based on the scintillation proximity principle. This relies on the excitation of a scintillant incorporated in a matrix, in the form of either *microbeads* ('SPA') or *microplates* (Flashplates™, Perkin Elmer Life and Analytical Sciences) (Sittampalam et al., 1997), to the surface of which the target molecule is also attached (Figure 8.6). Binding of the radioligand to the target brings it into close proximity to the scintillant, resulting in light emission, which can be quantified. Free radioactive ligand is too distant from the scintillant and no excitation takes place. Isotopes such as ^{3}H or ^{125}I are typically used, as they produce low-energy particles that are absorbed over short distances (Cook, 1996). Test compounds that bind to the target compete with the radioligand, and thus reduce the signal.

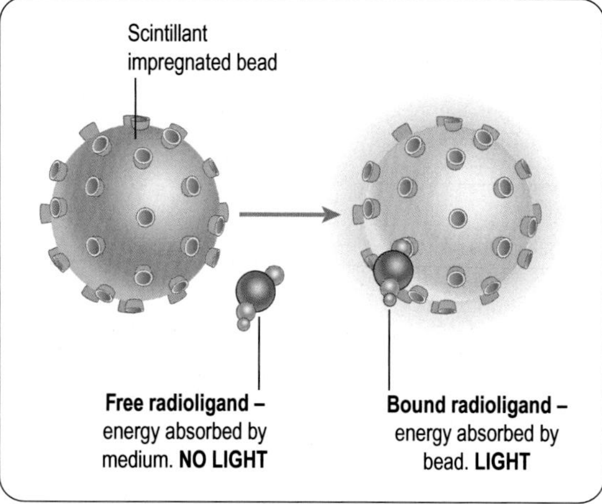

Fig. 8.6 Principle of scintillation proximity assays. *Reproduced with kind permission of GE Healthcare.*

With bead technology (Figure 8.8A), polymer beads of ~5 µm diameter are coated with antibodies, streptavidin, receptors or enzymes to which the radioligand can bind (Bosworth and Towers, 1989; Beveridge et al., 2000). Ninety-six- or 384-well plates can be used. The emission wavelength of the scintillant is in the range of 420 nm and is subject to limitations in the sensitivity due to both colour quench by yellow test compounds, and the variable efficiency of scintillation counting, due to sedimentation of the beads. The homogeneous platforms are also still subject to limitations in throughput associated with the detection technology via multiple photomultiplier tube-based detection instruments, with a 384-well plate taking in the order of 15 minutes to read.

The drive for increased throughput for radioactive assays led to development of scinitillants, containing europium yttrium oxide or europium polystyrene, contained in beads or multiwell plates with an emission wavlength shifted towards the red end of the visible light spectrum (~560 nm) and suited to detection on charge-coupled device (CCD) cameras (Ramm, 1999). The two most widely adopted instruments in this area are LEADseeker™ (GE Healthcare) and Viewlux™ (Perkin Elmer), using quantitative imaging to scan the whole plate, resulting in a higher throughput and increased sensitivity. Imaging instruments provide a read time typically in the order of a few minutes or less for the whole plate irrespective of density, representing a significant improvement in throughput, along with increased sensitivity. The problem of compound colour quench effect remains, although blue compounds now provide false hits rather than yellow. As CCD detection is independent of plate density, the use of imaging based radioactive assays has been adopted widely in HTS and adapted to 1536-well format and higher (see Bays et al., 2009, for example).

In the microplate form of scintillation proximity assays the target protein (e.g. an antibody or receptor) is coated on to the floor of a plate well to which the radioligand and test compounds are added. The bound radioligand causes a microplate surface scintillation effect (Brown et al., 1997). FlashPlate™ has been used in the investigation of protein–protein (e.g. radioimmunoassay) and receptor–ligand (i.e. radioreceptor assay) interactions (Birzin and Rohrer, 2002), and in enzymatic (e.g. kinase) assays (Braunwaler et al., 1996).

Due to the level of sensitivity provided by radioactive assays they are still widely adopted within the HTS setting. However, environmental, safety and local legislative considerations have led to the necessary development of alternative formats, in particular those utilizing fluorescent-ligands (Lee et al., 2008; Leopoldo et al., 2009). Through careful placement of a suitable fluorophore in the ligand via a suitable linker, the advantages of radioligand binding assays in terms of sensitivity can be realized without the obvious drawbacks associated with the use of radioisotopes. The use of fluorescence-based technologies is discussed in more detail in the following section.

Fluorescence technologies

The application of fluorescence technologies is widespread, covering multiple formats (Gribbon and Sewing, 2003) and yet in the simplest form involves excitation of a sample with light at one wavelength and measurement of the emission at a different wavelength. The difference between the absorbed wavelength and the emitted wavelength is called the *Stokes shift*, the magnitude of which depends on how much energy is lost in the fluorescence process (Lakowicz, 1999). A large Stokes shift is advantageous as it reduces optical crosstalk between photons from the excitation light and emitted photons.

Fluorescence techniques currently applied for HTS can be grouped into six major categories:

- Fluorescence intensity
- Fluorescence resonance energy transfer
- Time-resolved fluorescence
- Fluorescence polarization
- Fluorescence correlation
- AlphaScreen™ (amplified luminescence proximity homogeneous assay).

Fluorescence intensity

In fluorescence intensity assays, the change of total light output is monitored and used to quantify a biochemical reaction or binding event. This type of readout is frequently used in enzymatic assays (e.g. proteases, lipases). There are two variants: *fluorogenic assays* and *fluorescence quench assays*. In the former type the reactants are not fluorescent, but the reaction products are, and their formation can be monitored by an increase in fluorescence intensity.

In fluorescence quench assays a fluorescent group is covalently linked to a substrate. In this state, its fluorescence is quenched. Upon cleavage, the fluorescent group is released, producing an increase in fluorescence intensity (Haugland, 2002).

Fluorescence intensity measurements are easy to run and cheap. However, they are sensitive to fluorescent interference resulting from the colour of test compounds, organic fluorophores in assay buffers and even fluorescence of the microplate itself (Comley, 2003).

Fluorescence resonance energy transfer (FRET)

In this type of assay a *donor* fluorophore is excited and most of the energy is transferred to an *acceptor* fluorophore or a quenching group; this results in measurable photon emission by the acceptor. In simple terms, the amount of energy transfer from donor to acceptor depends on the fluorescent lifetime of the donor, the spatial distance between donor and acceptor (10–100 Å), and the dipole orientation between donor and acceptor. The transfer efficiency for a given pair of fluorophores can be calculated using the equation of Förster (Clegg, 1995).

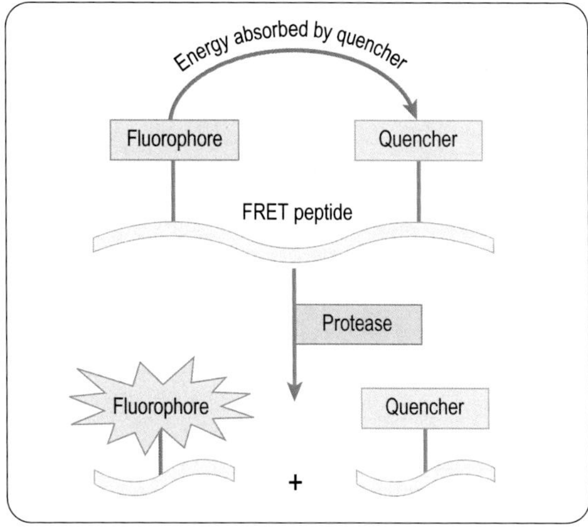

Fig. 8.7 Protease assay based on FRET. The donor fluorescence is quenched by the neighbouring acceptor molecule. Cleavage of the substrate separates them, allowing fluorescent emission by the donor molecule.

Usually the emission wavelengths of donor and acceptor are different, and FRET can be determined either by the quenching of the donor fluorescence by the acceptor (as shown in Figure 8.7) or by the fluorescence of the acceptor itself. Typical applications are for protease assays based on quenching of the uncleaved substrate, although FRET has also been applied for detecting changes in membrane potential in cell-based assays for ion channels (Gonzalez and Maher, 2002). With simple FRET techniques interference from background fluorescence is often a problem, which is largely overcome by the use of time-resolved fluorescence techniques, described below.

Time resolved fluorescence (TRF)

TRF techniques (Comley, 2006) use lanthanide chelates (samarium, europium, terbium and dysprosium) that give an intense and long-lived fluorescence emission (>1000 μs). Fluorescence emission is elicited by a pulse of excitation light and measured after the end of the pulse, by which time short-lived fluorescence has subsided. This makes it possible to eliminate short-lived autofluorescence and reagent background, and thereby enhance the signal-to-noise ratio. Lanthanides emit fluorescence with a large Stokes shift when they coordinate to specific ligands.

Typically, the complexes are excited by UV light, and emit light of wavelength longer than 500 nm.

Europium (Eu^{3+}) chelates have been used in immunoassays by means of a technology called DELFIA (dissociation-enhanced lanthanide fluoroimmuno assay). DELFIA is a heterogeneous time-resolved fluorometric assay based on *dissociative fluorescence enhancement*. Cell- and membrane-based assays are particularly well suited to the DELFIA system because of its broad detection range and extremely high sensitivity (Valenzano et al., 2000).

High sensitivity – to a limit of about 10^{-17} moles/well – is achieved by applying the dissociative enhancement principle. After separation of the bound from the free label, a reagent is added to the bound label which causes the weakly fluorescent lanthanide chelate to dissociate and form a new highly fluorescent chelate inside a protective micelle. Though robust and very sensitive, DELFIA assays are not ideal for HTS, as the process involves several binding, incubation and washing steps.

The need for homogeneous ('mix and measure') assays led to the development of LANCE™ (Perkin Elmer Life Sciences) and HTRF® (Homogeneous Time-Resolved Fluorescence; Cisbio). LANCE™, like DELFIA®, is based on chelates of lanthanide ions, but in a homogeneous format. The chelates used in LANCE™ can be measured directly without the need for a dissociation step, however in an aqueous environment the complexed ion can spontaneously dissociate and increase background fluorescence (Alpha et al., 1987).

In HTRF® (Figure 8.8) these limitations are overcome by the use of a *cryptate* molecule, which has a cage-like structure, to protect the central ion (e.g. Eu^{+}) from dissociation. HTRF® uses two separate labels, the donor (Eu)K and the acceptor APC/XL665 (a modified allophycocyanine from red algae) and such assays can be adapted for use in plates up to 1536-well format.

In both LANCE™ and HTRF®, measurement of the ratio of donor and acceptor fluorophore emission can be applied to compensate for non-specific quenching of assay reagents. As a result, the applications of both technologies are widespread, covering detection of kinase enzyme activity (Jia et al., 2006), protease activity (Karvinen et al., 2002), second messengers such as cAMP and inositiol triphosphate ($InsP_3$) (Titus et al., 2008; Trinquet et al., 2006) and numerous biomarkers such as interleukin 1β (IL-1β) and tumour necrosis factor alpha (TNFα) (Achard et al., 2003).

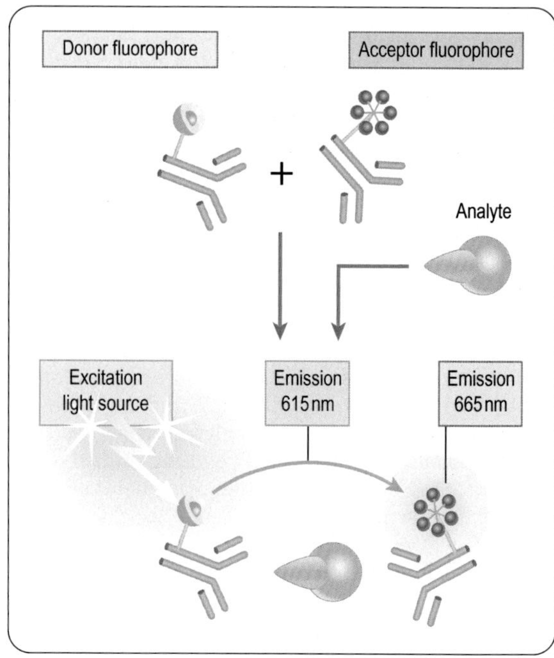

Fig. 8.8 HTRF assay type: the binding of a europium-labelled ligand (= donor) to the allophycocyanine (APC = acceptor)-labelled receptor brings the donor–acceptor pair into close proximity and energy transfer takes place, resulting in fluorescence emission at 665 nm.
Reproduced with kind permission of Cisbio.

Fluorescence polarization (FP)

When a stationary molecule is excited with plane-polarized light it will fluoresce in the same plane. If it is tumbling rapidly, in free solution, so that it changes its orientation between excitation and emission, the emission signal will be depolarized. Binding to a larger molecule reduces the mobility of the fluorophore so that the emission signal remains polarized, and so the ratio of polarized to depolarized emission can be used to determine the extent of binding of a labelled ligand (Figure 8.11; Nasir and Jolley, 1999). The rotational relaxation speed depends on the size of the molecule, the ambient temperature and the viscosity of the solvent, which usually remain constant during an assay.

The method requires a significant difference in size between labelled ligand and target, which is a major restriction to its application (Nosjean et al., 2006) and the reliance on a single, non-time resolved fluorescence output makes the choice of fluorphore important to minimize compound interference effects (Turek-Etienne et al., 2003). FP-based assays can be used in 96-well up to 1536-well formats.

Fluorescence correlation methods

Although an uncommon technique in most HTS departments, due the requirement for specific and dedicated instrumentation, this group of fluorescence technologies provide highly sensitive metrics using very low levels of detection reagents and are very amendable to ultra-high throughput screening (uHTS) (Eggeling et al., 2003). The most widely applied readout technology, *fluorescence correlation spectroscopy*, allows molecular interactions to be studied at the single-molecule level in real time. Other proprietary technologies such as fluorescence intensity distribution analysis (FIDA and 2-dimensional FIDA (Kask et al., 2000) also fall into this grouping, sharing the common theme of the analysis of biomolecules at extremely low concentrations. In contrast to other fluorescence techniques, the parameter of interest is not the emission intensity itself, but rather intensity fluctuations. By confining measurements to a very small detection volume (achieved by the use of confocal optics) and low reagent concentrations, the number of molecules monitored is kept small and the statistical fluctuations of the number contributing to the fluorescence signal at any instant become measurable. Analysis of the frequency components of such fluctuations can be used to obtain information about the kinetics of binding reactions.

With help of the confocal microscopy technique and laser technologies, it has become possible to measure molecular interactions at the single molecule level. Single molecule detection (SMD) technologies provide a number of advantages: significant reduction of signal-to-noise ratio, high sensitivity and time-resolution. Furthermore, they enable the simultaneous readout of various fluorescence parameters at the molecular level. SMD readouts include fluorescence intensity, translational diffusion (fluorescence correlation spectroscopy, FCS), rotational motion (fluorescence polarization), fluorescence resonance energy transfer, and time-resolved fluorescence. SMD technologies are ideal for miniaturization and have become amenable to automation (Moore et al., 1999). Further advantages include very low reagent consumption and broad applicability to a variety of biochemical and cell-based assays.

Single molecular events are analysed by means of confocal optics with a detection volume of approximately 1 fL, allowing miniaturization of HTS assays to 1 μL or below. The probability is that, at any given time, the detection volume will have a finite number of molecular events (movement, intensity, change in anisotropy), which can be measured and computed. The signal-to-noise ratio typically achieved by these methods is high, while interference from scattered laser light and background fluorescence are largely eliminated (Eigen and Rigler, 1994).

Fluorescence lifetime analysis (Moger et al., 2006) is a relatively straightforward assay methodology that overcomes many of the potential compound intereference effects achieved through the use of TRF, but without the requirement for expensive fluorophores. The technique utilizes the intrinsic lifetime of a fluorophore, corresponding to the time the molecule spends in the excited state. This time is altered upon binding of the fluorophore to a compound or protein and can be measured to develop robust assays that are liable to minimum compound intereference using appropriate detection instrumentation.

AlphaScreen™ Technology

The proprietary bead-based technology from Perkin Elmer is a proximity-based format utilizing a donor bead which,

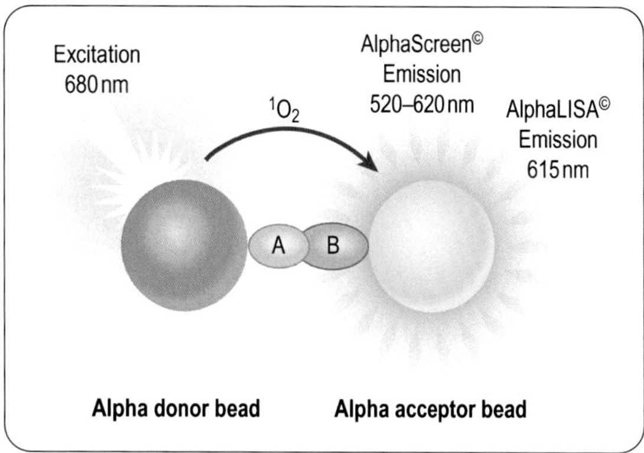

Fig. 8.9 Principle of AlphaScreen™ assays.
Reproduced with kind permission of Perkin Elmer.

when excited by light at a wavelength of 680 nm, releases singlet oxygen that is absorbed by an acceptor bead, and assuming it is in sufficiently close proximity (<200 nm) this results in the emission of light between 520 and 620 nm (Figure 8.9). This phenomenon is unusual in that the wavlength of the emitted light is shorter and therefore has higher energy than the excitation wavelength. This is of significance since it reduces the potential for compound inner filter effects; however, reactive functionality may still inhibit the energy transfer.

As with other bead-based technologies the donor and acceptor beads are available with a range of surface treatments to enable the immobilization or capture of a range of analytes. The range of immobolization formats and the distance over which the singlet oxygen can pass to excite the donor bead provide a suitable format for developing homogeneous antibody-based assays similar to enzyme-linked immunosorbent assays (ELISA) which are generally avoided in the HTS setting due to multiple wash, addition and incubation steps. These bead-based ELISA, such as AlphaLISA™ (Perkin Elmer), provide the required sensitivity for detection of biomarkers in low concentration and can be configured to low volume 384-well format without loss of signal window.

Cell-based assays

Readouts for cell-based assays

Readouts that can be used for cell-based assays are many and varied. In some cases, such as radioligand binding or enzyme activity, the readouts are essentially the same as those described above. Here we describe five cell-based readout technologies that have found general application in many types of assay, namely *fluorometric methods, reporter gene assays, yeast complementation assays, high-throughput electrophysiology assays* and more recently *label free detection platforms*. Some informative case histories of cell-based assays based on different readout principles have been presented by Johnston and Johnston (2002).

Fluorometric assays

Fluorometric assays are widely used to monitor changes in the intracellular concentration of ions or other constituents such as cAMP. A range of fluorescent dyes has been developed which have the property of forming reversible complexes with ions such as Ca^{2+} or Tl^{+} (as a surrogate for K^{+}). Their fluorescent emission intensity changes when the complex is formed, thereby allowing changes in the free intracellular ion concentration to be monitored, for example in response to activation or block of membrane receptors or ion channels, Other membrane-bound dyes are available whose fluorescence signal varies according to the cytoplasmic or mitochondrial membrane potential. Membrane-impermeable dyes which bind to intracellular structures can be used to monitor cell death, as only dying cells with leaky membranes are stained. In addition to dyes, ion-sensitive proteins such as the jellyfish photoprotein *aequorin* (see below), which emits a strong fluorescent signal when complexed with Ca^{2+}, can also be used to monitor changes in $[Ca^{2+}]_i$. Cell lines can be engineered to express this protein, or it can be introduced by electroporation. Such methods find many applications in cell biology, particularly when coupled with confocal microscopy to achieve a high level of spatial resolution. For HTS applications, the development of the Fluorescence Imaging Plate Reader (FLIPR™, Molecular Devices Inc., described by Schroeder and Negate, 1996), allowing the simultaneous application of reagents and test compounds to multiwell plates and the capture of the fluorescence signal from each well was a key advance in allowing cellular assays to be utilized in the HTS arena. Early instruments employed an argon laser to deliver the excitation light source with the emission measured using a CCD imaging device. In more recent models the laser has been replaced with an LED light source (www.moleculardevices.com) and overcomes some of the logistical considerations for deploying these instruments in some laboratories. Repeated measurements can be made at intervals of less than 1 s, to determine the kinetics of the cellular response, such as changes in $[Ca^{2+}]_i$ or membrane potential, which are often short-lasting, so that monitoring the time profile rather than taking a single snapshot measurement is essential.

Reporter gene assays

Gene expression in transfected eukaryotic cells can be quantified by linking a promoter sequence to a reporter gene, whose level of expression is readily monitored, and reflects the degree of activation or inhibition of the promoter (Naylor, 1999). Compounds activating or inhibiting the promoter itself, or interfering with a signal pathway connected to that promoter, can thus be detected. By using two different reporter constructs e.g. firefly and *Renilla* luciferase, different targets can be screened simultaneously (Kent et al., 2005). The principle of a reporter gene assay for GPCR activity, based on luciferase, is shown in Figure 8.10. Reporter readouts can also be duplexed with more

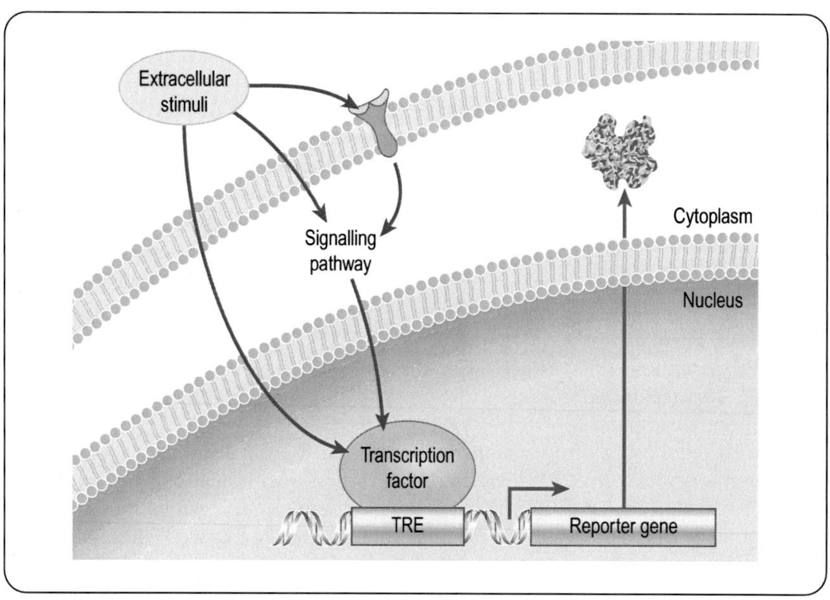

Fig. 8.10 Reporter gene assay principle for the detection of a ligand mediated signalling event in a cell based assay. Upon binding of a small molecule to the receptor the signalling cascade is initiated, resulting in the binding of a signalling mediator to a specific transcription factor response element, controlling the expression of the reporter protein.

immediate readouts of cell signalling, such as calcium sensitive dyes, to reduce the false positive liability associated with using a single assay readout (Hanson, 2006)

Commonly used reporter genes are CAT (chloramphenicol acetyltransferase), GAL (β-galactosidase), LAC (β-lactamase) (Zlokarnik et al., 1998), LUC (luciferase, Kolb and Neumann, 1996) and GFP (green fluorescence protein, Kain, 1999), usually employing a colorimetric or fluorescent readout and each having relative merits (Suto and Ignar, 1997). The number of reporter genes is dwarfed compared to the range of promoters that can be employed in this format, covering a diversity of signalling events.

Whilst having been widely deployed in the drug discovery process there are several limitations of reporter gene technology, not least because of the measurement of a response distal to the ligand interaction and the longer compound incubation times required, increasing the potential for cytotoxic events (Hill et al., 2001).

Yeast complementation assay

Yeast is a well-characterized organism for investigating mammalian systems, and the yeast two-hybrid assay is a powerful genetic screening technique for measuring the protein–protein and protein–DNA interactions that underlie many cellular control mechanisms (Tucker, 2002 and reviewed in Brückner et al., 2009). Widely applied in cell and systems biology to study the binding of transcription factors at the sequence level, it can also be used to screen small molecules for their interference with specific protein–protein and protein–DNA interactions, and has recently been adapted for other types of drug–target interactions (Fields and Song, 1989; Young et al., 1998; Serebriiskii et al., 2001). Conventional *in vitro* measurements, such as immunoprecipitation or chromatographic co-precipitation (Regnier, 1987; Phizicky and Fields, 1995), require the interacting proteins in pure form and at high concentrations, and therefore are often of limited use.

The yeast two-hybrid system uses two separated peptide domains of transcription factors: a DNA-specific binding part (DNB) and a transcription activation domain (AD). The DNB moiety is coupled to one protein (the 'bait'), and the AD moiety to another (the 'prey'). If the prey protein binds to the bait protein, the AD moiety is brought into close association with the reporter gene, which is thereby activated, producing a product (e.g. GAL or LAC, as described above, or an enzyme which allows the yeast to grow in the presence of cycloheximide). The addition of a test compound that blocks the specific protein–protein interaction prevents activation of the reporter gene. Serebriiskii et al. (2001) describe a project in which lead compounds able to block the activation of a specific N-type voltage-gated Ca^{2+} channel have been identified with a yeast two-hybrid assay. The bait and prey proteins contained domains of two different channel subunits which need to associate to form a functional channel.

High throughput electrophysiology assays

The progression of ion channels, and in particular voltage-gated ion channels, as druggable targets using screening approaches was, until recently, severely limited by the throughput of conventional electrophysiology techniques and lack of suitable higher throughput assay platforms. Although fluorescence methods using membrane potential sensitive dyes such as $DiBAC_4(3)$ and the FLIPR™ variants of this and the FRET based voltage sensor probes (Gonzalez and Maher, 2002) were widely used, the methodology could not provide accurate voltage control and the temporal resolution of the evoked responses was poor. The introduction of planar patch-clamp instruments, particularly systems such as IonWorks Quattro which record using multihole planar substrate consumables (Finkel et al., 2006, Southan and Clark, 2009) has to a certain extent overcome the throughput hurdle. The operating principle of this instrument is shown in Figure 8.11 and whilst the data point generation is not as high throughput so as to compete with fluorescence methods (a maximum of approximately 3000 data points per day per instrument compared with > 20 000 per day for a FLIPR™) it is sufficient for screening of targeted libraries, diverse compound decks up to around 100 000 compounds and the confirmation of a large number of hits identified in less physiologically relevant platforms.

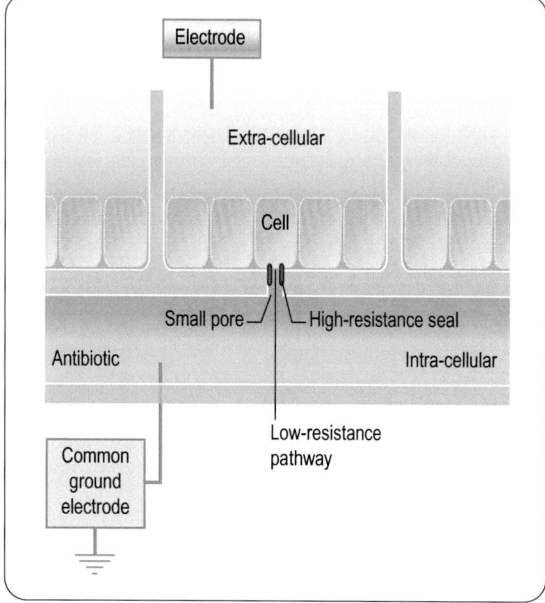

Fig. 8.11 Planar patch clamp, the underlying principle of high throughput electrophysiology.
Reproduced with kind permission of Molecular Devices.

Label free detection platforms

The current drive for the drug discovery process is to move towards as physiologically relevant systems as possible and away from target overexpression in heterologous expression systems and, in the case of G-protein coupled receptors, to avoid the use of promiscuous G-proteins where possible. The downside to this is that endogenous receptor expression levels tend to be lower and therefore more sensitive detection methods are required. Also, for the study of targets where the signalling mechanism is unknown, e.g. orphan GPCRs, multiple assay systems would need to be developed which would be time consuming and costly. Consequently, the application of assay platforms which detect gross cellular responses, usually cell morphology due to actin cytoskeleton remodelling, to physiological stimuli have been developed. These fall into two broad categories, those that detect changes in impedance through cellular dielectric spectroscopy (Ciambrone et al., 2004), e.g. CellKey™, Molecular Devices Corporation; xCelligence, Roche Diagnostics or the use of optical biosensors (Fang, 2006), e.g. Epic™, Corning Inc; or Octect, Fortebio. The application of these platforms in the HTS arena is still in its infancy largely limited by throughput and relatively high cost per data point compared to established methods. However, the assay development time is quite short, a single assay may cover a broad spectrum of cell signalling events and these methods are considered to be more sensitive than many existing methods enabling the use of endogenous receptor expression and even the use of primary cells in many instances (Fang et al., 2007; Minor, 2008).

High content screening

High content screening (HCS) is a further development of cell-based screening in which multiple fluorescence readouts are measured simultaneously in intact cells by means of imaging techniques. Repetitive scanning provides temporally and spatially resolved visualization of cellular events. HCS is suitable for monitoring such events as nuclear translocation, apoptosis, GPCR activation, receptor internalization, changes in $[Ca^{2+}]_i$, nitric oxide production, apoptosis, gene expression, neurite outgrowth and cell viability (Giuliano et al., 1997).

The aim is to quantify and correlate drug effects on cellular events or targets by simultaneously measuring multiple signals from the same cell population, yielding data with a higher content of biological information than is provided by single-target screens (Liptrot, 2001).

Current instrumentation is based on automated digital microscopy and flow cytometry in combination with hard and software systems for the analysis of data. Within the configuration a fluorescence-based laser scanning plate reader (96, 384- or 1536-well format), able to detect fluorescent structures against a less fluorescent background, acquires multicolour fluorescence image datasets of cells at a preselected spatial resolution. The spatial resolution is largely defined by the instrument specification and whether it is optical confocal or widefield. Confocal imaging enables the generation of high-resolution images by sampling from a thin cellular section and rejection of out of focus light; thus giving rise to improved signal : noise compared to the more commonly applied epi-fluorescence microscopy. There is a powerful advantage in confocal imaging for applications where subcellular localization or membrane translocation needs to be measured. However, for many biological assays, confocal imaging is not ideal e.g. where there are phototoxicity issues or the applications have a need for a larger focal depth.

HCS relies heavily on powerful image pattern recognition software in order to provide rapid, automated and unbiased assessment of experiments.

The concept of gathering all the necessary information about a compound at one go has obvious attractions, but the very sophisticated instrumentation and software produce problems of reliability. Furthermore, the principle of 'measure everything and sort it out afterwards' has its drawbacks: interpretation of such complex datasets often requires complex algorithms and significant data storage capacity. Whilst the complexity of the analysis may seem daunting, high content screening allows the study of complex signalling events and the use of phenotypic readouts in highly disease relevant systems. However, such analysis is not feasible for large number of compounds and unless the technology is the only option for screening in most instances HCS is utilized for more detailed study of lead compounds once they have been identified (Haney et al., 2006).

Biophysical methods in high-throughput screening

Conventional bioassay-based screening remains a mainstream approach for lead discovery. However, during recent years alternative biophysical methods such as nuclear magnetic resonance (NMR) (Hajduk and Burns, 2002), surface plasmon resonance (SPR) (Gopinath, 2010) and X-ray crystallography (Carr and Jhoti, 2002) have been developed and/or adapted for drug discovery. Usually in assays whose main purpose is the detection of low-affinity low-molecular-weight compounds in a different approach to high-throughput screening, namely *fragment-based screening*. Hits from HTS usually already have drug-like properties, e.g. a molecular weight of ~300 Da. During the following lead optimization synthesis programme an increase in molecular weight is very likely, leading to poorer drug-like properties with respect to solubility, absorption or clearance. Therefore, it may be more effective to screen small sets of molecular fragments (<10 000) of lower molecular weight (100–250 Da) which can then be chemically linked to generate high-affinity drug-like compounds. Typically, such fragments have much weaker binding affinities than drug-like compounds and are outside the sensitivity range of a conventional HTS assay. NMR-, SPR- or X-ray crystallography-based assays are better suited for the identification of weak binders as these methodologies lend themselves well to the area of fragment based screening. As the compound libraries screened are generally of limited size throughput is less important than sensitive detection of low-affinity interactions. Once the biophysical interactions are determined, further X-ray protein crystallographic studies can be undertaken to understand the binding mode of the fragments and this information can then be used to rapidly drive the fragment-to-hit or fragment-to-lead chemistry programme (Carr et al., 2005).

As discussed in Chapter 9, the chemical linkage of weak binding fragments can generate a high-affinity lead without violating the restrictions in molecular weight. The efficiency of this strategy has been demonstrated by several groups (Nienaber et al., 2000; Lesuisse et al., 2002).

Assay formats – miniaturization

Multiwell plates began to be used for screening in the early 1980s, before which time tube-based assays were routinely used in a low-throughput mode. The introduction of 96-well plates allowed the automation and miniaturization of biochemical experiments and was rapidly followed by the transition of many cell-based assays into the same density formats. The drive to increase throughput and reduce associated reagent costs has seen great advances in liquid handling and detection technologies since the 1990s with most vendors basing their approach on adaptation of the 96-well format to reduce the space between wells (the pitch) whilst maintaining an overall standard footprint and depth for the plate for the ease and constancy of instrument design (see Society for Laboratory Automation and Screening, www.slas.org/education/microplate.cfm). Reducing the pitch by one-half yields a four-fold increase in density to 384 wells per plate and a further two-fold reduction gives rise to 1536-well format plates. In both cases, the wells of these increased density plates can still be addressed using standard 96-well technology, although for liquid handling the reduced volumes and well area associated with the 1536-well formats present challenges for tip-based, displacement dispensing. To overcome this, the low-volume 384-well plate (Garyantes, 2002) has emerged as an important format, offering lower reagent usage per well whilst overcoming the issues of well access. In turn, the liquid-handling technologies to support 1536-well plates has developed significantly through the use of fixed tips or non-contact dispensing using piezo-electric dispensers or acoustic dispensing. These latter formats do not rely on tip-based technology and can dispense volumes as low as 2.5 nanolitres (Dunn and Feygin, 2000; Ellson et al., 2003).

Beyond the 96-, 384- and 1536-well arena there remains a drive for further increased density to 3456-well format (Kornienko et al., 2004) and micro-fluidics/lab-on-a-chip (Pihl et al., 2005) approaches to further reduce reagent usage.

Regardless of the microplate format adopted by a screening laboratory, the advances in microplates, liquid handling, plate stacking and handling devices, and sensitive reagents and detection instrumentation (such as CCD imagers) have advanced to the point where execution of a high throughput screen is rarely the bottleneck in drug discovery. Although as the density increases the time to develop a robust assay with low variability can also increase as the challenges of reagent evaporation and mixing are overcome.

Robotics in HTS

In many dedicated HTS facilities automation is employed to varying degrees to facilitate execution of the screen. This varies from the use of automated work stations with some manual intervention to the use of fully automated robotic platforms. During the assay development phases the key pieces of automation present in the automated platform will be used to ensure the assay is optimized correctly followed by transfer of the assay to a robotic workstation that can operate in high-throughput mode (typically up to 100 000 compounds per day at a single concentration). The robotic system consists of devices for storage, incubation and transportation of plates in different format; instruments for liquid transfer; and a series of plate readers for the various detection technologies. In many instances, these devices will be replicated on the same system to allow the screen to continue, albeit at lower throughput, should one device fail mid-run.

A typical robotic system is illustrated in Figure 8.12. Robotic arms and/or automated transport systems move plates between different devices. Plate storage devices ('hotels') and incubators are used for storage and incubation of microplates. Incubators can be cooled or heated; for mammalian cell cultivation they can also be supplied with CO_2 and are designed to facilitate automatic transfer of plates in and out. Compound plates are typically supplied with seals that can be perforated by the liquid handling devices to allow easy dilution and compound transfer to the assay plates. The assay plates themselves may either have removable lids or be sealed automatically once all reagents have been added. Stackers are sequential storage units for microtitre plates, connected to automated pipetting instruments and are equally common in laboratories where HTS is conducted without the large scale application of automation as they allow the scientists to walk away and return when the pipetting steps are complete. Various detection devices (enabling different modes of detection) are located at the output of the system before the assay plate, and usually the compound plate as well,

Detection devices
Liquid handling devices
Incubators
Temperature controlled storage
Bulk reagent dispensers/ dilutors
Plate sealer
Plate conveyor
(A)

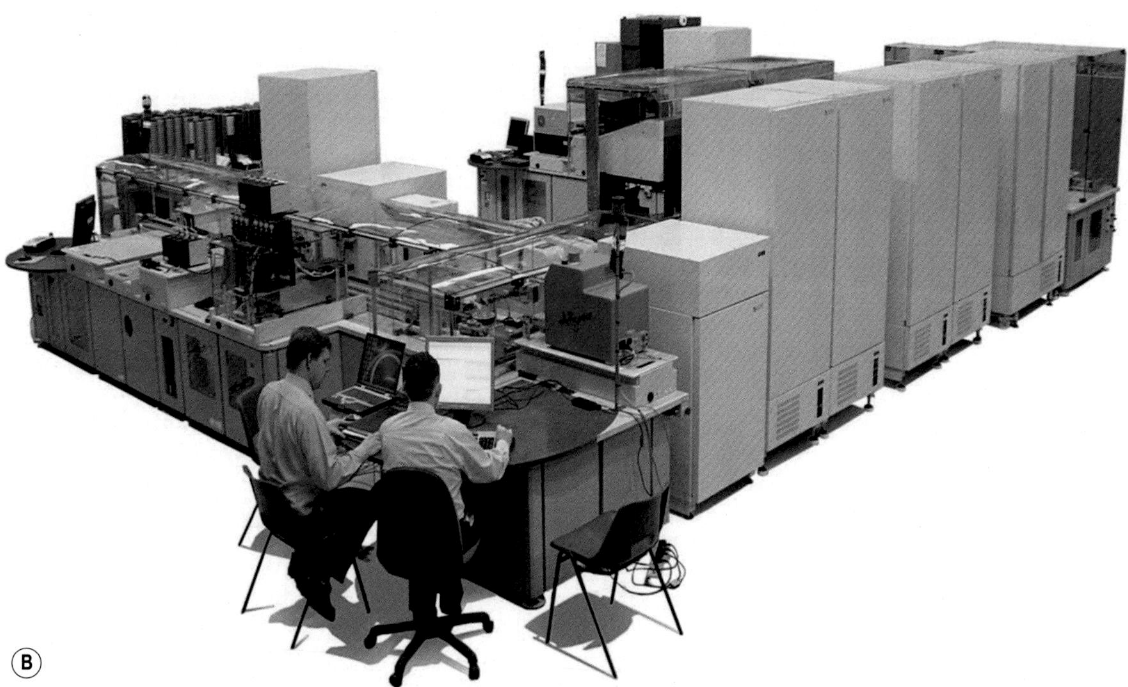
(B)

Fig. 8.12 Typical layout of fully automated high throughput screening platform. (A) Computer-aided design of the automated HTS work station and (B) photograph of the final installation.
Images supplied courtesy of the RTS Group, a leading supplier or laboratory automation, and Novartis.

are automatically discarded to waste. Central to the platform is the control (scheduling) software which controls the overall process including correct timing of different steps during the assay. This is critical, and ensures co-ordination of the use of the different devices (pipetters, incubators, readers etc.) to produce maximum efficiency. This software will also control recovery and/or continued operation of the platform, in the event of an error, without manual intervention. As one can imagine, programming and testing of the different process steps for individual screens can be a time-consuming part of the operation and frequently dedicated automation teams exist in large HTS departments to expedite this.

Before primary screening can start sample plates have to be prepared, which is usually done offline by separate automated liquid transfer systems (384-tip pipettes or acoustic dispensing devices). Compound storage plates, containing the library to be screened prepared as DMSO solutions, are delivered from the compound library warehouse and samples are further diluted with aqueous buffer to reach the desired compound and DMSO concentration for the assay. Samples are usually transferred to the assay plates by the robot during the assay run.

During the screening itself, all processes have to be monitored online to ensure the quality of the data obtained. The performance of the assay is continuously measured by calculating Z′ values for each plate (see earlier section). For this purpose, each screening plate includes high and low controls for quality analysis, in addition to the compounds for screening.

For the selection of positives a variety of methods may be applied based upon the control wells present on the assay plate. This hit threshold may be an arbitrary activity cut-off set across the screen or statistically based on a plate-by-plate or screen-wide basis and is then usually set at least three standard deviations away from the mean of the library signal (Brideau et al., 2003).

Data analysis and management

Owing to the large volume of data generated in HTS, efficient data management is essential. Software packages for HTS (e.g. ActivityBase, Spotfire, GeneData) are available to carry out the principal tasks:

- Storage of raw data
- Association of raw data with compound information
- Quality control
- Transformation of data into information
- Visualization
- Documentation
- Reporting.

In HTS each biochemical experiment in a single well is analysed by an automated device, typically a plate reader or other kind of detector. The output of these instruments comes in different formats depending on the type of reader. Where possible the HTS favours the use of a single 'end point' read rather than more time-consuming multiple or kinetic readings. However, the instrument itself may perform some initial calculations and these heterogeneous types of raw data are automatically transferred into the data management software. Assay plates are typically identified by a unique bar-code to relate the data to the compound plate layout. Ideally the plate reader will have an integral bar-code reader and the data file will be automatically named with the bar-code to provide an error-free association of the correct data file with the compounds tested.

In a next step raw data are translated into contextual information by calculating results. Data on percentage inhibition or percentage of control are normalized with values obtained from the high and low controls present in each plate. In secondary screening IC_{50}/EC_{50} and K_i values are also calculated. The values obtained depend on the method used (e.g. the fitting algorithm used for concentration–response curves) and have to be standardized for all screens within a company. Once the system captures the data it is then necessary to apply validation rules and techniques, such as trimmed means, to eliminate outliers (ideally using an automated algorithm) and to apply predetermined acceptance criteria to the data, for example, the signal-to-noise ratio, the Z′-value, or a test for gaussian distribution of the data. All plates that fail against one or more quality criteria are flagged and discarded.

The process may also involve a step to monitor visually the data that have been flagged, as a final check on quality. This is to ensure the system has performed correctly, i.e. no missed reagent dispense or patterns indicative of blocked dispenser tips or edge effects which may lead to false positives or negatives (Gunter et al., 2003). Whilst this inspection may be performed manually there are a number of software packages available, e.g. GeneData Assay Analyzer (www.genedata.com), which flag such errors and, in the case of edge effects, apply mathematical corrections to overcome them. Examples of validation data obtained in a typical screening of 100,000 compounds and some common data patterns revealed by tracking such parameters are shown in Figure 8.13. In addition to tracking high and low control values, most HTS departments also include quality-control plates at regular intervals throughout an assay run which contain standard compounds to allow target pharmacology to be monitored.

On completion of the screen it is advisable to plot a distribution histogram of the compound data against the control well populations and any other quality-control wells that have been included (Figure 8.14). The median of the test wells should be the same as the null control population and, if the assay is robust as demonstrated by the Z′ value, there will be good separation between the two control well populations. The variability of the null control population can be used to determine an

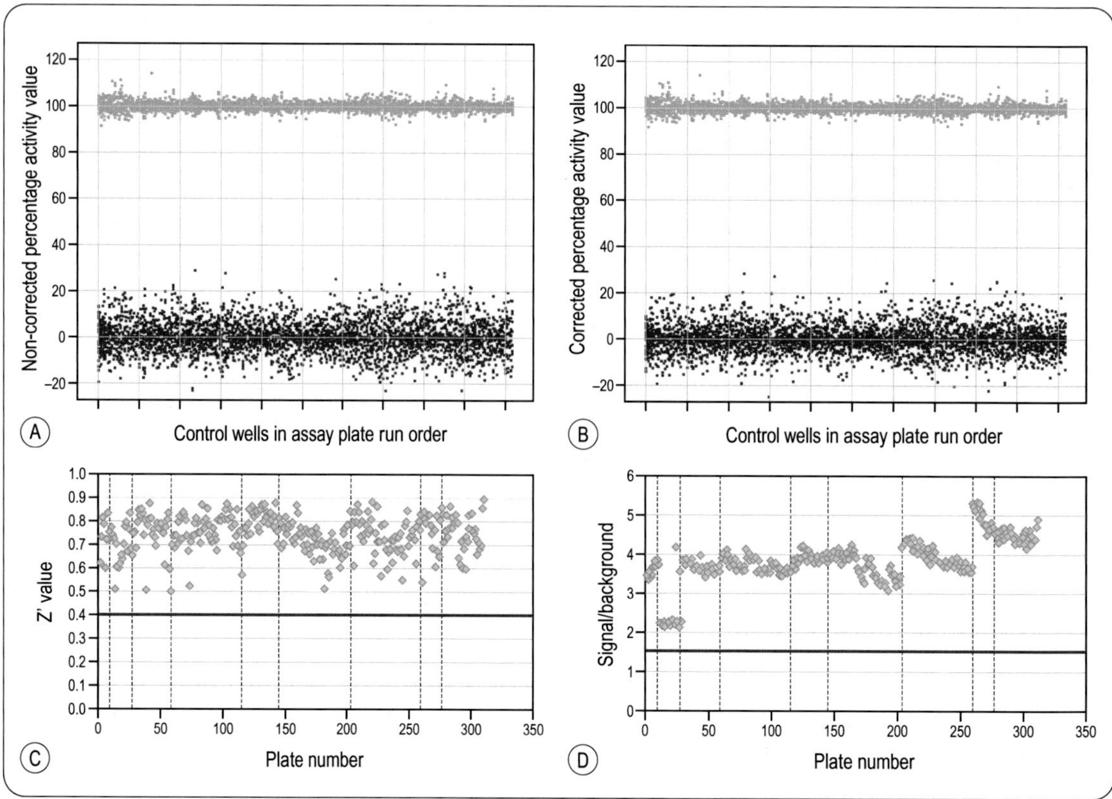

Fig. 8.13 Data validation checks in a typical screening assay. Distribution of high (green symbols) and low controls (red symbols) (% inhibition) in a set of screening plates. Each marker represents one well. Panel (A) shows the original data and (B) is the same data following treatment with GeneData Assay Analyzer to take account of spatially induced effects. Note the reduction in variability of the low control well data. (C) Z′ values and (D) signal to background ratios from an HTS campaign. The plate run order is shown on the x-axis and vertical dashed line divide each screening run, the horizontal lines at Z′ = 0.5 and signal-to-background = 1.5 represents the quality control pass levels and each data point represents on assay plate. The data demonstrate a decline in assay performance during each screening day. The marked change in rate of assay performance deterioration after plate 150 correlates with a change in the batch of a key assay component.
Data kindly supplied by BioFocus, with permission.

acceptable cut-off level for selecting the hit compounds for further progression.

In addition to registering the test data, all relevant information about the assay has to be logged, for example the supplier and batch of reagents, storage conditions, a detailed assay protocol, plate layout, and algorithms for the calculation of results. Each assay run is registered and its performance documented. If assay performance is charted any significant change in assay quality can be reviewed and if caused by reagent change readily identified

HTS will initially deliver hits in targeted assays. Retrieval of these data has to be simple, and the data must be exchangeable between different project teams to generate knowledge from the mass of data.

SCREENING LIBRARIES AND COMPOUND LOGISTICS

Compound logistics

In the drug discovery value chain the effective management of compound libraries is a key element and is usually handled by a dedicated compound logistics group, either within the screening organization or at a specialist outsourcing provider. The compound management facility is the central port for transshipment of compounds in lead discovery, not only for primary screening, but also during the hit-to-lead phase. It is the unit responsible for

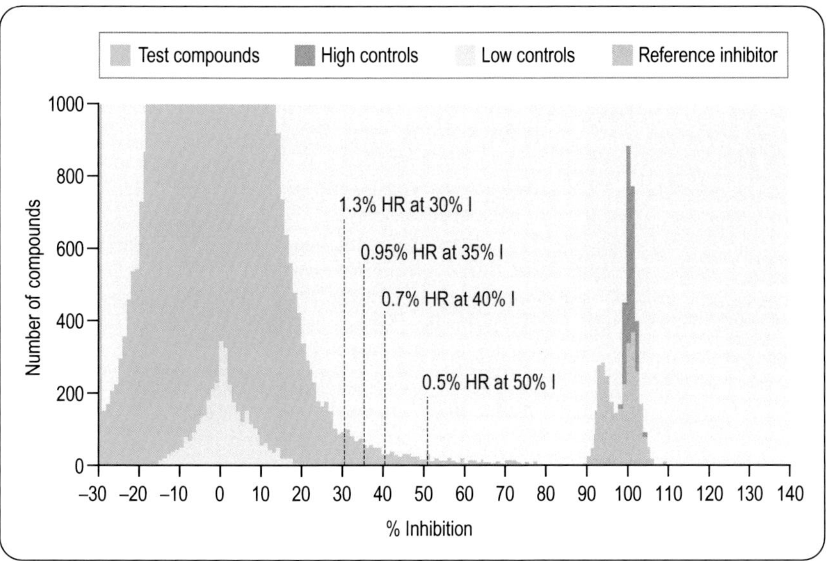

Fig. 8.14 Histogram analysis of compound activity against control well populations from a screen to identify antagonists of a G-protein coupled receptor. The median of the compound wells is in line with the null control population. The hit rate (% HR) associated with selecting each of the percentage inhibition value (% I) is as indicated. As the percentage inhibition is lowered the confidence in the reality of the hit is reduced; however, these compounds can provide useful information on the hit series being identified. Note the reference compound controls appear to fall into two populations. This is associated with the change in reagent batch as described in Figure 8.13.

Data kindly supplied by BioFocus, with permission.

registration of samples, their preparation, storage and retrieval. This facility has to ensure global compound accessibility, both individually and in different formats; maintain compound integrity (quality control and proper storage); guarantee error-free compound handling; guarantee efficient compound use; and guarantee a rapid response to compound requests.

Many pharmaceutical companies have greatly increased both the size and quality of their compound collection. Screening libraries frequently exceed 1,000,000 compounds and originate from many different sources with variable quality, although there has been great attention to how the assays themselves are impacted by poor compound quality, particularly solubility (Di and Kerns, 2006). This has necessitated both hardware and software automation of compound management in order to cope with the increasing demands of HTS and lead discovery.

Most advanced systems use fully automated robotics for handling compounds (Figure 8.15). Compounds used for screening are stored as liquids in microtitre plates in a controlled environment (temperature –4 °C to –20 °C; low humidity or storage under an inert atmosphere and control of freeze-thaw cycles) and numerous studies have been undertaken to identify the most appropriate conditions to maintain compound stability (e.g. Blaxill et al., 2009).

Splitting the collection into a number of copies in different formats secures a balance between fast response times to the various compound requests and optimal storage conditions. Different sets of compound libraries are needed, depending on the target and project specifications with the preferred storage format of the compound collection being dictated by the chosen screening plate density, i.e. 384- or 1536-well.

Because library sets are not static, as new compounds are continuously being added, samples in the repository need to be individually addressable to allow a flexible and quick rearrangement of existing libraries to more specific, focused collections. Advanced compound logistic systems store compound libraries in a single tube system so that individual tubes can be accessed without the need to take out a whole plate from the storage facility.

This functionality is a prerequisite for efficient 'cherry picking'. After primary screening, positive compounds have to be confirmed in secondary assays and concentration–response curves determined. The individual active compounds have to be located and reformatted in microtitre plates. With a large number of targets and projects running at any one time, a highly automated compound handling systems is needed to do this efficiently.

PROFILING

High-throughput screening, the subject of this chapter, has as its first objective the identification of a few 'validated

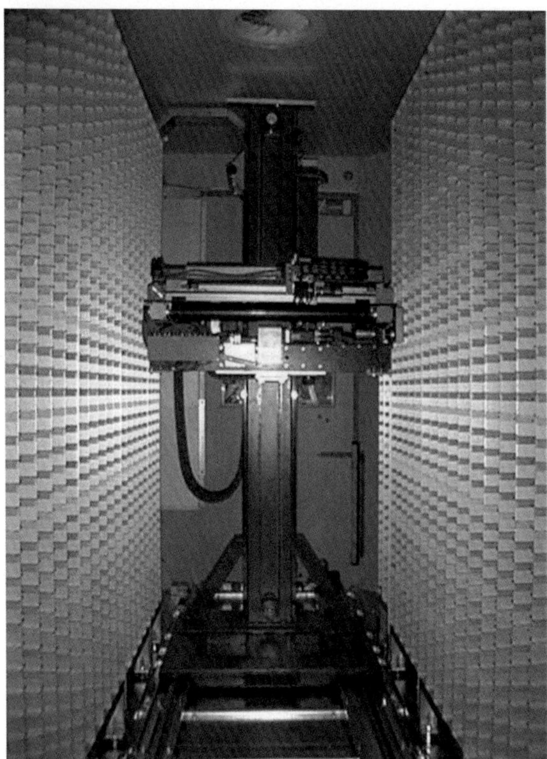

Fig. 8.15 Storage of a compound screening collection in 384-well plates at −4°C. A robot is able to move around and collect the plates or individual samples specified in the compound management software.

hits' (defined in Chapter 9) within large compound libraries. The decision as to whether a particular hit is worth pursuing as a chemical lead in a drug discovery project depends on several factors, important ones being its chemical characteristics and its pharmacodynamic and pharmacokinetic properties. These aspects, broadly covered by the term 'compound profiling', are discussed in detail in the next three chapters.

The technology involved in miniaturization, automation and assay readouts required for HTS has developed rapidly and continues to do so. As this technology evolves, the laboratory set-ups installed in HTS facilities are steadily broadening their capabilities beyond their primary function of identifying hits to apply HTS techniques to more diverse compound profiling assays relating not only to the target selectivity of compound libraries, but also to their pharmacokinetic characteristics. Increasingly, therefore, early compound profiling tasks on 'hit' compounds are being carried out in HTS laboratories where the necessary technological expertise is concentrated. Such assays are also very helpful in the 'lead identification' stage of a project, where focused synthetic compound libraries based on the initial hits need to be assessed. As this work generally involves testing small compound libraries, usually fewer than 1000 compounds at a time, in several different assays, small dedicated robotic workstations are needed, rather than the fast but inflexible factory-style robotic assemblies used for large-scale HTS.

In vitro pharmacokinetic assays (see Chapter 10), which are not generally project specific and can be automated to run in medium-throughput fashion, are very suitable for running in this environment. This extension of the work of HTS laboratories beyond the primary task of finding hits is a clear and continuing trend, for which the term 'high-throughput profiling' (HTP) has been coined. It brings the work of HTS laboratories into a close and healthy relationship with drug discovery teams. The highly disciplined approach to assay formats and data logging that is essential for HTS, but not second nature to many laboratory scientists, brings the advantage that profiling data collected over a wide range of projects and drug targets is logged in standard database formats, and is therefore a valuable company-wide tool for analysing structure–activity relationships. This necessity to handle and visualize such data has driven the development software packages such as Spotfire (spotfire.tibco.com).

In summary, it is clear that pharmacological profiling will be an increasing activity of HTS units in the future, and will help to add further value in the drug discovery chain.

REFERENCES

Achard S, Jean A, Lorphelin D, et al. Homogeneous assays allow direct 'in well' cytokine level quantification. Assay and Drug Development Technologies 2003;1(supplement 2): 181–5.

Alpha B, Lehn JM, Mathis G. Energy-transfer luminescence of europium(III) and terbium(III) with macrobicyclic polypyridine ligands. Angewandte Chemie 1987;99:259–61.

Bays N, Hill A, Kariv I. A simplified scintillation proximity assay for fatty acid synthase activity: development and comparison with other FAS activity assays. Journal of Biomolecular Screening 2009;14: 636–42.

Beske O, Goldbard S. High-throughout cell analysis using multiplexed array technologies. Drug Discovery Today 2002;7:S131–5.

Beveridge M, Park YW, Hermes J, et al. Detection of p56(lck) kinase activity using scintillation proximity assay in 384-well format and imaging proximity assay in 384- and 1536-well format. Journal of

Biomolecular Screening 2000;5:205–12.

Birzin ET, Rohrer SP. High-throughput receptor-binding methods for somatostatin receptor 2. Analytical Biochemistry 2002;307:159–66.

Blaxill Z, Holland-Crimmen S, Lifely R. Stability through the ages: the GSK experience. Journal of Biomolecular Screening 2009;14:547–56.

Bosworth N, Towers P. Scintillation proximity assay. Nature 1989;341:167–8.

Braunwaler AF, Yarwood DR, Hall T, et al. A solid-phase assay for the determination of protein tyrosine kinase activity of c-src using scintillating microtitration plates. Analytical Biochemistry 1996;234:23–6.

Brideau C, Gunter B, Pikounis B, et al. Improved statistical methods for hit selection in high-throughput screening. Journal of Biomolecular Screening 2003;8:634–47.

Brown BA, Cain M, Broadbent J, et al. FlashPlate technology. In: Devlin PJ, editor. High-throughput screening. New York: Marcel Dekker; 1997. p. 317–28.

Brückner A, Polge C, Lentze N, et al. Yeast two-hybrid, a powerful tool for systems biology. International Journal of Molecular Science 2009;10:2763–88.

Carr R, Congreve M, Murray C, et al. Fragment-based lead discovery: leads by design. Drug Discovery Today 2005;10:987–92.

Carr R, Jhoti H. Structure-based screening of low-affinity compounds. Drug Discovery Today 2002;7: 522–7.

Ciambrone G, Liu V, Lin D, et al. Cellular dielectric spectroscopy: a powerful new approach to label-free cellular analysis. Journal of Biomolecular Screening 2004;9:467–80.

Clegg RM. Fluorescence resonance energy transfer. Current Opinion in Biotechnology 1995;6: 103–10.

Clemons P. Complex phenotypic assays in high-throughput screening. Current Opinions in Chemical Biology 2004;8:334–8.

Comley J. Assay interference a limiting factor in HTS? Drug Discovery World Summer 2003;91.

Comley J. TR-FRET based assays – getting better with age. Drug Discovery World Spring 2006;22–37.

Congreve M, Chessari G, Tisi D, et al. Recent developments in fragment-based drug discovery. Journal of Medicinal Chemistry 2008;51: 3661–80.

Cook ND. Scintillation proximity assay: a versatile high-throughput screening technology. Drug Discovery Today 1996;1:287–94.

Di L, Kerns E. Biological assay challenges from compound solubility: strategies for bioassay optimization. Drug Discovery Today 2006;11:446–51.

Dunn D, Feygin I. Challenges and solutions to ultra-high-throughput screening assay miniaturization: submicroliter fluid handling. Drug Discovery Today 2000;5(Suppl. 12): S84–91.

Eggeling C, Brand L, Ullmann D, et al. Highly sensitive fluorescence detection technology currently available for HTS. Drug Discovery Today 2003;8:632–41.

Ehrlich P, Bertheim A. Berichte. 1912;4:756.

Eigen M, Rigler R. Sorting single molecules: application to diagnostics and evolutionary biotechnology. Proceedings of the National Academy of Sciences of the USA 1994;91:5740–7.

Ellson R, Mutz M, Browning B, et al. Transfer of low nanoliter acoustics – automation considerations. Journal of the Association for Laboratory Automation 2003;8:29–34.

Fang Y. Label-free cell-based assays with optical biosensors in drug discovery. Assay and Drug Development Technologies 2006;4:583–95.

Fang Y, Guangshan L, Ferrie A. Non-invasive optical biosensor for assaying endogenous G protein-coupled receptors in adherent cells. Journal of Pharmacological and Toxicological Methods 2007; 55:314–22.

Fields S, Song O. A novel genetic system to detect protein–protein interactions. Nature 1989;340:245–6.

Finkel A, Wittel A, Yang N, et al. Population patch clamp improves data consistency and success rates in the measurement of ionic currents. Journal of Biomolecular Screening 2006;11:488–96.

Fligge T, Schuler A. Integration of a rapid automated solubility classification into early validation of hits obtained by high throughput screening. Journal of Pharmaceutical and Biomedical Analysis 2006;42:449–54.

Garyantes TK. 1536-well assay plates: when do they make sense? Drug Discovery Today 2002;7: 489–90.

Ghosh S, Nie A, An J, et al. Structure-based virtual screening of chemical libraries for drug discovery. Current Opinion in Chemical Biology 2006;10:194–202.

Giuliano KA, de Basio RL, Dunlay RT, et al. High-content screening: a new approach to easing key bottlenecks in the drug recovery process. Journal of Biomolecular Screening 1997;2:249–59.

Gonzalez J, Maher M. Cellular fluorescent indicators and voltage/ ion probe reader (VIPR(tm)): tools for ion channel and receptor drug discovery. Receptors and Channels 2002;8:283–95.

Gopinath S. Biosensing applications of surface plasmon resonance-based Biacore technology. Sensors and Actuators B 2010;150:722–33.

Gribbon P, Sewing A. Fluorescence readouts in HTS: no gain without pain? Drug Discovery Today 2003;8:1035–43.

Gunter B, Brideau C, Pikounis B, et al. Statistical and graphical methods for quality control determination of high-throughput screening data. Journal of Biomolecular Screening 2003;8:624–33.

Hajduk PJ, Burns DJ. Integration of NMR and high-throughput screening. Combinatorial Chemistry High Throughput Screening 2002;5:613–21.

Hallis T, Kopp A, Gibson J, et al. An improved beta-lactamase reporter assay: multiplexing with a cytotoxicity readout for enhanced accuracy of hit identification. Journal of Biomolecular Screening 2007;12:635–44.

Haney S, LaPan P, Pan J, et al. High-content screening moves to the front of the line. Drug Discovery Today 2006;11:889–94.

Hanson B. Multiplexing Fluo-4 NW and a GeneBLAzer® transcriptional assay for high-thoughput screening of G-protein-coupled receptors. Journal of Biomolecular Screening 2006;11:644–51.

Hartshorn M, Murray C, Cleasby A, et al. Fragment-based lead discovery using X-ray crystallography. Journal of Medicinal Chemistry 2005;48:403–13.

Haugland RP. Handbook of fluorescent probes and chemical research, 9th edn. Molecular Probes. Web edition: www.probes.com/handbook, 2002.

Hemmilä I, Hurskainen P. Novel detection strategies for drug discovery. Drug Discovery Today 2002;7:S150–6.

Hill S, Baker G, Rees S. Reporter-gene systems for the study of G-protein-coupled receptors. Current Opinion in Pharmacology 2001;1:526–32.

Jia Y, Quinn C, Gagnon A, et al. Homogeous time-resolved fluorescence and its applications for kinase assays in drug discovery. Analytical Biochemistry 2006;356:273–81.

Johnston PA, Johnston PA. Cellular platforms for HTS: three case studies. Drug Discovery Today 2002;7:353–63.

Kain RK. Green fluorescent protein (GFP): applications in cell-based assays for drug discovery. Drug Discovery Today 1999;4:304–12.

Karvinen J, Hurskainen P, Gopalakrishnan S, et al. Homogeneous time-resolved fluorescence quenching assay (LANCE) for Caspase-3. Journal of Biomolecular Screening 2002;7:223–31.

Kask P, Palo K, Fay N, et al. Two-dimensional fluorescence intensity distribution analysis: theory and applications. Biophysics Journal 2000;78:1703–13.

Kent T, Thompson K, Naylor L. Development of a generic dual-reporter gene assay for screening G-protein-couped receptors. Journal of Biomolecular Screening 2005;10:437–46.

Kolb AJ, Neumann K. Luciferase measurements in high throughput screening. Journal of Biomolecular Screening 1996;1:85–8.

Kornienko O, Lacson R, Kunapuli P, et al. Miniaturization of whole live cell-based GPCR assays using microdispensing and detection systems. Journal of Biomolecular Screening 2004;9:186–95.

Kroeze W, Sheffler D, Roth B. G-protein-coupled receptors at a glance. Journal of Cell Science 2003;116: 4867–9.

Lakowicz JR. Principles of fluorescence spectroscopy. New York: Plenum Press; 1999.

Lee P, Miller S, Van Staden C, et al. Development of a homogeneous high-throughput live-cell G-protein-coupled receptor binding assay. Journal of Biomolecular Screening 2008;13:748–54.

Leopoldo M, Lacivita E, Berardi F, et al. Developments in fluorescent probes for receptor research. Drug Discovery Today 2009;14:706–12.

Lesuisse D, Lange G, Deprez P, et al. SAR and X-ray. A new approach combining fragment-based screening and rational drug design: application to the discovery of nanomolar inhibitors of Src SH2. Journal of Medicinal Chemistry 2002;45:2379–87.

Liptrot C. High content screening – from cells to data to knowledge. Drug Discovery Today 2001;6:832–4.

Minor L. Label-free cell-based functional assays. Combinatorial Chemistry and High Throughput Screening 2008;11:573–80.

Moger J, Gribon P, Sewing A, et al. The application of fluorescence lifetime readouts in high-throughput screening. Journal of Biomolecular Screening 2006;11:765–72.

Moore K, Rees S. Cell-based versus isolated target screening: how lucky do you feel? Journal of Biomolecular Screening 2001;6:69–74.

Moore KJ, Turconi S, Ashman S, et al. Single molecule detection technologies in miniaturized high throughput screening: fluorescence correlation spectroscopy. Journal of Biomolecular Screening 1999;4:335–54.

Muegge I, Oloff S. Advances in virtual screening. Drug Discovery Today: Technologies 2006;3:405–11.

Nasir MS, Jolley ME. Fluorescence polarization: an analytical tool for immunoassay and drug discovery. Combinatorial Chemistry High Throughput Screening 1999;2:177–90.

Naylor L. Reporter gene technology: the future looks bright. Biochemical Pharmacology 1999;58:749–57.

Nienaber VL, Richardson PL, Klighofer V, et al. Discovering novel ligands for macromolecules using X-ray crystallographic screening. Nature Biotechnology 2000;18:1105–8.

Nosjean O, Souchaud S, Deniau C, et al. A simple theoretical model for fluorescence polarization binding assay development. Journal of Biomolecular Screening 2006;11:949–58.

Phizicky EM, Fields S. Protein–protein interactions: methods for detection and analysis. Microbiology Review 1995;59:94–123.

Pihl J, Karlsson M, Chiu D. Microfluidics technologies in drug discovery. Drug Discovery Today 2005;10:1377–83.

Regnier FE. Chromatography of complex protein mixtures. Journal of Chromatography 1987;418: 115–43.

Ramm P. Imaging systems in assay screening. Drug Discovery Today 1999;4:401–10.

Rees D, Congreve M, Murray C, et al. Fragment-based lead discovery. Natures Reviews Drug Discovery 2004;3:660–72.

Russ A, Lampel S. The druggable genome: an update. Drug Discovery Today 2005;10:1607–10.

Schroeder KS, Negate BD. FLIPR, a new instrument for accurate high-throughput optical screening. Journal of Biomolecular Screening 1996;1:75–80.

Serebriiskii IG, Khazak V, Golemis EA. Redefinition of the yeast two-hybrid system in dialogue with changing priorities in biological research. Biotechniques 2001;30:634–55.

Sittampalam GS, Kahl SD, Janzen WP. High-throughput screening: advances in assay technologies. Current Opinion in Chemistry and Biology 1997;1:384–91.

Southan A, Clark G. Recent technological advances in electrophysiology based screening technology and the impact upon ion channel discovery research. High Throughput Screening: Methods and

Protocols (Methods in Molecular Biology) 2009;565:187–208.

Stahura F, Xue L, Godden J, et al. Methods for compound selection focused on hits and application in drug discovery. Journal of Molecular Graphics and Modelling 2002;20:439–46.

Sui Y, Wu Z. Alternative statistical parameter for high-thoughput screening assay quality assessment. Journal of Biomolecular Screening 2007;12:229–34.

Suto C, Ignar D. Selection of an optimal reporter gene for cell-based high throughput screening assays. Journal of Biomolecular Screening 1997;2:7–9.

Titus S, Neumann S, Zheng W, et al. Quantitative high-throughput screening using a live-cell cAMP assay identifies small-molecule agonists of the TSH receptor. Journal of Biomolecular Screening 2008;13:120–7.

Trinquet E, Fink M, Bazin H, et al. D-*myo*-Inositol 1-phosphate as a surrogate of D-*myo*-inositol 1,4,5-tris phosphate to monitor G protein-coupled receptor activation. Analytical Biochemistry 2006;358:126–35.

Tucker C. High-throughput cell-based assays in yeast. Drug Discovery Today 2002;7:S125–30.

Turek-Etienne T, Small E, Soh S, et al. Evaluation of fluorescent compound interference in 4 fluorescence polarization assays: 2 kinases, 1 protease and 1 phosphatase. Journal of Biomolecular Screening 2003;8:176–84.

Valenzano KJ, Miller W, Kravitz JN, et al. Development of a fluorescent ligand-binding assay using the AcroWell filter plate. Journal of Biomolecular Screening 2000;5:455–61.

Valler MJ, Green D. Diversity screening versus focussed screening in drug discovery. Drug Discovery Today 2000;5:286–93.

Waszkowycz B. Towards improving compound selection in structure-based virtual screening. Drug Discovery Today 2008;13: 219–26.

Young K, Lin S, Sun L, et al. Identification of a calcium channel modulator using a high throughput yeast two-hybrid screen. National Biotechnology 1998;16: 946–50.

Zhang JH, Chung TD, Oldenburg KR. A simple statistical parameter for use in evaluation and validation of high-throughput screening assays. Journal of Biomolecular Screening 1999;4:67–73.

Zlokarnik G, Negulescu PA, Knapp TE, et al. Quantitation of transcription and clonal selection of single living cells with beta-lactamase as reporter. Science 1998;279:84–8.

Chapter 9

The role of medicinal chemistry in the drug discovery process

P Beswick, A Naylor

INTRODUCTION

Clinically the unmet need for novel and safe drugs is becoming more significant due to increasing longevity in the developed world and the consequential increased prevalence of age-related diseases such as cancer and dementia. Whilst few would dispute that the role of the medicinal chemist is pivotal to the discovery of new medicines to address this growing need, and will continue to be so for the foreseeable future, the environment in which the medicinal chemist operates has changed dramatically over the last 5–10 years. Despite many years of rising investment in R&D, the productivity of major Pharma, in terms of New Chemical Entities (NCEs) delivered to the patient, has not improved over the past 10 years. In 2009 only nineteen NCEs were approved by the FDA, two less than in 2008 (Hughes, 2010) (Figure 9.1; see also Chapter 22). The approval of six biological licence applications in 2009, compared with three in 2008, is perhaps the first indication of the greater emphasis which Pharma is placing on the discovery of biological therapeutic agents. However, the challenges and current limitations of such treatments are such that small molecule discovery is likely to remain the mainstay of therapeutic innovation for at least the next 20 years (but see also Chapter 22).

Whilst a detailed discussion of the reasons behind Pharma's poor level of productivity is beyond the scope of this chapter (see Chapter 22), it is clear that the high level of attrition in the clinic, due to lack of clinical efficacy and insufficient safety margins, is a major component and it is appropriate to consider what role the medicinal chemist might play in addressing this challenge in the future. The high level of attrition in the clinic due to lack of sufficient efficacy reflects an inadequate understanding of disease pathophysiology in man and the poor predictability of many of the preclinical animal models of human disease. Thus there is a pressing need to improve the quality of validation of novel targets, placing less emphasis on preclinical in vivo models and single gene 'knock-outs', and a greater emphasis on cellular pathways, genetically associated targets and innovative clinical trial design. This approach will require the availability of selective chemical tools with which to validate targets in human tissue and thus the role of the medicinal chemist in the future may incorporate a greater component of chemical biology. The increasing trend towards academic target and drug discovery is also likely to place greater emphasis on chemical biology skills.

Despite stringent toxicity evaluation during the discovery phase, an unacceptable level of failure due to safety issues remains. The present situation is arguably worse than 20 years ago as there has been a trend towards molecules failing later in the safety evaluation process, incurring greater cost and time. If significant impact is to be made on this source of attrition it will be important for the medicinal chemist to develop a rational understanding of possible structural and physicochemical determinants of toxicity in much the same way as the determinants of oral bioavailability have been recognized. However, this objective is likely to be much more challenging due to the diverse and complex nature of the multiple pathologies. Preliminary studies to evaluate this approach have been recently reported and will be discussed later in the chapter.

It is clear that addressing the challenges described above and raising productivity will require long-term investment and persistence. However, due to the immediate financial pressures, the industry has responded to the productivity challenge by minimizing costs, shifting focus to cheaper sources of chemistry, predominantly in the Far East, and in-licensing assets. Thus today's medicinal chemist is required to optimally integrate a network of both internal

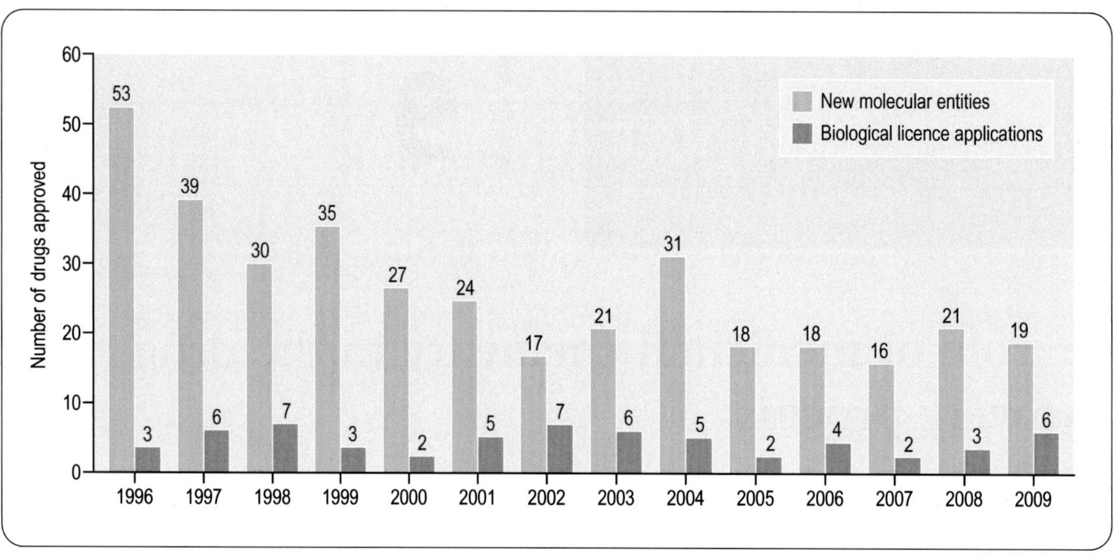

Fig. 9.1 Recent trends in small molecule approvals and biological licence applications – *reproduced with the kind permission of Nature publishing.*

and external resources to prosecute the identification of development candidates.

Whilst medicinal chemistry is facing unprecedented pressures due to the volatility of the sector, it is clear that small molecule therapeutics will be required for the foreseeable future and that, whatever infrastructure evolves within the industry, the medicinal chemist will have a key role to play. This chapter will discuss some of the recent scientific advances in the field which will enable the medicinal chemist to rise to the challenges ahead.

TARGET SELECTION AND VALIDATION

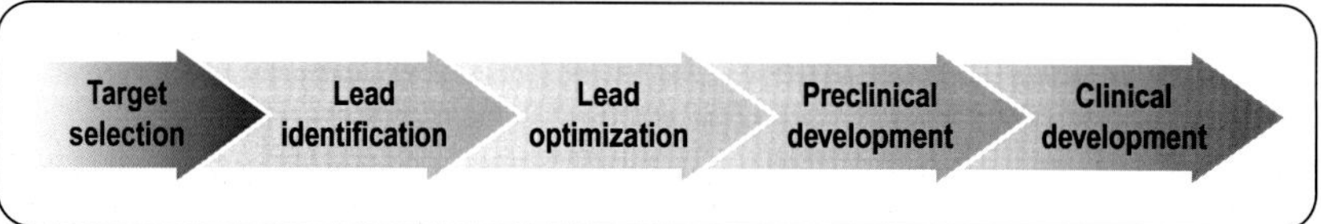

A key challenge in increasing the industry's productivity will be the selection of targets which have compelling validation in terms of both efficacy and safety in the human context and, which, consequently, have a greater probability of achieving a successful clinical proof of concept. The role of the medicinal chemist has previously focused primarily on ensuring the quality of preclinical candidate molecules in terms of potency, selectivity and physicochemical properties such as those highlighted initially by Lipinski et al. (Lipinski CA, 1997) and, more recently, by others (Leeson PD and Springthorpe B, 2007). As a result, the level of attrition due to poor ADME properties fell dramatically between 1991 and 2000 (Kola I and Landis J, 2004), but the level of clinical success with new mechanisms remains poor. However, chemists are now increasingly becoming engaged, along with their biology and clinical counterparts, in the process of selecting and prioritizing future protein targets. In particular the development of an in-depth understanding of the structural biology of the target and the biophysics of its interaction with low-molecular-weight ligands is a critical component at the outset of a project and very much in the chemist's domain. The necessity for a rigorous analysis of potential targets cannot be over-emphasized since this occurs at the start of the 12–15-year period of intensive effort and investment required to achieve the launch of a new medicine into large scale clinical usage. The post genomic era has provided the industry with a plethora of potential drug targets; however, the selection of tractable targets with a high probability of delivering safe and effective treatments represents a huge challenge requiring a multidisciplinary approach.

Whilst a detailed discussion of the complex facets of target validation is beyond the scope of this chapter (see Chapter 6), it is clear that targets with strong genetic associations, such as the voltage-gated sodium channel $NaV_{1.7}$ (Dib-Hajj SD et al., 2007), with potential utility in the treatment of pain, and the chemokine CCR_5 receptor (Westby M and van der Ryst E, 2005), which has led to the discovery of treatments for HIV infection, exemplify an aspirational level of target validation.

Whilst genetic disease-association data provide strong evidence of target involvement, target modulation, ideally within a human cellular pathway, provides compelling validation, and the identification of early chemical probes in addition to subsequent lead molecules will be an important challenge for the medicinal chemist in the future.

Frye has recently described (Frye SV, 2010) essential features of a quality chemical probe which are summarised below:

Molecular profiling. Sufficient *in vitro* potency and selectivity data to confidently associate its *in vitro* profile to its cellular or *in vivo* profile.
Mechanism of action. Activity in a cell-based or cell-free assay influences a physiologic function of the target in a dose-dependent manner.
Identity of the active species. Has sufficient chemical and physical property data to interpret results as due to its intact structure or a well-characterized derivative.
Proven utility as a probe. Cellular activity data available to confidently address at least one hypothesis about the role of the molecular target in a cell's response to its environment.
Availability. Is readily available to the academic community with no restrictions on use.

The first four criteria attempt to describe ideal properties of a probe whilst the last point addresses a more philosophical viewpoint on the sharing of precompetitive information. Further evolution of this 'wish list' will inevitably take place in the future.

It is well known that target classes are associated with different levels of tractability with respect to the probability of being able to identify quality lead molecules. For example the G-protein coupled receptor (GPCR) superfamily is generally considered to be one of the most tractable target classes with approximately 40% of prescription drugs in current practice producing efficacy via modulation of a GPCR. In contrast, voltage-gated ion channels are generally regarded as one of the more challenging variety of protein targets to modulate, particularly with respect to subunit specificity. Progress in this area was for many years limited by lack of suitable screening platforms to facilitate drug discovery; however, recent technological developments offer the potential to more fully explore this target class (Kaczorowski GJ et al., 2008).

Various criteria for the selection and prioritization of targets are utilized within major Pharma in the process of building sustainable portfolios of viable potential targets for the discovery scientists to address. A recent illustration (Wehling M, 2009) has highlighted one such approach which objectively applies weighted scores to available target information.

With the emergence of exciting new insights into disease pathologies, the importance of rigorous target selection will become even more important in the future. The availability of the human genome sequence coupled with impressive advances in biology is uncovering challenging targets for the medicinal chemist to address. As an example, epigenetic phenomena are increasingly being recognized as a potentially important area in the development of chronic diseases (Gluckman PD et al., 2008) and the discovery and characterization of specific histone-modifying enzyme subfamilies (Cole PA, 2008) offers the medicinal chemist the opportunity to design specific enzyme modulators with which to regulate gene expression. The availability of selective chemical probes for specific domains within these enzyme classes will be a critical factor in the identification and selection of the most relevant targets. The promise of this area is illustrated by the successful discovery of the histone deacetylase (HDAC) inhibitor Vorinostat (McGuire C and Lee J, 2010; Figure 9.2).

Historically natural products have been considered as a source of both new drugs and potential targets. More recently this approach has suffered demise due to its disappointing productivity. However, there have been a number of recent success stories which are illustrated by the following examples. Ziconotide (Prialt®); (Schmidtko A et al., 2010) is a potent and selective N-type calcium channel blocker approved by the FDA in December 2004 for the treatment of severe chronic pain. Ziconotide has subsequently demonstrated efficacy in patients with refractory pain, i.e. pain which has proven difficult to control using conventional analgesics. Ziconotide is a synthetic peptide derived from a toxin extracted from the marine snail *Conus magus*. The success of ziconotide has highlighted the potential of natural toxins in drug

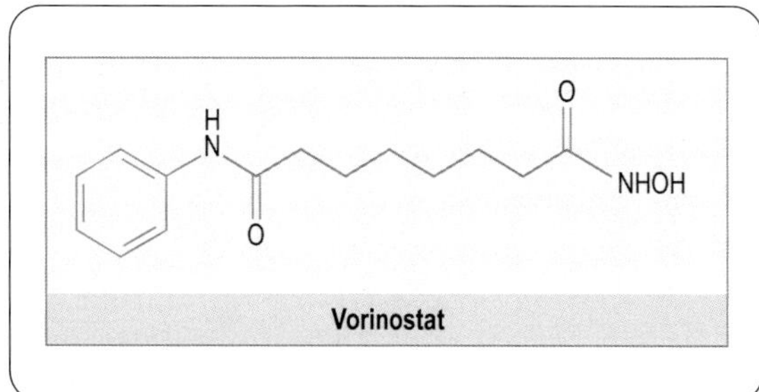

Fig. 9.2

discovery and has stimulated renewed interest from a number of groups in the area (Halai R and Craik DJ, 2009). Peptides offer high levels of both potency and selectivity which make them valuable tools for target validation and the toxins of a number of venomous species have proved to be a rich source of such molecules. The identification of the endogenous peptide hormone ghrelin (Helstroem PM, 2009), and subsequent understanding of its function, has highlighted the potential clinical value of ghrelin receptor agonists in a number of conditions such as gastroparesis (Ejskjaer N et al., 2009) and postoperative ileus (Popescu I, Fleschner PR et al., 2010) in which the ghrelin receptor agonist TZP-101 (Figure 9.3) has recently demonstrated clinical efficacy. Several of the major disease challenges facing society, such as Alzheimer's disease, cancer and heart disease, etc., have been shown to be associated, at least in part, with aberrant protein folding and/or protein–protein interactions and the identification of both small molecule and peptidic therapeutics to address these pathologies will require significant innovation.

Encouragingly great strides have recently been made in our understanding of the factors which cause proteins to misfold, primarily through the use of biophysical and computational techniques that enable systematic and quantitative analysis of the effects of a range of different perturbations in proteins (Luheshi LM et al., 2008). Recent advances in the design of small molecule inhibitors which inhibit protein–protein interactions has been amply demonstrated by the discovery of the serum amyloid P cross-linking agent CPHPC (Pepys MB et al., 2002; Figure 9.4) and the C-reactive protein inhibitor 1,6-bis(phosphocholine)-hexane (Pepys MB et al., 2006; Figure 9.5).

It is clear from the above selected examples that there is likely to be a plethora of novel biological targets to challenge the innovation of medicinal chemists for the foreseeable future.

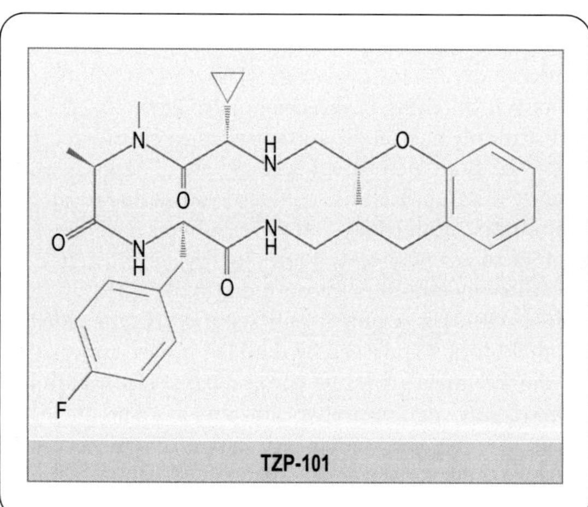

Fig. 9.3

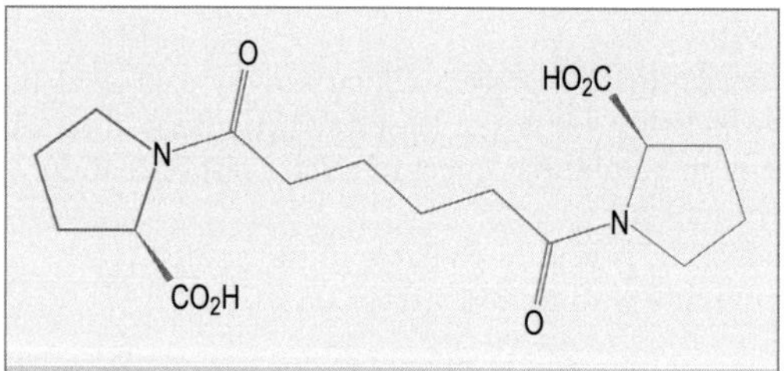

CPHPC

Fig. 9.4

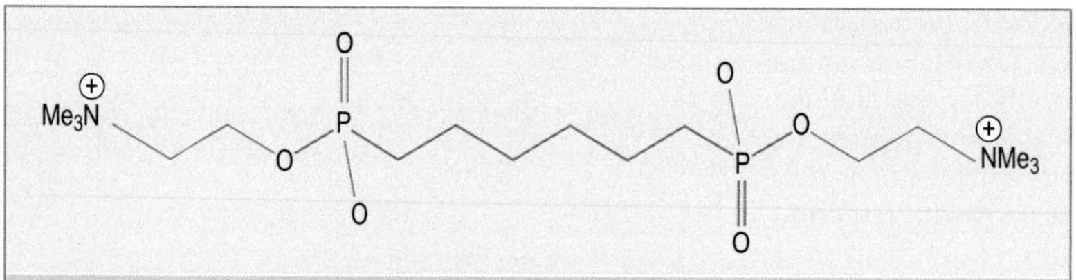

1,6-bis(phosphocholine)hexane

Fig. 9.5

LEAD IDENTIFICATION/GENERATION

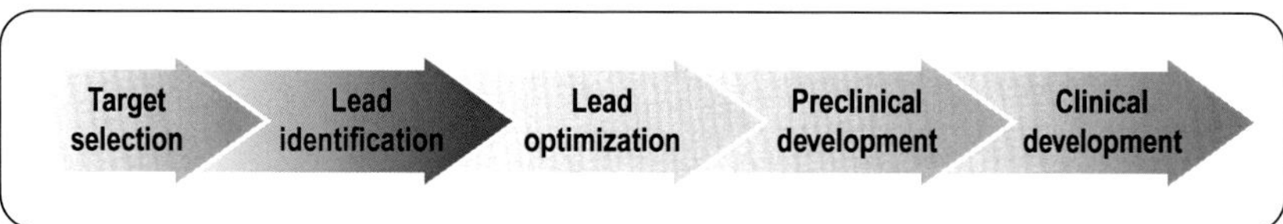

The identification of high-quality lead molecules is a critical phase in the discovery of drug candidates since decisions made at this point in the process are likely to have a significant impact on the outcome of the project as it sets the framework for future lead optimization and development (Bleicher KH et al., 2003).

Reducing attrition has already been alluded to as a major challenge in the discovery of new therapeutic agents and the lead generation phase is the earliest point in the drug discovery process where the incorporation of appropriate physicochemical properties can be addressed. It is important to establish a clear target lead profile at this early stage of the process which takes into account the critical properties required of the ultimate preclinical candidate and extrapolates back into an appropriate minimum acceptable profile for a lead series. Such a profile should not simply take into account target potency and selectivity but should also include consideration of a wide range of physicochemical characteristics which would facilitate favourable ADMET properties later in the process.

The initial aim at the lead identification/generation stage is to identify 'hits' which are molecules that interact with the chosen biological target in an initial screen, often carried out at a high concentration, to elicit a measurable response in a reproducible assay. Once validated by establishing the molecular integrity of the hit molecule(s), and confirming the robustness of the biological response, a 'validated hit' may be further investigated to establish whether it possesses the potential to be regarded as a lead series.

Several strategies have been adopted to identify these early hits as listed below:

- Existing drugs
- Natural ligands
- Natural products
- Focused screens
- Rational structure-based design
- Knowledge-based design
- Fragment screening
- Virtual screening
- High-throughput screening (including phenotypic screens).

The widespread use of high-throughput screening has generally been reported to have enabled the identification of leads for approximately 50% of the projects addressed by this approach (Fox S et al., 2006), although a more recent review suggests that, over the past 3 years, the success rate may have increased to approximately 60% (Macarron R et al., 2011). However, it is noteworthy that, despite the massive growth in the numbers of compounds screened over the past 20 years, no corresponding increase in the number of successful registered NCEs has resulted. It has been argued that, in view of increasing development times, it is still too early to evaluate the true success of high-throughput screening (Macarron R et al., 2011). Nevertheless, there has been greater focus on improving the 'drug and lead-like' properties and the structure/property diversity of screening collections. 'Drug-likeness' can be broadly defined as the overall profile of biophysicochemical properties of a molecule which facilitate its access to and effective mode of interaction at the site of action at a biologically relevant and safe concentration for sufficient duration to elicit the desired therapeutic effect. Leeson and Springthorpe discuss the importance of considering the properties conferring 'drug-likeness', particularly lipophilicity, in a recent survey of selected development candidates in leading drug companies (Leeson PD and Springthorpe B, 2007). An analysis of the structural relationship of launched drugs to their corresponding lead molecules revealed that in general the structure of the marketed molecule was very closely related to the lead series (Proudfoot JR, 2002). Thus one could infer that the apparent disappointing success rate of high-throughput screening has been related to the lack of 'drug likeness' in the compound collections and significant effort is now being devoted to address this.

Major companies have, therefore, filtered their screening collections to exclude compounds which do not possess physicochemical properties that are generally accepted to confer 'drug-like' attributes (Bleicher KH et al., 2003). However, it should be noted that, although the discovery of drug-like preclinical development candidates requires the initial identification of quality leads, the properties which confer 'drug-likeness' and those associated with 'lead-likeness' are not the same (Rishton GM, 2003). It is, therefore, important to understand the components conferring 'lead-likeness' when assessing screening collections. A publication from the Astra-Zeneca group addressed the design of lead-like combinatorial libraries and suggested that leads suitable for further optimization are most likely to be relatively polar, low molecular weight (MW =

200–350) and of relatively low lipophilicity (clogP ca.1.0–3.0) (Oprea TI et al., 2001). The authors point out that when beginning from such a tractable low-molecular-weight lead molecule, subsequent optimization to increase potency and selectivity is likely to increase molecular weight and lipophilicity to values in the order of the accepted 'drug-likeness' parameters.

Whilst significant progress is being made in improving the quality of compound collections with respect to the enrichment of 'lead-like' components and the elimination of potentially toxic or undesirable functionality, improving chemical diversity is an ongoing preoccupation since the concept of diversity is open to a variety of interpretations. Whilst in its original conception combinatorial chemistry aimed to generate large numbers of molecules providing a high level of diversity, the early libraries tended to be bolstered with molecules having significant molecular complexity and only modest diversity due to the limitations of the synthetic methodologies which could be utilized in a high-throughput mode. Furthermore, compound collections with less than optimal physicochemical properties were previously employed in high-throughput screening campaigns. Thus more attention is now being paid to the generation of focused libraries containing subsets of compounds having so-called 'privileged scaffolds' for specific target classes. This has in turn shifted the emphasis from combinatorial synthesis to rapid automated synthesis of small quantities of target compounds.

High-throughput screening (Chapter 8) continues to be a valuable strategy where there is little information around the structure of the biological target or its ligands; however, where such knowledge exists, it has generally been more successful to utilize this information to identify potential molecular starting points. For example, structural information on ligands which are known to interact with a target can be used to construct a pharmacophore, which may be used in an initial virtual screening programme of proprietary or commercial compound collections to enrich the sample set of compounds ultimately selected for actual screening. A critical review assessing the past effectiveness of virtual screening and proposing considerations for future improvements has recently appeared (Schneider G, 2010). Computational tools are widely used to generate in silico pharmacophores, using either molecular or electronic overlays. The introduction of electronic field overlay technology has allowed chemists to interrogate electronic properties in a relatively accessible manner. Similarly the latter technology may be usefully applied to 'scaffold hopping' where a structurally distinct compound class has been derived from an active series via application of a field pharmacophore (Cheeseright TJ et al., 2008). An extreme example of utilizing structural information is where an existing known drug molecule is used as the starting point to discover an improved agent (Naik P et al., 2010).

Although the majority of high-throughput screens are aimed at known biological targets with supporting target validation in the disease of interest, there has been significant activity in establishing screens based on the cell phenotype, i.e. where biochemical pathways are targeted as opposed to specific proteins within the pathway. The major challenge associated with this approach is the subsequent identification of the specific molecular target or targets with which the agents interact to produce the desired cellular response (Hart CP, 2005). Whilst in some cases further optimization of leads has been carried using the phenotypic assay itself, because of the numerous variables involved, e.g. multiple targets and cellular distribution, etc., precise SAR can be difficult to obtain from the phenotypic assay. Thus a detailed analysis and elucidation of the mechanism of action is often required to enable rapid progress to be achieved using a protein specific assay.

Over the past few years fragment-based drug discovery has become an established technique for lead generation, often in conjunction with other strategic approaches (Whittaker M et al., 2010). Fragment-based screening consists of screening a chemical library of low-molecular-weight compounds, usually at high concentration, using sensitive assay methods. In addition to biochemical assays such campaigns often incorporate biophysical methodology such as NMR, surface plasmon resonance (SPR), isothermal titration calorimetry (ITC) and X-ray crystallography (Carr R and Jhoti H, 2002; Rees DC et al., 2004; Orita M et al., 2009). The considerable progress achieved with in silico design of fragment libraries using a variety of techniques has recently been reviewed (Konteatis ZD, 2010). Essentially the fragment-based approach aims to identify ligands for the target protein which have relatively low affinity but high ligand/ligand-lipophilicity efficiency. Ligand efficiency (LE) is a measure of the binding energy of a molecule normalized by its size. This is often calculated by dividing the pKi or IC_{50} by the molecular weight or number of heavy atoms. Similarly ligand-lipophilicity efficiency (LLE) can be calculated by determining the difference between the pKi or pIC_{50} value and the clogP, which provides a measure of the binding energy of a molecule normalized by its lipophilicity (Smith GF, 2009). Thus compounds with high LE and LLE interact highly efficiently with the biological target. Subsequent optimization is then focused on increasing potency whilst maintaining high LE/LLE, thus avoiding the pitfall of increasing potency by increasing size and lipophilicity which often leads to promiscuous 'off-target' interactions and subsequent toxicity. Although the concepts of LE and LLE have been particularly applied in fragment-based design they are now widely applied across all lead generation strategies. There are now numerous examples of a fragment-base approach being employed in drug discovery projects and several have been reviewed recently (Congreve M, Chessari G et al., 2008).

In stark contrast to the fragment-based approach to lead generation, natural products have been, and arguably continue to be, a fruitful source of lead molecules and drugs over the past 25–30 years (Newman DJ and Cragg JM,

2007). However, despite the demonstrable historical successes of natural product research, major Pharma has largely reduced its investment in natural product screening in favour of the small molecule library approaches described above. The anticipation that combinatorial chemistry/automated synthesis would provide an excess of small molecule leads for most biological targets was partly responsible for the demise of this strategy. Furthermore the technical challenges associated with the deconvolution of multicomponent natural product mixtures and subsequent chemical simplification of large and complex structures has also deterred continued investment in this field. Nevertheless a number of smaller companies have recognized this as an opportunity and are pursuing this strategy for lead identification and it has recently been argued that the technical challenges associated with this approach have been lessened (Harvey AI, 2008; Harvey AI, 2010).

Despite the relative demise of natural product screening over the past few years, natural products have inspired the development of new strategies in the identification of privileged structures from which small molecule libraries have been constructed. Herbert Waldmann has received notable acclaim for his biology-oriented synthesis (BIOS) strategy which encompasses the development of small molecular entities derived from natural product and drug families, the so-called 'structural classification of natural products' (SCONP) (Keiser M et al., 2008) and an associated 'scaffold hunter' approach (Wetzel S et al., 2009).

X-ray crystallography has been effectively applied over many years to optimize small molecule ligands primarily for soluble enzyme targets. With the introduction of fragment-based screening high-throughput X-ray crystallography has over the past decade also assumed an important role in the identification of lead molecules (Carr R and Jhoti H, 2002). Similarly, NMR is proving to be an effective, accessible, complementary technique in identifying ligand-protein interactions particularly for membrane bound proteins such as GPCRs, for which detailed X-ray structures are relatively rare (Bartoschek S et al., 2010).

Recent developments in the acquisition of bioengineered protein and subsequent X-ray crystal structures of stabilized GPCRs (Tate GC and Schertler GFX, 2009) may provide exciting future opportunities for medicinal chemists to actively use ligand-bound co-crystal structures of GPCRs in an analogous fashion to the enzyme co-crystallization structures which have greatly facilitated the discovery of selective enzyme inhibitors.

Industry pressure to improve productivity and efficiency in the identification of new chemical entities has added stimulus to the exploration of new technologies in the identification of lead molecules. In particular miniaturization and automation of chemical synthesis and biological screening assays are currently under intense focus (Lombardi D and Dittrich PS, 2010).

The identification of screening platforms which obviate the requirement for artificial labels or reporter systems is also receiving considerable attention (Shiau AK et al., 2008). Biophysical methods such as surface-plasmon resonance and impedance-based technologies are developing rapidly and will become more widely used, particularly since these approaches are less likely to identify false positives which result from labelling artefacts and aggregation phenomena (Giannetti AM et al., 2008). The successful development of these new technologies has the potential to transform the lead identification process and address, in part, the challenge of improving productivity.

LEAD OPTIMIZATION

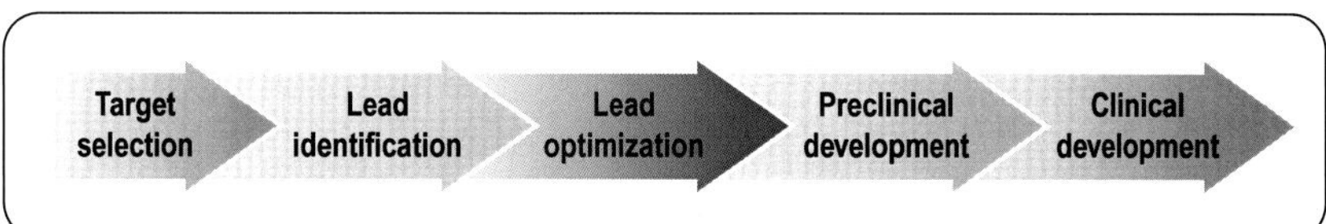

The lead optimization stage of drug discovery is at the pivotal interface between lead identification and the early development phase of a molecule. The ultimate aim of the lead optimization phase is the identification of a compound which possesses the required properties of the targeted preclinical development candidate. Thus the medicinal chemist must be cognizant of the wide range of parameters which will need to be optimized in the lead thus ensuring a high probability of success during subsequent development. It is important that the desired candidate profile is clearly defined as early as possible, ideally before the initiation of a programme, thus giving the medicinal chemist and the programme team a clear focus. From the candidate profile a focused screening strategy can be developed and should only contain screens which facilitate decision-making. Careful consideration should be given to the components and order of assays within the screening cascade which should include higher throughput assays, for which high attrition can be expected, early in the triage and lower throughput and more discerning assays, including those involving animals, later in the cascade. A major consideration in constructing an effective screening cascade is the choice of selectivity assays which need to be included. The selectivity panel normally consists of proteins both within the target family and selected 'off-target' proteins which, if modulated, would result in undesirable toxicity or side effects, discussed in more detail below.

In addition to fulfilling potency and selectivity criteria a potential development candidate should possess appropriate ADME properties to deliver acceptable exposure of the compound at the target site by the preferred route of administration allowing data obtained from subsequent in vivo profiling in preclinical disease models to be interpreted with confidence and facilitate predictions for future clinical efficacy. Much of this section will focus on molecules intended for oral administration, but a brief discussion on the different requirements of drugs intended for administration *via* other routes will also be included.

A number of excellent reviews have recently appeared which describe the lead optimization process in detail (Baringhaus KH and Matter H 2005; Lindsley GW et al., 2009). This section will focus on recent discoveries and developments that have enhanced or have the potential to further improve the traditional process.

The process commences with the careful selection of lead series which, as previously stated, is of great importance since this selection has consequences for the future lengthy and expensive discovery and development programme. It is essential that great attention is paid to selecting robust leads with the appropriate physicochemical properties. Recent analyses (Kola I and Landis J, 2004; Keserü GM and Makara GM, 2009) have clearly shown that leads chosen from the 'wrong' area of chemical space have a much higher probability of failure than those from the 'correct' area. Often failure occurs late in development and can be extremely costly. Far too often medicinal chemists have been seduced by high levels of potency in 'non drug-like' lead molecules only to find that the physical properties of the molecule are incompatible with the desired candidate profile.

Lipinski has highlighted (Lipinski CA et al., 1997) the importance of the physical properties of a molecule and, whilst this paper is often quoted, the guidelines contained within are too often disregarded.

It is important to measure key physical properties such as logD, solubility and pKa (where appropriate), etc., of novel compounds throughout the drug discovery process to ensure that molecules continue to reside within 'drug-like' chemical space and to regularly analyse data to investigate potential correlations between physicochemical properties, ADME parameters and biological activities (see also Chapter 10).

In addition to having the desired physicochemical properties a lead molecule should also have the following characteristics: (a) be a member of a distinct structural series with confirmed structure–activity relationships, (b) show evidence of the desired selectivity profile, (c) have activity in cellular systems if necessary, (d) have acceptable metabolic stability in vitro, (e) be free of any structural toxicity alerts, and (f) not have any major cytotoxicity issues. It is highly advantageous for a lead to demonstrate some evidence of oral exposure even at this early stage.

It is important also to consider how many lead series should be investigated in the early stages of the optimization process and the requisite level of structural diversity in order to mitigate against failure of a particular series. Ideally three structurally distinct lead series would be selected for lead optimization at the commencement of the process.

A lead molecule will have a predefined level of potency at the chosen target together with the initial target selectivity for both related targets and common 'off-target' liabilities which are considered important to avoid. The primary assays in most screening cascades focus on activity at the target protein and selectivity to allow the medicinal chemist to quickly optimize these important parameters early in the process. At this stage rudimentary structure–activity relationships will have already been established during the lead identification phase providing an insight as to which moieties of the lead compound may be modified to achieve the desired result. Furthermore the availability of other information such as protein X-ray crystal structures or docking predictions from target protein homology models can provide strategic guidance for the optimization process. In addition to considering selectivity within the target protein family it is important to consider selectivity more broadly (Bass AS et al., 2009) since a growing number of 'liability targets' are being identified as being potentially responsible for safety issues which are often only detected later in the development process.

Screening compounds against recombinant proteins has become widely accepted since this allows the configuration of robust high-throughput assays, which perform consistently over time. However, caution should be exercised when interpreting data generated from such assays since the biological activity data from these assays do not necessarily correlate well with activity from native tissue systems (Eglen RM et al., 2008). It is therefore important, where feasible, to periodically interrogate the relationship between activities derived from each assay system. Ideally the native tissue used should be closely related to the target tissue and from the relevant disease situation wherever possible.

A further consideration when designing a screening cascade is the potential for species differences to exist in which the biological activity at the target protein varies between different species. Species differences can lead to problems in the extrapolation of in vitro to in vivo data and the interpretation of data from in vivo efficacy and safety studies (Swanson R and Beasley JR, 2010). Whilst an indication of potential species differences can be obtained by performing a bioinformatics analysis early in the project, differences in activity can occur even when there is a high degree of homology between proteins. It is therefore important to consider the incorporation of animal orthologue assays in the screening cascade which would typically be the species of choice for the primary animal model.

Much of the focus in lead optimization is on optimization of ADME parameters which are clearly important to (a) select the most appropriate compounds for evaluation in in vivo disease models, (b) ensure that the drug is optimally delivered to its intended site of action, (c) allow a prediction of the human pharmacokinetics and estimation of clinical dose, (d) minimize the potential for drug–drug interactions, (e) avoid selecting compounds with the potential to form reactive metabolites and thus reduce the potential for idiosyncratic toxicity, and (f) provide confidence that safety studies can be performed in several species.

Several in vitro ADME screens feature early in virtually all screening strategies. The introduction of cytochrome P450 (CYP450) inhibition assays has allowed potent inhibitors of these key metabolizing enzymes to be identified early in the optimization process. The elucidation of crystal structures of a number of CYP450 enzymes has alerted medicinal chemists to specific chemical modifications with which to mitigate such liabilities from candidate molecules, thus reducing the risk of drug–drug interactions in the clinic (Ekroos M and Sjögren T, 2006; Foti RS et al., 2010). For most CYP450 isoforms a strong correlation exists between the lipophilicity of a compound and its CYP450 inhibitory potential (Lewis DFV et al., 2007).

In addition to determining the potential of a molecule to inhibit CYP450 enzymes, it is also important to assess the potential of a compound to induce CYP450 expression. CYP450 induction can potentially lead to increased clearance of the compound on chronic dosing and toxicity due to the possible formation of reactive oxygen species. For some years the pregnane X receptor (PXR), a nuclear hormone receptor assay has been used to determine the potential of a compound to induce CYP3A4. More recently, additional assays have become available for mechanisms by which other CYP isoforms are induced (Chu V et al, 2009) and could enter more routine use in the future. Currently such CYP450 induction assays are not commonly included early in the screening cascade unless the particular liability has been identified, but are employed in the later stages of lead optimization, particularly if the level of systemic exposure falls following chronic dosing.

Much attention is currently being given to the role of transporter proteins (Chu V et al, 2009), which have been implicated in the unfavourable disposition of drugs, either by active efflux from target tissue, potentially limiting efficacy, or through accumulation leading to toxicity and potential drug–drug interactions (Lai Y et al, 2010). Currently only P-glycoprotein (Pgp) assays are used in routine screening, but assays for many other transporters are being developed and are anticipated to be in routine use as screening assays in the near future.

The assessment of potential metabolic instability is also an important early evaluation in a screening cascade. Thus, typically compounds are incubated with human and/or rodent liver microsomes and their metabolic stability is expressed as the percentage of compound remaining after a given time or, more commonly, as an intrinsic clearance parameter (Nagai N, 2010). For a more thorough evaluation of in vitro metabolic turnover human and rodent hepatocytes may be used which possess the capacity to carry out both phase 1 and 2 metabolic processing. In addition an assessment of plasma protein binding is often included since the degree to which a molecule binds to plasma proteins can influence both the efficacy and the tissue distribution of the compound (Chang G et al, 2010).

As molecules progress to the later stages of lead optimization an understanding of the route and specific sites of metabolism of the compounds can be important information to assist the medicinal chemist to further improve the metabolic stability of the compound. For example, the introduction of blocking groups at sites of metabolism or electron withdrawing substituents at appropriate sites on the molecule, which will reduce electrophilicity, can significantly reduce the rate of metabolic turnover. An early assessment of the potential of a compound to form reactive and, therefore, potentially toxic metabolites is also valuable and can be achieved by using a combination of time-dependent CYP450 inhibition (Howard M et al, 2010) and trapping experiments, typically with either glutathione or cyanide (Riley RJ et al., 2007). For molecules with the potential for reactive metabolite formation additional in vitro and in vivo studies to detect covalent binding to tissue protein, using radiolabelled compound, may be required (Evans DC et al., 2004).

A preclinical pharmacokinetic study (see Chapter 10) is often the first occasion at which a compound is tested in an in vivo experiment. These studies are normally performed in rats since this is the species of choice for the majority of disease models and for rodent safety assessment studies. Compounds targeted as oral therapies are administered by both intravenous (i.v.) and oral (p.o.) routes, each experiment providing valuable information for the medicinal chemist. An i.v. pharmacokinetic study allows the clearance (the rate by which the drug is eliminated from the system) of the drug to be measured together with the volume of distribution (a measure of how well the drug distributes into tissue). Both the clearance and the volume of distribution determine the half-life of the drug. A p.o. study is used to determine the circulating levels that can be achieved after a given p.o. dose. Studies frequently use both i.v. and p.o. routes of administration to gain a full profile of a compound and allow the absolute bioavailability to be determined (White RE, 2009; Chapter 10).

The volume of distribution is a parameter which quantifies the distribution of the drug between the plasma and body tissue, and ideal molecules should have low clearance from the blood and a volume of distribution indicative of distribution into total body water (i.e. > 1). It is thus important to understand the properties which affect the volume of distribution of a compound. Common factors which can affect this parameter are plasma protein binding, the physical properties (particularly the presence or absence of either an acidic or basic centre) and the involvement of transporters (Grover A and Benet LZ, 2009). Common strategies to increase the volume of distribution include the introduction of a basic centre to increase the pKa, if appropriate, and to increase the LogD. However, unless the lead molecule is hydrophilic in nature, increasing lipophilicity can result in increased metabolism and CYP450 inhibition as discussed above and thus the identification of the optimal properties is often a trade-off of physicochemical properties. In addition to blocking sites of metabolism to reduce clearance, reducing the lipophilicity of a molecule is often effective at reducing the rate of metabolism. Drugs which are specifically aimed at targets within the central nervous system (CNS) require more stringent control of their physicochemical properties to facilitate passive permeation of the blood–brain barrier which is comprised of endothelial tight junctions. In comparison with Lipinski guidelines, molecules designed to cross the blood–brain barrier would typically have a lower molecular weight (<450), lower clogP (1–3), reduced hydrogen bond acceptors (<6) and donors (<2) and lower total polar surface area (TPSA) (<75A^2). The blood–brain barrier also contains efflux transporters such as P-glycoprotein which serve to prevent access of substrates into the CNS. The free fraction of the compound, i.e. that proportion which is not bound to plasma protein, has also been reported to have a profound effect on both access to the CNS and subsequent distribution to the site of action (Jeffrey P and Summerfield S, 2010).

The desired pharmacokinetic profile of a drug will depend on the site of action and the nature of the target. Most commonly used drugs are required to penetrate tissue to reach their target protein and to be present at therapeutically efficacious concentrations for long enough to support once, or at most twice, daily dosing.

The majority of discovery programmes have targeted orally well-absorbed molecules with high metabolic stability to maintain high circulating blood levels for sufficient time to deliver the required duration of action. Thus the duration of action for these agents is related to their pharmacokinetic properties, particularly the rate of clearance from the plasma. An alternative approach has been to identify molecules which have an extended residence time, due to a slow 'off rate', at the target protein which is significantly longer than the time over which an efficacious plasma concentration of the compound is maintained. In such cases there is a clear mismatch between the pharmacokinetic and pharmacodynamic half-lives for the compounds, thus obviating the need to maintain high drug levels in the plasma over an extended time period to produce an efficacious response. A potential key advantage of these so-called 'tight binders' is that they may possess an improved safety profile (Packeu A et al., 2010), as the total body burden of drug is reduced.

Molecules which fulfil the targeted potency, selectivity and ADME properties will usually progress to in vivo studies in animal models to assess their potential for in vivo efficacy. The relevance of animal models for both efficacy and, in some cases, safety is a matter of much debate within the drug discovery community. With an increasing number of compounds failing to demonstrate clinical efficacy, despite having shown excellent results in preclinical models of disease, it is clear that the animal models are not totally predictive and a better understanding of the translation of data from animal model to human disease for a particular mechanism is required. Within areas where validated predictive models exist for specific mechanisms in vivo data can be very powerful both in aiding the selection of advanced molecules as potential development candidates and in predicting the efficacious clinical dose through the use of pharmacokinetic/pharmacodynamic (PK/PD) studies which correlate the systemic exposure of the compound with the degree of efficacy.

In addition to the optimization of ADME properties during the lead optimization phase, compounds are also evaluated for potential toxicity with subsequent chemical modification being applied to mitigate potential risks. A detailed discussion of toxicological evaluation in drug discovery is beyond the scope of this section (see Chapter 15); however, it is pertinent to mention the function of such assays in the process. Cytotoxicity assays are commonly used alongside cellular functional screens to identify molecules which produce biological activity by virtue of cellular toxicity. An area of intense current interest is that of the potential for compounds to produce adverse cardiovascular effects in the clinic, since cardiovascular toxicity is responsible for a significant number of drug withdrawals. An increasing number of targets, currently confined to ion channels, have been identified in recent years and are now commonly included in 'off-target' selectivity panels during lead optimization, the most well characterized of these being the hERG channel (Hancox JC et al., 2008; see also Chapter 15). The panel of cardiac liability channels being incorporated into screening cascades is increasing with many groups routinely including other channels such as Nav1.5, Kv1.5, Cav1.2, KCNQ1 (hmink) amongst others (Cao X et al., 2010). Later in the optimization phase, when potential candidates have been identified, assays to detect genotoxicity are routinely employed. Typically compounds are tested in both a bacterial mutagenicity assay such as the Ames test initially and also in a mammalian screen such as the mouse micronucleus assay (Reifferscheid G and

Buchinger S, 2010). Prior to being accepted into preclinical development it is usual to conduct a preliminary in vivo safety study, typically dosing for 7 or 14 days, to provide an initial assessment of the maximum tolerated dose in preparation for subsequent more precise regulatory safety studies.

Much of this section has focused on the lead optimization process for oral drugs and it is important to recognize other routes of administration where the molecule profiles will be significantly different, particularly with respect to ADME and physical properties. Other common routes of administration are inhaled or intranasal, intravenous and topical.

For inhaled drugs, whose site of action is in the lung, a poorly soluble molecule which is highly metabolized in the circulation and of low membrane permeability is often the preferred profile. This profile is aimed at ensuring maximum residence time in the lung for optimal efficacy and minimal systemic exposure thus reducing the potential for any side effects (Ritchie TJ et al., 2009). A similar profile is desirable for topical drugs for application to the skin (Sloan KB et al., 2006).

For intravenously administered drugs a very different profile is required where a highly soluble molecule is preferred (Shi Y et al., 2009) to allow a low dose volume to be employed. In the latter case the focus of optimization is generally on the identification of highly potent agents (to facilitate low dose), with high metabolic stability and an acceptable duration of action. For drugs projected to be administered via routes other than the oral route, considerations such as Lipinski guidelines, which address oral bioavailability, are inappropriate.

ADDRESSING ATTRITION

Attrition is currently the major issue facing scientists engaged in the drug discovery process. During the 1990s the pharmaceutical industry took great steps to identify the reasons responsible for the high attrition rate in development and introduced measures to overcome the issues (Kola I and Landis J, 2004). The incorporation of both in vitro and in vivo ADME assays in discovery screening cascades significantly reduced the subsequent level of attrition due to poor pharmacokinetic properties during clinical evaluation between 1990 and 2000. However, in 2000 an increased number of molecules were failing due to toxicity (Kola I and Landis J, 2004). Ten years later the level of attrition due to toxicity is still high in the discovery phase and much effort is currently being devoted to identifying the key reasons responsible for this.

Of more concern is the level of late stage attrition, i.e. that occurring subsequent to the discovery and development phase and a worrying number of registered drugs continue to be withdrawn from the market at an unacceptable level. In the last 10 years 17 drugs have been withdrawn (http://en.wikipedia.org/wiki/List_of_withdrawn_drugs) due to adverse drug reactions. Furthermore, adverse drug reactions have been estimated to account for approximately 5% of deaths amongst hospital patients and 3% of the general population (Wester K et al., 2008). The most common toxicities are associated with the liver, the cardiovascular system, skin and blood. Significant efforts are being made to understand the reasons responsible for these toxicities and thus to develop assays capable of identifying molecules possessing the potential to cause these adverse events.

There are four main factors which can give rise to organ toxicities: the overall physical properties of a drug molecule, the primary pharmacology, the secondary or 'off-target' pharmacology and the presence of structural elements known to cause toxicity. The medicinal chemist needs to consider all of these factors when designing potential drug molecules.

Medicinal chemists have long been aware of the relationship between physical properties and 'drug likeness' (Lipinski CA et al., 1997); however, recent reviews (Leeson PD and Springthorpe B, 2007) suggest that a significant percentage of compounds being prepared by major pharmaceutical companies are too highly lipophilic and it has been proposed that high lipophilicity is likely to be a major cause of toxicity. A study by Pfizer (Price DA et al., 2009) which investigated potential correlations between physical properties and observed in vivo toxicity for 245 of their preclinical development compounds showed a marked correlation between cLogP and toxicity and an inverse correlation between total polar surface area (TPSA). They concluded that ideally a molecule should have a cLogP < 3 and TPSA > 75 to reduce the probability of producing toxicity. The importance of reducing lipophilicity cannot be over-emphasized as it has been shown to influence all parameters that the medicinal chemist needs to control in discovering an orally bioavailable drug including solubility, membrane permeability, plasma protein binding, metabolism (Waring MJ, 2010) and the potential to cause drug–drug interactions (Lewis D and Ito Y, 2010). High lipophilicity has been postulated to increase the probability for promiscuous binding of the compound to 'off-target' proteins thus increasing the likelihood of toxicity (Leeson PD and Springthorpe B, 2007).

Adverse drug reactions have been characterized into three groups (Pirmohamed M et al., 1998). Type A (augmented) adverse reactions are the so-called target-mediated toxicities and are related to the pharmacological effect of the drug and such adverse events are predictable and dose-related. Type B (idiosyncratic) adverse reactions are unpredictable, often non-dose related, less common, but frequently more severe than Type A. Type C (chemical) adverse reactions are related to structural elements in the drug molecule and may be predictable from the molecular structure.

Type A, augmented or target-mediated, toxicity is an important factor to take into account, particularly when choosing a target or during a target validation exercise. If interacting with the target is likely to cause an adverse event then the implications of the adverse event in the context of the disease requires careful consideration based on the potential benefit of the entity versus its risk. For example many anticancer agents are cytotoxic and would not be considered suitable treatments for less serious conditions.

Type B, idiosyncratic toxicity is a growing area of considerable interest (Ulrich RG, 2007) and the major cause of drug withdrawals. This type of toxicity is often severe and can result in hospitalization and, in extreme cases, death. Recent data suggest that some of the mechanisms responsible are becoming better understood, but there is still a need for much further work. In particular the formation of reactive metabolites which may bind covalently to cellular protein and precipitate an immunological response is currently a leading hypothesis to explain at least some of the idiosyncratic toxicity (Kaplowitz N, 2005). The potential for a compound to form reactive metabolites can be assessed by a combination of time-dependent CYP450 inhibition studies and electrophile trapping experiments with an agent such as glutathione (Kalgutkar AS and Didiuk MT, 2009) followed, if necessary, by detailed covalent protein binding studies (Evans D et al., 2004). The major organs affected by idiosyncratic toxicity are the heart, liver, kidneys and skin (Caldwell, 2006). It is important that any potential for idiosyncratic toxicity should be considered in the context of the predicted efficacious plasma concentration of the drug and the targeted indication. Empirically it is assumed that if the dose is 10 mg or less then the probability of idiosyncratic toxicity is reduced significantly (Uetrecht J, 2001).

Cardiovascular toxicity still remains one of the major causes of drug withdrawal and the recent removal of clobutinol from clinical usage as a result of cardiac QT interval prolongation (Takahara A et al., 2009) highlights the need to study potential drug molecules carefully to assess the risk of this phenomenon. The hERG channel, a potassium channel involved in the repolarization phase of the heart, has been known for some time to be associated with cardiac QT interval prolongation and there is a good correlation between compounds which have high hERG binding activity and clinical arrhythmogenic activity, particularly the torsade des pointes syndrome (Polak S et al., 2009). A variety of assays are available to assess the potential of compounds to inhibit the hERG channel, but it is important to choose the most appropriate in vitro assay and not to rely on data from one assay in isolation (Pollard CE et al., 2010). It is advisable, for advanced compounds, to obtain data in both in vitro and in vivo assays to allow an informed decision on the potential progression of the molecule (see Chapter 14). The hERG channel is one of several ion channels (Witchel HJ, 2010) involved in the repolarization phase of the heart, interference with any of which could lead to an adverse cardiovascular effect. Many groups are now screening compounds against a panel of cardiac ion channels throughout the discovery process (see Lead optimization section).

A number of medicinal chemistry strategies have been adopted to reduce the potential for hERG inhibition, which include reducing lipophilicity, modulating the pKa to reduce π-cationic interactions and reducing the potential for π-π interactions. The relative success of these strategies has been recently reviewed (Jamieson C et al., 2006). There is currently no available X-ray crystal structure of the hERG channel; however, the value of homology models using known potassium channel structures to guide structural modifications has been effectively demonstrated in the discovery of the CCR5 receptor antagonist, maraviroc (Price DA et al., 2006).

Drug-induced liver injury is also a major cause of compound attrition, often through the formation of reactive metabolites and this will be discussed later in this section. A greater understanding is emerging on the possible role of drug–transporter interactions in the development of hepatotoxicity (Lai Y et al., 2010) which may result in cellular accumulation, impaired efflux, alteration of nutrient transport and altered drug disposition leading to drug–drug interactions. For example the toxicity of troglitazone has been partially attributed to its interaction with the bile salt export pump (BSEP) (Funk C et al., 2001). The number of known transporters is currently growing and assays are being developed to assess the potential of drugs to cause toxicity through interaction with these proteins (Greer MI et al., 2010).

Another area of current growing interest, which has been implicated in liver toxicity, and, indeed, toxicity in other organs, is the potential of a drug to impair mitochondrial function (Dykens JA and Will Y, 2010). This is a complex and developing area which is beyond the scope of this chapter, however 80% of drugs which have received FDA 'Black Box Warnings' for hepatotoxicity and cardiovascular toxicity have been shown to inhibit mitochondrial function (Dykens JA and Will Y, 2007). Assay systems are currently available and a suggested protocol for their use in drug discovery has been published (Dykens JA and Will Y, 2010).

Recent studies have suggested biomarkers that are potentially predictive of liver injury that could be used both preclinically and clinically. Two such biomarkers are the high mobility group box1 and keratin 18 proteins (Antoine DJ et al., 2009).

Whilst renal toxicity has not been responsible for a large number of drug withdrawals, it is still a major cause for concern. Interaction with transporter proteins has recently been implicated in the renal toxicity of a number of substances. Rosuvastatin (Crestor®) was shown to cause proteinuria at a dose of 80 mg in Phase 3 clinical trials. This phenomenon has subsequently been shown to be due to a combination of the target pharmacology of the drug (inhibition of protein endocytosis) and the fact that it is a substrate for the organic anion transporter 3 (OAT3), which causes it to accumulate in the kidney (Windass AS et al., 2007). Until recently there has been a lack of predictive biomarkers for renal toxicity; however, a recent study by an international consortium, has identified seven biomarkers which can be used both preclinically and in human studies (Hewitt P and Herget T, 2009).

Type C or structural-based toxicity is clearly an area that the medicinal chemist should particularly consider before embarking on a chemical modification. Structural alerts, of which the chemist should be aware, can be divided into four groups, chemically reactive functionality, structural elements which present a risk following metabolic activation, DNA binders and CYP450 inhibitors. There are several excellent reviews in the recent literature covering this area (Blagg J, 2006; Kalgutkar AS and Didiuk MT, 2009) in detail and describe many structural features which should be given careful consideration before incorporation within a drug molecule. The medicinal chemist is advised to read these carefully and to be aware of new toxicophores as they appear in the literature.

Despite the increasing volume of information, the theoretical prediction of toxicity is still imprecise. It is, therefore, important to incorporate 'predictive' assays early in screening strategies. Despite recent progress, current in vitro safety testing is conducted in animal cells or, at best, in recombinant human cell lines. It would be preferable to conduct these studies in native human cells and recent advances in stem cell research facilitate this opportunity in the future (Balls M, 2010). Whilst toxicity is a major cause of compound failure, the failure of potential drug molecules to demonstrate efficacy upon clinical evaluation is a more difficult issue to address since the factors which contribute to these failures are complex. Inadequate target validation, poor predictability of animal models, poor clinical trial design and patient selection are potential causes. Whilst the medicinal chemist cannot address all of these issues, it is important that potent, selective and safe molecules with appropriate physical properties are identified for such studies to ensure that it is the mechanism of action of the drug that is being tested and not the quality of the molecule. Greater involvement of the medicinal chemist at the initial target identification and validation stage may provide better tool or probe compounds (see Target selection and validation section) with which to validate novel targets.

SUMMARY

The environment in which drug discovery is taking place is currently undergoing considerable change and will continue to do so for some time to come. The downsizing of major Pharma and the increased focus on academic drug discovery are attempts to deal with the escalating costs, high attrition rate and patent expiries which are threatening the viability of the current discovery model (see Chapter 22).

This chapter is intended to convey the message that the medicinal chemist has an extremely important role to play in all aspects of the discovery process to address the challenges of increasing efficiency and productivity and reducing attrition. Whilst traditionally the medicinal chemist has not become engaged with the drug discovery process until the lead identification phase, there is a compelling argument for their involvement at the target selection and validation stage. The identification of high-quality chemical probes as early as possible will enable robust target validation and the selection of those biological targets which are more likely to succeed.

Furthermore, an increasing array of technological advances are becoming available which will enable the chemist to develop a detailed understanding of the biophysics associated with compound-target engagement, which can be effectively incorporated into the design of suitable preclinical candidates.

Whilst significant progress has been made over the past 10–15 years in reducing attrition due to poor ADME properties, toxicity remains to be a major source of attrition and the chemist has an important role to play in reducing the late-stage attrition due to compound-related toxicity. Whilst the current predictive packages are imperfect, there is a developing understanding of the impact of chemical structure and physicochemical properties on toxicity. It is anticipated that an increasing number of screening assays will become available for incorporation into project screening cascades which will help to identify potential risks as early as possible in the discovery process.

Thus, whilst the industry is entering uncharted territory, there is an unprecedented opportunity for the medicinal chemist to make a major contribution to the future success of the discovery of new and important medicines to meet the growing level of unmet clinical need.

REFERENCES

Antoine DJ, Williams DP, Kipar A, et al. High-mobility group box-1 protein and keratin-18, circulating serum proteins informative of acetaminophen-induced necrosis and apoptosis in vivo. Toxicological Sciences 2009; 112:521–31.

Balls M. Adult human stem cells and toxicity – realising the potential. Alternatives to Laboratory Animals 2010;38:91.

Baringhaus KH, Matter H. Efficient strategies for lead optimization by simultaneously addressing affinity, selectivity and pharmacokinetic parameters. Methods and Principles in Medicinal Chemistry 2005;

23(Chemoinformatics in Drug Discovery):333–79.

Bartoschek S, Klabunde T, Defossa E, et al. Drug design for G-protein-coupled receptors by a ligand-based NMR method. Angewandte Chemie, International Edition 2010;49:1426–9, S1426/1–S1426/5.

Bass AS, Cartwright ME, Mahon C, et al. Exploratory drug safety – a drug discovery strategy to reduce attrition in development. Journal of Pharmacological and Toxicological Methods 2009;60:69–78.

Blagg J. Structure-activity relationships for in vitro and in vivo toxicity. Annual Reports in Medical Chemistry 2006;41:358.

Bleicher KH, Boehm HJ, Mueller K, et al. A guide to drug discovery: hit and lead generation: beyond high-throughput screening. Nature Reviews Drug Discovery 2003;2:369–78.

Caldwell GW, Yan Z. Screening for reactive intermediates and toxicity assessment in drug discovery. Current Opinion in Drug Discovery & Development 2006;9:47–60.

Cao X, Lee YT, Holmqvist M, et al. Cardiac ion channel safety profiling on the IonWorks Quattro automated patch clamp system. Assay and Drug Development Technologies 2010;8:766–80.

Carr R, Jhoti H. Structure-based screening of low-affinity compounds. Drug Discovery Today 2002;7:522–7.

Chang G, Steyn SJ, Umland JP, et al. Strategic use of plasma and microsome binding to exploit in vitro clearance in early drug discovery. ACS Medicinal Chemistry Letters 2010;1:50–3.

Cheeseright TJ, Mackey MD, Melville JL, et al. FieldScreen: virtual screening using molecular fields. Application to the DUD data set. Journal of Chemical Information and Modeling 2008;48:2108–17.

Chu V, Einolf HJ, Evers R, et al. In vitro and in vivo induction of Cytochrome P450: A survey of the current practices and recommendations: a pharmaceutical research and manufacturers of America perspective. Drug MetAbolism and Disposition 2009;37:1339.

Cole PA. Chemical probes for histone-modifying enzymes. Nature Chemical Biology 2008;4: 590–7.

Congreve M, Chessari G, Tisi D, et al. Recent developments in fragment-based drug discovery. Journal of Medicinal Chemistry 2008;51:3661–80.

Dib-Hajj SD, Cummins TR, Black JA, et al. From genes to pain: Nav1.7 and human pain disorders. Trends in Neurosciences 2007;30:555–63.

Dykens JA, Will Y. The significance of mitochondrial toxicity testing in drug development. Drug Discovery Today 2007;12:777–85.

Dykens JA, Will Y. Drug-induced mitochondrial dysfunction: an emerging model of idiosyncratic drug toxicity. International Drug Discovery 2010;5:32–6.

Eglen RM, Gilchrist A, Reisine T. The use of immortalized cell lines in GPCR screening: the good, bad and ugly. Combinatorial Chemistry & High Throughput Screening 2008;11:560–5.

Ejskjaer N, Vestergaard ET, Hellström PM, et al. Ghrelin receptor agonist (TZP-101) accelerates gastric emptying in adults with diabetes and symptomatic gastroparesis. Alimentary Pharmacology and Therapeutics 2009;29:1179–87.

Ekroos M, Sjögren T. Structural basis for ligand promiscuity in cytochrome P 450 3A4. Proceedings of the National Academy of Sciences of the United States of America 2006;103:13682–7.

Evans DC, Watt AP, Nicoll-Griffith DA, et al. Drug-protein adducts: an industry perspective on minimizing the potential for drug bioactivation in drug discovery and development. Chemical Research in Toxicology 2004;17:3–16.

Foti RS, Wienkers LC, Wahlstrom JL. Application of cytochrome P450 drug interaction screening in drug discovery. Combinatorial Chemistry & High Throughput Screening 2010;13:145–58.

Fox S, Farr-Jones S, Sopchak L, et al. High-throughput screening: update on practices and success. Journal of biomolecular screening 2006;11:864–9.

Frye SV. The art of the chemical probe. Nature Chemical Biology 2010;6:159–61.

Funk C, Ponelle C, Scheuermann G, et al. Cholestatic potential of troglitazone as a possible factor contributing to troglitazone-induced hepatotoxicity: in vivo and in vitro interaction at the canalicular bile salt export pump (BSEP) in the rat. Molecular Pharmacology 2001;59:627–35.

Giannetti AM, Koch BD, Browner MF. Surface plasmon resonance based assay for the detection and characterization of promiscuous inhibitors. Journal of Medicinal Chemistry 2008;51:574–80.

Gluckman PD, Hanson MA, Cooper C, et al. In utero and early-life conditions and adult health and disease – in reply. New England Journal of Medicine 2008;359:61–3.

Greer ML, Barber J, Eakins J, et al. Cell based approaches for evaluation of drug induced liver injury. Toxicology 2010;268:125.

Grover A, Benet LZ. Effects of drug transporters on volume of distribution. AAPS Journal 2009;11:250–61.

Halai R, Craik DJ. Conotoxins: natural product drug leads. Natural Product Reports 2009;26:526–36.

Hancox JC, McPate MJ, El Harchi A, et al. The hERG potassium channel and hERG screening for drug-induced torsades de pointes Pharmacology & Therapeutics 2008;119:118–32.

Hart CP. Finding the target after screening the phenotype. Drug Discovery Today 2005;10:513–9.

Harvey AL. Natural products in drug discovery. Drug Discovery Today 2008;13:894–901.

Harvey AL, Clark RL, Mackay SP, et al. Current strategies for drug discovery through natural products. Expert Opinion on Drug Discovery 2010;5:559–68.

Helstroem PM. Faces of ghrelin – research for the 21st century. Neurogastroenterology and Motility 2009;21:2.

Hewitt P, Herget T. Value of new biomarkers for safety testing in drug development. Expert Review of Molecular Diagnostics 2009;9:531–6.

Howard ML, Hill JJ, Galluppi GR, et al. Plasma protein binding in drug discovery and development. Combinatorial Chemistry & High Throughput Screening 2010;13:170–87.

Hughes B. 2009 FDA drug approvals. Nature Reviews Drug Discovery 2010;9:89–92.

Jamieson C, Moir EM, Rankovic Z, et al. Medicinal chemistry of hERG optimizations: highlights and hang-ups. Journal of Medicinal Chemistry 2006;49:5029–46.

Jeffrey P, Summerfield S. Assessment of the blood–brain barrier in CNS drug discovery. Neurobiology of Disease 2010;37:33–7.

Kaczorowski GJ, McManus OB, Priest BT, et al. Ion channels as drug targets: the next GPCRs. Journal of General Physiology 2008;131:399–405.

Kalgutkar AS, Didiuk MT. Structural alerts, reactive metabolites, and protein covalent binding: how reliable are these attributes as predictors of drug toxicity? Chemistry & Biodiversity 2009;6:2115–37.

Kaplowitz N. Idiosyncratic drug hepatotoxicity. Nature Reviews Drug Discovery 2005;4:489–99.

Keiser M, Wetzel S, Kumar K, et al. Biology-inspired synthesis of compound libraries. Cellular and Molecular Life Sciences 2008;65:1186–201.

Keserü GM, Makara GM. The influence of lead discovery strategies on the properties of drug candidates. Nature Reviews Drug Discovery 2009;8:203–12.

Kola I, Landis J. Opinion: can the pharmaceutical industry reduce attrition rates? Nature Reviews Drug Discovery 2004;3:711–6.

Konteatis ZD. In silico fragment-based drug design. Expert Opinion on Drug Discovery 2010;5:1047–65.

Lai Y, Sampson KE, Stevens JC. Evaluation of drug transporter interactions in drug discovery and development. Combinatorial Chemistry & High Throughput Screening 2010;13:112–34.

Leeson PD, Springthorpe B. The influence of drug-like concepts on decision-making in medicinal chemistry. Nature Reviews Drug Discovery 2007;6:881–90.

Lewis D, Ito Y. Human CYPs involved in drug metabolism, structures, substrates and binding affinities. Expert Opinion on Drug Metabolism and Toxicology 2010;6:661–74.

Lewis DFV, Lake BG, Dickins M. Quantitative structure-activity relationships (QSARs) in inhibitors of various cytochromes P450: the importance of compound lipophilicity. Journal of Enzyme Inhibition and Medicinal Chemistry 2007;22:1–6.

Lindsley CW, Weaver D, Bridges TM, et al. Lead optimization in drug discovery. Wiley Encyclopedia of Chemical Biology 2009;2:511–9.

Lipinski CA, Lombado F, Dominy BW, et al. Experimental and computational approaches to estimate solubility and permeability in drug discovery and development settings. Advanced Drug Delivery Reviews 1997;23:3–25.

Lombardi D, Dittrich PS. Advances in microfluidics for drug discovery. Expert Opinion on Drug Discovery 2010;5:1081–94.

Luheshi LM, Crowther DC, Dobson CM. Protein misfolding and disease: from the test tube to the organism. Current Opinion in Chemical Biology 2008;12:25–31.

Macarron R, Banks MN, Bojanic D, et al. Impact of high-throughput screening in biomedical research. Nature Reviews Drug Discovery 2011;10:188–95.

McGuire C, Lee J. Brief review of vorinostat. Clinical Medicine Insights: Therapeutics 2010;2:83–8.

Nagai N. Drug interaction studies on new drug applications – current situation and regulatory view in Japan. Drug Metabolism and Pharmacokinetics 2010;25:3–15.

Naik P, Murumkar P, Giridhar R, et al. Angiotensin II receptor type 1 (AT1) selective nonpeptidic antagonists – a perspective. Bioorganic & Medicinal Chemistry 2010;18:8418–56.

Newman DJ, Cragg JM. Natural products as sources of new drugs over the last 25 years. Journal of Natural Products 2007;70:461–77.

Oprea TI, Davis AM, Teague SJ, et al. Is there a difference between leads and drugs? A historical perspective. Journal of Chemical Information and Computer Sciences 2001;41:1308–15.

Orita M, Warizaya M, Amano Y, et al. Advances in fragment-based drug discovery platforms. Expert Opinion on Drug Discovery 2009;4:1125–44.

Packeu A, Wennerberg M, Balendran A. Estimation of the dissociation rate of unlabelled ligand-receptor complexes by a 'two-step' competition binding approach. British Journal of Pharmacology 2010;161:1311–28.

Pepys MB, Herbert J, Hutchinson WL, et al. Targeted pharmacological depletion of serum amyloid P component for treatment of human amyloidosis. Nature (London, United Kingdom) 2002;417:254–9.

Pepys MB, Hirschfield GM, Tennent GA, et al. Targeting C-reactive protein for the treatment of cardiovascular disease. Nature (London, United Kingdom) 2006;440:1217–21.

Pirmohamed M, Breckenridge AM, Kitteringham NR, et al. Adverse drug reactions. British Medical Journal (Clinical Research Edition) 1998;316:1295–8.

Polak S, Wisniowska B. Brandys Collation, assessment and analysis of literature in vitro data on hERG receptor blocking potency for subsequent modeling of drugs cardiotoxic properties. Journal of Applied Toxicology 2009;29(3): 183–206.

Pollard CE, Abi Gerges N, Bridgland-Taylor MH, et al. An introduction to QT interval prolongation and non-clinical approaches to assessing and reducing risk. British Journal of Pharmacology 2010;159:12–21.

Popescu I, Fleshner PR, Pezzullo JC, et al. The ghrelin agonist TZP-101 for management of postoperative ileus after partial colectomy: a randomized, dose-ranging, placebo-controlled clinical trial. Diseases of the Colon and Rectum 2010;53:126–34.

Price DA, Armour D, de Groot M, et al. Overcoming HERG affinity in the discovery of the CCR5 antagonist maraviroc. Bioorganic & Medicinal Chemistry Letters 2006;16:4633–7.

Price DA, Blagg J, Jones L, et al. Physicochemical drug properties associated with toxicological outcomes – a review. Expert Opinion on Drug Metabolism & Toxicology 2009;5:921–31.

Proudfoot JR. Drugs, leads, and drug-likeness: an analysis of some recently launched drugs. Bioorganic & Medicinal Chemistry Letters 2002;12:1647–50.

Rees DC, Congreve M, Murray CW, et al. Fragment-based lead discovery. Nature Reviews Drug Discovery 2004;3:660–72.

Reifferscheid G, Buchinger S. Cell-based genotoxicity testing. Genetically modified and genetically engineered bacteria in environmental genotoxicology. Advances in Biochemical Engineering/ Biotechnology 2010;118(Whole Cell Sensing Systems II) 85–112.

Riley RJ, Grime K, Weaver R. Time-dependent CYP inhibition. Expert Opinion on Drug Metabolism & Toxicology 2007;3:51–66.

Rishton GM. Reactive compounds and in vitro false positives in HTS. Drug Discovery Today 2003;8: 86–96.

Ritchie TJ, Luscombe CN, Macdonald SJ. Analysis of the calculated physicochemical properties of respiratory drugs: can we design for inhaled drugs yet? Journal of Chemical Information and Modeling 2009;49:1025–32.

Schmidtko A, Lötsch J, Freynhagen R, et al. Ziconotide for treatment of severe chronic pain. Lancet 2010;375:1569–77.

Schneider G. Virtual screening: an endless staircase? Nature Reviews Drug Discovery 2010;9:273–6.

Shi Y, Merdan T, Li LC. Recent advances in intravenous delivery of poorly water-soluble compounds. Expert Opinion on Drug Delivery 2009;6:1261–82.

Shiau AK, Massari ME, Ozbal CC. Back to basics: label-free technologies for small molecule screening. Combinatorial Chemistry & High Throughput Screening 2008;11:231–7.

Sloan KB, Wasdo SC, Rautio J. Design for optimized topical delivery: prodrugs and a paradigm change. Pharmaceutical Research 2006;23:2729–47.

Smith GF. Medicinal chemistry by the numbers: the physicochemistry, thermodynamics and kinetics of modern drug design. Progress in Medicinal Chemistry 2009;48:1–29.

Source http://en.wikipedia.org/wiki/ List_of_withdrawn_drugs

Swanson R, Beasley JR. Pathway-specific, species, and sub-type counterscreening for better GPCR hits in high throughput screening. Current Pharmaceutical Biotechnology 2010;11:757–63.

Takahara A, Sasaki R, Nakamura M, et al. Clobutinol delays ventricular repolarisation in the guinea pig heart – comparison UIT cardiac effects of hERG K+ channel inhibitor E-4031. Journal of Cardiovascular Pharmacology 2009;54:552–9.

Tate CG, Schertler GFX. Engineering G protein-coupled receptors to facilitate their structure determination. Current Opinion in Structural Biology 2009;19: 386–95.

Uetrecht J. Prediction of a new drug's potential to cause idiosyncratic reactions. Current Opinion in Drug Discovery & Development 2001;4:55–9.

Ulrich RG. Idiosyncratic toxicity: a convergence of risk factors. Annual Review of Medicine 2007;58:17–34.

Waring MJ. Lipophilicity in drug discovery. Expert Opinion on Drug Discovery 2010;5:235–48.

Wehling M. Assessing the translatability of drug projects: what needs to be scored to predict success? Nature Reviews Drug Discovery 2009;8: 541–6.

Westby M, van der Ryst E. CCR5 antagonists: host-targeted antivirals for the treatment of HIV infection. Antiviral Chemistry & Chemotherapy 2005;16(6):339–54.

Wester K, Jönsson AK, Spigset O, et al. Incidence of fatal adverse drug reactions: a population based study. British journal of Clinical Pharmacology 2008;65:573–9.

Wetzel S, Klein K, Renner S, et al. Interactive exploration of chemical space with scaffold hunter. Nature Chemical Biology 2009;5: 581–3.

White RE. Pharmacokinetics of drug candidates. Wiley Encyclopedia of Chemical Biology 2009;3:652–61.

Whittaker M, Law RJ, Ichihara O, et al. Fragments: past, present and future. Drug Discovery Today: Technologies 2010;7:E163–E171.

Windass AS, Lowes S, Wang Y, et al. The contribution of organic anion transporters OAT1 and OAT3 to the renal uptake of rosuvastatin. Journal of Pharmacology and Experimental Therapeutics 2007;322:1221–7.

Witchel HJ. Emerging trends in ion channel-based assays for predicting the cardiac safety of drugs. IDrugs 2010;13:90–6.

Chapter | 10 |

Metabolism and pharmacokinetic optimization strategies in drug discovery

P Ballard, P Brassil, K H Bui, H Dolgos, C Petersson, A Tunek, P J H Webborn

INTRODUCTION

Optimization of drug metabolic and pharmacokinetic properties is an integral component of the modern drug discovery process. The objective of the drug metabolism and pharmacokinetics (DMPK) discipline in drug discovery is to aid design and selection of candidate drugs with properties that yield the required efficacy and safety for effective clinical use. The roles of DMPK at the various stages of drug discovery are summarized in Table 10.1. DMPK in vitro and in vivo information are used throughout the drug discovery process to facilitate target validation and safety assessment, and to guide the conversion of early screening hits and leads into drug candidates. Indeed, the frontloading of DMPK in drug discovery has resulted in a reduction of drug attrition rate due to undesirable DMPK properties from approximately 40% in 1990 to 10% in 2000 (Kola and Landis, 2004).

To help drug hunting teams focus on the key issues and goals, in a multitude of screening options, it is important to prescribe, as early as possible, a candidate drug target profile in terms of efficacy, potency, safety and ease of use. DMPK plays a central role in defining this target profile. For instance to be commercially attractive in terms of ease of use, a compound has to be orally active, has a convenient dosing regimen and be able to be administered without effect from food and other medications. The physicochemical and DMPK attributes that will allow a compound to meet this target profile would be: good solubility and permeability, high oral bioavailability, low clearance and reasonable half-life (if PD half-life is not much longer than PK half life), and absence of 'drug–drug interaction' potential. Likewise to be orally active, a compound should have good oral bioavailability and able to reach the target organ at high enough concentration to engage the target.

In this chapter, strategies to optimize key DMPK challenges using appropriate in silico, in vitro and in vivo DMPK tools during drug discovery are presented. The rational use of these strategies will help 'drug hunting' projects to advance drug candidates with attractive DMPK target profile and with low potential for failure in development due to DMPK issues. In addition, as prediction of human PK and safe and effective dose is probably the most important activity in drug discovery to ensure that the candidate drug has the attribute to test the biological hypothesis in patients, strategy to integrate information in discovery to holistically predict PK properties in man will be discussed.

OPTIMIZATION OF DMPK PROPERTIES

Optimization principles are described for six key DMPK areas:

- Absorption and bioavailability
- Avoiding PK-based drug–drug interactions
- Achieving/avoiding CNS exposure
- Clearance
- Role of metabolite identification:
  - Active metabolites
  - Minimizing risk for reactive metabolites.

The following sections summarize current understanding/available tools and suggest best practice for each of the above. Each section introduces the challenges, outlines tactics for dealing with them and identifies areas requiring caution.

Table 10.1 Roles of drug metabolism and pharmacokinetics (DMPK) in various phases of drug discovery

Discovery phase	DMPK roles
Target identification	Selection and characterization of tool compounds Partner with in vivo pharmacology and toxicology in target validation and safety assessment activities
Hit identification	In silico and in vitro DMPK profiling to help prioritize hit series
Lead identification	Identify DMPK liabilities of lead series Determine whether if DMPK properties in lead series are optimizable (DMPK liabities not linked to pharmacophore) Develop structure (DMPK) property relationship (SPR) Develop 'in vitro in vivo' correlation (IVIVC) Guide selection of lead series Contribute to development of PD assay and develop early PK/PD understanding Contribute to development of PD assays and develop early PK/PD understanding
Lead optimization	Guide optimization of DMPK properties toward target profile Comprehensive DMPK characterization of candidate compounds Develop biomarker based and/or efficacy/disease related PK/PD models Prediction of human PK Prediction of efficacious human dose Integration of predicted profile to calculate key margins against side effects

Absorption and oral bioavailability

Introduction

As the preferred route of administration for most indications is oral, it is important to characterize oral bioavailability (F) of a compound during drug discovery. In addition, F must be optimized, as a low F is often associated with poor and variable exposure and lack of efficacy. F is defined as the percentage of dosed drug that reaches the systemic circulation compared to the IV route. As shown below, it can be considered to be dependent on three serial steps: the fraction of dosed drug absorbed (f_a), the fraction escaping intestinal metabolism (f_g) and the fraction extracted by the liver as it passes from the portal vein to the systemic circulation (f_h) (see Rowland and Tozer, 1989):

$$F = f_a \times f_g \times f_h$$

f_a is influenced by a number of factors including the gastrointestinal (GI) solubility (dose, particle size, pH solubility profile and formulation), the effective permeability (both passive permeability and active transport processes) and GI stability. f_g and f_h are affected by metabolic enzymes in the intestinal wall and liver, respectively. In addition, f_h can be influenced by transporters if a drug is excreted unchanged into the bile. Both metabolic and active transport processes are saturable, generally obeying Michaelis–Menten kinetics. Hence, f_a, f_g and f_h can all be non-linear if relevant concentrations are above the Michaelis–Menten constant (K_m) for the particular enzyme/transporter–drug interaction.

In humans, the combinations of high to low solubility and permeability have led compounds to be characterized according to the Biopharmaceutical Classification System (Amidon et al., 1995). Class 1 compounds, with high solubility and permeability, generally have very good absorption properties. Those in Class 4, with poor solubility and permeability, are likely to present significant formulation challenges and/or variable and poor exposure. It can be important to characterize the maximum absorbable dose (MAD) of a compound relative to its predicted therapeutic dose, as this will determine the risk of being able to deliver an efficacious dose to humans and guide whether high exposure in safety studies is achievable.

Table 10.2 gives guidance on acceptable pharmaceutical properties for typical oral drug candidates.

Tactics

In theory, it is relatively simple to obtain good absorption and to ensure that solubility and permeability fall within the right ranges. However, the reality is more complex. From an in vivo perspective, the product of absorption and intestinal metabolism is often assessed by accounting for first-pass hepatic clearance in bioavailability estimations:

$$f_a \times f_g = F/f_h$$

If f_a x f_g is low, it is important to understand the relative contribution of both f_a and f_g to F so that this can be designed out of the project. Generally it is simplest to

Table 10.2 Pharmaceutical development candidate drug target profile (CDTP)

Property	CDTP	Impact on pivotal safety studies and initial clinical evaluations if not met	Impact of not meeting on later drug development timelines
Crystallinity	Crystalline	Significant risk of non-robustness of manufacture and performance of drug substance with the potential for variable exposure in safety and clinical studies due to physical instability Crystalline material required for assessment of formulation approaches and exposure	Significant issues with robustness of manufacture, performance and ease of handling of both drug substance and drug product Potential of compromising clinical studies due to physical instability as drug substance and in drug product requiring additional time and resources
Thermal property	No melt or other event < 80°C		
Hygroscopicity	< 2% uptake at 25 °C/80% relative humidity		
Chemical stability	>90% (in solution formulation after at least 1 day at room temperature)	Insufficient stability for SA studies. More time and resources needed to understand degradation and mitigate in line with the formulation strategy (storage, pack or formulation) for safety and first time in man studies	Consideration of the learning in phase 1 and assess impact and options in line with the formulation strategy. Risk of short shelf-life of the product
Maximum absorbable dose (MAD)	MAD ≥ predicted dose to man	Significant risk for not reaching required exposures in early clinical and safety studies. More time and resources needed to develop enhancing formulations as well as a risk of failure	High risk for not reaching clinically relevant exposures using conventional formulations. Strategy with non-conventional formulations will require more time and resources in development. Obvious risk of development failure
Predicted fraction absorbed (fa) at predicted dose to man	Fa ≥ 50 %		

estimate the likely f_a and if this does not account for the poor f_a x f_g value, f_g should be investigated. Poor absorption can be a result of slow dissolution rate, low solubility in the GI tract, poor effective permeability (passive or active efflux), or instability in GI fluids or in the wall of the GI tract. If absorption is adequate but bioavailability is poor, hepatic clearance (metabolic or biliary elimination) and/or intestinal metabolism may need to be optimized.

When maximizing the chances of good absorption, the starting point is to ensure that the physicochemical properties of the compound/series are in the optimal space as described by Lipinski and others (Lipinski et al., 1997; Wenlock et al., 2003; Johnson et al., 2009; Waring, 2009). Generally, this requires minimizing the number of H-bond donors and acceptors, restricting lipophilicity in the range $LogD_{7.4}$ 0 to 3, and limiting molecular weight to <500. Both the solubility and passive permeability of a compound should be assessed prior to any in vivo study. Predictive models for these should be assessed for suitability in each project and considered in compound design if either is an issue for a chemical series.

The primary in vitro tool for assessing absorption is the cell based Caco-2 permeability assay, although MDCK-MDR1, PAMPA (parallel artificial membrane permeability assay), or in silico predictions may also provide valuable information about efflux transporter risk and permeability. This permeability assessment, in combination with a solubility measurement (ideally using crystalline material), is used to estimate f_a using commercially available modelling tools like GastroPlus (www.simulations-plus.com) or SIMCYP (www.simcyp.com). For actively transported (efflux or uptake) compounds, bi-directional permeability assays can be used as a guide to possible in vivo effects. However, it should be noted that it is often difficult to extrapolate the results from these in vitro transport assays to accurately quantify effects in vivo. Because of its reasonable throughput, the Caco-2 assay can be positioned as an early screen if absorption or permeability/efflux is found to be an issue in the project. If further evaluation of absorption or efflux is warranted, it is possible to use more physiological models such as sections of intestinal tissue in an Ussing Chamber (Ungell et al., 1998), or transfected cell lines over-expressing particular

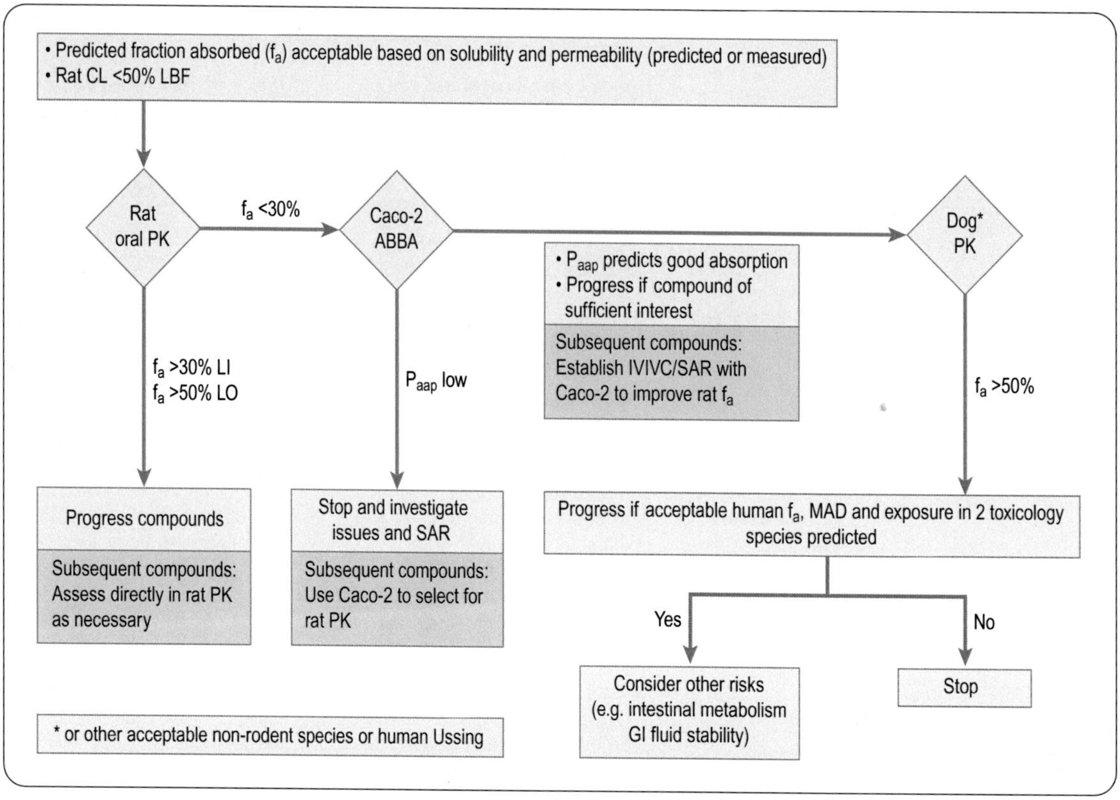

- Predicted fraction absorbed (f_a) acceptable based on solubility and permeability (predicted or measured)
- Rat CL <50% LBF

Rat oral PK

f_a <30%

Caco-2 ABBA

Dog* PK

- P_{aap} predicts good absorption
- Progress if compound of sufficient interest

Subsequent compounds: Establish IVIVC/SAR with Caco-2 to improve rat f_a

f_a >30% LI
f_a >50% LO

P_{aap} low

f_a >50%

Progress compounds

Subsequent compounds: Assess directly in rat PK as necessary

Stop and investigate issues and SAR

Subsequent compounds: Use Caco-2 to select for rat PK

Progress if acceptable human f_a, MAD and exposure in 2 toxicology species predicted

Yes

No

Consider other risks (e.g. intestinal metabolism GI fluid stability)

Stop

* or other acceptable non-rodent species or human Ussing

Fig. 10.1 Absorption troubleshooting decision tree. Caco-2 ABBA, transport assays; CL, clearance; f_a, fraction of dose absorbed; GI, gastro-intestinal; IVIVC, in vitro to in vivo correlation; LBF, liver blood flow; LI, lead identification; LO, optimization; MAD, maximum absorbable dose; Papp, apparent permeability; SAR, structure–activity relationship.

efflux transporters (e.g. P-gp in the MDCK-MDR1 cell line). The Ussing Chamber technique can help in understanding cross-species differences and, because the tissue used is enzymatically competent (metabolic and transporters), the output represents the product of f_a and f_g.

Compounds with low hepatic clearance in the rat, good solubility and high effective permeability should exhibit good oral absorption and bioavailability in that species. However, if this is not the case, the troubleshooting decision tree in Figure 10.1 can be used to help determine the cause(s) of poor absorption, identify assays to aid in optimizing compound design and understand if the compound is of sufficient quality to progress in the value chain, despite its non-optimal absorption properties.

Table 10.3 is an aid to selecting the assays and techniques to use in the decision tree (Figure 10.1), to explain potential issues and risks, and the parameter (f_a, f_g and/or f_h) the assays impact on.

Cautions

- As scaling factors for intestinal microsomes or other subcellular intestinal fractions are currently not available, it is difficult to make an accurate quantitative assessment of the contribution of intestinal metabolism to in vivo f_a. However, attempts have been made to use CL_{int} from human liver microsomes or S9 fraction to estimate the relative contributions of f_a and f_g to F (Gertz et al., 2010).
- It is often very difficult to pinpoint why compounds have poor absorption characteristics and, therefore, to resolve this design issue. Thus, it is often reasonable to prioritize series with good f_a x f_g, in early discovery even if other properties (e.g. potency, clearance) are less attractive.
- Typically, oral doses are formulated as suspensions which, on many occasions, may be derived from amorphous material. However, it is important to assess absorption periodically using crystalline material, as physical form may have substantial effects on absorption profiles.
- Particularly for compounds likely to proceed into development, it is important to determine the effect of the polymorphic solid states on absorption. It is also important to ensure that the formulations used are discussed with Pharmaceutical Development (see

Table 10.3 Assays and techniques used when troubleshooting absorption

Assay/technique	Potential issue/risk addressed	Impacted
Intestinal microsomes or S9 fraction	Assess cross species differences in intestinal metabolism. Nature and source of metabolites can give key information about potential for gut metabolism, as CYP3A and UGTs account for most gut metabolites	f_g
Absorption profiling on Caco-2 cells	Varying apical to basolateral pH gradient Concentration dependency Use of proteins (e.g. BSA) at various percentages in apical chamber Use of efflux transporter inhibitors	f_a
PAMPA	Passive permeability	f_a
High dose PK studies	Saturation of efflux or metabolism	f_a, f_g, f_h
Ussing chamber technique	Effective permeability (including transporters) Intestinal tissue metabolism	f_a, f_g
GI stability test	Degradation of drug in stomach or intestinal lumen is possible explanation (usually the case if predicted F much greater than measured F)	f_a
Human metabolic phenotyping	Gut metabolism	f_g, f_h
In situ/in vivo portal vein cannulation preparation	Determine amount of drug and metabolites passing through intestine	f_a, f_g
SIMCYP; GastroPlus	Predict absorption rate and extent (software methods)	f_a
Transfected cell lines; vesicles expressing specific transporters; Caco-2 efflux assay with and without specific transporter inhibitors	Determine involvement of specific efflux transporters	f_a, f_h
Knock-out (KO) animals; chemical KO with inhibitors	Determine involvement of specific efflux transporters	f_a, f_g, f_h

Chapter 16), and are appropriate for safety and early clinical development studies.

- If in vitro and in vivo (rat and dog) assessments of f_a do not agree, the risk of an inaccurate estimate of absorption in man will increase. Sometimes other species have been investigated to mitigate this risk, but we caution that there can, for example, be marked discrepancies in f_a x f_g between cynomolgus monkeys and humans (Takahashi et al., 2009).

Avoidance of PK based drug–drug interactions

Introduction

Aid in the design and selection of candidate drugs with a low potential for PK-based drug–drug interactions (DDI) is a key role of discovery DMPK. There are four main forms of PK-based DDI, in which the compound may be a perpetrator or be a victim of DDI:

- Competitive (reversible) cytochrome P450 (CYP) inhibition
- Mechanism based/time dependent CYP inhibition
- Uptake and efflux transporter inhibition
- CYP induction.

CYP, notably CYP3A4 and CYP2D6, based DDI is the most important and most common, and may occur in the liver or intestine. Transporter based DDI is mainly related to renal clearance, although specific issues can arise with CNS compounds and hepatic uptake of statins. The science and regulatory guidance to support risk assessment of CYP-based DDI are well established, but is less advanced for transporter-related issues (Bjornsson et al., 2003; US Food and Drug Administration, 1997, 2006; Huang et al., 2008; International Transporter Consortium, 2010).

Tactics

Competitive (reversible) CYP inhibition

Two main types of CYP inhibition assays with different capabilities are in general use. Fluorescence based assays are relatively cheap and have enhanced throughput, but in a small but significant number of cases can lead to misrepresenting DDI risk (Bell et al., 2008). They are best used for initial profiling of large numbers of compounds, with the data being acceptable in the early phase such as lead generation. LCMS based assays are more expensive, have lower throughput, but are more predictive. They should be used in optimization cycles once CYP inhibition issues have been identified, and for generating compound profiles during more advanced project phases.

Inhibition of the five major CYP isoforms 1A2, 2C9, 2C19, 2D6 and 3A4, should be evaluated in the earliest phases, while later it would be prudent to assess potential interactions with isoforms 2B6, 2C8 and 3A5.

Reduction of CYP inhibition potential is facilitated by the fact that strong QSAR relationships are often obtained. Various computational models that allow prediction of CYP DDI risk are available within most drug development companies. It is well established that lipophilicity, aromaticity and charge type are major drivers for inhibiting various CYP enzymes (Gleeson et al., 2007).

The risk of DDIs based on Phase 2 metabolism (e.g. glucuronidation and sulphation) is usually small, resulting in less than a two-fold increase in area under the concentration versus time curve (AUC), and they are rarely observed, possibly due in part to the nature of the enzymatic reaction (high V_{max} and moderate to high K_m values). Such DDIs are not generally evaluated in lead optimization (Williams et al., 2004). Evidence suggesting the need to do so at this stage should prompt re-evaluation of the risk.

The decision tree in Figure 10.2 can be used to assess the potential DDI risk of a competitive CYP inhibitor. Hits identified in a fluorescence-based assay should be confirmed with an LCMS-based assay using druglike substrates as probes for the different CYP isoforms. Although the ratio $C_{max}/K_{i,u}$ can be used to obtain a preliminary estimate of the DDI risk, more accurate evaluation should be conducted using PBPK modelling (e.g. SIMCYP platform) to predict the potential clinical risk (expanded below in 'Prediction of DDI risk'").

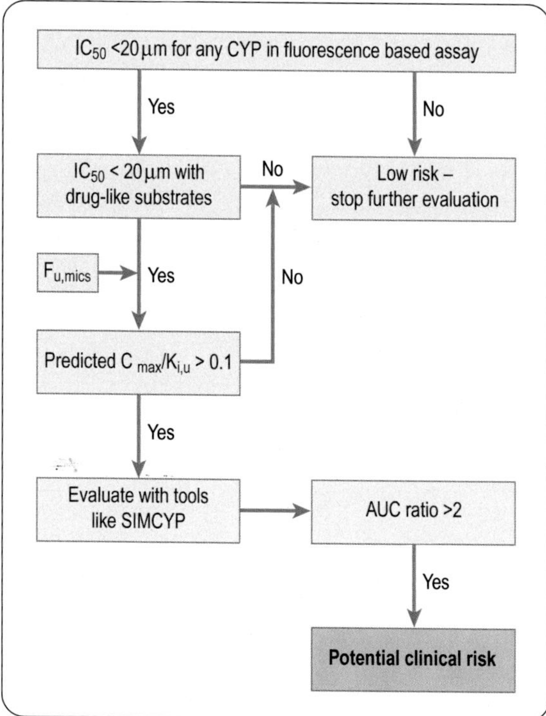

Fig. 10.2 Decision tree for reversible DDI CYP inhibition. AUC, area under the concentration-time curve; C_{max}, maximum concentration; CYP, cytochrome P450; DDI, drug-drug interaction; $f_{u,mics}$, fraction unbound in microsomes); IC_{50}, concentration producing 50% inhibition; $K_{i,u}$, unbound dissociation rate constant; SIMCYP, software platform.

Mechanism-based/time-dependent CYP inhibition

The inhibition of CYP enzymes may be irreversible (due to irreversible or covalent binding to the prosthetic haem or the enzyme) or quasi-irreversible (due to the formation of transient complexes with the iron of the haem prosthetic group). Time-dependent inhibition (TDI) methods can be used to determine this (Riley et al., 2007; Fowler and Zhang, 2008). During early phases of drug discovery, a medium throughput screening assay can be used to screen for TDI. However, for selecting candidates at later phases, the method employed should provide accurate determination of K_{inact} and K_i to properly evaluate the DDI risks of compounds in which preliminary screening indicated the potential for TDI. A positive TDI finding also suggests that the compound or its metabolites may be reactive, and further evaluation should be conducted as specified by reactive metabolite strategies.

A decision tree to help evaluate the potential DDI risk of a TDI CYP inhibitor is shown in Figure 10.3. If a compound is found to be at risk for CYP inhibition (IC_{50} <20 µM) or is flagged to have a potential liability for reactive metabolites, it should be screened for TDI. If it is found to have potential TDI risk based on screening data, K_i and K_{inact} values should be generated to help accurately predict the risk using prediction tools like SIMCYP.

Uptake and efflux transporter inhibition

Uptake transporter inhibition assays are emerging as being of real value (Ward, 2008), but they are highly

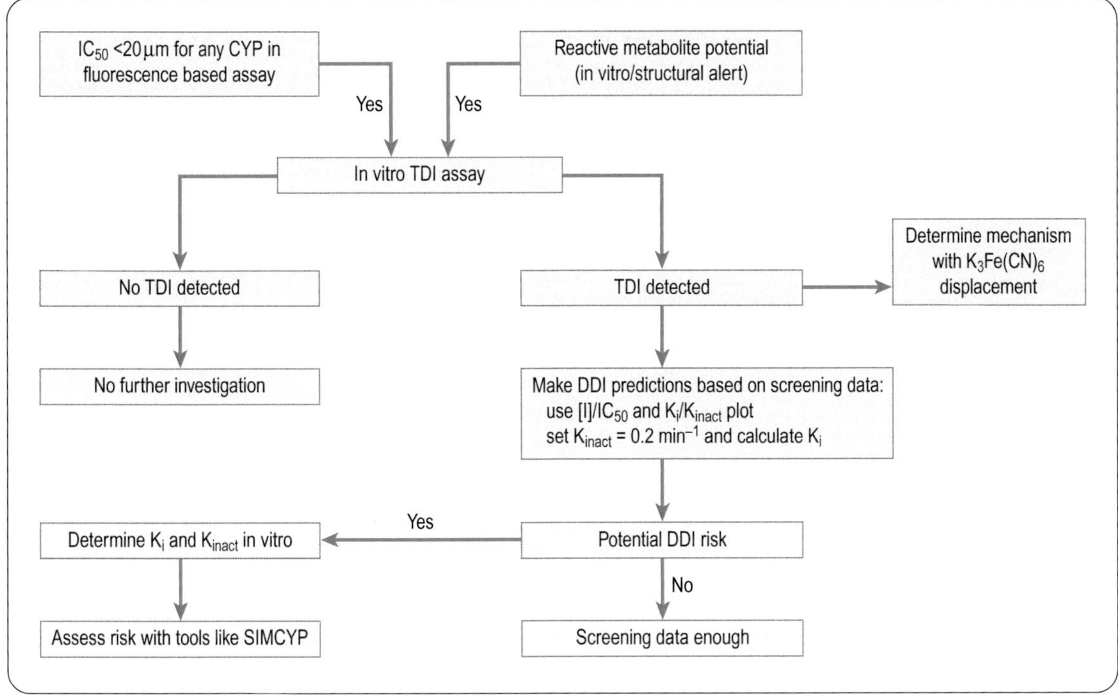

Fig. 10.3 Decision tree to assess time dependent inhibition (TDI) risk. CYP, cytochrome P450; DDI, drug–drug interaction; K_i, dissociation rate constant; K_{inact}, inactivation rate constant; [I], inhibitor concentration; IC_{50}, concentration producing 50% inhibition; SIMCYP, assay method; TDI, time dependent inhibition.

dependent on chemotype (e.g. acids being primarily transported by organic anion transporters (OATs)) and likely co-medications (e.g. OCT2 and metformin). Acids and zwitterions should be assessed for inhibition of OATP1B1 during drug discovery. Other inhibition assays (OAT1, OAT3, OATP1B1, OCT1 and OCT2) should be used on a case-by-case basis.

Efflux transporters are believed to serve a protective function, and prevent molecules perceived as foreign from gaining entry in cells or tissues. Of the various efflux transporters, P-glycoprotein (P-gp) is the most prevalent and well understood. As specific locations of the P-gp transporter include small intestine enterocytes, hepatocytes, the kidney and the blood–brain barrier, P-gp can affect oral bioavailability, biliary and renal clearance, and brain uptake of compounds that are substrates of P-gp. In addition, compounds that modulate P-gp can influence the clearance and distribution of drugs that are substrates of P-gp. The bi-directional transport assay using either Caco-2 (P-gp, BCRP, and MRP2) or MDCK-MDRI (specifically for P-gp) cells is widely available. Evaluation of the potential to inhibit P-gp should be evaluated in early discovery using a bi-directional transport assay with a probe P-gp substrate (e.g. digoxin). If a compound is found to be a P-gp inhibitor, its potential impact for P-gp inhibition in the liver or in the gut can be estimated based on its estimated local exposure and the IC_{50}.

Determination of clearance mechanism and CYP phenotyping

The potential for a compound to be a victim of a DDI with a co-medication is greatly reduced if there are multiple clearance mechanisms, particularly involving metabolism by multiple CYP enzymes. This should be a consideration if the therapeutic window is low or if the clinical/marketing disadvantage of the interaction would be significant. Quantitative assessment of multiple clearance mechanisms and phenotyping of CYP metabolism should be established for any candidate drug. Methods for phenotyping the individual CYP enzymes responsible for a drug's metabolism include the use of (1) specific chemicals or antibodies as specific enzyme inhibitors, (2) individual human recombinant CYPs, and (3) a bank of human liver microsomes characterized for CYP activity prepared from individual donor livers. At nomination of a candidate drug, human phenotyping work should include all eight major CYPs (1A2, 2B6, 2C8, 2C9, 2C19, 2D6, 3A4/3A5), and be followed by other enzymes if necessary. Another way to investigate clearance mechanisms in vitro is a so-called 'fractional Clint' assay. In such an assay the rate of parent disappearance is measured in human hepatocytes with and without the presence of an enzyme inhibitor. Most common is the addition of ketoconazole to block out the CYP3A4 contribution to metabolism. The remaining rate of metabolism in such an assay can be attributed non-CYP3A4 pathways like phase 2 enzymes, other CYPs or any other possible mechanism.

CYP induction mediated risk for DDI

Induction of specific CYP enzymes may not only change a drug's metabolic profile but also have toxicological consequences as CYP enzymes are also involved in the metabolism and synthesis of important endogenous compounds. Although close collaboration with Safety Assessment (see Chapter 15) is needed to evaluate the full impact of CYP induction, it is DMPK's primary responsibility to predict the DDI potential caused by CYP induction in man. This should be done during optimization with the use of HepaRG cells which are a good surrogate of primary human hepatocytes for AhR-mediated CYP1A induction and PXR- and CAR-mediated CYP3A4 and CYP2B6 induction. If higher throughput is needed during the optimization phase, the PXR reporter gene assay may be used to minimize PXR-dependent CYP3A4 induction liability.

Prediction of DDI risk

Once inhibition (of CYP enzymes and/or transporters) potential has been assessed in vitro, a risk assessment is made by examining the data in relation to the likely clinical exposures. At candidate drug nomination, a thorough evaluation of CYP-based DDI risk (both reversible and irreversible) should be made using PBPK modelling (e.g. SIMCYP platform). PBPK modelling can be used to estimate relevant concentration of inhibitors at the inlet to the liver or in the gut and to assess DDI risks in various patient populations.

During early drug discovery, a simple criterion can be used to determine if CYP inhibition presents little or no risk. For this purpose, an IC_{50} of >20 μM provides a reasonable cut-off. Should the predicted therapeutic exposures be very low, then a lower cut-off might be rationally adopted.

To assess CYP induction potential, the E_{max} and EC_{50} obtained from human hepatocytes (e.g. HepaRG cells) induction assays, can be used in conjunction with predicted human exposure (free C_{max} or free liver inlet concentration) to calculate a relative induction score. This is then compared against the relative induction scores of known inducers to estimate the percent human AUC change.

A compound is likely to be a victim of clinically relevant DDI with a co-medication if it has a narrow therapeutic

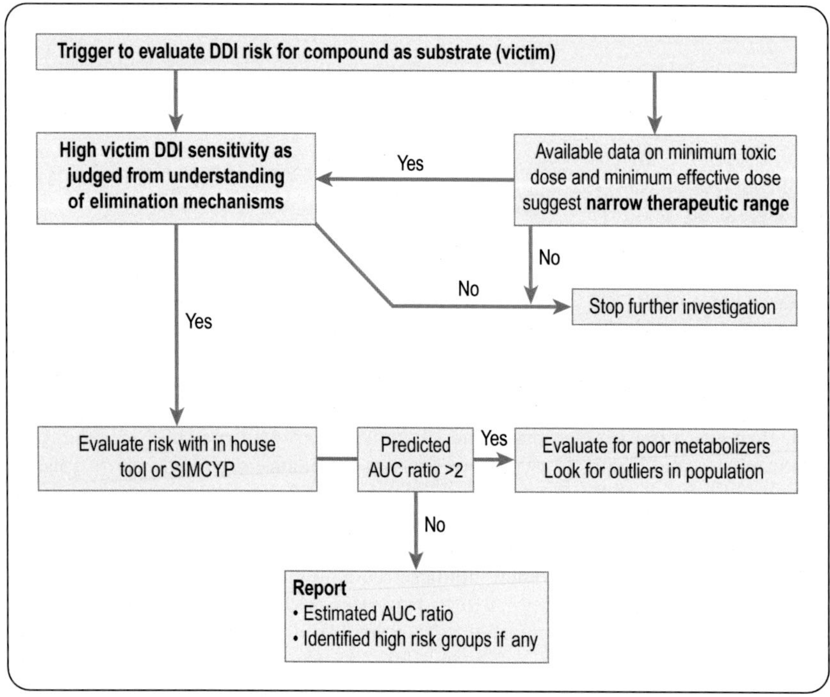

Fig. 10.4 Decision tree to assess risk as a drug–drug interaction (DDI) victim. AUC, area under the concentration-time curve; CYP, cytochrome P450; f_m, fraction metabolized; f_u, fraction unbound; SIMCYP, software platform.

window and is a sensitive substrate to an inhibited enzyme/transporter, as indicated by high values of fraction metabolized (f_m), fraction of CYP metabolized ($f_{m,CYP}$), and fraction unbound (f_u), and by plasma and hepatic extraction. This risk can be reduced by ensuring that the clearance mechanism in question represents <50% of total clearance (resulting in less than a two-fold change in the AUC of the victim compound). At candidate drug nomination, software tools such as SIMCYP could be used to evaluate the impact of known inhibitors or inducers on the relevant candidate compounds if their clearance is driven mainly by a single enzyme or transporter. Figure 10.4 is a decision tree to help in assessing the potential risk that a compound will be a DDI victim. A compound is deemed to have this potential risk if it has a narrow therapeutic window or is cleared predominantly by a single CYP enzyme. A simple Excel based DDI template or SIMCYP should be used to estimate the risk. If the CYP enzyme involved is polymorphic, evaluate the impact of polymorphism to identify high-risk populations.

Cautions

- Software tools such as SIMCYP can be used to estimate the potential and magnitude of DDI, particularly in populations at most risk. DDI risk is currently best assessed by relating IC_{50} to free drug concentrations at the sites of action (liver or gut). However, because of the current regulatory position, it may be necessary to conduct clinical studies where the perceived risk is based on total drug concentrations.
- CYP based DDI due to CYP3A4 inhibition may have an impact on the bioavailability of co-medications through inhibition of intestinal CYP3A4. Although the area is complex, SIMCYP has the capability of assessing likely clinical impact.
- Animal studies are of little value for assessing CYP DDI risk. However, they may be of use in developing an understanding of potential transporter mediated DDI.

Central nervous system uptake

Introduction

The brain is a protected organ, being separated from the systemic circulation by three barriers: the blood–brain barrier formed primarily by cerebrovascular endothelial cells between the blood and brain tissue, the choroid plexus epithelium between the blood and ventricular cerebrospinal fluid (CSF), and the arachnoid epithelium between the blood and subarachnoid CSF. These barriers, which exhibit low paracellular permeability and express multiple drug transporters, restrict the entry of compounds with either very low transcellular (passive) permeability and/or, more importantly, compounds with high affinity for efflux transporters.

The quantitation of CNS exposure is necessary for both CNS and peripherally targeted (i.e. that require restriction from the CNS) therapies as a means to estimate the unbound brain concentration required for efficacy and CNS-mediated side effects. Unless other information is available, the unbound concentration is assumed to be the relevant exposure measure for both desired and undesired pharmacological effects. The reason for this is that measurement of total concentration can be very misleading, being to a large extent driven by non-specific binding to brain tissue and thus strongly correlated with physicochemical properties (e.g. lipophilicity and charge). The tactics below therefore focus on assessing unbound concentration in the brain relative to the free concentration in blood or plasma.

Tactics

Screening cascades for both CNS targeted and CNS-restricted compounds should contain an efflux/permeability assay (Di et al., 2008). MDCK-MDR1 or Caco-2 cells may be used (Table 10.2) and MDCK-MDR1 may offer better sensitivity for P-gp substrates, while Caco-2 cells, which are a constitutive system, have the advantage of identifying substrates of several efflux mechanisms not necessarily limited to P-gp.

Peripheral restriction can be obtained either by efflux or very low passive permeability. The latter is often difficult to combine with oral pharmacological activity, as it requires extreme physical properties (e.g. very low/negative LogP).

Efflux ratios obtained in vitro should be used for risk assessment in the early phases and once validated in vivo, can be used for progression of compounds through the screening cascade. The ratio may be optimized using in silico models (Fridén et al., 2009b) or simple rule sets. Roughly, P-gp substrates can be estimated by the 'rule of fours' (Didziapetris et al., 2003), where compounds with a sum of nitrogen and oxygen atoms ≥8, molecular weight >400 and acid pK_a >4 are likely to be P-gp substrates, whereas compounds with a sum of nitrogen and oxygen atoms ≤4, molecular weight <400 and base pK_a <8 are likely to be non-substrates. Additionally, it has been suggested that LogP should be >2 to allow for sufficient passive permeability, i.e. lower sensitivity to efflux (Hitchcock and Pennington, 2006).

Commencing during lead generation, it is important to establish an in vitro/in vivo correlation using in vivo experiments to determine the ratio $C_{u,br}/C_{u,pl}$ (Table 10.4). The fraction unbound in brain may be determined ex vivo using brain binding assays such as the brain homogenate or brain slice (Fridén et al., 2009a; Wan et al., 2007) methods and, together with determined total brain concentration in vivo, enables the calculation of $C_{u,br}$.

Table 10.4 Assay and CNS measurement attributes at various milestones for compounds requiring CNS access or restriction

Phase	Assay/study	Attribute if access required to CNS	Attribute required for CNS restriction
Hit to lead	Bidirectional Caco-2 assay	Profile hit series for permeability/efflux liabilities	Profile hit series for permeability/ efflux liabilities
		Prioritize and select hit series based on absence of liabilities	Prioritize and select hit series based on absence of liabilities
Lead identification	Bidirectional Caco-2 assay	Determine optimization feasibility	Determine optimization feasibility
Early		Evaluate usefulness of in silico tools and develop project specific in silico model	Evaluate usefulness of in silico tools and develop project-specific in silico model
		Develop series-specific CNS penetrant tool compounds	
Late	Protein and brain binding assay	Estimate free brain concentration to help develop PD model and establish IVIVC	Estimation of free brain concentration to help develop a PD model and establish IVIVC
	In vivo CNS distribution study	Estimate free brain concentration to help develop PD model and establish IVIVC	Estimation of free brain concentration to help develop a PD model and establish IVIVC
Lead optimization	Bi-directional Caco-2 assay Protein and brain binding assays	Optimize away from efflux substrates Optimize free ratio $C_{u,br}/C_{u,pl}$ at steady state towards unity, build IVIVC	Optimize away towards efflux substrates Optimize free ratio $C_{u,br}/C_{u,pl}$ at steady state away from unity, build IVIVC Continue to build IVIVC
	In vivo CNS distribution study In vivo P-gp inhibitor/KO studies	Continue to build IVIVC Understand impact of efflux in vivo Establish IVIVC	
Milestones	**Assay/study**	**Attribute if access required to CNS**	**Attribute required for CNS restriction**
CD nomination	Bi-directional Caco-2 assay	Assess risk of involvement of efflux transporters in human	Assess risk of involvement of efflux transporters in human (DDI focus)
	In vivo P-gp inhibitor/KO studies	Assess risk of involvement of efflux transporters in human	Assess risk of involvement of efflux transporters in human (DDI focus)
	In vitro mechanistic studies	Evaluate species difference in efflux if tools exist	Evaluate species difference in efflux if tools exist
	Protein and brain binding assays	For central targets, free brain concentrations should be <3 times free plasma concentrations at steady state*	
	In vivo CNS distribution study	Understand potential interspecies differences in plasma protein binding	Knowledge of pharmacodynamics for CNS related side effects to establish required ratio
	Microdialysis/CSF	To determine rates, and better understand pharmacodynamics and translation to man	To determine rates, and better understand pharmacodynamics and translation to man

*Measurement of free ratios is a composite of one in vivo and two in vitro experiments. Total experimental error may be as high as three-fold.

CSF, cerebrospinal fluid; DDI, drug–drug interaction; IVIVC, in vitro to in vivo correlation; KO, knock-out; PD, pharmacodynamic

Initial brain distribution studies may be performed with single compounds or cassettes using subcutaneous or oral administration, preferably at steady state or with more than one time point. Samples generated in pharmacodynamic models may also be used. In late stages, longer intravenous infusion studies may be used to generate a ratio closer to steady state.

Failure to establish in vitro/in vivo correlations may provide a trigger for investigations using:

- In vitro/in vivo interaction studies with inhibitors
- CNS distribution studies in alternative species to gain an understanding of differences in transporter expression/specificity
- In vitro studies (e.g. alternate cell lines) with over-expression of animal transporters or additional human transporters
- In vivo studies in knock-out (KO)/polymorph animals.

In vivo intracerebral microdialysis may be useful for indications where the rate of CNS distribution is critical, and for simultaneous studies of biomarkers/effect and CNS compound levels. Because this method enables direct and repeated measurement of extracellular fluid, it is possible to determine both the rate and extent of CNS penetration. The utility of the technique is limited by the physicochemical properties of the compounds studied.

Although the concentration in CSF may differ from that in extracellular fluid, sampling of CSF in animals could be used since it may offer translatability of CNS distribution in man. In addition, associations between in vitro potency and unbound plasma EC_{50}s of robust PD endpoints such as receptor occupancy should be made, to confirm CNS distribution.

Cautions

- It is important to note that a relevant brain to plasma ratio will only be generated at steady state like conditions, so the $C_{u,br}/C_{u,pl}$ may be very different in steady state and non-steady state conditions. For CNS acting compounds, it is therefore critical not only to appreciate any acute/steady state differences in CNS distribution, but also to consider the steady state CNS distribution kinetics at pharmacodynamic endpoints using human dose estimates. For peripheral targets where CNS restriction is important, high $C_{u,br}/C_{u,pl}$ ratios may be unacceptable.
- There are indications that levels in CSF overestimate free levels in brain, especially for efflux substrates (Fridén et al., 2009b), although the latter has been challenged (Doran et al., 2005). The translatability of CSF concentrations from animal to human is also somewhat limited because CSF samples in animals are usually collected from the cisterna magna (proximal part of CSF) while those in man are collected from the more distal lumbar region. Very few data are available regarding the distribution of compounds within CSF.
- It may be difficult to assess free levels of acidic compounds in CNS with standard methodologies (Fridén et al., 2010), because the high plasma protein binding and low tissue binding of such compounds result in inaccurate data due to blood contamination of the brain tissue. The brain homogenate binding method has limited use for drugs that reside predominantly in the interstitial space or compounds that are accumulated intracellularly. In such cases, the brain slice method may provide a better alternative.

Clearance optimization

Introduction

Optimization of clearance is one of the major challenges in drug discovery because clearance must be suitably low in order to achieve an appropriate half-life and bioavailability, and therefore dose, in man. However, human clearance cannot be optimized directly because it is never measured preclinically, which presents two key challenges. Firstly, there is the need to identify the key elimination processes that determine clearance, and secondly, those processes must be optimized through appropriate use of human in vitro systems and/or animal data.

Identification of the likely key clearance mechanism(s) in man is supported by a detailed understanding of elimination kinetics in animals and demonstration of the ability of human in vitro tools to predict hepatic clearance in man. This puts emphasis on animal kinetics in all phases of drug discovery to select the appropriate tools and models for both compound optimization and human PK prediction.

There are advantages in having elimination via multiple clearance mechanisms, notably for mitigation of DDI risks. This extends to metabolism by multiple enzymes, which helps mitigate against significant metabolism (>70%) by highly variable enzyme activities in a population (i.e. CYP3A4 – see Rawden et al., 2005) and against polymorphic enzyme metabolism (e.g. CYP2D6 – see Zhou, 2009a, 2009b, and CYP2C19 – see Damle et al., 2009). The severity of variability of human PK depends on therapeutic area and on margins to side effects.

Tactics for optimizing clearance are highly dependent on the nature of the clearance mechanism, as outlined below in sections dealing with metabolic, renal and biliary clearance, respectively.

Optimization of metabolic clearance

Introduction

Optimizing metabolic clearance is one of the most common and challenging activities in drug discovery projects, because high metabolic clearance can be associated with various metabolic pathways. These include CYP mediated (NADPH dependent) oxidation or reduction in the liver and, to a lesser extent, in other organs such as the small intestine (Galetin et al., 2008). In addition, FMOs (Cashman, 2008) and MAO can be involved in oxidative metabolism (Bortolato et al., 2008). High metabolic clearance can also be associated with direct or phase 2 conjugation via UGTs, sulphotransferases, or glutathione-S-transferases (Jana and Mandlekar, 2009). Although less common, whole blood and tissue amidases, esterases, various amine oxidases (diamine oxidase, semi-carbazine sensitive amine oxidase), adenosine deaminase, and alcohol and aldehyde dehydrogenase may come into play, depending on the chemotype in question (Cossum, 1988). During project work, metabolic clearance can be efficiently screened with available front-line metabolic tools (i.e. microsomes and hepatocytes). Differential results between microsomes and hepatocytes can highlight the involvement of phase 2 processes or the involvement of uptake transporters (Soars et al., 2009). Whole blood and/or plasma stability can easily be screened where appropriate when the chemotype dictates.

High metabolic clearance is known to be associated with physicochemical properties of molecules such as a high $LogD_{7.4}$ (i.e. $LogD_{7.4}$ values >2.5), where lipophilicity can correlate with metabolic liability (Van de Waterbeemd et al., 2001).

Failure to clarify and control metabolic clearance is a major issue in discovery because it can:

- result in very high total body clearance, low oral bioavailability or short half-life
- result in an inability to deliver an oral therapeutic drug level
- lead to excessively long discovery timelines
- ultimately lead to the demise of a project that cannot find an alternative chemotype.

Tactics

In order to optimize metabolic clearance it is essential to understand the enzymatic source of the instability and to exclude other clearance mechanisms. It is also necessary to have an in vivo assessment of clearance in selected compounds to establish that the in vitro system is predictive of the in vivo metabolic clearance.

Addressing high rates of metabolism requires an understanding of metabolic soft spots and their impact on clearance. For instance, reductions of electron density or removal of metabolically labile functional groups are successful strategies to reduce CYP-related clearance. Knowing where in the structure catalysis takes place also gives information about how the compound is oriented in the active site of a CYP. As a result, the site of metabolism could be blocked for catalysis, or other parts of the molecule could be modified to reduce the affinity between the substrate and CYPs. Such knowledge should, therefore, be used to assist in the rational design of novel compounds.

For more lipophilic compound series, CYP3A4 is usually the CYP responsible for most of the metabolism. The rate of such metabolism is sometimes difficult to reduce with specific modifications of soft spots. Commonly, the overall lipophilicity of the molecules needs to be modified. Once a project has established a means to predict lipophilicity and pKa, correlations with clearance measurements in microsomes or hepatocytes can be established, and in turn, used in early screening phases to improve metabolic stability and to influence chemical design.

Screening of compounds in rat or human microsomes or hepatocytes is an effective way to determine improvements in metabolic clearance. Once alternative clearance mechanisms have been ruled out, total body clearance greater than hepatic blood flow may indicate an extrahepatic metabolic clearance mechanism. While not always warranted, this can be investigated with a simple plasma or blood stability assay if the offending chemotype contains esters, amide linkages, aldehydes or ketones.

Softwares that predict sites of metabolism can be used to guide experiments to identify potential labile sites on molecules. In addition, structure-based design has taken a major step forward in recent years with the crystallization and subsequent elucidation of major CYP isoform structures. In silico methods based on molecular docking can facilitate an understanding of metabolic interactions with CYP's 3A4, 2D6 and 2C9. Although most of the tools, software and modelling expertise to perform structure-based design reside within computational chemistry, there is an increasing role for DMPK personnel in this process. Sun and Scott (2010) provide a review of the 'state of the art' in structure-based design to modify clearance.

Cautions

In theory, scaling to in vivo from metabolic stability in vitro, should in most cases underpredict clearance since almost always other mechanisms, more or less, contribute to overall clearance in vivo. Where common in vitro models (e.g. hepatocytes) significantly underestimate in vivo hepatic clearance and where the chemotype is either a carboxylic acid or a low $LogD_{7.4}$ base, poor scaling may be due to the compound being a substrate for hepatic uptake transporters (e.g. OATPs) which can significantly influence clearance. In such instances, a hepatic uptake experiment may prove useful to predict in vivo clearance (see Soars et al., 2007 for methodologies). In other instances, carbonyl-containing compounds metabolized by carbonyl reductases in microsomes have been shown to significantly underestimate clearance when in vitro reactions are driven by direct addition of NADPH, *versus* the addition of an NADPH regenerating system (Mazur et al., 2009).

Reductions in in vivo clearance may not be due to increased metabolic stability, but driven by increased plasma protein binding. Either may be used to reduce plasma clearance, but the implications of both need to be appreciated.

Optimization of renal clearance

Introduction

Renal clearance is most commonly a feature of polar, low $LogD_{7.4}$ (<~1) compounds due to their low plasma protein binding, lack of passive permeability (and inability to facilitate re-absorption in the distal tubule), and the high expression in the kidney of a number of transporter proteins (e.g. OATs and OCTs). Passively cleared compounds are generally well predicted from animal data because $CL_r = GFR \times f_u$ (where CL_r is renal clearance, GFR glomerular filtration rate, f_u the fraction unbound). Hence, simple, related, allometric relationships can be readily established.

By introducing the potential for large interspecies differences, transporters significantly complicate the issue, making prediction of renal clearance in man more difficult. While there are in vitro assays for animal and human transporters (e.g. OATs) that can generate useful QSAR information; their utility for human PK prediction is yet to be fully established.

Tactics

Reducing renal clearance in order to reduce total body clearance is generally achieved by increasing lipophilicity through modulation of LogP or pKa. All data are amenable to QSAR analysis, and particularly those from cell lines expressing individual transporter proteins.

Based on a few descriptors, a relatively simple diagram (Figure 10.5) can be used to classify drugs as having high (>1 mL/min/kg), medium (>0.1 to <1 mL/min/kg) or low (≤0.1 mL/min/kg) renal clearance (Paine et al., 2010).

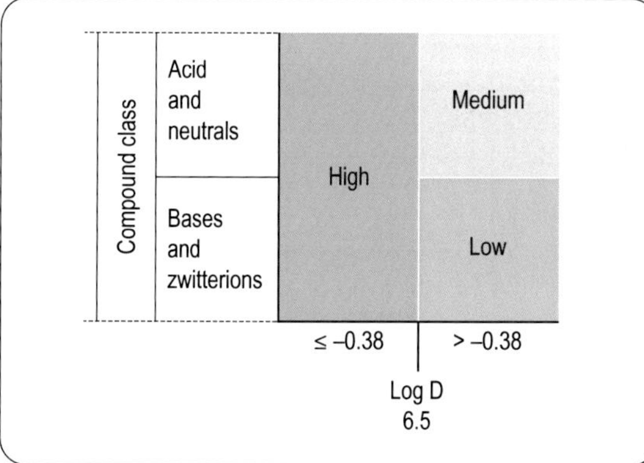

Fig. 10.5 Simple diagram to classify compounds for risk of renal clearance. Low renal clearance is defined as ≤ 0.1 mL/min/kg, moderate as >0.1 to <1 mL/min/kg, and high as 1> mL/min/kg

For acids and zwitterions, early determination of renal clearance in rat and dog is recommended as part of establishing the primary clearance mechanism of a compound. Once these data are available two possible scenarios exist: firstly, a simple allometric relationship can be used to predict human renal clearance or secondly, if such a relationship is not apparent, this prediction should be based on f_u and renal blood flow corrected dog data. On balance, there are enough examples to suggest that for acids and zwitterions, human renal clearance is best predicted from the dog (McGinnity et al., 2007).

Cautions

Accurately predicting renal clearance of acids and zwitterions (i.e. within three-fold) is important, as volumes of distribution tend to be low and acceptable half-lives are at risk.

The potential for renal DDI of renal transporter substrates should be considered.

Optimization of biliary clearance

Introduction

The biliary clearance of compounds involves active secretion from hepatocytes by ATP-dependent transporter proteins (primarily P-gp, MRP2 and BCRP) into the biliary canaliculus, and drainage into the small intestine. It is commonly a feature of acidic and zwitterionic compounds and can be very efficient, resulting in hepatic blood flow limited clearances. This efficiency is partly a consequence of many biliary transporter substrates also being substrates of sinusoidal uptake transporters (e.g. OATPs).

Biliary clearance is a major issue in discovery because it:

- can result in very high drug clearance and low bioavailability
- can result in low systemic exposure and small safety margins
- is difficult to optimize chemically and predict across species
- is often the synergistic product of two transporter systems in series (uptake and efflux).

Tactics

Regardless of the compound, no specific investigation of biliary clearance is recommended if total clearance is well predicted from in vitro metabolic systems, although bile collected for other reasons can be used to confirm that biliary clearance is low.

In an extensive evaluation of biliary clearance, Yang et al. (2009) showed molecular weight to be a good predictor of biliary clearance in anionic (but not cationic or neutral) compounds, with a threshold of 400 Da in rat and 475 Da in man.

If total clearance is not well predicted from in vitro metabolic systems, a biliary elimination study in the rat should be considered. High biliary clearance in the rat presents a significant hurdle to a discovery project, as much of time and resource can be spent establishing SARs in the rat, and in considering likely extrapolations to the dog and man. High biliary clearance is considered a major defect in high clearance chemotypes at candidate drug nomination. Tactics for resolving biliary clearance include the following:

- Consider molecular weight and ionic charge as determinants of biliary CL
- Track progress in rat and dog using intravenous PK studies without bile collection
- Make use of in vitro hepatic uptake or uptake transporter models
- If rat and dog provide ambiguous data, an intravenous PK study in another non-rodent species (possibly a non-human primate) may help establish a higher species trend
- Consider assessing efflux in sandwiched cultured rat and human hepatocytes. An emerging body of literature supports this approach, although quantification is challenging (Li et al., 2009).

Cautions

Vesicle-based efflux transporter systems are available, but they are not usually of use in detecting/monitoring substrates. Vesicle-based transporter assays have greater utility in screening of inhibition potential (Yamazaki et al., 1996).

Biliary secretion does not necessarily result in the elimination of compounds from the body, as there is the potential for re-absorption from the GI tract, which can lead to overestimation of V_{ss}.

Role of metabolite identification studies in optimization

Introduction

Knowledge of the metabolites formed from a compound/compound series is often highly beneficial or even essential during drug discovery, because knowing the sites of metabolism facilitates rational optimization of clearance and aids in understanding DDI, particularly time-dependent DDI. As these issues are considered elsewhere (sections on clearance optimization and avoidance of PK-based drug–drug interactions), they are not discussed further here. However, two other major areas of drug discovery which are dependent on metabolite identification and on understanding metabolite properties are considered below:

- Assessment of pharmacologically active metabolites
- Avoiding/assessing risk from reactive metabolites.

Active metabolites

Introduction

Active metabolites can influence PD and influence PKPD relationships (Gabrielsson and Green, 2009), one example being their major effect on the action of many statins (Garcia et al., 2003). Knowledge about the SAR for potency should be kept in mind during drug optimization when evaluating pathways of biotransformation. Active metabolites with equal or better potency, more favourable distribution and/or longer half-lives than the parent can have profound effects on PKPD relationships. Time–response studies will indicate the presence of such metabolites provided an appropriate PD model is available. Failure to discover the influence of such metabolites may lead to erroneous dose predictions. Assuming similar potency, metabolites with shorter half-lives than the parent will have more limited effects on dose predictions and are difficult to reveal by PKPD modelling. The presence of circulating active metabolites of candidate drugs can be beneficial for the properties of a candidate, but also adds significant risk, complexity and cost in development.

Prodrugs are special cases where an inactive compound is designed in such a way as to give rise to pharmacologically active metabolite(s) with suitable properties (Smith, 2007). The rationale for attempting to design oral prodrugs is usually that the active molecule is not sufficiently soluble and/or permeable. Remarkably successful prodrugs include omeprazole, which requires only a chemical conversion to activate the molecule (Lindberg et al., 1986), and clopidogrel (Testa, 2009) which is activated through CYP3A4. Both omeprazole and clopidogrel became the world's highest selling drugs.

Tactics

In vitro metabolite identification studies, combined with the SAR, may suggest the presence of an active metabolite. Studies of plasma metabolite profiles from PKPD animals may support their hypothesized presence and relevance. Disconnect between the parent compound's plasma profile and its PD in PKPD studies may be a trigger for in vitro metabolite identification studies.

If active metabolites cannot be avoided during compound optimization, or are considered beneficial for efficacy, their ADME properties should be determined. Advancing the metabolite rather than the parent compound is an option to be considered.

The decision tree in Figure 10.6 highlights ways to become alerted to the potential presence of active metabolites, and suitable actions to take.

Cautions

Using preclinical data to predict exposure to an active metabolite in man is usually accompanied by considerable uncertainty (Anderson et al., 2009). Plasma and tissue concentrations of metabolites in man are dependent on a number of factors. Species differences in formation, distribution and elimination need to be included in any assessment.

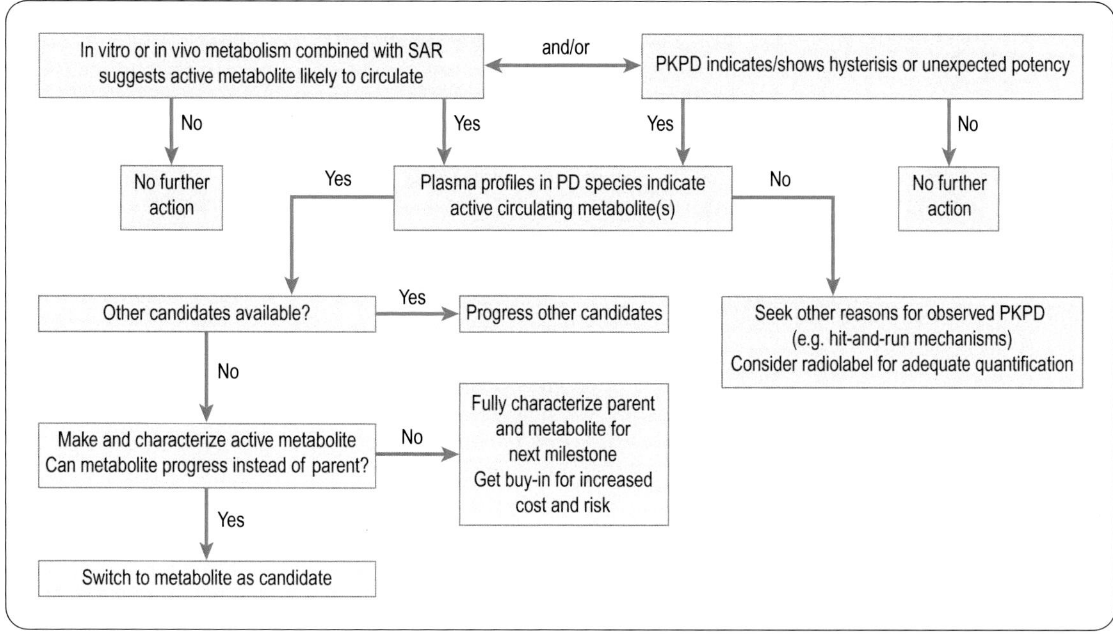

Fig. 10.6 Active metabolite decision tree. PKPD, pharmacokinetics-pharmacodynamics; SAR, structure–activity relationship.

Minimizing risk for reactive metabolites during drug discovery

Introduction

Many xenobiotics are converted by drug metabolizing enzymes to chemically reactive metabolites which may react with cellular macromolecules. The interactions may be non-covalent (e.g. redox processes) or covalent, and can result in organ toxicity (liver being the most common organ affected), various immune mediated hypersensitivity reactions, mutagenesis and tumour formation. Mutagenesis and carcinogenesis arise as a consequence of DNA damage, while other adverse events are linked to chemical modification of proteins and in some instances lipids. Avoiding, as far as possible, chemistry giving rise to such reactive metabolites is, therefore, a key part of optimization in drug discovery.

Tactics

Minimizing the reactive metabolite liability in drug discovery is based on integrating DMPK and safety screening into the design-make-test-analyse process. A number of tools are available to assist projects in this work (Thompson, et al., 2011 submitted to Chem-Biol Interact, and references therein):

- **Search tools/databases**: this includes in silico tools to (1) identify substructures associated with potential reactive metabolite formation, (2) identify potential bacterial mutagenicity, and (3) learn how to avoid/design away from reactive metabolite formation.
- **Trapping studies** in human liver microsomes to enable the detection of reactive metabolites. Agents used to trap unstable reactive intermediates are glutathione (for soft electrophiles) and radiolabelled potassium cyanide ($K^{14}CN$) (for iminium ions) as first-line assays. Structural information can be obtained from further analysis of GSH and CN adduct mass spectrometry data. For very reactive aldehydes, i.e. α,β-unsaturated aldehyde, methoxylamine can be used as trapping reagent.
- **Metabolite identification** in human liver microsomes or hepatocytes. Interpretation of the metabolite patterns may give information about existence of putative short-lived intermediates preceding the observed stable metabolites (e.g. dihydrodiols are likely to be result of hydration of epoxides).
- **Time-dependent inhibition** (TDI) studies in human liver microsomes to flag the likelihood of a mechanism based inhibitor (mainly inhibition of CYPs).
- **Formation and degradation of acyl glucuronides** from carboxylic acids in activated human liver microsomes. This gives an overall estimate of the acylating capability of acyl glucuronides.

If it proves difficult or not possible to optimize away from reactive metabolite signals using the screen assays listed above, yet compounds in the series for other reasons are regarded as sufficiently promising, then a reactive metabolite risk assessment will have to be undertaken. Such assessment includes covalent binding to human hepatocytes in vitro and/or to rat in vivo. Predicted dose to man and fraction of the dose being predicted to be metabolized over the reactive metabolite pathway will have to be taken into account. Other experimental systems which might be used for assaying metabolite-mediated cytotoxicity are cell systems devoid of, or overexpressing, various CYPs. Details of such an assessment are beyond the scope of this review but are discussed by Thompson et al., 2011 (Chem-Biol Interact, submitted).

Caution

Although reactive metabolites, beyond reasonable doubt, constitute a risk worthwhile to screen away from, the underlying science of potential toxicity is complex; e.g. overall covalent binding to proteins is a crude measure indeed. It is likely covalent binding to some proteins might give rise to antigenic conjugates, while binding to other proteins will be quite harmless. Formation of glutathione adducts as such is not alarming, particularly when catalysed by glutathione transferases. The relevance of trapping with an unphysiological agent like cyanide could be even more challenged. Simply quantifying covalent binding in vivo or in vitro may be misleading, but since the science of estimating risks associated with different patterns of binding is still in its infancy, there is little choice.

Despite these and other fundamental shortcomings in the reactive metabolite science, most pharmaceutical companies invest significant resources into screening away from chemistry giving rise to such molecular species. Taking a compound with such liabilities into man will require complex, and probably even more costly and time-consuming risk assessment efforts.

HUMAN PK AND DOSE PREDICTION

The overriding goal of in silico, in vitro, and in vivo DMPK methods conducted at all stages of drug discovery is to help design and select compounds with acceptable human pharmacokinetics. Hence the prediction of human PK is an important component of modern drug discovery and is employed throughout the drug discovery process. In the early stages, it is used to estimate how far project chemistry is from its target profile and to identify the most critical parameters for optimization. At candidate selection, accurate PK and dose prediction is required to determine not only whether the drug candidate meets the target profile but also to estimate safety margins, compound requirements for early development phases and potential DDI risk.

The prediction of human PK involves two distinct stages – firstly, the estimation of individual kinetic parameters, and secondly, the integration of these processes into a model to simulate a concentration-time profile (see Figure 10.7).

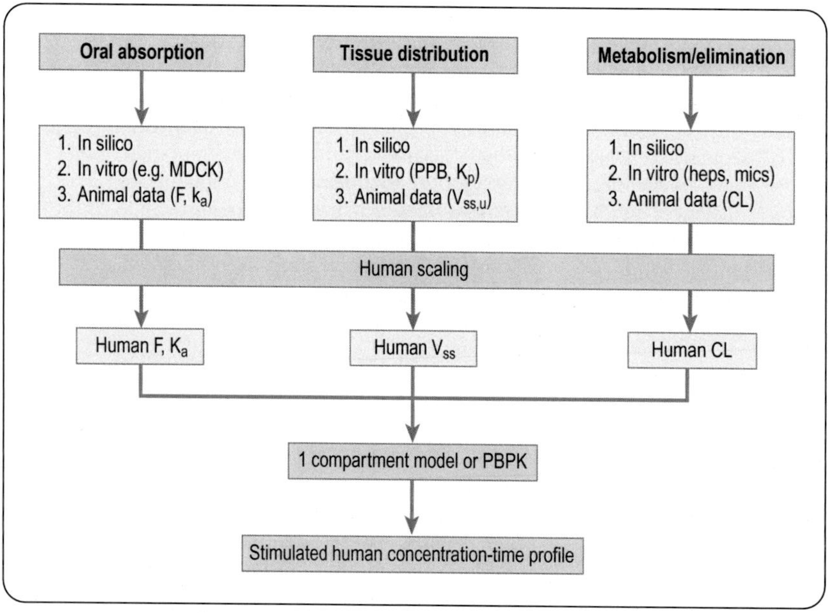

Fig. 10.7 Process for predicting human pharmacokinetics.

To predict the human PK profile following oral administration, the following fundamental PK parameters must be determined: (a) absorption rate (k_a) and bioavailability (F), (b) volume of distribution (V_{ss}), and (c) clearance (CL, total, hepatic, renal and other routes). Methods used to predict individual PK parameters can be classified into two approaches: empirical or mechanistic. Mechanistic methods are based on knowledge of the underlying mechanisms or processes that define the PK parameters while empirical methods rely on little or no a priori knowledge. Data required for these methods can be in silico, in vitro, or in vivo data and in general, methods that integrate and use both in vitro and in vivo data. PBPK (physiologically based pharmacokinetic) models utilising measured parameters (in vivo or in vitro) tend to be more accurate than methods that rely on in silico predictions.

Prediction of absorption rate and oral bioavailability

Although frequently ignored in scaling, accurate prediction of oral absorption rates (k_a) is required to predict C_{max} and to project the potential for drug–drug interactions. Oral absorption rate is heavily dependent on the final physical form of the compound and the prediction of this parameter in the early phase of discovery may be of limited value. k_a can be scaled empirically using k_a values determined from preclinical species. k_a values are usually obtained from rat or dog, i.v. and p.o. PK studies via de-convolution analysis. Oral absorption determined in the rat was usually found to be in good agreement to that in human. However, in the dog, oral absorption rates for hydrophilic compounds were usually much faster than in human (Chiou et al., 2000a). Hence, if there is discrepancy in the absorption rate between the two species, the value from the rat should be used for the prediction.

k_a can also be predicted mechanistically using various variations of a physiologically based transit model originally developed by Amidon et al. (Yu and Amidon, 1999). The model is termed compartment absorption and transit (CAT) model and characterizes the fraction of compound absorbed per unit time (based on its dissolution rate, pH solubility profile, effective permeability, intestinal metabolism and efflux, etc.) as the compound moves through the different compartments of the GI tract. This approach is used in a number of commercially available tools such as GastroPlus and SIMCYP and can be used to estimate fraction of the dose absorbed and (f_a), and the fraction escaping intestinal metabolism (f_g), in addition to k_a.

As mentioned earlier in the optimizing oral bioavailability section, oral bioavailability is a composite product of (f_a), (f_g) and hepatic 'first-pass' extraction (f_h). Hepatic extraction is a function of hepatic clearance and hepatic blood flow and can be estimated using the following equation:

$$f_h = 1 - CL_h/Q$$

where CL_h is the hepatic clearance and Q is the hepatic blood flow.

Prediction of clearance

Clearance is a primary pharmacokinetic parameter that is used to characterize drug disposition. Total or systemic clearance, the sum of all individual organ clearance responsible for overall elimination of a drug, can be predicted empirically using allometry. Allometric scaling is based on the empirical observations that organ sizes and physiological processes in the mammalian body are proportional to body weight by the following equation:

$$Y = aW^b$$

where Y is the parameter of interest, W the body weight, and a and b are the coefficient and exponent of the allometric equation, respectively. For rates, flows and clearance processes, the exponent should be 0.75. If the calculated exponent deviates significantly from the above, the prediction may not be accurate (Mahmood, 2007).

For individual organ clearance, allometry is useful for flow-dependent clearance processes, e.g. renal and high hepatic CL. However, for low CL compounds that exhibit large species differences in metabolism, hepatic clearance and hence total clearance cannot be reliably predicted by allometry. Hepatic clearance can be mechanistically scaled using an in vitro and in vivo correlation (IVIVC) approach. With this approach, intrinsic in vitro clearance is measured using in vitro metabolic stability assays (microsomes or hepatocytes). The measured in vitro clearance values are scaled to clearance by the whole liver and then converted to an hepatic clearance using a liver model that incorporates blood flow (a well-stirred model most often used). If IVIVC predicts clearance in animal species, it is likely that the method is applicable for human predictions. Historically, the method for predicting intrinsic hepatic metabolic clearance does so to within a factor of 3, unless confounded by transporter or other mechanistic effects that are not incorporated in the modelling. For any chemical series, a key component of gaining confidence in the use of IVIVC to predict human clearance comes from establishing the ability of analogous tools to predict metabolic clearance in the rat and dog. It is important to establish such relationships and this requires an accurate estimation of the metabolic, and other clearance mechanisms in each species, as well as prediction of all significant clearance mechanisms in man.

Prediction of volume of distribution

Volume of distribution (V) is a primary PK parameter that relates drug concentration measured in plasma or blood to the amount of drug in the body and is used to characterize drug distribution. It is a key parameter as it is a primary determinant (together with clearance) of drug half-life. Higher volume compounds will have longer half-lives. In a simple system:

$$T1/2 = \ln(2) * V/CL$$

Volume of distribution is a measure of the relative affinity of the compound for plasma/blood constituents and tissue constituents. In general, for moderately lipophilic compounds, acids have a high affinity for albumin and, therefore, have a low volume of distribution (0.1–0.5 L/kg), based have a high affinity for tissues and, therefore, have high volumes (>3 L/kg), while neutral compounds have volumes around 1 L/kg. Correcting V for plasma protein binding yields a very useful parameter 'unbound volume':

$$Vu = V/fu$$

Unbound volume is a measure of the average tissue affinity of a compound, but more importantly should be relatively constant across species. If this consistency is observed in preclinical species, human predictions are relatively straightforward, and a sound basis for the use of more sophisticated tools (e.g. physiologically based (PBPK) models, see below) to predict complex distribution profiles is established.

In PBPK modelling, the body is portrayed as a series of compartments that represent tissues and organs. The compartments are arranged to reflect anatomical layout and are connected by arterial and venous pathways. Each tissue (i) has an associated blood flow rate (Q), volume (Vt) and a tissue partition coefficient (Kp) and the rate of change of the drug in each tissue is mathematically described by a differential equation.

The total volume of distribution is the sum of the volume of distribution of all the organs. The volume of distribution in each organ is simply the actual volume of the organ multiplied by its corresponding tissue distribution coefficient (Kp). Kp can be determined experimentally in animals for each organ; however, this is very resource intensive and impractical. There are two approaches for estimating Kp in various organs. In silico estimation of Kp can be done using various tissue composition methods. This is the approach used in commercial software packages such as GastroPlus and SIMCYP. The other approach was developed by Arundel (1997) using rat V_{ss} data and is based on the observation that Kps are constant for a given V_{ss} and that they can be predicted from V_{ss} (Arundel, 1997). With the tissue composition methods, partitions to various components in the tissue (neutral lipid, acidic phospholipids, lipoproteins, tissue albumin) are estimated by logD and pKa of the compound (Poulin and Theil, 2000; Rodgers et al., 2005; Rodgers and Rowland, 2006). A key assumption is that unbound tissue Kps are constant across species. This underpins the assumption described above, that the unbound volume of distribution is constant across species.

Prediction of plasma concentration time profile

To accurately estimate C_{max} and C_{min}, which are important exposure parameters for assessing safety and efficacy, the plasma concentration-time profile has to be accurately predicted.

For compounds displaying mono-exponential decreases in plasma concentrations over time, the concentration-time profile in man can be predicted using the following equation:

$$C(t) = \frac{\mathrm{FDka}}{\mathrm{V}\left(\mathrm{ka} - \frac{\mathrm{CL}}{\mathrm{V}}\right)\left(e^{-\frac{\mathrm{CL}}{\mathrm{V}}*\mathrm{t}} - e^{-\mathrm{ka}*\mathrm{t}}\right)}$$

where C is the concentration at time t, F is bioavailability, D is the dose, ka is the absorption rate, CL is the clearance, and V is the volume of distribution.

For compound showing biphasic or multi-exponential concentration time profile in animals, PBPK modelling is the recommended approach to simulate the profile in man.

Prediction of human efficacious dose

Estimation of the likely therapeutic dose and dosing frequency in patients, requires not only the prediction of the human pharmacokinetics, but also a robust understanding of the concentration-time-response relationship. The quality of the prediction depends on how well the PD effect scales from animals to man and the linkage between the effect and the clinical outcome. The linkage between the effect and the clinical outcome is based on a series of translational biomarkers. The different types of biomarkers are classified (Figure 10.8, adapted from Danhof et al., 2005). The classification is based on the mechanism of drug action and the relationship to the disease process. In general, the closer the relationship of the biomarker is to the disease process, the more relevant and predictive is the biomarker.

SUMMARY

To be a successful drug candidate, a compound, in addition to having good efficacy and safety profile, has to have acceptable DMPK properties. This chapter highlights the

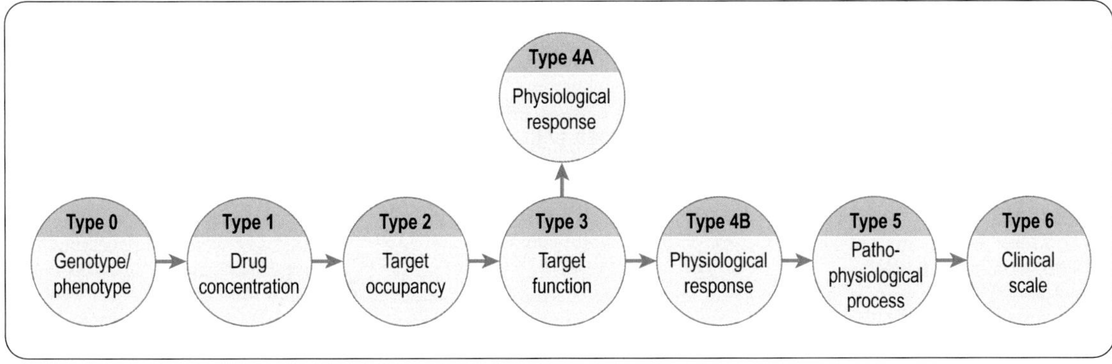

Fig. 10.8 Classification of biomarkers useful to quantify a project's therapeutic model.

roles of DMPK in drug discovery and provides strategies to resolve key DMPK challenges such as improving oral bioavailability, optimizing clearance, avoiding drug–drug interaction, achieving or avoiding CNS exposure, and avoiding risks from metabolites. In addition, approaches used to scale individual PK parameters and strategy to integrate these parameters to predict human pharmacokinetics and dose are discussed in the chapter. The proposed strategy is based on best practices within AstraZeneca as well as current science, technology and understanding of DMPK. It is our hope that the proposed integrated strategy, which focus DMPK efforts toward the optimization and prediction of DMPK properties in human will provide a sound basis to efficiently progress drug discovery projects.

ACKNOWLEDGMENTS

The authors wish to thank Lovisa Afzelius, Tommy B. Andersson, Madeleine Antonsson, Ulf Bredberg, Anne Cooper, Doug Ferguson, C. Edwin Garner, Ken Grime, Anshul Gupta, Lena Gustavsson, Ramon Hendrickx, Suzanne Iversson, Owen Jones, Etienne Lessard, Stefan Lundquist, Yan Li, Nektaria Markoglou, Jan Neelisen, Ken Page, Stuart Paine, Jan Paulson, Denis Projean, Maria Ribadeneira, Caroline Rivard, Ralf Schmidt, Patricia Schroeder, Anna-Karin Sternbeck, Per Strandberg, Richard Thompson, Anna-Lena Ungell, and Lucas Utley for their inputs to the strategy.

REFERENCES

Arundel P. A multi-compartment model generally applicable to physiologically based pharmacokinetics. 3rd IFAC Symposium: modelling and control in biological systems, Warwick, UK, March 23rd–26th, 1997.

Amidon GL, Lennernas H, Shah VP, et al. A theoretical basis for a biopharmaceutic drug classification: the correlation of in vitro drug product dissolution and in vivo bioavailability. Pharmacology Research 1995;12:413–20.

Anderson S, Luffer-Atlas D, Knadle MP. Predicting circulating human metabolites: how good are we? Chemical Research Toxicology 2009;22:243–56.

Bell L, Bickford S, Nguyen PH, et al. Evaluation of fluorescence- and mass spectrometry-based CYP inhibition assays for use in drug discovery. Journal of Biomolecular Screening 2008;13(5):343–53.

Bjornsson T, Callaghan J, Einolf JH, et al. The conduct of in vitro and in vivo drug-drug interaction studies: a PhRMA perspective. Journal of Clinical Pharmacology 2003;43:443–69.

Bortolato M, Chen K, Shih JC. Monoamine oxidase inactivation: from pathophysiology to therapeutics. Adverse Drug Delivery Review 2008;60: 1527–33.

Cashman JR. Role of flavin-containing monooxygenase in drug development. Expert Opinion on Drug Metabolism and Toxicology 2008;4:1507–21.

Chiou WL, Ma C, Chung SM, et al. Similarity in the linear and non-linear oral absorption of drugs between human and rat. International Journal of Clinical Pharmacolology Therapy 2000a;38:532–9.

Chiou W, Jeong Y, Chung S, et al. Evaluation of dog as an animal model to study the fraction of oral dose absorbed for 43 drugs in humans. Pharmacology Research 2000b;17:135–40.

Cossum PA. Role of the red blood cell in drug metabolism. Biopharmaceutics and Drug Disposition 1988;9:321–36.

Damle BD, Uderman H, Biswas P, et al. Influence of CYP2C19 polymorphism on the pharmacokinetics of nelfinavir and its active metabolite. British Journal of Clinical Pharmacology 2009;68:682–9.

Danhof M, Alvan G, Dahl SG, et al. Mechanism-based pharmacokinetic-pharmacodynamic modeling – a new classification of biomarkers. Pharmaceutical Research 2005;22:1432–7.

Di L, Kerns H, Carte G. Strategies to assess blood–brain barrier penetration. Expert Opinion on Drug Discovery 2008;3:677–87.

Didziapetris R, Japertas P, Avdeef A, et al. Classification analysis of P-glycoprotein substrate specificity. Journal of Drug Targeting 2003;11:391–406.

Doran A, Obach RS, Smith BJ, et al. The impact of P-glycoprotein on the disposition of drugs targeted for indications of the central nervous system: evaluation using the MDR1A/1B knockout mouse model. Drug Metabolism and Disposition 2005;33:165–74.

Fowler S, Zhang H. In vitro evaluation of reversible and irreversible cytochrome P450 inhibition: current status on methodologies and their utility for predicting drug-drug interactions. AAPS Journal 2008;10:410–24.

Fridén M, Ducrozet F, Middleton B, et al. Development of a high-throughput brain slice method for studying drug distribution in the central nervous system. Drug Metabolism and Disposition 2009a;37:1226–33.

Fridén M, Ljungqvist H, Middleton B, et al. Improved measurement of drug exposure in brain using drug-specific correction for residual blood. Journal of Cerebral Blood Flow and Metabolism 2010;30:150–61.

Fridén M, Winiwarter S, Jerndal G, et al. Structure-brain exposure relationships in rat and human using a novel data set of unbound drug concentrations in brain interstitial and cerebrospinal fluids. Journal of Medicinal Chemistry 2009b;52:6233–43.

Gabrielsson J, Green AR. Quantitative pharmacology or pharmacokinetic pharmacodynamic integration should be a vital component in integrative pharmacology. Journal of Pharmacology and Experimental Therapeutics 2009;331:767–74.

Galetin A, Gertz M, Houston JB. Potential role of intestinal first-pass metabolism in the prediction of drug-drug interactions. Expert Opinion on Drug Metabolism and Toxicology 2008;4:909–22.

Garcia MJ, Reinoso RF, Sanchez Navarro A, et al. Clinical pharmacokinetics of statins. Methods and Findings in Experimental and Clinical Pharmacology 2003;25:457–81.

Gertz M, Harrison A, Houston JB, et al. Prediction of human intestinal first-pass metabolism of 25 CYP3A substrates from in vitro clearance and permeability data. Drug Metabolism and Disposition 2010;38:1147–58.

Gleeson P, Davis A, Chohan K, et al. Generation of in silico cytochrome P450 1A2, 2C9, 2C19, 2D6, 3A4 inhibition QSAR models. Journal of Computer Aided Molecular Design 2007;21:559–73.

Hitchcock S, Pennington L. Structure-brain exposure relationships. Journal of Medicinal Chemistry 2006;49:7559–83.

Huang S, Strong J, Zhang L, et al. New era in drug interaction evaluation: US Food and Drug Administration update on CYP enzymes, transporters, and the guidance process. Journal of Clinical Pharmacology 2008;48:662–70.

International Transporter Consortium. Membrane transporters in drug development. Nature Reviews. Drug Discovery 2010;9:215–36.

Jana S, Mandlekar S. Role of phase II drug metabolizing enzymes in cancer chemoprevention. Current Drug Metabolism 2009;10: 595–616.

Johnson TW, Dress KR, Edwards M. Using the golden triangle to optimise clearance and oral absorption. Bioorganic and Medicinal Chemistry Letters 2009;19:5560–1554.

Kola I, Landis J. Can the pharmaceutical industry reduce attrition rates? Nature Reviews. Drug Discovery 2004;3:711–5.

Li N, Bi YA, Duignan DB, et al. Quantitative expression profile of hepatobiliary transporters in sandwich cultured rat and human hepatocytes. Molecular Pharmacology 2009;6:1180–9.

Lindberg P, Nordberg P, Alminger T, et al. The mechanism of action of the gastric acid secretion inhibitor omeprazole. Journal of Medicinal Chemistry 1986;29:1327–9.

Lipinski CA, Lombardo F, Dominy BW, et al. Experimental and computational approaches to estimate solubility and permeability in drug discovery and development settings. Advanced Drug Delivery Reviews 1997;23:3–25.

Mahmood I. Application of allometric principles for the prediction of pharmacokinetics in human and veterinary drug development. Advanced Drug Delivery Reviews 2007;59:1177–92.

Mazur CS, Kenneke JF, Goldsmith MR, et al. Contrasting influence of NADPH and a NADPH-regenerating system on the metabolism of carbonyl-containing compounds in hepatic microsomes. Drug Metabolism and Disposition 2009;37:1801–5.

McGinnity DF, Collington J, Austin RP, et al. Evaluation of human pharmacokinetics, therapeutic dose and exposure predictions using marketed oral drugs. Current Drug Metabolism 2007;8:463–79.

Paine SW, Barton P, Bird J, et al. A rapid computational filter for predicting the rate of human renal clearance. Journal of Molecular Graphics and Modelling 2010;29:529–37. Epub 2010 Oct 20.

Poulin P, Theil FP. A priori prediction of tissue:plasma partition coefficients of drugs to facilitate the use of physiologically-based pharmacokinetic models in drug discovery. Journal of Pharmaceutical Sciences 2000;89:16–35.

Rawden HC, Carlile DJ, Tindall A, et al. Microsomal prediction of in vivo clearance and associated interindividual variability of six benzodiazepines in humans. Xenobiotica 2005;35:603–25.

Riley R, Grime K, Weaver R. Time-dependent CYP inhibition. Expert Opinion on Drug Metabolism and Toxicology 2007;3:51–66.

Rodgers T, Leahy D, Rowland M. Physiologically based pharmacokinetic modeling 1: predicting the tissue distribution of moderate-to-strong bases. Journal of

Pharmaceutical Sciences 2005;94:1259–76.

Rodgers T, Rowland M. Physiologically based pharmacokinetic modelling 2: predicting the tissue distribution of acids, very weak bases, neutrals and zwitterions. Journal of Pharmaceutical Sciences 2006;95:1238–57.

Rowland M, Tozer TN. Clinical pharmacokinetics – concepts and applications. 2nd ed. London: Lea and Febiger; 1989.

Smith DA. Do prodrugs deliver? Current Opinion on Drug Discovery and Development 2007;10:550–9.

Soars MG, Grime K, Sproston JL, et al. Use of hepatocytes to assess the contribution of hepatic uptake to clearance in vivo. Drug Metabolism and Disposition 2007;35:859–65.

Soars MG, Webborn PJ, Riley RJ. Impact of hepatic uptake transporters on pharmacokinetics and drug-drug interactions: use of assays and models for decision making in the pharmaceutical industry. Molecular Pharmacology 2009;6:1662–77.

Sun H, Scott DO. Structure-based drug metabolism predictions for drug design. Chemical Biology and Drug Design 2010;75:3–17.

Takahashi M, Washio T, Suzuki N, et al. The species differences of intestinal drug absorption and first-pass metabolism between cynomolgus monkeys and humans. Journal of Pharmaceutical Sciences 2009;98:4343–53.

Testa B. Drug metabolism for the perplexed medicinal chemist. Chemistry and Biodiversity 2009;6:2055–70.

Thompson RA, Isin EM, Yan L, et al. Risk assessment and mitigation strategies for reactive metabolites in drug discovery and development. Chemico-Biological Interactions 2011;192:65–71.

Ungell AL, Nylander S, Bergstrand S, et al. Membrane transport of drugs in different regions of the intestinal tract of the rat. Journal of Pharmaceutical Sciences 1998;87:360–6.

US Food and Drug Administration. Draft Guidance for Industry: Drug Interaction Studies – Study Design, Data Analysis and Implications for Dosing and Labeling, 2006. Available from: URL: http://www.fda.gov/downloads/Drugs/GuidanceComplianceRegulatoryInformation/Guidances/ucm072101.pdf.

US Food and Drug Administration. Guidance for Industry: Drug Metabolism/Drug Interactions in the Drug Development Process: Studies in vitro, 1997. Available from: URL: http://www.fda.gov/downloads/Drugs/GuidanceComplianceRegulatoryInformation/Guidances/ucm072104.pdf.

Van de Waterbeemd H, Smith DA, Jones BC. Lipophilicity in PK design: methyl, ethyl, futile. Journal of Computer Aided Molecular Design 2001;15(3):273–86.

Wan H, Rehngren M, Giordanetto F, et al. High-throughput screening of drug-brain tissue binding and in silico prediction for assessment of central nervous system drug delivery. Journal of Medicinal Chemistry 2007;50:4606–15.

Ward P. Importance of drug transporters in pharmacokinetics and drug safety. Toxicology Mechanisms and Methods 2008;18:1–10.

Waring MJ. Defining optimum lipophilicity and molecular weight ranges for drug candidates – molecular weight dependent lower logD limits based on permeability. Bioorganics and Medicinal Chemistry Letters 2009;19:2844–51.

Wenlock MC, Austin RP, Barton P, et al. A comparison of physiochemical property profiles of development and marketed oral drugs. Journal of Medicinal Chemistry 2003;46:1250–6.

Williams J, Hyland R, Jones B, et al. Drug-drug interactions for UDP-glucuronosyltransferase substrates; a pharmacokinetic explanation for typically observed low exposure (AUCi/AUC) ratios. Drug Metabolism and Disposition 2004;32:1201–8.

Yamazaki M, Kobayashi K, Sugiyama Y. Primary active transport of pravastatin across the liver canalicular membrane in normal and mutant Eisai hyperbilirubinemic rats. Biopharmaceutics and Drug Disposition 1996;17:607–21.

Yang X, Gandhi YA, Duignan DB, et al. Prediction of biliary excretion in rats and humans using molecular weight and quantitative structure-pharmacokinetic relationships. AAPS Journal 2009;11:511–25.

Yu LX, Amidon GL. A compartmental absorption and transit model for estimating oral absorption. International Journal of Pharmaceutics 1999;186:119–25.

Zhou SF. Polymorphism of human cytochrome P450 2D6 and its clinical significance: part I. Clinical Pharmacokinetics 2009a;48:689–723.

Zhou SF. Polymorphism of human cytochrome P450 2D6 and its clinical significance: part II. Clinical Pharmacokinetics 2009b;48:761–804.

Chapter |11|

Pharmacology: its role in drug discovery

H P Rang

INTRODUCTION

Pharmacology as an academic discipline, loosely defined as the study of the effects of chemical substances on living systems, is so broad in its sweep that it encompasses all aspects of drug discovery, ranging from the molecular details of the interaction between the drug molecule and its target to the economic and social consequences of placing a new therapeutic agent on the market. In this chapter we consider the more limited scope of 'classical' pharmacology, in relation to drug discovery. Typically, when a molecular target has been selected, and lead compounds have been identified which act on it selectively, and which are judged to have 'drug-like' chemical attributes (including suitable pharmacokinetic properties), the next stage is a detailed pharmacological evaluation. This means investigation of the effects, usually of a small number of compounds, on a range of test systems, up to and including whole animals, to determine which, if any, is the most suitable for further development (i.e. for nomination as a drug candidate). Pharmacological evaluation typically involves the following:

- **Selectivity screening**, consisting of in vitro tests on a broad range of possible drug targets to determine whether the compound is sufficiently selective for the chosen target to merit further investigation
- **Pharmacological profiling**, aimed at evaluating in isolated tissues or normal animals the range of effects of the test compound that might be relevant in the clinical situation. Some authorities distinguish between *primary pharmacodynamic studies*, concerning effects related to the selected therapeutic target (i.e. therapeutically relevant effects), and *secondary pharmacodynamic studies*, on effects not related to the target (i.e. side effects). At the laboratory level the two are often not clearly distinguishable, and the borderline between secondary pharmacodynamic and safety pharmacology studies (see below) is also uncertain. Nevertheless, for the purposes of formal documentation, the distinction may be useful
- **Testing in animal models of disease** to determine whether the compound is likely to produce therapeutic benefit
- **Safety pharmacology**, consisting of a series of standardized animal tests aimed at revealing undesirable side effects, which may be unrelated to the primary action of the drug. This topic is discussed in Chapter 15.

The pharmacological evaluation of lead compounds does not in general follow a clearly defined path, and often it has no clearcut endpoint but will vary greatly in its extent, depending on the nature of the compound, the questions that need to be addressed and the inclinations of the project team. Directing this phase of the drug discovery project efficiently, and keeping it focused on the overall objective of putting a compound into development, is one of the trickier management tasks. It often happens that unexpected, scientifically interesting data are obtained which beg for further investigation even though they may be peripheral to the main aims of the project. From the scientists' perspective, the prospect of opening up a new avenue of research is highly alluring, whether the work contributes directly to the drug discovery aims or not. In this context, project managers need to bear in mind the question: Who needs the data and why? – a question which may seem irritatingly silly to a scientist in academia but totally obvious to the commercial mind. The same principles apply, of course, to all parts of a drug discovery and development project, but it tends to be at

Table 11.1 Characteristics of pharmacological test systems

Test system attribute	Molecular/cellular assays	In vitro pharmacology	Whole animal pharmacology (normal animals)	Whole animal disease models
Throughput	High (thousands/day)	Moderate (*c.* 10/day)	Low (<10/day)	Generally low or very low, depending on nature of model
Quantitative precision	Good	Good, but may be subject to environmental and physiological variation	Relatively poor, due to uncontrolled pharmacokinetic and physiological factors	As for whole animal pharmacology, plus added variability of disease model phenotype
Cost	Low	Fairly low depending on number and cost of animals needed	High, depending on number and cost of animals needed	High, depending on number and cost of animals needed
Flexibility of experimental design	Generally inflexible. Washout effects, repeat dose effects, etc., difficult to study	Highly adaptable	Adaptable, but limitations imposed by pharmacokinetics	
Suitability for chronic experiments	Unsuitable	Unsuitable	Depends on model. Suitable if repeated non-invasive readouts are feasible. Possible, but expensive for one-off terminal readouts	As for whole animal, provided disease phenotype remains stable
Species dependence	Often performed on human cell lines or cloned human targets	Rarely possible with human tissues	Animal studies may not be applicable to humans	Animal studies may not be applicable to human
Usefulness for predicting therapeutic efficacy	OK for me-too drugs. Poor for drugs acting through novel mechanisms	OK for me-too drugs. Poor for drugs acting through novel mechanisms	As above	Variable, depending on characteristics of model
Usefulness for predicting side effects	Useful if broad selectivity screen is performed	Sometimes useful	Generally useful as basis for 'safety pharmacology' screening	Usually not informative

the stage of pharmacological evaluation that conflicts first arise between scientific aspiration and commercial need.

An important principle in pharmacological evaluation is the use of a *hierarchy* of test methods, covering the range from the most reductionist tests on isolated molecular targets to much more elaborate tests of integrated physiological function. Establishing and validating such a series of tests appropriate to the particular target and indication being addressed is one of the most important functions of pharmacologists in the drug discovery team. In general, assays become more complicated, slow and expensive, and more demanding of specialist skills as one moves up this hierarchy.

The strengths and weaknesses of these test systems are summarized in Table 11.1.

Pharmacological characterization of a candidate compound often has to take into account active metabolites, based on information from drug metabolism and pharmacokinetics (DMPK) studies (see Chapter 10). If a major active metabolite is identified, it will be necessary to synthesize and test it in the same way as the parent compound in order to determine which effects (both wanted and unwanted) relate to each. Particular problems may arise if the metabolic fate of the compound shows marked species differences, making it difficult to predict from animal studies what will happen in humans.

Although most of the work involved in pharmacological characterization of a candidate drug takes place before clinical studies begin, it does not normally end there. Both ongoing toxicological studies and early trials in man may reveal unpredicted effects that need to be investigated pharmacologically, and so the discovery team needs to remain actively involved and be able to perform experiments well into the phase of clinical development. They cannot simply wave the compound goodbye once the discovery phase is completed.

SCREENING FOR SELECTIVITY

The selectivity of a compound for the chosen molecular target needs to be assessed at an early stage. Compounds selected for their potency, for example on a given amine receptor, protease, kinase, transporter or ion channel, are very likely to bind also to related – or even unrelated – molecular targets, and thereby cause unwanted side effects. Selectivity is, therefore, as important as potency in choosing potential development candidates, and a 'selectivity screen' is usually included early in the project. The range of targets included in such a screen depends very much on the type of compound and the intended clinical indication. Ligands for monoamine receptors and transporters form a large and important group of drugs, and several contract research organizations (e.g. CEREP, MDL) offer a battery of assays – mainly binding assays, but also a range of functional assays – designed to detect affinity for a wide range of receptors, transporters and channels. In the field of monoamine receptors, for example, it is usually important to avoid compounds that block or activate peripheral muscarinic receptors, adrenergic receptors or histamine (particularly H_1) receptors, because of the side effects that are associated with these actions, and a standard selectivity test battery allows such problems to be discovered early. Recently, several psychotropic and anti-infective drugs have been withdrawn because of sudden cardiac deaths, probably associated with their ability to block a particular type of potassium channel (known as the *hERG channel*; see Chapter 16) in myocardial cells. This activity can be detected by electrophysiological measurements on isolated myocardial cells, and such a test is now usually performed at an early stage of development of drugs of the classes implicated in this type of adverse reaction.

Interpretation of binding assays

Binding assays, generally with membrane preparations made from intact tissues or receptor-expressing cell lines, are widely used in drug discovery projects because of their simplicity and ease of automation. Detailed technical manuals describing the methods used for performing and analysing drug binding experiments are available (Keen, 1999; Vogel, 2002). Generally, the aim of the assay is to determine the dissociation constant, K_D, of the test compound, as a measure of its affinity for the receptor. In most cases, the assay (often called a *displacement assay*) measures the ability of the test compound to inhibit the binding of a high-affinity radioligand which combines selectively with the receptor in question, correction being made for 'non-specific' binding of the radioligand.

In the simplest theoretical case, where the radioligand and the test compound bind reversibly and competitively to a homogeneous population of binding sites, the effect of the test ligand on the amount of the radioligand specifically bound is described by the simple mass-action equation:

$$B/B_{max} = ([A]/K_A)/([A]/K_A + [L]/K_L + 1) \qquad (1)$$

where B = the amount of radioligand bound, after correcting for non-specific binding, B_{max} = the maximal amount of radioligand bound, i.e. when sites are saturated, [A] = radioligand concentration, K_A = dissociation constant for the radioligand, [L] = test ligand concentration, and K_L = dissociation constant for the test ligand.

By testing several concentrations of L at a single concentration of A, the concentration, $[L]_{50}$, needed for 50% inhibition of binding can be estimated. By rearranging equation 1, K_L is given by:

$$K_L = [L]_{50}/([A]/K_A + 1) \qquad (2)$$

This is often known as the Cheng–Prusoff equation, and is widely used to calculate K_L when $[L]_{50}$, [A] and K_A are known. It is important to realize that the Cheng–Prusoff equation applies only (a) at equilibrium, (b) when the interaction between A and L is strictly competitive, and (c) when neither ligand binds cooperatively. However, an $[L]_{50}$ value can be measured for any test compound that inhibits the binding of the radioligand by whatever mechanism, irrespective of whether equilibrium has been reached. Applying the Cheng–Prusoff equation if these conditions are not met can yield estimates of K_L that are quite meaningless, and so it should strictly be used only if the conditions have been shown experimentally to be satisfied – a fairly laborious process. Nevertheless, Cheng–Prusoff estimates of ligand affinity constants are often quoted without such checks having been performed. In most cases it would be more satisfactory to use the experimentally determined $[L]_{50}$ value as an operational measure of potency. A further important caveat that applies to binding studies is that they are often performed under conditions of low ionic strength, in which the sodium and calcium concentrations are much lower than the physiological range. This is done for technical reasons, as low $[Na^+]$ commonly increases both the affinity and the B_{max} of the radioligand, and omitting $[Ca^{2+}]$ avoids clumping of the membrane fragments. Partly for this reason, ligand affinities estimated from binding studies are often considerably higher than estimates obtained from functional assays

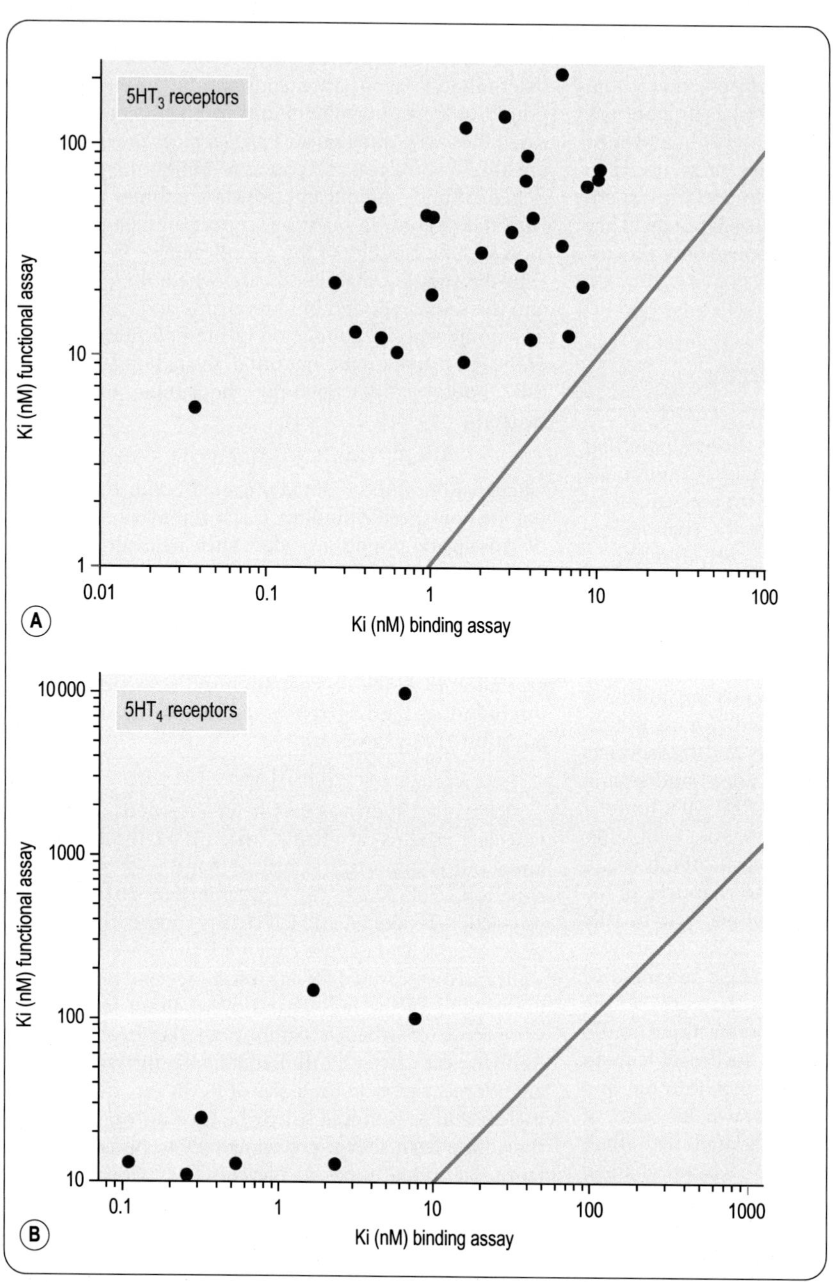

Fig. 11.1 Correlation of binding and functional data for 5HT receptor ligands. (A) $5HT_3$ receptors, (B) $5HT_4$ receptors.
Data from Heidempergher et al., 1997.
Data from Yang et al., 1997.

(Hall, 1992), although the effect is not consistent, presumably because ionic bonding, which will be favoured by the low ionic strength medium, contributes unequally to the binding of different ligands. Consequently, the correlation between data from binding assays and functional assays is often rather poor (see below). Figure 11.1 shows data obtained independently on $5HT_3$ and $5HT_4$ receptors; in both cases the estimated K_D values for binding are on average about 10 times lower than estimates from functional assays, and the correlation is very poor.

PHARMACOLOGICAL PROFILING

Pharmacological profiling aims to determine the pharmacodynamic effects of the new compound – or more often of a small family of compounds – on in vitro model systems, e.g. cell lines or isolated tissues, normal animals, and animal models of disease. The last of these is particularly important, as it is intended to give the first real pointer to therapeutic efficacy as distinct from pharmacodynamic activity. It is valuable to assess the activity of the compounds in a series of assays representing increasingly complex levels of organization. The choice of test systems depends, of course, on the nature of the target. For example, characterization of a novel antagonist of a typical G-protein-coupled receptor might involve the following:

- Ligand-binding assay on membrane fragments from a cell line expressing the cloned receptor
- Inhibition of agonist activity in a cell line, based on a functional readout (e.g. raised intracellular calcium)
- Antagonism of a selective agonist in an isolated tissue (e.g. smooth muscle, cardiac muscle). Such assays will normally be performed with non-human tissue, and so interspecies differences in the receptor need to be taken into account. Sometimes specific questions have to be asked about effects on human tissues for particular compounds and then collecting viable tissues to use becomes a major challenge
- Antagonism of the response (e.g. bronchoconstriction, vasoconstriction, increased heart rate) to a selective receptor agonist in vivo. Prior knowledge about species specificity of the agonist and antagonist is important at this stage.

Pharmacological profiling is designed as a hypothesis-driven programme of work, based on the knowledge previously gained about the activity of the compound on its specific target or targets. In this respect it differs from safety pharmacology (see below), which is an open-minded exercise designed to detect unforeseen effects. The aim of pharmacological profiling is to answer the following questions:

- Do the molecular and cellular effects measured in screening assays actually give rise to the predicted pharmacological effects in intact tissues and whole animals?
- Does the compound produce effects in intact tissues or whole animals not associated with actions on its principal molecular target?
- Is there correspondence between the potency of the compound at the molecular level, the tissue level and the whole animal level?
- Do the in vivo potency and duration of action match up with the pharmacokinetic properties of the compound?
- What happens if the drug is given continuously or repeatedly to an animal over the course of days or weeks? Does it lose its effectiveness, or reveal effects not seen with acute administration? Is there any kind of 'rebound' after effect when it is stopped?

In vitro profiling

Measurements on isolated tissues

Studies on isolated tissues have been a mainstay of pharmacological methodology ever since the introduction of the isolated organ bath by Magnus early in the 20th century. The technique is extremely versatile and applicable to studies on smooth muscle (e.g. gastrointestinal tract, airways, blood vessels, urinary tract, uterus, biliary tract, etc.) as well as cardiac and striated muscle, secretory epithelia, endocrine glands, brain slices, liver slices, and many other functional systems. In most cases the tissue is removed from a freshly killed or anaesthetized animal and suspended in a chamber containing warmed oxygenated physiological salt solution. With smooth muscle preparations the readout is usually mechanical (i.e. tension, recorded with a simple strain gauge). For other types of preparation, various electrophysiological or biochemical readouts are often used. Vogel (2002) and Enna et al. (2003) give details of a comprehensive range of standard pharmacological assay methods, including technical instructions.

Studies of this kind have the advantage that they are performed on intact normal tissues, as distinct from isolated enzymes or other proteins. The recognition molecules, signal transduction machinery and the mechanical or biochemical readout are assumed to be a reasonable approximation to the normal functioning of the tissue. There is abundant evidence to show that tissue responses to GPCR activation, for example, depend on many factors, including the level of expression of the receptor, the type and abundance of the G proteins present in the cell, the presence of associated proteins such as receptor activity-modifying proteins (RAMPs; see Morfis et al., 2003), the state of phosphorylation of various constituent proteins in the signal transduction cascade, and so on. For compounds acting on intracellular targets, functional activity depends on permeation through the membrane, as well as affinity for the target. For these reasons – and probably also for others that are not understood – the results of assays on isolated tissues often differ significantly from results found with primary screening assays. The discrepancy may simply be a quantitative one, such that the potency of the ligand does not agree in the two systems, or it may be more basic. For example, the *pharmacological efficacy* of a receptor ligand, i.e. the property that determines whether it is a full agonist, a partial agonist, or an antagonist, often depends on the type of assay used (Kenakin, 1999), and this may have an important bearing

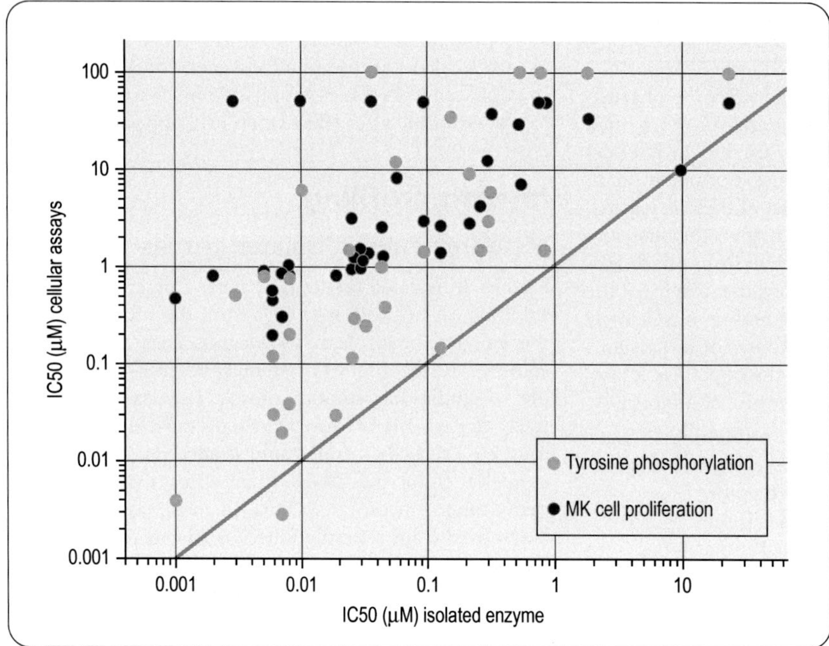

Fig. 11.2 Correlation of cellular activity of EGFR receptor kinase inhibitors with enzyme inhibition.
Data from Traxler et al., 1997.

on the selection of possible development compounds. Examples that illustrate the poor correlation that may exist between measurements of target affinity in cell-free assay systems, and functional activity in intact cell systems, are shown in Figures 11.1 and 11.2. Figure 11.1 shows the relationship between binding and functional assay data for $5HT_3$ and $5HT_4$ receptor antagonists. In both cases, binding assays overestimate the potency in functional assays by a factor of about 10 (see above), but more importantly, the correlation is poor, despite the fact that the receptors are extracellular, and so membrane penetration is not a factor. Figure 11.2 shows data on tyrosine kinase inhibitors, in which activity against the isolated enzyme is plotted against inhibition of tyrosine phosphorylation in intact cells, and inhibition of cell proliferation for a large series of compounds. Differences in membrane penetration can account for part of the discrepancy between enzyme and cell-based data, but the correlation between intracellular kinase inhibition and blocking of cell proliferation is also weak, which must reflect other factors.

It is worth noting that these examples come from very successful drug discovery projects. The quantitative discrepancies that we have emphasized, though worrying to pharmacologists, should not therefore be a serious distraction in the context of a drug discovery project.

A very wide range of physiological responses can be addressed by studies on isolated tissues, including measurements of membrane excitability, synaptic function, muscle contraction, cell motility, secretion and release of mediators, transmembrane ion fluxes, vascular resistance and permeability, and epithelial transport and permeability. This versatility and the relative technical simplicity of many such methods are useful attributes for drug discovery. Additional advantages are that concentration–effect relationships can be accurately measured, and the design of the experiments is highly flexible, allowing rates of onset and recovery of drug effects to be determined, as well as measurements of synergy and antagonism by other compounds, desensitization effects, etc.

The main shortcomings of isolated tissue pharmacology are (a) that tissues normally have to be obtained from small laboratory animals, rather than humans or other primates; and (b) that preparations rarely survive for more than a day, so that only short-term experiments are feasible.

In vivo profiling

As already mentioned, experiments on animals have several drawbacks. They are generally time-consuming, technically demanding and expensive. They are subject to considerable ethical and legal constraints, and in some countries face vigorous public opposition. For all these reasons, the number of experiments is kept to a bare minimum, and experimental variability is consequently often a problem. Animal experiments must, therefore, be used very selectively and must be carefully planned and designed so as to produce the information needed as efficiently as possible. In the past, before target-directed approaches were the norm, routine in vivo testing was often used as a screen at a very early stage in the drug discovery process, and many important drugs (e.g. thiazide diuretics, benzodiazepines, ciclosporin) were discovered on the basis of their effects in vivo. Nowadays, the use of in vivo methods is much more limited, and will probably decline further in response to the pressures on time and costs, as alternative in vitro and in silico methods are developed, and as public attitudes to animal experimentation harden. An additional difficulty is the decreasing number of pharmacologists trained to perform in vivo studies[1].

Imaging technologies (Rudin and Weissleder, 2003; see also Chapter 18) are increasingly being used for pharmacological studies on whole animals. Useful techniques include magnetic resonance imaging (MRI), ultrasound imaging, X-ray densitometry tomography, positron emission tomography (PET) and others. They are proving highly versatile for both structural measurements (e.g. cardiac hypertrophy, tumour growth) and functional measurements (e.g. blood flow, tissue oxygenation). Used in conjunction with radio-active probes, PET can be used for studies on receptors and other targets in vivo. Many of these techniques can also be applied to humans, providing an important bridge between animal and human pharmacology. Apart from the special facilities and equipment needed, currently the main drawback of imaging techniques is the time taken to capture the data, during which the animal must stay still, usually necessitating anaesthesia. With MRI and PET, which are currently the most versatile imaging techniques, data capture normally takes a few minutes, so they cannot be used for quick 'snapshots' of rapidly changing events.

A particularly important role for in vivo experiments is to evaluate the effects of long-term drug administration on the intact organism. 'Adaptive' and 'rebound' effects (e.g. tolerance, dependence, rebound hypertension, delayed endocrine effects, etc.) are often produced when drugs are given continuously for days or weeks. Generally, such effects, which involve complex physiological interactions, are evident in the intact functioning organism but are not predictable from in vitro experiments.

The programme of in vivo profiling studies for characterization of a candidate drug depends very much on the drug target and therapeutic indication. A comprehensive catalogue of established in vivo assay methods appropriate to different types of pharmacological effect is given by Vogel (2002). Charting the appropriate course through the plethora of possible studies that might be performed to characterize a particular drug can be difficult.

[1]The rapid growth in the use of transgenic animals to study the functional role of individual gene products has recently brought in vivo physiology and pharmacology back into fashion, however.

Box 11.1 **Pharmacological profiling of beraprost**

In vitro studies

Binding to PGI_2 receptors of platelets from various species, including human

PGI_2 agonist activity (cAMP formation) in platelets

Dilatation of arteries and arterioles in vitro, taken from various species

Increased red cell deformability (hence reduced blood viscosity and increased blood flow) in blood taken from hypercholesterolaemic rabbits

In vivo studies

Increased peripheral blood flow in various vascular regions (dogs)

Cutaneous vasodilatation (rat)

Reduced pulmonary hypertension in rat model of drug-induced pulmonary hypertension (measured by reduction of right ventricular hypertrophy)

Reduced tissue destruction (gangrene) of rat tail induced by ergotamine/epinephrine infusion

Reduction of vascular occlusion resulting from intra-arterial sodium laureate infusion in rats

Reduction of vascular occlusion and thrombosis following electrical stimulation of femoral artery in anaesthetized dogs and rabbits

Reduction of vascular damage occurring several weeks after cardiac allografts in immunosuppressed rats

A typical example of pharmacological profiling is summarized in Box 11.1. The studies were carried out as part of the recent development of a cardiovascular drug, *beraprost* (Melini and Goa, 2002). Beraprost is a stable analogue of prostaglandin I_2 (PGI_2) which acts on PGI_2 receptors of platelets and blood vessels, thereby inhibiting platelet aggregation (and hence thrombosis) and dilating blood vessels. It is directed at two therapeutic targets, namely occlusive peripheral vascular disease and pulmonary hypertension (a serious complication of various types of cardiovascular disease, drug treatment or infectious diseases), resulting in hypertrophy and often contractile failure of the right ventricle. The animal studies were, therefore, directed at measuring changes (reduction in blood flow, histological changes in vessel wall) associated with peripheral vascular disease, and with pulmonary hypertension. As these are progressive chronic conditions, it was important to establish that long-term systemic administration of beraprost was effective in retarding the development of the experimental lesions, as well as monitoring the acute pharmacodynamic effects of the drug.

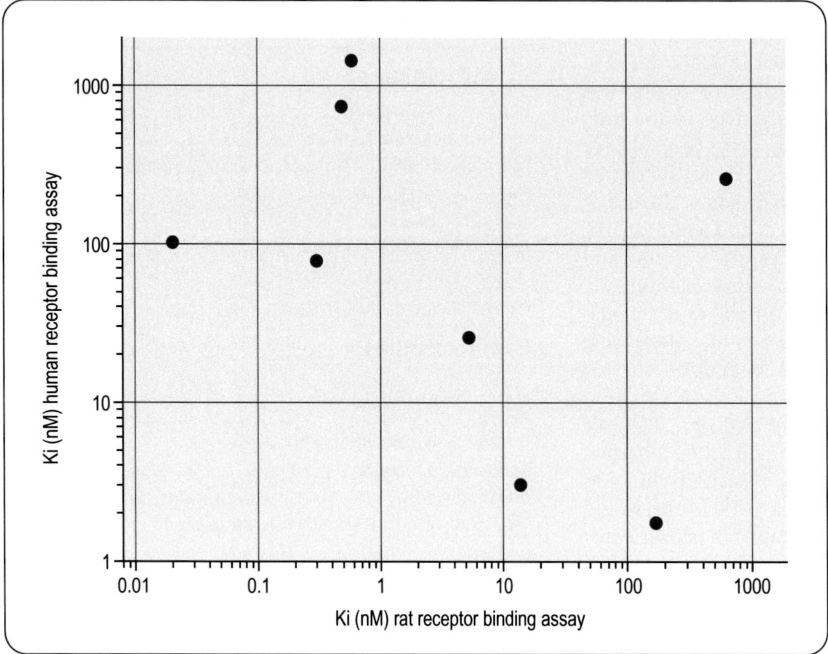

Fig. 11.3 Species differences in bradykinin B_2 receptors.
Data from Dziadulewicz et al., 2002.

Species differences

It is important to take species differences into account at all stages of pharmacological profiling. For projects based on a defined molecular target – nowadays the majority – the initial screening assay will normally involve the human isoform. The same target in different species will generally differ in its pharmacological specificity; commonly, there will be fairly small quantitative differences, which can be allowed for in interpreting pharmacological data in experimental animals, but occasionally the differences are large, so that a given class of compounds is active in one species but not in another. An example is shown in Figure 11.3, which compares the activities of a series of bradykinin receptor antagonists on cloned human and rat receptors. The complete lack of correlation means that, for these compounds, tests of functional activity in the rat cannot be used to predict activity in man.

Species differences are, in fact, a major complicating factor at all stages of drug discovery and preclinical development. The physiology of disease processes such as inflammation, septic shock, obesity, atherosclerosis, etc., differs markedly in different species. Most importantly (see Chapter 10), drug metabolism often differs, affecting the duration of action, as well as the pattern of metabolites, which can in turn affect the observed pharmacology and toxicity.

Species differences are, of course, one of the main arguments used by animal rights activists in opposing the use of animals for the purpose of drug discovery. Their claim – misleading when examined critically (see Understanding Animal Research website) – is that animal data actually represent disinformation in this context. While being aware of the pitfalls, we should not lose sight of the fact that non-human data, including in vivo experiments, have actually been an essential part of every major drug discovery project to date. The growing use of transgenic animal models has led to an increase, rather than a decrease, in animal experimentation, as even breeding such animals is counted as an experiment for statistical purposes.

ANIMAL MODELS OF DISEASE

The animal models discussed earlier were used to investigate the pharmacodynamic effects of the drug and to answer the question: How do the effects observed at the molecular and cellular levels of organization translate into physiological effects in the whole animal?

The next, crucial, question is: Can these physiological effects result in therapeutic benefit? Animal experiments can never answer this conclusively – only clinical trials can do that – but the use of animal models of human disease provides a valuable link in the chain of evidence, and there is strong pressure on drug discovery teams to produce data of this sort as a basis for the important decision to test a new compound in man. Despite the immense range and diversity of animal models that have been described, this is often the most problematic aspect of a drug discovery project, particularly where a novel target or mechanism is involved, so that there is no mechanistic precedent among established drugs. The magnitude of the difficulties varies considerably among different therapeutic areas. Many inflammatory conditions, for example, are straightforward to model in animals, as are some cancers. Animal models of hypertension generally predict very well the ability of compounds to lower blood pressure in man. Endocrine disorders involving over- or undersecretion of particular hormones can also be simply modelled in animals. Psychiatric disorders are much more difficult, as the symptoms that characterize them are not observable in animals. In most therapeutic areas there are certain disorders, such as migraine, temporal lobe epilepsy, asthma or irritable bowel syndrome, for which animal models, if they exist at all, are far from satisfactory in predicting clinical efficacy.

Here we consider, with a few selected examples, the main experimental approaches to generating animal models, and the criteria against which their 'validity' as models of human disease need to be assessed.

Types of animal model

Animal models of disease can be divided broadly into acute and chronic physiological and pharmacological models, and genetic models.

Acute physiological and pharmacological models are intended to mimic certain aspects of the clinical disorder. There are many examples, including:

- Seizures induced by electrical stimulation of the brain as a model for epilepsy (see below)
- Histamine-induced bronchoconstriction as a model for asthma
- The hotplate test for analgesic drugs as a model for pain
- Injection of lipopolysaccharide (LPS) and cytokines as a model for septic shock
- The elevated maze test as a model for testing anxiolytic drugs.

Chronic physiological or pharmacological models involve the use of drugs or physical interventions to induce an ongoing abnormality similar to the clinical condition. Examples include:

- The use of alloxan to inhibit insulin secretion as a model for Type I diabetes
- Procedures for inducing brain or coronary ischaemia as models for stroke and ischaemic heart disease
- 'Kindling' and other procedures for inducing ongoing seizures as models for epilepsy
- Self-administration of opiates, nicotine or other drugs as a model for drug-dependence
- Cholesterol-fed rabbits as a model for hypercholesterolaemia and atherosclerosis
- Immunization with myelin basic protein as a model for multiple sclerosis
- Administration of the neurotoxin MPTP, causing degeneration of basal ganglia neurons as a model of Parkinson's disease
- Transplantation of malignant cells into immunodeficient animals to produce progressive tumours as a model for certain types of cancer.

Details of these and many other examples of physiological and pharmacological models can be found in Vogel (2002). As discussed above, species differences need to be taken into account in the selection of animal models, and in the interpretation of results. In *septic shock*, for example, rodents show a much larger elevation of nitric oxide (NO) metabolites than do humans, and respond well to NO synthesis inhibitors, which humans do not. Rodents and rabbits transgenically engineered to favour cholesterol deposition nevertheless develop atherosclerosis only when fed high-cholesterol diets, whereas humans often do so even on low-cholesterol diets. Genetically obese mice are deficient in the hormone *leptin* and lose weight when treated with it, whereas obese humans frequently have high circulating leptin concentrations and do not respond to treatment with it. It is often not clear whether such discrepancies reflect inherent species differences, or simply failure of the model to replicate satisfactorily the predominant human disease state (see Validity criteria below).

Genetic models

There are many examples of spontaneously occurring animal strains that show abnormalities phenotypically resembling human disease. In addition, much effort is going into producing transgenic strains with deletion or over-expression of specific genes, which also exhibit disease-like phenotypes.

Long before genetic mapping became possible, it was realized that certain inbred strains of laboratory animal were prone to particular disorders, examples being spontaneously hypertensive rats, seizure-prone dogs, rats insensitive to antidiuretic hormone (a model for diabetes insipidus), obese mice and mouse strains exhibiting a range of specific neurological deficits. Many such strains have been characterized (see Jackson Laboratory website, www.jaxmice.jax.org) and are commercially available, and are widely used as models for testing drugs.

The development of transgenic technology has allowed inbred strains to be produced that over- or under-express particular genes. In the simplest types, the gene abnormality is present throughout the animal's life, from early development onwards, and throughout the body. More recent technical developments allow much more control over the timing and location of the transgene effect. For reviews of transgenic technology and its uses in drug discovery, see Polites (1996), Rudolph and Moehler (1999), Törnell and Snaith (2002) and Pinkert (2002).

The genetic analysis of disease-prone animal strains, or of human families affected by certain diseases, has in many cases revealed the particular mutation or mutations responsible (see Chapters 6 and 7), thus pointing the way to new transgenic models. Several diseases associated with single-gene mutations, such as *cystic fibrosis* and *Duchenne muscular dystrophy*, have been replicated in transgenic mouse strains. Analysis of the obese mouse strain led to the identification of the leptin gene, which is mutated in the *ob/ob* mouse strain, causing the production of an inactive form of the hormone and overeating by the mouse. Transgenic animals closely resembling *ob/ob* mice have been produced by targeted inactivation of the gene for leptin or its receptor. Another example is the discovery that a rare familial type of Alzheimer's disease is associated with mutations of the amyloid precursor protein (APP). Transgenic mice expressing this mutation show amyloid plaque formation characteristic of the human disease. This and other transgenic models of Alzheimer's disease (Yamada and Nabeshima, 2000) represent an important tool for drug discovery, as there had hitherto been no animal model reflecting the pathogenesis of this disorder.

The number of transgenic animal models, mainly mouse, that have been produced is already large and is growing rapidly. Creating and validating a new disease model is, however, a slow business. Although the methodology for generating transgenic mice is now reliable and relatively straightforward, it is both time-consuming and labour-intensive. The first generation of transgenic animals are normally hybrids, as different strains are used for the donor and the recipient, and it is necessary to breed several generations by repeated back-crossings to create animals with a uniform genetic background. This takes 1–2 years, and is essential for consistent results. Analysis of the phenotypic changes resulting from the transgene can also be difficult and time-consuming, as the effects may be numerous and subtle, as well as being slow to develop as the animal matures. Despite these difficulties, there is no doubt that transgenic disease models are playing an increasing part in drug testing, and many biotechnology companies have moved into the business of developing and providing them for this purpose. The fields in which transgenic models have so far had the most impact are cancer, atherosclerosis and neurodegenerative diseases, but their importance as drug discovery tools extends to all areas.

Producing transgenic rat strains proved impossible until recently, as embryonic stem (ES) cells cannot be obtained from rats. Success in producing gene knockout strains by an alternative method has now been achieved (Zan et al., 2003), and the use of transgenic rats is increasing, this being the favoured species for pharmacological and physiological studies in many laboratories.

The choice of model

Apart from resource limitations, regulatory constraints on animal experimentation, and other operational factors, what governs the choice of disease model?

As discussed in Chapter 2, naturally occurring diseases produce a variety of structural biochemical abnormalities, and these are often displayed separately in animal models. For example, human allergic asthma involves: (a) an immune response; (b) increased airways resistance; (c) bronchial hyperreactivity; (d) lung inflammation; and (e) structural remodelling of the airways. Animal models, mainly based on guinea pigs, whose airways behave similarly to those of humans, can replicate each of these features, but no single model reproduces the whole spectrum. The choice of animal model for drug discovery purposes, therefore, depends on the therapeutic effect that is being sought. In the case of asthma, existing bronchodilator drugs effectively target the increased airways resistance, and steroids reduce the inflammation, and so it is the other components for which new drugs are particularly being sought.

A similar need for a range of animal models covering a range of therapeutic targets applies in many disease areas.

Validity criteria

Obviously an animal model produced in a laboratory can never replicate exactly a spontaneous human disease state, so on what basis can we assess its 'validity' in the context of drug discovery?

Three types of validity criteria were originally proposed by Willner (1984) in connection with animal models of depression. These are:

- Face validity
- Construct validity
- Predictive validity.

Face validity refers to the accuracy with which the model reproduces the phenomena (symptoms, clinical signs and pathological changes) characterizing the human disease.

Construct validity refers to the theoretical rationale on which the model is based, i.e. the extent to which the aetiology of the human disease is reflected in the model. A transgenic animal model in which a human disease-producing mutation is replicated will have, in general, good construct validity, even if the manifestations of the human disorder are not well reproduced (i.e. it has poor face validity).

Predictive validity refers to the extent to which the effect of manipulations (e.g. drug treatment) in the model is predictive of effects in the human disorder. It is the most pragmatic of the three and the most directly relevant to the issue of predicting therapeutic efficacy, but also the most limited in its applicability, for two main reasons. First, data on therapeutic efficacy are often sparse or non-existent, because no truly effective drugs are known (e.g. for Alzheimer's disease, septic shock). Second, the model may focus on a specific pharmacological mechanism, thus successfully predicting the efficacy of drugs that work by that mechanism but failing with drugs that might prove effective through other mechanisms. The knowledge that the first generation of antipsychotic drugs act as dopamine receptor antagonists enabled new drugs to be identified by animal tests reflecting dopamine antagonism, but these tests cannot be relied upon to recognize possible 'breakthrough' compounds that might be effective by other mechanisms. Thus, predictive validity, relying as it does on existing therapeutic knowledge, may not be a good basis for judging animal models where the drug discovery team's aim is to produce a mechanistically novel drug. The basis on which predictive validity is judged carries an inevitable bias, as the drugs that proceed to clinical trials will normally have proved effective in the model, whereas drugs that are ineffective in the model are unlikely to have been developed. As a result, there are many examples of tests giving 'false positive' expectations, but very few false negatives, giving rise to a commonly held view that conclusions from pharmacological tests tend to be overoptimistic.

Some examples

We conclude this discussion of the very broad field of animal models of disease by considering three disease areas, namely epilepsy, psychiatric disorders and stroke. Epilepsy-like seizures can be produced in laboratory animals in many different ways. Many models have been described and used successfully to discover new antiepileptic drugs (AEDs). Although the models may lack construct validity and are weak on face validity, their predictive validity has proved to be very good. With models of psychiatric disorders, face validity and construct validity are very uncertain, as human symptoms are not generally observable in animals and because we are largely ignorant of the cause and pathophysiology of these disorders; nevertheless, the predictive validity of available models of depression, anxiety and schizophrenia has proved to be good, and such models have proved their worth in drug discovery. In contrast, the many available models of stroke are generally convincing in terms of construct and face validity, but have proved very unreliable as predictors of clinical efficacy. Researchers in this field are ruefully aware that despite many impressive effects in laboratory animals, clinical successes have been negligible.

Epilepsy models

The development of antiepileptic drugs, from the pioneering work of Merritt and Putnam, who in 1937 developed phenytoin, to the present day, has been highly dependent on animal models involving experimentally induced seizures, with relatively little reliance on knowledge of the underlying physiological, cellular or molecular basis of the human disorder. Although existing drugs have significant limitations, they have brought major benefits to sufferers from this common and disabling condition – testimony to the usefulness of animal models in drug discovery.

Human epilepsy is a chronic condition with many underlying causes, including head injury, infections, tumours and genetic factors. Epileptic seizures in humans take many forms, depending mainly on where the neural discharge begins and how it spreads.

Some of the widely used animal models used in drug discovery are summarized in Table 11.2. The earliest models, namely the *maximal electroshock (MES) test* and the *pentylenetetrazol-induced seizure (PTZ) test*, which are based on acutely induced seizures in normal animals, are still commonly used. They model the seizure, but without distinguishing its localization and spread, and do not address either the chronicity of human epilepsy or its aetiology (i.e. they score low on face validity and construct validity). But, importantly, their predictive validity for conventional antiepileptic drugs in man is very good, and the drugs developed on this basis, taken regularly to reduce the frequency of seizures or eliminate them altogether, are of proven therapeutic value. Following on from these acute seizure models, attempts have been made to replicate the processes by which human epilepsy develops and continues as a chronic condition with spontaneous seizures, i.e. to model *epileptogenesis* (Löscher, 2002; White, 2002) by the use of models that show greater construct and face validity. This has been accomplished in a variety of ways (see Table 11.2) in the hope that such models would be helpful in developing drugs capable of preventing epilepsy. Such models have thrown considerable light on the pathogenesis of epilepsy, but have not so far contributed significantly to the development of improved antiepileptic drugs. Because there are currently no drugs known to prevent epilepsy from progressing, the predictive validity of epileptogenesis models remains uncertain.

Psychiatric disorders

Animal models of psychiatric disorders are in general problematic, because in many cases the disorders are defined by symptoms and behavioural changes unique to humans, rather than by measurable physiological, biochemical or structural abnormalities. This is true in conditions such as schizophrenia, Tourette's syndrome and autism, making face validity difficult to achieve. Depressive symptoms, in contrast, can be reproduced to

Table 11.2 Epilepsy and epileptogenesis models

Model	Procedure	Face validity	Construct validity	Predictive validity
Acute seizure models				No acute seizure models show 'treatment-resistance' to conventional antiepileptic drugs, though this occurs in ~30% of human cases
Maximal electroshock model	Acute seizures evoked by whole-brain stimulation. Measure: proportion of mice responding with seizures	Weak. No spontaneous seizures. No neuropathological changes	Weak. Production of seizures not related to epileptogenesis	Good. Predictive of activity of drugs against partial seizures and generalized tonic–clonic seizures (with some false positives). Poor prediction of drugs effective in absence seizures
Pentylenetetrazole (PTZ)-induced seizure model	Seizures induced by s.c. injection of the convulsant drug PTZ. Measure: proportion of mice responding with seizures	As above	As above	Quite good as predictor of efficacy in absence seizures. Unreliable for other clinical types
Epileptogenesis models				
Kindling model	Weak electrical stimulation of amygdala repeated over several days. Evoked full-blown seizures develop gradually	Moderate, though spontaneous seizures are rarely produced. Histological, electrophysiological and biochemical changes similar to human epilepsy	Uncertain	Moderate, but model is generally more drug-responsive than human epilepsy
Post-seizure models	Various procedures (e.g. injection of kainate, lithium or other agents into brain, sustained stimulation of amygdala or other pathways) evoke sustained seizures, with ongoing spontaneous seizures appearing days or weeks later. Can be used to test drug effects on fully kindled seizures, or on the kindling process	Good. Spontaneous seizures, latent period after initial trigger. Replicates histological and other changes, including neurodegeneration	Probably good for some clinical forms of epilepsy	As MES for anti-seizure drugs. Uncertain for antiepileptogenic drugs, of which there are no proven clinical examples
Surgical procedures	Cortical undercutting. Isolated region of cortex gradually develops spontaneous seizure activity	Good as model of post-traumatic epilepsy. Replicates histological and other changes	Probably good for post-traumatic epilepsy	As above

some extent in animal models (Willner and Mitchell, 2002), and face validity is therefore stronger. The aetiology of most psychiatric conditions is largely unknown[2], making construct validity questionable.

Models are therefore chosen largely on the basis of predictive validity, and suffer from the shortcomings mentioned above. Nonetheless, models for some disorders, particularly depression, have proved very valuable in the discovery of new drugs. Other disorders, such as autism and Tourette's syndrome, have proved impossible to model so far, whereas models for others, such as schizophrenia (Lipska and Weinberger, 2000; Moser et al., 2000), have been described but are of doubtful validity. The best prediction of antipsychotic drug efficacy comes from pharmacodynamic models reflecting blockade of dopamine and other monoamine receptors, rather than from putative disease models, with the result that drug discovery has so far failed to break out of this mechanistic straitjacket.

Stroke

Many experimental procedures have been devised to produce acute cerebral ischaemia in laboratory animals, resulting in long-lasting neurological deficits that resemble the sequelae of strokes in humans (Small and Buchan, 2000). Interest in this area has been intense, reflecting the fact that strokes are among the commonest causes of death and disability in developed countries, and that there are currently no drugs that significantly improve the recovery process. Studies with animal models have greatly advanced our understanding of the pathophysiological events. Stroke is no longer seen as simple anoxic death of neurons, but rather as a complex series of events involving neuronal depolarization, activation of ion channels, release of excitatory transmitters, disturbed calcium homeostasis leading to calcium overload, release of inflammatory mediators and nitric oxide, generation of reactive oxygen species, disturbance of the blood–brain barrier and cerebral oedema (Dirnagl et al., 1999). Glial cells, as well as neurons, play an important role in the process. Irreversible loss of neurons takes place gradually as this cascade builds up, leading to the hope that intervention after the primary event – usually thrombosis – could be beneficial. Moreover, the biochemical and cellular events involve well-understood signalling mechanisms, offering many potential drug targets, such as calcium channels, glutamate receptors, scavenging of reactive oxygen species and many others. Ten years ago, on the basis of various animal models with apparently good construct and face validity and a range of accessible drug targets, the stage seemed to be set for major therapeutic advances. Drugs of many types, including glutamate antagonists, calcium and sodium channel blocking drugs, anti-inflammatory drugs, free radical scavengers and others, produced convincing degrees of neuroprotection in animal models, even when given up to several hours after the ischaemic event. Many clinical trials were undertaken (De Keyser et al., 1999), with uniformly negative results. The only drug currently known to have a beneficial – albeit small – effect is the biopharmaceutical 'clot-buster' tissue plasminogen activator (TPA), widely used to treat heart attacks. Stroke models thus represent approaches that have revealed much about pathophysiology and have stimulated intense efforts in drug discovery, but whose predictive validity has proved to be extremely poor, as the drug sensitivity of the animal models seems to be much greater than that of the human condition. Surprisingly, it appears that whole-brain ischaemia models show better predictive validity (i.e. poor drug responsiveness) than focal ischaemia models, even though the latter are more similar to human strokes.

[2]Many psychiatric disorders have a strong genetic component in their aetiology, and much effort has gone into identifying particular susceptibility genes. Success has so far been very limited, but the expectation is that, in future, success in this area will enable improved transgenic animal models to be developed.

Good laboratory practice (GLP) compliance in pharmacological studies

GLP comprises adherence to a set of formal, internationally agreed guidelines established by regulatory authorities, aimed at ensuring the reliability of results obtained in the laboratory. The rules (see *GLP Pocketbook*, 1999; EEC directives 87/18/EEC, 88/320/EEC, available online: pharmacos.eudra.org/F2/eudralex/vol-7/A/7AG4a.pdf) cover all stages of an experimental study, from planning and experimental design to documentation, reporting and archiving. They require, among other things, the assignment of specific GLP-compliant laboratories, certification of staff training to agreed standards, certified instrument calibration, written standard operating procedures covering all parts of the work, specified standards of experimental records, reports, notebooks and archives, and much else. Standards are thoroughly and regularly monitored by an official inspectorate, which can halt studies or require changes in laboratory practice if the standards are thought not to be adequately enforced. Adherence to GLP standards carries a substantial administrative overhead and increases both the time and cost of laboratory studies, as well as limiting their flexibility.

The regulations are designed primarily to minimize the risk of errors in studies that relate to safety. They are, therefore, not generally applied to pharmacological profiling as described in this chapter. They are obligatory for toxicological studies that are required in submissions for regulatory approval. Though not formally required for safety pharmacology studies, most companies and contract research organizations choose to do such work under GLP conditions.

REFERENCES

Current protocols in pharmacology. New York: John Wiley and Sons. [Published as looseleaf binder and CD-ROM, and regularly updated.)

De Keyser J, Sulter G, Luiten PG. Clinical trials with neuroprotective drugs in ischaemic stroke: are we doing the right thing? Trends in Neurosciences 1999;22:535–40.

Dirnagl U, Iadecola C, Moskowitz MA. Pathobiology of ischaemic stroke: an integrated view. Trends in Neurosciences 1999;22:391–7.

Dziadulewicz EK, Ritchie TJ, Hallett A, et al. Nonpeptide bradykinin B_2 receptor antagonists: conversion of rodent-selective bradyzide analogues into potent orally active human bradykinin B_2 receptor antagonists. Journal of Medicinal Chemistry 2002;45:2160–72.

Enna S, Williams M, Ferkany JW, et al., editors. Current protocols in pharmacology. Hoboken, NJ: Wiley; 2003.

GLP Pocketbook. Contains the *Good Laboratory Practice (GLP) Regulations 1999* and the *Guide to the GLP Regulations*. London: MCA Publications; 1999.

Hall JM. Bradykinin receptors: pharmacological properties and biological roles. Pharmacology and Therapeutics 1992;56:131–90.

Heidempergher F, Pillan A, Pinciroli V, et al. Phenylimidazolidin-2-one derivatives as selective 5-HT3 receptor antagonists and refinement of the pharmacophore model for 5-HT3 receptor binding. Journal of Medicinal Chemistry 1997;40: 3369–80.

Keen M, editor. Receptor binding techniques. Totowa, NJ: Humana Press; 1999.

Kenakin T. The measurement of efficacy in the drug discovery agonists selection process. Journal of Pharmacologic and Toxicologic Methods 1999;42:177–87.

Lipska BK, Weinberger DR. To model a psychiatric disorder in animals: schizophrenia as a reality test. Neuropsychopharmacology 2000;23:223–39.

Löscher W. Animal models of epilepsy for the development of antiepileptogenic and disease-modifying drugs. A comparison of the pharmacology of kindling and post-status epilepticus models of temporal lobe epilepsy. Epilepsy Research 2002;50:105–23.

Melini EB, Goa KL. Beraprost: a review of its pharmacology and therapeutic efficacy in the treatment of peripheral arterial disease and pulmonary hypertension. Drugs 2002;62:107–33.

Morfis M, Christopoulos A, Sexton PM. RAMPs: 5 years on, where to now? Trends in Pharmacological Sciences 2003;24:596–601.

Moser PC, Hitchcock JH, Lister S, et al. The pharmacology of latent inhibition as an animal model of schizophrenia. Brain Research Reviews 2000;33:275–307.

Pinkert CA. Transgenic animal technology. 2nd ed. San Diego, CA: Academic Press; 2002.

Polites HG. Transgenic model applications to drug discovery. International Journal of Experimental Pathology 1996;77:257–62.

Research Defense Society website: www.rds-online.org.uk/ethics/arclaims – a reasoned rebuttal of the view put forward by opponents of animal experimentation that the use of such experiments in drug discovery is at best unnecessary, if not positively misleading.

Rudin M, Weissleder R. Molecular imaging in drug discovery and development. Nature Reviews Drug Discovery 2003;2:122–31.

Rudolph U, Moehler H. Genetically modified animals in pharmacological research: future trends. European Journal of Pharmacology 1999;375: 327–37.

Small DL, Buchan AM. Stroke: animal models. British Medical Bulletin 2000;56:307–17.

Törnell J, Snaith M. Transgenic systems in drug discovery: from target identification to humanized mice. Drug Discovery Today 2002;7: 461–70.

Traxler P, Bold G, Frei J, et al. Use of a pharmacophore model for the design of EGF-R tyrosine kinase inhibitors: 4-(phenylamino) pyrazolo[3,4-d]pyrimidines. Journal of Medicinal Chemistry 1997;40:3601–16.

Vogel WH, editor. Drug discovery and evaluation: pharmacological assays. Heidelberg: Springer-Verlag; 2002.

White HS. Animal models of epileptogenesis. Neurology 2002;59:S7–14.

Willner P. The validity of animal models of depression. Psychopharmacology 1984;83:1–16.

Willner P, Mitchell PJ. The validity of animal models of predisposition to depression. Behavioural Pharmacology 2002;13:169–88.

Yamada K, Nabeshima T. Animal models of Alzheimer's disease and evaluation of anti-dementia drugs. Pharmacology and Therapeutics 2000;88:93–113.

Yang D, Soulier J-L, Sicsic S, et al. New esters of 4-amino-5-chloro-2-methoxybenzoic acid as potent agonists and antagonists for 5-HT4 receptors. Journal of Medicinal Chemistry 1997;40:608–21.

Zan Y, Haag JD, Chen KS, et al. Production of knockout rats using ENU mutagenesis and a yeast-based screening assay. Nature Biotechnology 2003;21:645–51.

Chapter **12**

Biopharmaceuticals

H LeVine

INTRODUCTION

The term 'biopharmaceutical' was originally coined to define therapeutic proteins produced by genetic engineering, rather than by extraction from normal biological sources. Its meaning has broadened with time, and the term now encompasses nucleic acids as well as proteins, vaccines as well as therapeutic agents, and even cell-based therapies. In this chapter we describe the nature of biopharmaceuticals, and the similarities and differences in discovery and development between biopharmaceuticals and conventional small-molecule therapeutic agents. The usual starting point for biopharmaceuticals is a naturally occurring peptide, protein or nucleic acid. The 'target' is thus identified at the outset, and the process of target identification and validation, which is a major and often difficult step in the discovery of conventional therapeutics (see Chapter 6), is much less of an issue for biopharmaceuticals. Equally, the process of lead finding and optimization (Chapters 7, 8, 9) is generally unnecessary, or at least streamlined, because nature has already done the job. Even if it is desirable to alter the properties of the naturally occurring biomolecule, the chemical options will be much more limited than they are for purely synthetic compounds. In general, then, biopharmaceuticals require less investment in discovery technologies than do conventional drugs. Toxicity associated with reactive metabolites – a common cause of development failure with synthetic compounds – is uncommon with biopharmaceuticals. On the other hand, they generally require greater investment in two main areas, namely *production methods* and *formulation*. Production methods rely on harnessing biological systems to do the work of synthesis, and the problems of yield, consistency and quality control are more complex than they are for organic synthesis. Formulation problems arise commonly because biomolecules tend to be large and unstable, and considerable ingenuity is often needed to improve their pharmacokinetic properties, and to target their distribution in the body to where their actions are required.

It is beyond the scope of this book to give more than a brief account of the very diverse and rapidly developing field of biopharmaceuticals. More detail can be found in textbooks (Buckel, 2001; Ho and Gibaldi, 2003; Walsh, 2003). As the field of biopharmaceuticals moves on from being mainly concerned with making key hormones, antibodies and other signalling molecules available as therapeutic agents, efforts – many of them highly ingenious – are being made to produce therapeutic effects in other ways. These include, for example, using antisense nucleic acids, ribozymes or RNAi (see below and Chapter 6) to reduce gene expression, the use of catalytic antibodies to control chemical reactions in specific cells or tissues, and the development of 'DNA vaccines'. So far, very few of these more complex 'second-generation' biopharmaceutical ideas have moved beyond the experimental stage, but there is little doubt that the therapeutic strategies of the future will be based on more sophisticated ways of affecting biological control mechanisms than the simple 'ligand → target → effect' pharmacological principle on which most conventional drugs are based.

RECOMBINANT DNA TECHNOLOGY: THE ENGINE DRIVING BIOTECHNOLOGY

The discovery of enzymes for manipulating and engineering DNA – the bacterial restriction endonucleases, polynucleotide ligase and DNA polymerase – and the invention of the enabling technologies of DNA sequencing and copying of DNA sequences by using the polymerase chain reaction (PCR) allowed rapid determination of the amino acid sequence of a protein from its mRNA message. Versatile systems for introducing nucleic acids into target cells or tissues and for the control of host nucleic acid metabolism brought the potential for correction of genetic defects and for new therapeutic products for disorders poorly served by conventional small-molecule drugs. The importance of these discoveries for the biological sciences was indicated by the many Nobel Prizes awarded for related work. No less critical was the impact that these reagents and technologies had on applied science, especially in the pharmaceutical industry. The business opportunities afforded by biotechnology spawned thousands of startup companies and profoundly changed the relationship between academia and industry. The mainstream pharmaceutical industry, with its 20th-century focus on small-molecule therapeutic agents, did not immediately embrace the new methodologies except as research tools in the hands of some discovery scientists. Entrepreneurs in biotechnology startup firms eventually brought technology platforms and products to large pharmaceutical companies as services or as products for full-scale development. This alliance allowed each party to concentrate on the part they did best.

Biotechnology products were naturally attractive to the small startup companies. Because the protein or nucleic acid itself was the product, it was unnecessary to have medicinal chemists synthesize large collections of organic small-molecule compounds to screen for activity. A small energetic company with the right molecule could come up with a profitable and very useful product. The niche markets available for many of the initial protein or nucleic acid products were sufficient to support a small research-based company with a high-profit-margin therapeutic agent.

THE EARLY DAYS OF PROTEIN THERAPEUTICS

Along with plant-derived natural products, proteins and peptides were some of the first therapeutic agents produced by the fledgling pharmaceutical industry in the latter half of the 19th century, before synthetic chemistry became established as a means of making drugs. Long before antibiotics were discovered, serum from immune animals or humans was successfully used to treat a variety of infectious diseases. Serotherapy was the accepted treatment for *Haemophilus influenzae* meningitis, measles, diphtheria, tetanus, hepatitis A and B, poliovirus, cytomegalovirus and lobar pneumonia. Antisera raised in animals were used to provide passive protection from diphtheria and tetanus infection.

Extracts of tissues provided hormones, many of which were polypeptides. After its discovery in 1921, insulin extracted from animal pancreas replaced a starvation regimen for treating diabetes. The size of the diabetic population, and the activity in humans of the hormone isolated from pancreas of pigs and cows, permitted early commercial success. Generally, however, the low yield of many hormones and growth factors from human or animal sources made industrial scale isolation difficult and often uneconomic. Nevertheless, several such hormones were developed commercially, including *follicle-stimulating hormone* (FSH) extracted from human urine to treat infertility, *glucagon* extracted from pig pancreas to treat hypoglycaemia, and *growth hormone*, extracted from human pituitary to treat growth disorders. Some enzymes, such as *glucocerebrosidase*, extracted from human placenta and used to treat an inherited lipid storage disease (Gaucher's disease), and *urokinase*, a thrombolytic agent extracted from human urine, were also developed as commercial products.

Some serious problems emerged when proteins extracted from human or animal tissues were developed for therapeutic use. In particular:

- Repeated dosage of non-human proteins generated an immune response in some patients against the foreign sequences, which differed by several amino acids from the human sequence. Such immune responses could cause illnesses such as serum sickness, or loss of efficacy of the protein.
- Human tissue was in short supply and was subject to potential contamination with infectious agents. Growth hormone extracted from human cadaver pituitary glands was contaminated with prions that cause Creutzfeld–Jakob disease, a dementing brain-wasting disease similar to bovine spongiform encephalitis (BSE) and sheep scrapie. Human blood plasma-derived products have been tainted with hepatitis B virus and HIV.
- Many agents (e.g. cytokines) cannot be extracted in sufficient quantities to be used therapeutically.
- Batch-to-batch variability was considerable, requiring standardization by bioassay in many cases.

The recombinant DNA revolution and the subsequent development of biotechnology resolved many of these issues. Many vaccines and antisera, however, are still prepared from blood products or infectious organisms, rather than by recombinant DNA methods.

CURRENTLY AVAILABLE CLASSES OF BIOPHARMACEUTICALS

The major classes of biopharmaceuticals currently on the market include hormones, cytokines, growth factors, antibodies, enzymes, vaccines and nucleotide-based agents. Examples of therapeutic proteins, including antibodies, enzymes and other proteins approved for clinical use, are presented in Table 12.1. Others not included in the compilation include therapeutic preparations such as serum albumin, haemoglobin and collagen, which are not drugs in the conventional sense.

In addition to the 'mainstream' biopharmaceuticals considered here are numerous speciality products for niche markets that are under investigation or in development by small 'boutique' companies.

Growth factors and cytokines

The production, differentiation and survival of the various types of blood cell are tightly regulated by an interacting network of hormones, cytokines and growth factors. Species-specific activities of many of these chemical mediators, and their very low abundance, highlighted the need for biopharmaceutical products.

The most common uses of haemopoietic factors are for the treatment of various types of neutropenia, where specific white cell levels are depressed as a result of infection, immune disorders, recovery from chemotherapy or reaction to various drug regimens. They are especially useful in aiding recovery from the dose-limiting side effects of cancer chemotherapy. *Granulocyte colony-stimulating factor (G-CSF)* and *granulocyte-macrophage colony-stimulating factor (GM-CSF)* are used for this purpose to improve patient quality of life and allow the continuation of chemotherapy.

Erythropoietin (EPO), normally secreted by the kidney to stimulate the production of red blood cells, is the most successful biotechnology product so far marketed. EPO boosts red cell counts and reduces transfusion requirements for patients rendered anaemic by cancer chemotherapy or renal disease. Various forms of EPO with clearance profiles – and hence duration of action – modified by linkage with polyethylene glycol (PEGylation) or alteration of its glycosylation (see below and Chapter 17) are also available. Off-label use of EPO by athletes to improve performance has caused controversy.

Interferons are a complex group of proteins that augment immune effector cell function. *Interferon-α* was the first recombinant biotherapeutic agent approved by the FDA for cancer treatment. Recombinant interferons have been approved for melanoma, hepatitis C, Karposi's sarcoma, T-cell lymphoma, chronic myelogenous leukaemia, multiple sclerosis and severe malignant osteopetrosis. Mechanism-based side effects have thus far restricted their utility to these severe disorders.

Hormones

Hormone replacement or augmentation is a commonly accepted medical practice in certain diseases of deficiency or misregulation. *Insulin* isolated from biological sources is administered to diabetics to control blood glucose levels. Immunological reaction to non-human (porcine or bovine) insulin preparations, which occur in a significant number of patients, are avoided by recombinant products incorporating parts of the human insulin sequence. A variety of human insulin and glucagon preparations are now on the market.

Human growth hormone (somatotropin) was originally developed for treating paediatric growth failure and Turner's syndrome. Originally, growth hormone was extracted from human pituitary tissue post mortem, but this material carried a significant risk of transmitting Creutzfeld-Jakob disease, a fatal neurodegenerative condition now known to be transmitted by a prion, an abnormal protein found in affected nervous tissue, whose existence was unsuspected when human-derived growth hormone was introduced as a therapeutic agent. The production of human growth hormone by recombinant methods rather than extraction avoids this serious problem as well as providing a much more abundant source. Growth hormone has acquired notoriety since the potential for misuse to produce taller and stronger athletes was realized.

Human gonadotropin-releasing *hormones* have been extensively used in fertility management as well as in treating endometriosis and precocious puberty. Originally isolated from urine, there are now numerous recombinant products on the market.

Coagulation factors

Coagulation factors are a group of plasma proteins required for proper haemostasis. Deficiencies are associated with genetic lesions and occur as complications of viral infections such as hepatitis C and HIV. They were initially treated with plasma-derived concentrates, which carried a significant risk of viral and prion contamination. *Recombinant factor VIII* (Recombinate, Kogenate) and *factor IX* (BeneFix) avoid this risk and are now widely used.

Antithrombotic factors

To reduce blood coagulation, when conventional heparin or warfarin therapy is contraindicated, recombinant *thrombin inhibitors* (Leprudin, Bivalirudin) and *antiplatelet gpIIb/IIIa antagonists* (Eptifibatide) are now available. In conditions such as stroke, coronary thrombosis and pulmonary embolism early treatment with thrombolytic agents to relieve the vascular block is highly beneficial. *Streptokinase* and *urokinase* are proteases that process plasminogen to plasmin, activating its thrombolytic activity to dissolve fibrin clots. Newer products include *tissue plasminogen activator* (tPA) and TNKase, which catalyse the same reaction but in a fibrin-dependent fashion, so that plasmin production is concentrated in the region of the clot. These proteins are also less immunogenic than the

Table 12.1 Examples of approved therapeutic proteins produced by recombinant technology

Product	Trade name	Date approved	Indications
Blood clotting factors and plasminogen activators			
Human factor VIII	Kogenate, Recombinate	1992	Haemophilia A
Human factor IX	Benefix	1997	Haemophilia B
Human tissue plasminogen activator (tPA)	Activase	1987	Heart attacks, stroke
Haemopoietic factors			
Erythropoietin	Epogen, Procrit	1989	Anaemia
Granulocyte-macrophage colony-stimulating factor (GM-CSF)	Leukine	1991	Neutropenia
Hormones			
Human insulin	Humulin, Novolin, Protropin	1982	Diabetes mellitus
Human glucagons	GlucaGen	1998	Hypoglycaemia
Human growth hormone	Humatrope, Nutropin	1987	Growth hormone deficiency
Human thyroid-stimulating hormone (TSH)	Thyrogen	1998	Thyroid deficiency
Human follicle-stimulating hormone (FSH)	Gonal F, Follistim	1995	Infertility
Interferons and interleukins			
Human interferon-α	Intron A, Viraferon	1986	Hepatitis B and C
Human interferon-β	Betaferon	1995	Multiple sclerosis
Human interferon-γ	Actimmune	1990	Chronic inflammatory disease
Modified human interleukin-2	Proleukin	1992	Renal carcinoma
Modified human interleukin-11	Neumega	1997	Thrombocytopenia
Monoclonal antibodies			
Abciximab (against platelet GPIIb/IIIa)	ReoPro	1994	Blood clot prevention
Trastuzumab (against human EGF receptor)	Herceptin	1998	Breast cancer
Infliximab (against TNF-α)	Remicade	1998	Crohn's disease, arthritis
Rituximab (against CD20 lymphocyte antigen)	Rituxan	1997	Non-Hodgkin's lymphoma
Others			
Hirudin	Revasc, Refludan	1998	Prevention of thrombosis
Human β-cerebrosidase	Cerezyme	1994	Gaucher's disease (lipid storage disorder)
DNase	Pulmozyme	1993	Cystic fibrosis

bacterial streptokinase, which is important in cases where repeated administration of the thrombolytic agent is required.

Another regulator of coagulation is the serine protease *protein C*. The activated form of protein C breaks down the clotting factors Va and VIIIa and plasminogen activator inhibitor-1, tipping the balance in the favour of thrombolysis. These enzymes are important bio-pharmaceutical products that have no small-molecule counterpart.

Therapeutic antibodies

Monoclonal antibodies

A breakthrough in high-quality reproducible and scalable production of antibodies came with the development by Kohler and Milstein in 1975 of monoclonal antibodies. Fusion of primed T cells from an immunized mouse with an immortalized mouse myeloma (B-cell) line that secretes immunoglobulin light chains provided a cell-culture system that could produce unlimited quantities of antibody with defined specificity. Single-cell clones secreted antibody against a single epitope of the antigen. The initial immunization could, for toxic or scarce immunogens, be replaced by in vitro stimulation of isolated mouse thymocytes for fusion with the myeloma cells.

The technology for antibody production has now gone mouseless. It has moved into the realm of molecular biology, in which bacteriophages, gene libraries in plasmids and bacterial hosts are engineered to produce either whole antibodies or derivatives of antibodies with desired properties. 'Humanizing' the antibodies, or replacing the rodent constant domains with human sequences (chimerization), limits hypersensitivity reactions to foreign protein. Chimerization increases the half-life of the antibodies in human plasma up to six-fold and improves their function within the human immune network. The human Fc domain reacts with Fc receptors on human cells more avidly. Chimeric antibodies with human constant regions also interact optimally with human complement proteins, and are thus more effective in destroying target cells in patients than are their rodent counterparts.

Antibody selection by phage display

Phage display technology (Benhar, 2001) is a useful way to identify antigen combining regions to produce monoclonal antibodies that bind to therapeutically relevant antigens. Bacteriophages (or phages) are viruses that replicate in bacteria, *Escherichia coli* being the organism of choice in most cases. For antibody selection (Figure 12.1) a large DNA library, encoding millions of different putative antigen-binding domains, is incorporated into phage DNA, so that each phage particle encodes a single antigen combining region. The mixed phage population is added to *E. coli* cultures, where the phage replicate, each phage

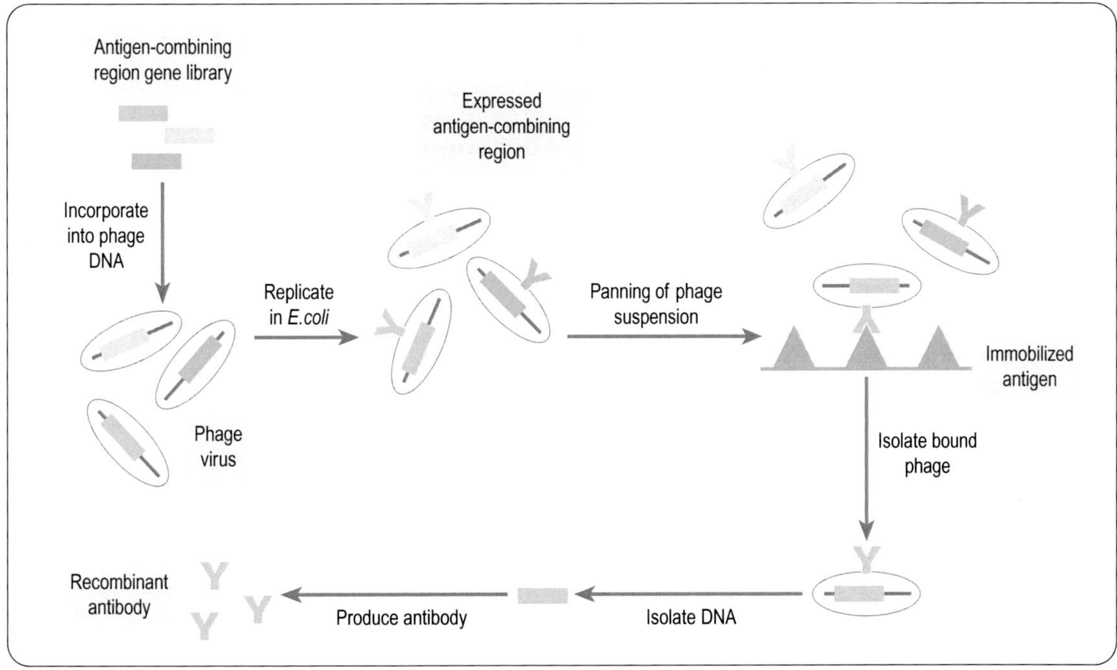

Fig. 12.1 Antibody selection by phage display technique.

particle expressing copies of a single antigen combining region on its surface. The phage suspension is applied to plates coated with the antigen of interest ('panning') and those phage particles expressing antigen combining regions recognizing the antigen stick to the plates. The adherent phages are isolated, allowing the antigen combining region-encoding DNA to be identified and inserted into the DNA sequence encoding an appropriate full-size antibody scaffold to produce a specific antibody, or into a reduced size, simplified monomeric framework to produce a single-chain (sFv) antibody.

Uses of antibodies as therapeutic agents

Cancer immunotherapy

Although high-affinity mouse monoclonal antibodies to target antigens can be reproducibly produced in industrial quantities, and bind to specific human targets, they generally function poorly in recruiting human effector functions. The therapeutic potency of these antibodies can be enhanced by taking advantage of the targeting selectivity of antibodies (see Chapter 17) for the purposes of drug delivery. Linking other agents, such as cytotoxic drugs, biological toxins, radioisotopes or enzymes to activate prodrugs to targeting antibodies enhances their delivery to the target cells and reduces side effects by directing the toxic agents to the tumour and minimizing clearance. Bispecific antibodies with one H-L chain pair directed against a target cell antigen and the other against a soluble effector such as a complement component, or against a cell surface marker of an effector cell type, have also been developed to bring the components of the reaction together. A number of these are in clinical trials for a variety of different malignancies, but have in general proved less successful than had been expected on the basis of animal studies.

Antibody use in transplantation and immunomodulation

The major obstacle in the transplantation of cells, tissues or organs is the body's recognition of foreign material. A strong immune response to rid the body of the non-self antigens leads to rejection of the transplant. Selective immunological suppression can ablate components of the antitransplant response. Fab fragments of antibodies to a number of surface antigens on T-cells are used to partially block T-cell responses to donor cells. Fab fragments are required because the Fc portion of the complete antibody targets the cell for destruction, resulting in unwanted complete immunosuppression.

Even human antibodies face disadvantages as therapeutics. Because of their size (MW ~150 kDa), their ability to penetrate into tissues, such as solid tumours, is limited. Engineered versions lacking the Fc region, which is largely responsible for hypersensitivity responses of patients treated with monoclonal antibodies, have replaced the $(Fab)_2$ fragments generated by proteolysis from the intact antibody. Single sFv chains containing the H and L variable regions are the smallest antibodies containing a high-affinity antigen-combining site. Still in the experimental stage, 'di-antibodies' with two H-L units connected by a 15-amino acid linker $(Gly_4Ser)_3$ peptide have greatly increased affinity for antigen (see also Chapter 13).

Catalytic antibodies

Antibodies can be used to enhance the chemical reactivity of molecules to which they bind. Such catalytic antibodies ('abzymes') created with transition state analogs as immunogens specifically enhance substrate hydrolysis by factors of 10^2–10^5 over the rate in their absence, and this principle has been applied to the development of therapeutic agents (Tellier, 2002). Both esterase and amidase activities have been reported. Catalytic turnover of substrates by abzymes is low in comparison to true enzymes, as high-affinity binding impedes the release of products. Attempts to improve catalytic efficiency and to identify therapeutic uses for catalytic antibodies have engrossed both academic and biotech startup laboratories. Targets being approached with these antibodies include cocaine overdose and drug addiction, bacterial endotoxin, and anticancer monoclonal antibody conjugated with a catalytic antibody designed to activate a cytotoxic prodrug. Attempts are also being made to develop proteolytic antibodies containing a catalytic triad analogous to that of serine proteases, designed to cleave gp120 (for treatment of HIV), IgE (for treatment of allergy), or epidermal growth factor receptor (for treatment of cancer).

Therapeutic enzymes

Enzymes can be useful therapeutic agents as replacements for endogenous sources of activity that are deficient as a result of disease or genetic mutation. Because enzymes are large proteins they generally do not pass through cellular membranes, and do not penetrate into tissues from the bloodstream unless assisted by some delivery system. Lysosomal hydrolases such as cerebrosidase and glucosidase have targeting signals that allow them to be taken up by cells and delivered to the lysosome. Genetic lysosomal storage diseases (Gaucher's, Tay–Sachs) are treated by enzyme replacement therapy. However, penetration of the enzymes into the nervous system, where the most severe effects of the disease are expressed, is poor. Cystic fibrosis, a genetic disorder characterized by deficits in salt secretion, is treated with digestive enzyme supplements and an inhaled DNase preparation (dornase-α) to reduce the extracellular viscosity of the mucous layer in the lung to ease breathing. All of these are produced as recombinant proteins.

Vaccines

Using the immune system to protect the body against certain organisms or conditions is a powerful way to provide long-term protection against disease. Unlike with small-molecule pharmaceuticals, which are administered when needed, once immunity is present subsequent exposure to the stimulus automatically activates the response. Most current vaccines are against disease-causing organisms such as bacteria, viruses and parasites. More complex conditions where the antigens are not so well defined are also being addressed by immunization. Vaccines are being tested for cancer, neurodegenerative diseases, contraception, heart disease, autoimmune diseases, and alcohol and drug addiction (Rousseau et al., 2001; Biaggi et al., 2002; BSI Vaccine Immunology Group, 2002; Kantak, 2003). Immune induction is complex. Pioneering experiments with attenuation of disease organisms showed that illness was not required for immunity. The goal in immunization is to retain enough of the disease-causing trait of an antigen to confer protection without causing the disease. For infectious agents, various methods of killing or weakening the organism by drying or exposure to inactivating agents still dominate manufacturing processes. Isolation of antigens from the organisms, or modifying their toxins, can be used in some cases. Vaccine production of isolated antigen 'subunit' vaccines benefits from protein engineering.

Novel approaches to presenting antigens are expected to have an impact on vaccination. An example is the *phage display* technique (Benhar, 2001), described earlier as a technique for antibody selection. The same approach can be used to provide the protein antigen in a display framework that enhances its immunogenicity and reduces the requirement for immune adjuvants (of which there are few approved for human use). Viruses encoding multiple antigens ('vaccinomes') can also be employed.

Genetic vaccination (Liu, 2003) employs a DNA plasmid containing the antigen-encoding gene, which is delivered to the host tissue by direct injection of DNA, or by more exotic techniques such as attaching the DNA to microparticles which are shot into tissues at high speed by a 'gene gun', or introduced by other transfection methods (Capecchi et al., 2004; Locher et al., 2004; Manoj et al., 2004). When the DNA is transcribed, the mRNA translated and the protein expressed in the host tissue, eukaryotic sequences will undergo appropriate post-translational modification, which does not occur with conventional protein vaccines. In general, partial sequences of pathogen-derived proteins are fully immunogenic, despite lacking the toxicity of full-length transcripts. The first human trial for a genetic vaccine against HIV took place in 1995, and others quickly followed, including hepatitis, influenza, melanoma, malaria, cytomegalovirus, non-Hodgkin's lymphoma, and breast, prostate and colorectal tumours. Initial results have been promising. At the time of writing, recombinant vaccines against hepatitis A and B (e.g. Twinrix), papillomavirus virus for genital warts and cervical cancer (Gardisil), and against Haemophilus b/meningococcal protein for meningitis (Comvax) are approved. Single or multiple proteins from an organism can be included, and proteins that interfere with the immune response (common in many infectious agents) excluded.

GENE THERAPY

The development and present status of gene therapy are discussed in Chapter 3. Here we focus on the technical problems of gene delivery and achieving expression levels sufficient to produce clinical benefit, which are still major obstacles.

Introduction of genetic material into cells

Nucleic acid polymers are large, highly charged polyanions at physiologic pH. The mechanism by which such cumbersome hydrophilic molecules traverse multiple membrane lipid bilayers in cells is poorly understood, although a variety of empirical techniques for getting DNA into cells have been devised by molecular biologists. Eukaryotic cells use many strategies to distinguish between self and foreign DNA to which they are continually exposed. Some mechanisms apparently interfere with the incorporation and expression of engineered genes in gene therapy and other DNA transfer applications. Despite advances in technology, expression of foreign genes in cells or animals in the right place, at the right moment, in the right amount, for a long enough time remains difficult. Doing so in a clinical situation where so many more of the variables are uncontrollable is yet more challenging. The high expectations of gene therapies, which conceptually seemed so straightforward when the first trials were started, have run aground on the shoals of cellular genetic regulatory mechanisms. Effective gene therapy awaits the selective circumventing of these biological controls to deliver precise genetic corrections.

Delivery of nucleic acids

A potential gene therapy requires three major components: the payload to accomplish the mission, a targeting system to direct the vehicle and its payload to the correct body compartment in the correct cell population, and finally gene regulatory element(s), such as promoters/enhancers, to control the time and place of expression of the payload sequence(s). Table 12.2 compares the properties of some gene therapy vectors that have been used in clinical trials.

Table 12.2 Gene therapy vectors

	Naked DNA	Liposome-encapsulated DNA	Adenovirus	Adenoassociated virus (AAV)	Retrovirus
Genetic material (max size insert)	DNA or RNA (≥50 kb)	DNA (≥50 kb)	DNA (7.5 kb)	DNA (5 kb)	RNA (8 kb)
Efficiency	Low	Low	Very high	Medium	High (low in vivo)
Transform non-dividing cells	Possibly, weak integration	Possibly, weak integration	Yes, transient expression, non-integrating	Yes, site-specific integration	No, transient integration
Safety issues	None, good safety profile	None, good safety profile	Viral recombination, immune reactions	Viral recombination, immune reactions	Viral recombination, tumorogenesis

To be clinically useful, a vehicle must elude host immunological or toxicological responses, must persist in the body, and must avoid sequestration in non-target organs such as the liver or kidney. Ideally, for clinical use one would want the ability to modulate or remove the genetic modification in case of adverse effects – the equivalent of discontinuing administration of a traditional drug. In practice, major difficulties are experienced in obtaining sufficient expression of the desired product for long enough to measure a positive clinical outcome.

Strategies for nucleic acid-mediated intervention

There are several points of attack for nucleic acid therapeutics. Most diseases are not due to an identified gene mutation, but rather reflect secondary cellular malfunction, often in response to events entirely external to the cell being targeted. Overexpressing proteins or fragments, either normal or mutated so as to compete with the normal protein for participation in cellular functions – known as the '*dominant negative*' strategy – is a commonly used approach.

RNA metabolism can be modulated in many different ways, including:

- Antisense RNA
- Small interfering mRNA (siRNA)
- RNA decoys for viral RNA-binding proteins
- Specific mRNA-stabilizing proteins
- Interference with mRNA splicing to induce exon skipping or to correct abnormal splicing
- Sequence-specific cleavage by catalytic RNAs such as hammerhead and hairpin ribozymes. Bacterial introns that code for a multifunctional reverse transcriptase/RNA splicing/DNA endonuclease/integrase protein can be altered to target specific DNA sequences
- MicroRNA (miRNA) regulation.

Transcription of DNA into mRNA can also be controlled either through transcription factors or through antisense oligonucleotide triplex formation. Direct interference with genomic DNA through quadruplex formation is another strategy. These oligonucleotide sequences can be provided by biologically derived vector systems or by chemical synthesis. Short double- and single strand oligonucleotide sequences are readily taken up by cells. Produced as single strands by automated solid-phase chemical synthesis, these short, single-stranded 8–20-nucleotide sequences can be chemically modified on the base, sugar, or phosphate linker to enhance their stability against nuclease degradation and cellular penetration (Figure 12.2).

Table 12.3 lists a number of clinical trials with nucleic acid-based therapeutics that are at different stages of completion.

RNA interference – gene silencing by RNAi

RNAi is a technique for reducing the expression of or silencing specific genes. Its usefulness as an experimental tool, particularly for identifying potential drug targets, is discussed in Chapter 6, and it also has considerable potential as a means of silencing genes for therapeutic purposes. It is similar to antisense modulation of mRNA, but extends further into the command and control of cellular nucleic acids. Short double-stranded RNA (21–23 nucleotides) is used to silence homologous gene activity. Specific *RNA-induced silencing complexes* (RISC) guide multiple activities that target mRNA for degradation, block translation, or block gene transcription by methylation of chromatin (Denli and Hannon, 2003).

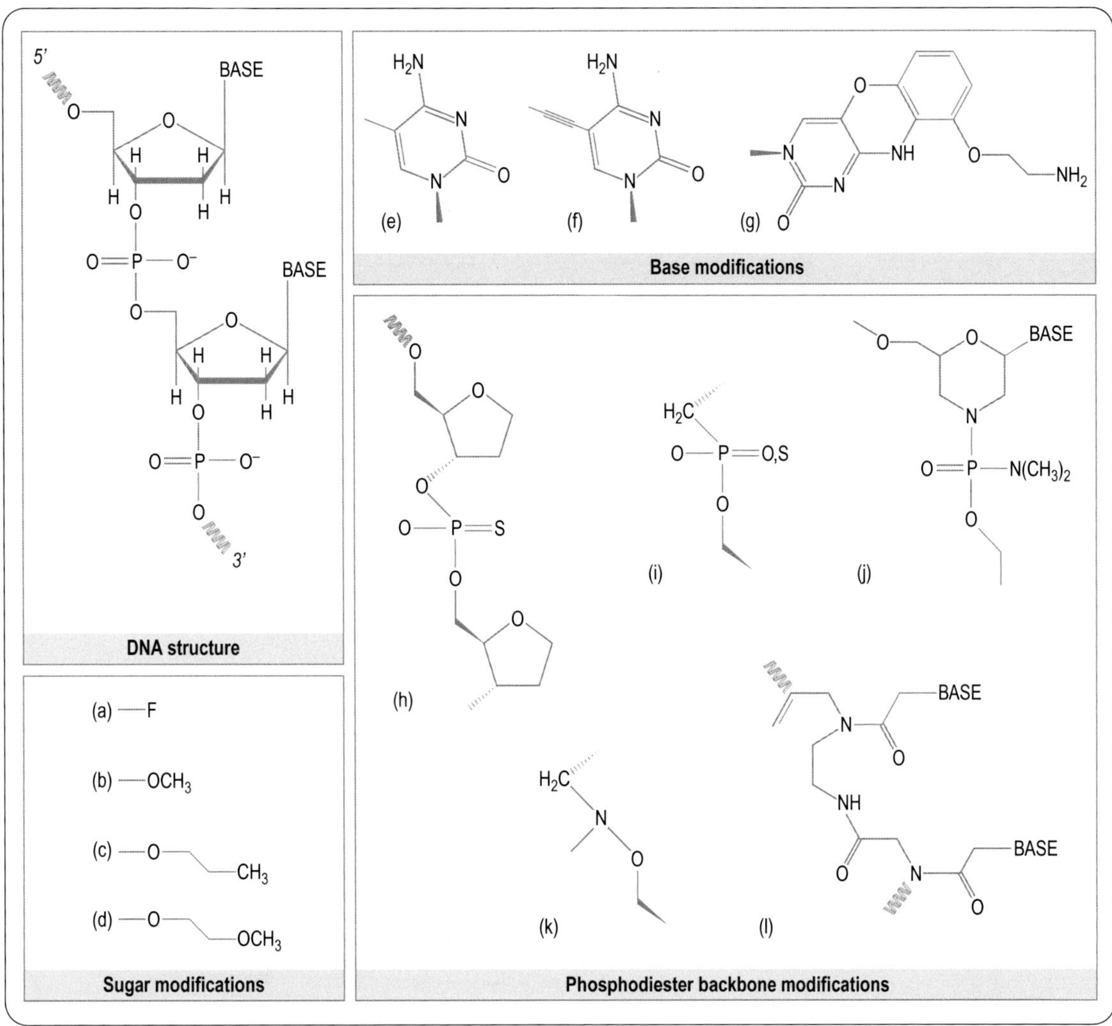

Fig. 12.2 Chemical modification of nucleotides. Key for modifications: Sugar modifications: (a) fluoro-, (b) methoxy-, (c) methoxyethyl-, (d) propoxy-. Base modifications: (e) 5-methyl cytosine, (f) 5-propyne cytosine, (g) tricyclic cytosine. Phosphodiester backbone modifications: (h) phosphorothioate, (i) mopholino-, (j) methylene- (on PDF), (k) methylene-methylimino, (l) peptide nucleic acid (PNA).

Examples of genes that have been targeted by RNAi include:

- Viruses such as HIV-1, poliovirus, respiratory syncytial virus and hepatitis C
- Oncogenes and tumour suppressors, such as Ras, bcl-abl, p53, p53bp and p73Dn
- Cell surface receptors for HIV-1-CD4, CCR5 and CXCR4, and the IL2 receptor α CD25 (Dykxhoorn et al., 2003).

Although RNA interference is highly efficient as a gene-silencing technique under laboratory conditions, most of the difficulties with antisense or expression technology still remain to be overcome. Unlike single-stranded antisense oligonucleotides, the double-stranded siRNAs are unable to penetrate cell membranes effectively without assistance. They are also highly susceptible to plasma degradation. Unfortunately, the same chemical modifications in the phosphodiester backbone used to stabilize antisense oligonucleotides reduces or eliminates silencing activity of interfering RNA constructs. Modification of the 2′ position of uridines and cytosines with fluorine increases plasma half-life and preserves their inhibitory capacity.

Although initial results suggested a high degree of specificity for siRNA in down-regulating a target molecule and the technique is widely used in cell culture studies, there

Table 12.3 Clinical trials with antisense oligonucleotides

Agent	Target	Indication	Company
ISIS 2302	ICAM-1	Crohn's disease, ulcerative colitis, rheumatoid arthritis, psoriasis, renal transplant	ISIS Pharmaceuticals/Boehringer Ingelheim
ISIS 2105*	HPV 6 and 11 E2 gene product	Genital warts	ISIS Pharmaceuticals
ISIS 2922 (Formivirsen)	CMV IE2 gene	CMV retinitis	ISIS Pharmaceuticals
GEM 132	CMV UL36 gene	CMV retinitis	Hybridon
CGP 64128A/ISIS 2531	Protein kinase C-α	Miscellaneous cancers	Novartis/ISIS Pharmaceuticals
CGP 69846A/ISIS 5132	c-*raf* kinase	Miscellaneous cancers	Novartis/ISIS Pharmaceuticals
GEM 91*	HIV gag protein	AIDS	Hybridon
Genta 3139	Bcl-2 protein	Non-Hodgkin's lymphoma	Genta
LR3280	c-*myc*	Restenosis	Lynx Therapeutics
OL(1)p53	P53	Haemopoetic malignancy	University of Nebraska/Lynx Therapeutics
	c-*myb*	Chronic myelogenous leukaemia	University of Pennsylvania/Lynx Therapeutics

*Trials terminated.
Source: Bennett CF, Dean NM, Monia BP (1998) In: Harvey A L (ed) Advances in drug discovery techniques. Chichester: John Wiley; 174.

is a surprising tolerance of mismatching leading to effects on unintended targets (Lin et al., 2005). Even if microarray analysis indicates that two siRNAs to the same protein give similar expression patterns, siRNAs with multiple mismatches in the centre of the sequence can operate as microRNAs (miRNA) that can inhibit expression of off-target proteins by arresting their translation without altering cellular mRNA levels, or affect mRNA stability (Saxena et al., 2003). Despite these challenges, several companies are moving ahead with siRNA candidates in clinical trials (Table 12.3), and other products in this class are in the pipeline for approval for testing. RNAi will probably dominate the next wave of gene therapeutics moving into clinical trials.

miRNAs are naturally occurring small RNA species that have been shown to have profound regulatory effects on the genome. Multiple genes may be regulated by a single miRNA and each gene may also be connected to multiple miRNAs, creating a vast network of interactions that may provide fine control to multiple processes from tissue development to a variety of disease states. They operate analogously to siRNA, but with a twist. The RISC complex differs in that noncomplementary nucleotides create bulges in the double-stranded nucleotide preventing the miRNA:RISC complex from continuing along the siRNA pathway. Instead, mRNA translation is affected and the mRNA is destabilized. Targeting microRNAs as a therapeutic strategy is in the very early stages of evaluation. Successful development faces both the known challenges of chemical matter and delivery as well as additional safety and efficacy hurdles because of the web of interactions among the genome and individual miRNAs (Seto, 2010).

COMPARING THE DISCOVERY PROCESSES FOR BIOPHARMACEUTICALS AND SMALL MOLECULE THERAPEUTICS

The approach to discovering new protein/peptide therapeutics differs in many ways from the drug discovery approach for synthetic compounds described in other chapters in this section.

Protein/peptide drug discovery usually starts with known biomolecules, which it may be desirable to trim down to smaller domains with desired activities. Alternatively, native proteins are often optimized for desirable properties by mutation or other kinds of modification. These modifications can also provide the basis for patent protection. Unlike small-molecule synthesis, where the possibilities are virtually limitless, there is a finite number of natural proteins and a limited range of feasible modifications that may be introduced to improve their biological properties. The race to protect important proteins as starting points for therapeutics is critical for the future application of biotechnology.

The production of biotechnology-based therapeutics also involves technologies and facilities quite different from those used for producing synthetic compounds.

Manufacture of biopharmaceuticals

Expression systems

Full-size proteins, including a number of hormones, growth factors and mediators, are produced recombinantly by inserting the cDNA version of the mRNA sequence coding for the protein of interest into specially designed plasmid vectors that orchestrate the expression of the desired protein product in the cell type of choice (Figure 12.3). The characteristics of different expression systems are compared in Table 12.4.

These vectors contain a selection marker to maintain the vector in the host cell along with regulatory DNA sequences that direct the host cell transcriptional machinery to produce mRNA from the inserted cDNA sequence, with appropriate initiation and termination codons and a ribosome-binding site. A polyA$^+$ tail is added to eukaryotic expression systems to stabilize the mRNA. mRNA transcription, and hence protein production, is controlled by an induction element, so that protein is produced only when required. This is important, as some expressed proteins are toxic to growing and dividing host cells. Other sequences, such as protein export signal peptides, hexahistidine tags, immunologic epitopes, or fusion with protein partners such as glutathione S-transferase, thioredoxin, maltose-binding protein or IgG Fc, facilitate secretion or provide handles for the detection/purification of the expressed protein. Purification tags are particularly useful in eukaryotic expression systems, which express exogenous proteins at lower levels than do bacterial systems, where the expressed protein can be 10–50% of the total cellular protein. The tags are designed to be removed from the protein once it has been purified.

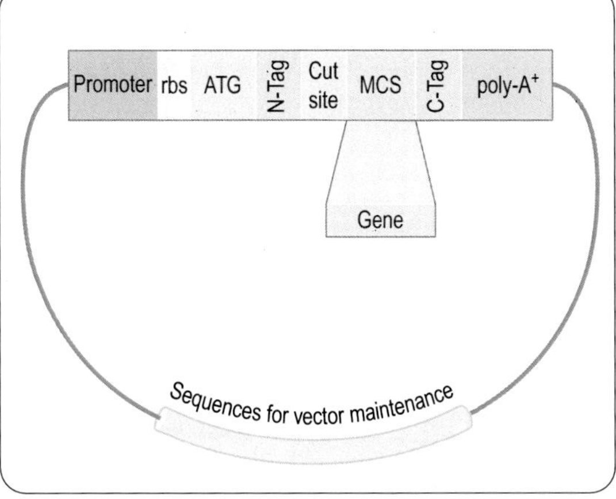

Fig. 12.3 Generic vector for protein expression. The cDNA for the protein to be expressed is cloned into restriction sites in the multiple cloning site (MCS) of an expression vector which contains appropriate sequences for maintenance in the chosen host cell. Expression of the gene is controlled by inducible promoter. A ribosome-binding site (rbs) optimized for maximum expression directs translation, beginning at the ATG initiation codon. Either N-terminal or C-terminal tags (N-, C-Tag) can be used to aid in purification or stabilization of the protein, and a protease cut site may be used to remove the tag after purification. A translation terminator codon is followed (in eukaryotic cells) by a poly-A$^+$ tail to stabilize the mRNA.

Table 12.4 Comparison of protein expression systems

Property	Similarity to human situation				
	E. coli	Yeast	*Aspergillus*	Insect	Mammalian cell culture
Folding	Some	Some	Some	Yes	Yes
Subunit assembly	No	Yes	?	Yes	Yes
Secretion	Some	Yes	Yes	Yes	Yes
Modifications:*					
acetylation	Yes	Yes	Probably	Probably	Yes
myristoylation	No	Yes	?	Yes	Yes
phosphorylation	No	Yes	?	Yes	Yes
glycosylation	No	Incomplete	Incomplete	Incomplete	Yes

*Co-transfection of appropriate enzymes into cells expressing the protein of interest can provide post-translational modifications.

Bacterial protein expression, usually in *Escherichia coli*, is the system of choice for high expression levels of many proteins, and because scale-up technology is well developed. However, not every protein is amenable to bacterial expression. Proteins that contain disulfide bonds or are comprised of multiple subunits are problematic, as are proteins containing critical carbohydrate, lipid or other post-translational modifications. In some cases the enzymes responsible for post-translational modification, such as fatty acylation, can be co-transfected with the desired protein. Highly expressed proteins are frequently produced as insoluble inclusion bodies in the bacterial cytoplasm or periplasmic space. Active proteins must be recovered from these inclusion bodies after denaturation and in vitro refolding. Intrinsic membrane-bound proteins can pose additional problems.

Eukaryotic microbial systems include *Saccharomycetes cerevisiae* and *Picha pastoralis* – yeasts that perform many mammalian post-translational modifications, including partial glycosylation. Insect cells, notably from *Spodoptera frugiperda* (Sf9), are infected with engineered baculovirus expression vectors carrying the protein of interest. This is a particularly efficient system for membrane protein expression. Many G-protein-coupled receptors, a large class of integral membrane proteins that includes many targets for currently marketed drugs, are often produced in these cells for use in screening assays for receptor ligands.

Cultured mammalian cells are used to express proteins on a research or production scale where faithful post-translational modification is required. Favourites include fibroblasts, anchorage-independent lymphocytes, Chinese hamster ovary (CHO) cells, and human embryonic kidney (HEK) cells. Mammalian cells grow more slowly and are more fastidious than the bacteria, yeasts or insect cells, and are therefore more expensive for production. Human cells are used in situations where there is some mammalian species dependence of bound carbohydrate. This can be particularly important for growth factors and the large glycoprotein hormones, as their glycosylation modulates the activity and stability of the protein product in vivo. Potential contaminating human pathogens in the human cell lines used for expression must be controlled. So must non-primate mammalian pathogens, as the possibility of transfer to humans cannot be ignored.

The use of transgenic animals and plants as 'factories' for genetically engineered proteins is discussed below.

Engineering proteins

Nature has devoted millions of years to optimizing protein structures for their biological roles. The natural configuration may not, however, be optimal for pharmaceutical applications. Recombinant DNA methods can be used to re-engineer the protein structure so as to better fulfil the requirements for a pharmaceutical agent.

Site-directed mutagenesis

Changes in the sequence of a protein at the level of a single amino acid can change the biochemical activity or the stability of the protein. It can also affect interactions with other proteins, and the coupling of those interactions to biological function. Stabilizing proteins to better withstand the rigours of industrial production and formulation is commercially important. Microorganisms adapted to extreme environments have evolved modified forms of enzymes and other functional proteins, such as increased disulfide (cystine) content and more extensive core interactions, to withstand high temperatures. Similar tricks are used to stabilize enzymes for use at elevated temperatures, such as in industrial reactors, or in the home washing machine with enzyme-containing detergents. Other mutations alter the response of the protein to environmental conditions such as pH and ionic strength. Mutations to add or remove glycosylation signal sequences or to increase resistance to proteolytic enzymes may be introduced to alter immunogenicity or improve stability in body fluids. Protein activation by conformational changes due to phosphorylation, binding of protein partners or other signals may sometimes be mimicked by amino acid changes in the protein. The solubility of a protein can often be improved, as can the ability to form well-ordered crystals suitable for X-ray structure determination.

Fused or truncated proteins

Sometimes the full-size form of a protein or peptide is too difficult or expensive to produce or deliver to the target. Domains of proteins can often be stripped to their essentials, so that they retain the required characteristics of activity or targeting specificity. They may require fusion with a partner for proper folding or stability, the partner being removed as part of purification.

Ligands and receptor-binding domains can be attached to the active biomolecule in order to target it to specific sites. Pathogens and infectious agents, in addition to appropriating intracellular targeting motifs, have evolved protein sequences that enable them to penetrate the cell membrane to access the machinery for their propagation. Some of these sequences can be incorporated into biopharmaceuticals in order to deliver peptides and proteins into cells. Hydrophobic portions of Kaposi fibroblast growth factor, Grb2 SH2 domain, and human integrin α and β subunits have been employed in this way as cell-penetrating agents. The fusion sequence (1–23) of HIV-1 gp41 has been used to deliver synthetic antisense oligonucleotides and plasmid DNA into cells. Amphipathic sequences containing periodic arrangements of polar and hydrophobic residues, such as those found in the fusion peptide of the influenza haemagglutinin-2 protein, promote fusion with cell membranes and the delivery of associated agents. Polycationic sequences in penetratin (residues 43–58 from the Antp protein), HIV-1 tat protein

(47–57), and the HIV-1 transcription factor VP22 (267–300), permeabilize membranes and increase the uptake of associated material.

Protein production

Although relatively small quantities of highly potent biologicals are normally required, production often presents problems. Only synthetic peptides and oligonucleotides and their derivatives can be produced by a scalable chemical synthesis. The others require large-scale fermentation or cell culture. The proteins and nucleic acids are then isolated and purified from the cells or media. Biotechnological process development is a complex field (Sofer and Zabriskie, 2000; Buckel, 2001; Gad, 2007). High-level production of recombinant proteins can result in heterogeneity because of the misincorporation of amino acids such as norvaline into the product, depending on the culture conditions, the nutrient composition of the medium and the producing organism. Post-translational modifications depend on the cultured organism and the subcellular localization of the protein. In cultured eukaryotic cells proteins undergo many kinds of post-translational modification, including glycosylation, sulfation, phosphorylation, lipidation, acetylation, γ-carboxylation and proteolytic processing. These and other modifications increase the heterogeneity of the product, affecting its biological half-life, immunogenicity and activity. The most homogeneous preparation consistent with retention of the important biological properties is standardized for production and a reproducible analytical profile is established. Nevertheless, protein products are invariably less homogeneous in composition than synthetic compounds, and the quality criteria for approval of clinical materials have to be adjusted to take account of this.

Formulation and storage conditions are critical because the protein primary amino acid sequences naturally display a variety of chemical instabilities. A major degradation route of protein products is through unfolding of the polypeptide chain and aggregation. Proteins have a finite half-life in an organism, governed partly by built-in chemical and conformational instabilities. Adsorption to surfaces of glass or plastic containers, particulates and air–liquid interfaces is often a cause of product loss.

The chemical reactivity of the various amino acid residues contributes to protein loss and heterogeneity. Succinimide formation, isomerization and racemization, as well as peptide bond cleavage, tend to occur at aspartate residues, to an extent that depends somewhat on the surrounding amino acid sequence. Examples include hACTH, soluble CD4, OKT-3 monoclonal antibody, hGH-releasing factor, IL-1β and hEGF. Oxidation, particularly at methionine residues, is catalysed by transition metal ions, pH, light, and various oxygen free radicals. Examples are relaxin A, hIGF-I and enkephalin analogs. Disulfide exchange (cysteine/cystine) can generate inappropriate folding or intermolecular bond formation, thereby promoting aggregation and precipitation of protein. Examples are interferon, and the acidic and basic forms of FGF. Beta-elimination at cystine, cysteine, serine and threonine leads to dehydroalanine formation and reaction with nucleophilic side chains. Anhydride formation between the α amino group on a protein and the C terminus is a major degradation pathway for insulin stored between pH3 and pH5. Sometimes peroxides contaminate the excipients and stabilizing agents, such as the polyethylene glycols or the surfactants Polysorbate 20 and Polysorbate 80 used in product formulation (see Chapter 16).

The first therapeutic proteins produced on an industrial scale were antibodies, which initially relied on immunization of large animals such as horses. Monoclonal technology paved the way for the production of murine antibodies in cell culture. With the ability to produce human antibody proteins and derivatives through molecular biological manipulation, the organism used to manufacture the protein is chosen on the basis of economics and requirements for post-translational modification. The characteristics of some commonly used organisms for protein production are summarized in Table 12.4.

Eukaryotic and prokaryotic microorganisms and eukaryotic cells in culture are the most common source of therapeutic proteins. Prokaryotic expression is generally the first choice, whereas higher organisms produce protein products that are most similar to human material and thus are more likely to be biologically active and pharmacokinetically stable. The production of proteins on a commercial scale by eukaryotic cell culture is, however, extremely expensive. The cells grow slowly (18–24 hours doubling time, compared with about 20 minutes for bacteria) and most require a serum source or expensive growth factor/hormone cocktails in the culture medium.

'Pharming' of protein expression in whole animals or plants is used for large-scale production of proteins for some therapeutics and for industrial applications. Transgenic farm animals – goats, cows, sheep and rabbits – have been engineered to secrete human proteins into their milk (van Berkel et al., 2002). Annual milk yields range from about 8 L (rabbit) to 8–10 000 L (cow). Expression levels of from 1 to 20 g of product per litre of milk have been achieved in favourable instances, allowing small herds of transgenic animals to do the work of large fermentation facilities. Many biopharmaceuticals are under development by specialized biotechnology companies (Table 12.5). The first drug produced in genetically engineered livestock (Atryn in goat milk) was approved by the FDA in February 2009. Thirty or more such products are expected to be registered in the next decade.

Plants can be directed to concentrate antibodies and other proteins in their leaves, seeds or fruit (Giddings et al., 2000; Daniell et al., 2001; Powledge, 2001; Streatfield and Howard, 2003), and are beginning to be used for the commercial production of antibodies and vaccines.

Table 12.5 Biopharmaceuticals produced in transgenic farm animals. (These products are in development; none have yet reached the market)

Protein	Indication	Host
Antithrombin III	Inflammation	Goat
α_1-Antitrypsin	Inflammation, inherited deficiency	Cow, goat, sheep
α-Glucosidase	Glycogen storage disease type II	Rabbit
h-Chorionic gonadotropin	Infertility	Cow, goat
Factor VIII	Haemophilia	Pig
Factor IX	Haemophilia	Pig
Factor XI	Haemophilia	Sheep
Fibrinogen	Burns, surgery	Pig, sheep
Lactoferrin	GI bacterial infection	Cow
Monoclonal antibody	Colon cancer	Goat
Protein C	Deficiency, adjunct to tPA	Pig, sheep
Serum albumin	Surgery, burns, shock	Cow, goat
Tissue plasminogen activator (tPA)	Infarction, stroke	Goat

Monoclonal antibodies expressed in plants – 'plantibodies' – have been produced in maize, tobacco and soybeans. Antibodies produced against *Streptococcus mutans*, the main cause of tooth decay in humans, have demonstrated efficacy against dental caries. CaroRX is in Phase II clinical trials for topical application for tooth decay. Other proteins, such as mouse and human interferon, human growth hormone, haemoglobin, human serum albumin and human epidermal growth factor, are also being targeted. Merispace, a recombinant mammalian gastric lipase, is being produced in corn for oral administration to counteract lipid maladsorption in cystic fibrosis and chronic pancreatitis Vaccine production for both animals and humans appears to be a most promising application of 'pharming'. By splicing the gene for the antigen into a modified plant virus (cowpea mosaic virus), companies such as Agricultural Genetics (Cambridge, UK) have produced effective vaccines for animals against mink enterovirus, HIV-1 and foot and mouth disease, obtaining up to 200 doses of vaccine from a single cowpea (black-eyed pea) leaf. Other companies are pursuing vaccines for hepatitis A and B, cold and wart viruses and *Plasmodium* (malaria). Splicing the antigen genes directly into the plant genome has been successful for hepatitis B, Norwalk, cholera and rabies virus vaccines.

Feeding antigen-producing plants to animals has shown promise for inducing immune protection (Judge et al., 2004), despite the differences in the type of immune response from oral exposure and the standard humoral administration. The oral route would be ideal for human vaccines, particularly in countries where refrigeration is uncertain. Although antigen expressed in potato for use in humans was effective in animals, the cooking required for human consumption of the vegetable destroyed the immunogenicity of the antigen. Current efforts are developing the technology for human foods that are eaten raw and which are suitable for tropical climates, such as tomato and banana (Korban et al., 2002).

There are many developments in plant-derived biopharmaceuticals for human use, but none has yet become commercially available. Widespread environmental and other concerns among the general public about transgenic crop production are a significant impediment, especially outide of the United States.

PHARMACOKINETIC, TOXICOLOGICAL AND DRUG-DELIVERY ISSUES WITH PROTEINS AND PEPTIDES

The main source of the bias against biologicals (proteins) as therapeutic agents in major pharmaceutical companies comes from the difficulties in delivering these expensive, large, highly charged molecules to the target in sufficient concentrations for long enough to achieve pharmacologic effects. The complexities faced in taking small molecules through preclinical development into clinical trials are compounded with biologicals. More detailed expositions of pharmacokinetics, toxicology and the delivery of therapeutic proteins are available (Frokjaer and Hovgaard, 2000; Sofer and Zabriskie, 2000; Ho and Gibaldi, 2003; Walsh, 2003; Steffansen et al., 2010).

Figure 12.4 illustrates the pathways that govern the distribution and elimination of a pharmacological agent. Factors that assume particular importance for biopharmaceuticals are (a) the choice of formulation and route of administration so as to achieve consistent absorption, (b) control of distribution by targeting to the required site of action, and (c) protection against rapid inactivation or elimination.

Absorption of protein/peptide therapeutics

Mucosal delivery

Peptide and protein drugs are in general poorly absorbed by mouth because of their high molecular weight, charge,

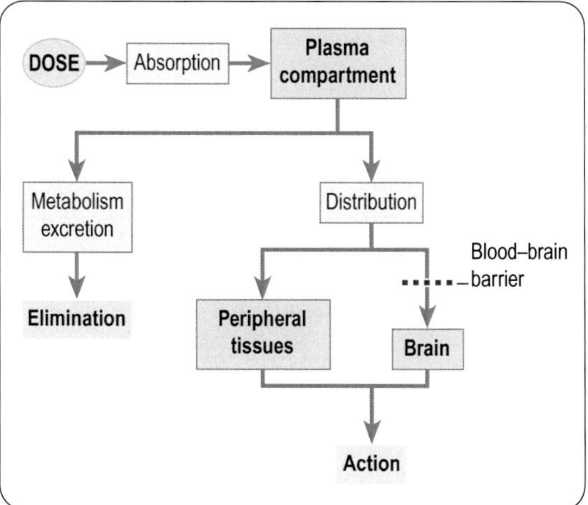

Fig. 12.4 Simplified scheme showing the processes involved in drug absorption, distribution and elimination. Pink boxes, body compartments; grey boxes, transfer processes.

Table 12.6 Physical properties of some therapeutic proteins

Protein	Molecular wt (Da)	Isoelectric point
Somatostatin	1600	10.4
Insulin	6000	5.6
Human growth hormone	20 000	5.3
t-PA	60 000	9.1
Human serum albumin	66 000	5.3
IgG	150 000	Variable
Factor VIII	270 000	7.4
Typical small-molecule drug	<500	Variable

and susceptibility to proteolytic enzymes. The main barriers to absorption of proteins are their size and charge (Table 12.6).

Large hydrophilic and charged molecules do not readily pass the cellular lipid bilayer membrane. Small peptides can be absorbed if they are relatively hydrophobic, or if specific transporters exist. Proteins can be transported by *transcytosis*, in which proteins enter cells at the basal surface via receptor-mediated endocytosis or fluid-phase pinocytosis into vesicles, are transported across the cell through the cytosol, and then released by exocytosis at the apical membrane. However, much of the protein is degraded by the lysosomal system during transit.

Formulations have been devised to optimize the stability and delivery of protein and peptide therapeutics (Frokjaer and Hovgaard, 2000). Protection from proteolysis is a major concern for many routes of administration. Various entrapment and encapsulation technologies have been applied to the problem (see Chapter 16). The greater the protection, though, the less rapidly the protein is released from the preparation. Hydrogels, hydrophilic polymers formed around the protein, avoid proteolysis but limit absorption. Microcapsule and microsphere formulations are made by enclosing the active compound within a cavity surrounded by a semipermeable membrane or within a solid matrix. The surface area for absorption is much greater than that provided by hydrogel or solid matrix formulations.

A variety of penetration-enhancing protocols have been applied to increase the rate and amount of protein absorption. These include surfactants (sodium dodecyl sulfate, polyoxyethylene fatty acyl ethers), polymers (polyacrylic acid, chitosan derivatives), certain synthetic peptides (occulin-related peptides), bile salts (sodium deoxycholate, sodium glycocholate, sodium taurocholate), fatty acids (oleic acid, caprylic acid, acyl carnitines, acylcholines, diglycerides), and chelating agents (EDTA, citric acid, salicylates, *N*-amino acyl β-diketones).

The nasal mucosal route of administration is emerging as an acceptable and reasonably effective method of drug delivery. Some peptide drugs, such as *nafarelin, oxytocin, lypressin, calcitonin* and *desmopressin*, are effective as nasal sprays, although the fraction absorbed in humans is generally low (≤10%). Pulmonary administration is surprisingly effective when ~3 μm particles of the therapeutic are dispersed deep in the lung. The vast alveolar surface area and blood supply allow even macromolecules to be absorbed.

Transdermal delivery across the stratum corneum, the outermost, least-permeable skin layer, is being increasingly used for proteins and other drugs. Transport of drug molecules across the skin is facilitated by transient disruption of epithelial barrier function with sonic energy (sonophoresis), electric current (iontophoresis) or electric field (electroporation). Table 12.7 compares different routes of non-parenteral dosing for the relative proteolytic activity to which a protein drug would be exposed.

Parenteral delivery

Oral or mucosal absorption of native, full-length proteins is inefficient even with enhancing strategies. Thus, many protein therapeutics are delivered parenterally by intravenous, intramuscular or subcutaneous injection. With intramuscular and subcutaneous administration sustained-release formulations can be used to increase the duration of action.

Table 12.7 Exposure of protein/peptide drugs to protease activity by different routes of administration

Oral	Very high
Rectal	High
Buccal	Medium
Nasal	Medium
Vaginal	Medium
Transdermal	Low
Pulmonary	Low
Ocular	Low

The blood–brain barrier is impermeable to most proteins and peptides, but possesses transporters that facilitate the entry of some, such as apolipoprotein E, transferrin and insulin. Linking active peptides to an antibody directed against the transferrin receptor has been shown in experimental animals to allow neurotrophic factors such as *nerve growth factor* (NGF) to enter the brain and produce neurotrophic effects when given systemically and this strategy may prove applicable for human use.

Elimination of protein/peptide therapeutics

Most therapeutic proteins are inactivated by proteolysis, producing short peptides and amino acids which then enter dietary pathways. Unlike small-molecule drugs, metabolites of protein therapeutics are not considered to be a safety issue. The rate and extent of degradation of protein therapeutics before excretion depend on the route of administration. Breakdown occurs in both plasma and tissues. Attempts to minimize these losses include the use of glycosylated proteins, which more closely resemble the native protein, or chemical modification of the protein with polyethylene glycol (PEG) chains or other entities. PEGylation can increase the plasma half-life of a protein between three- and several hundredfold. Besides reducing proteolysis, PEGylation can shield antigenic sites, enhance protein solubility and stability, and prevent rapid uptake by organs. With small peptides, cyclization or the inclusion of D-amino acid residues, particularly at the N terminus, can be used to protect against exoproteolysis, though this approach is of course applicable only to synthetic peptides and not to biopharmaceuticals.

The kidney is an important organ for the catabolism and elimination of small proteins and peptides. Proteins of 5–6 kDa, such as insulin, are able freely to pass the glomerular filter of the kidney. Passage through the glomerulus decreases to about 30% for proteins of 30 kDa, and to less than 1% for 69 kDa proteins. Some proteins, such as calcitonin, glucagon, insulin, growth hormone, oxytocin, vasopressin and lysozyme, are reabsorbed by the proximal tubules via luminal endocytosis, and then are hydrolysed in lysosomes. Linear peptides less than 10 amino acids long are hydrolysed by proteases on the surface of brush border membranes of the proximal tubules.

Liver metabolism is highly dependent on specific amino acid sequences in proteins. Cyclic peptides, small (<1.4 kDa) and hydrophobic peptides are taken up by carrier-mediated transport and degraded. Large proteins use energy-dependent carrier-mediated transport, including receptor-mediated endocytosis and transcytotic pathways (polymeric IgA), and are targeted to lysosomes.

SUMMARY

In the late 1970s recombinant DNA technology boosted biotechnology into a prominence it has not relinquished. Apart from fears about human genetic modification, the outlook has been positive for the production of new and better biopharmaceuticals. Whereas the traditional pharmaceutical companies were slow to embrace the new technology, a number of small biotech companies sprang up which have provided the innovative driving force for the protein and gene product industry. The genomic revolution is the latest manifestation of the technology, stimulating efforts to mine the information coming out of the various species genome projects for new products and therapies.

Recombinant DNA technology allows the production of individual proteins and peptides on a large scale regardless of their natural abundance. There are many advantages to recombinant production. Human sequence proteins reduce potential immunological problems and avoid potential infectious agents in materials isolated from natural sources. Proteins are expressed in a variety of cellular systems, determined by the properties of the molecule required. Bacterial systems are used wherever possible because of the high level of expression that can be obtained and the simplicity and availability of production. Bacteria, however, do not provide many of the post-translational modifications required for human protein stability and function, such as glycosylation, lipid modification, phosphorylation, sulfation and disulfide bond formation. Protein aggregation often occurs, and even though denaturation and refolding are successful for many proteins, some are problematic. In these cases eukaryotic systems, including various yeast species and cultured insect and mammalian cells, are used. Transgenic farm animals and plants are also coming into their own as protein 'factories'.

Antibodies in the form of animal sera were the first widely used protein therapeutics. Although immunization is still used as a prophylactic and as a therapeutic, recombinant DNA technology is used to produce both immunogen and antibodies. Hypersensitivity reactions are reduced by producing altered antibodies with the required epitope specificity. They are 'chimerized' (human constant domain) or 'humanized' (rodent complementarity-determining region (CDR)), with human Fc portions for optimal interaction with the human complement system. Single-chain and multichain antibodies can be expressed intracellularly to attack previously sequestered antigens. These immunological agents are also used to target infectious organisms, deliver radioisotopes or cytotoxic agents to cancer cells, and to moderate tissue rejection in transplantation.

Proteins and enzymes have been engineered to hone their therapeutic usefulness. Protein structure can be stabilized or modified to slow degradation or increase uptake, and multiple functions can be built into the same molecule. Recombinant vaccine production of cloned protein domains uses these modifications to increase immunogenicity and avoid exposure to infectious agents. Delivery of synthetic vectors coding for antigenic epitopes into host tissues promotes endogenous antigen expression.

The biggest obstacle to the use of proteins and peptides as therapeutics is the delivery to the site of action of sufficient agent to create a biological effect. Formulating proteins and peptides to penetrate epithelial barriers in a biologically active form is difficult. Because of their size, charge and instability in the gastrointestinal tract, special delivery systems often must be used to achieve efficacious blood levels. Penetration through the blood–brain barrier can be even more challenging. Small-molecule drugs of <500 Da molecular weight have a much better record in this regard. Once in the blood, proteins are often rapidly eliminated by a variety of mechanisms, although there are modifications that can slow degradation.

Even though protein and peptide therapeutics faces significant pharmacokinetic and pharmacodynamic liabilities, much work is still being done on agents for which small molecules are not available to perform the same function.

Nucleic acids can be delivered into cells in a variety of ways. Complexation of the highly charged DNA with lipophilic cations, or derivitization of nucleic acid bases, sugars or the phosphodiester backbone can be efficient in cell culture, but less so in whole organisms. Ingenious schemes of antisense, RNAi, ribozyme, decoy sequences and RNA splicing inhibition are used to attain therapeutic effects. Viruses, nature's DNA delivery machines, modified to eliminate their pathogenic capacity, are used in organisms to introduce the therapeutic gene into target cells. The inserted DNA directs the synthesis of a protein in the host cell, in the case of a growth factor deficiency in the brain providing a secreted product for the support of surrounding cells. Numerous gene therapy clinical trials are in progress, but the need to avoid side effects and host suppression of viral-based therapeutics has slowed progress.

REFERENCES

Benhar I. Biotechnological applications of phage and cell display. Biotechnology Advances 2001;19:1–33.

Biaggi E, Rousseau RF, Yvon E, et al. Cancer vaccines: dream, reality, or nightmare? Clinical and Experimental Medicine 2002;2:109–18.

BSI Vaccine Immunology Group. Vaccination against non infectious disease (BSI Vaccine Immunology Group/BSACI session). Immunology 2002;107(Suppl 1):67–70.

Buckel P, editor. Recombinant protein drugs. Basel: Birkhauser Verlag; 2001.

Capecchi B, Serruto D, Adu-Bobie J, et al. The genome revolution in vaccine research. Current Issues in Molecular Biology 2004;6:17–27.

Daniell H, Streatfield SJ, Wycoff K. Medical molecular farming: production of antibodies, biopharmaceuticals and edible vaccines in plants. Trends in Plant Science 2001;6:219–26.

Denli AM, Hannon GJ. RNAi: an ever growing puzzle. Trends in Biochemical Sciences 2003;28:196–201.

Dykxhoorn DM, Novina CD, Sharp PA. Killing the messenger: short RNAs that silence gene expression. Nature Reviews Molecular Cell Biology 2003;4:457–67.

Frokjaer S, Hovgaard L. Pharmaceutical formulation: development of peptides and proteins. Philadelphia, PA: Taylor & Francis; 2000.

Gad SC, editor. Handbook of Pharmaceutical Biotechnology. Hoboken, NJ: John Wiley and Sons; 2007.

Giddings G, Allison G, Brooks D, et al. Transgenic plants as factories for biopharmaceuticals. Nature Biotechnology 2000;18:1151–5.

Ho RJY, Gibaldi M. Biotechnology and biopharmaceuticals. Transforming proteins and genes into drugs. Hoboken, NJ: Wiley-Liss; 2003.

Judge NA, Mason HS, O'Brien AD. Plant cell-based intimin vaccine given orally to mice primed with intimin reduces time of *Escherichia coli* O157:H7 shedding in feces. Infection and Immunity 2004;72:168–75.

Kantak KM. Anti-cocaine vaccines: antibody protection against relapse. Expert Opinion in Pharmacotherapy 2003;4:213–18.

Korban SS, Krasnyanski SF, Buetow DE. Foods as production and delivery vehicles for human vaccines. Journal of the American College of Nutrition 2002;21:212S–17S.

Lin X, Ruan X, Anderson MG, et al. SiRNA-mediated off-target gene silencing triggered by a 7 nt complementation. Nucleic Acids Res 2005;33:4527–35.

Liu MA. DNA vaccines: a review. Journal of Internal Medicine 2003;253:402–10.

Locher CP, Soong NW, Whalen RG, et al. Development of novel vaccines using DNA shuffling and screening strategies. Current Opinion in Molecular Therapy 2004;6:34–9.

Manoj S, Babiuk LA, van Drunen Littel-van den Hurk S. Approaches to enhance the efficacy of DNA vaccines. Critical Reviews in Clinical Laboratory Science 2004;41:1–39.

Powledge TM. Tobacco pharming. A quest to turn the killer crop into a treatment for cancer. Scientific American 2001;285:25–6.

Rousseau RF, Hirschmann-Jax C, Takahashi S, et al. Cancer vaccines. Hematology/Oncology Clinics of North America 2001;15:741–73.

Saxena S, Jonsson ZO, Dutta A. Small RNAs with imperfect match to endogenous mRNA repress translation. Implications for off-target activity of small inhibitory RNA in mammalian cells. J Biol Chem 2003;278:44312–19.

Seto AG. The road toward microRNA therapeutics. Int J Biochem Cell Biol 2010;42:1298–305.

Sofer G, Zabriskie DW. Biopharmaceutical process validation, vol. 25. New York: Marcel Dekker; 2000.

Steffansen B, Brodin B, Nielson CU. Molecular biopharmaceuticals: aspects of drug characterization, drug delivery, and dosage form evaluation. Chicago: Pharmaceutical Press; 2010.

Streatfield SJ, Howard JA. Plant production systems for vaccines. Expert Review on Vaccines 2003;2:763–75.

Tellier C. Exploiting antibodies as catalysts: potential therapeutic applications. Transfusion Clinique et Biologique 2002;9:1–8.

van Berkel PH, Welling MM, Geerts M, et al. Large scale production of recombinant human lactoferrin in the milk of transgenic cows. Nature Biotechnology 2002;20:484–7.

Walsh G. Biopharmaceuticals, biochemistry, and biotechnology. 2nd ed. Chichester: John Wiley; 2003.

Chapter 13

Scaffolds: small globular proteins as antibody substitutes

D Grabulovski, J Bertschinger

INTRODUCTION

An emerging field in pharmaceutical biotechnology is represented by the generation of novel binding molecules based on small globular domains serving as protein frameworks ('scaffolds'). In this approach, certain amino acid residues of the surface of a single domain are combinatorially mutated to produce a protein library, which can then be screened for binding specificities of interest. Thus, the concept of a universal binding site from the antibody structure is transferred to alternative protein frameworks with suitable biophysical properties. On one hand these new proteins provide further insights into the processes of molecular recognition, on the other hand they also have commercial applications, as therapeutic agents, diagnostic reagents or affinity ligands.

SCAFFOLDS

Monoclonal antibodies (mAbs) are an increasingly important class of therapeutic agents as discussed in preceding chapters. Over 25 recombinant antibodies are currently on the market, the top 10 best-selling of these products earned over $32 billion in global sales during 2008, and five mAb products (rituximab, infliximab, bevacizumab, trastuzumab and adalimumab) were included in the top 15 best-selling prescription drugs for that year (Reichert, 2010). The future prospects for therapeutic antibodies are clearly bright, the annual growth rate estimated to be 12% during 2010–2012. However, even antibody blockbusters suffer from certain drawbacks: human immunoglobulin G (IgG) antibody is a complex molecule composed of four protein chains with attached carbohydrates. A full-size IgG antibody is a Y-shaped complex of two identical light chains, each with a variable and constant domain, and two heavy chains, each with one variable and three constant domains (Fig. 13.1H). Therefore, full-size IgGs are always bivalent molecules and elicit effector functions through their Fc part, which may not be ideal for certain applications. With regards to expression, there is the requirement for a rather expensive mammalian cell production system and, in addition, antibodies depend on disulfide bonds for stability. Through the versatile techniques of genetic engineering, smaller antibody fragments have been produced to overcome some of the limitations of full-size IgGs (Holliger and Hudson, 2005), but some antibody fragments tend to aggregate and display limited solubility. Finally, the success, and consequently the extensive use, of antibodies has led to a complicated patent situation for antibody technologies and applications. Therefore, several research groups and small and medium-sized companies have recently focused on the development of small globular proteins as scaffolds for the generation of a novel class of versatile binding proteins.

As therapeutics, globular proteins with engineered binding properties might be particularly interesting, (i) if the neutralization of a target protein is the desired pharmacological effect (in contrast to a full length antibody, where the Fc portion may stimulate immune processes), (ii) as fusion proteins, for the targeted delivery of bioactive molecules to sites of disease, (iii) as receptor-binding drugs, thus interfering with the cell-signalling and (iv) as enzyme inhibitors.

Common to all approaches of finding a suitable scaffold are the following steps (Nygren and Uhlen, 1997; Smith 1998; Binz and Pluckthun, 2005):

- Choosing a small protein (domain) that is well expressed in bacteria or yeast and has good biophysical properties (stability, solubility)

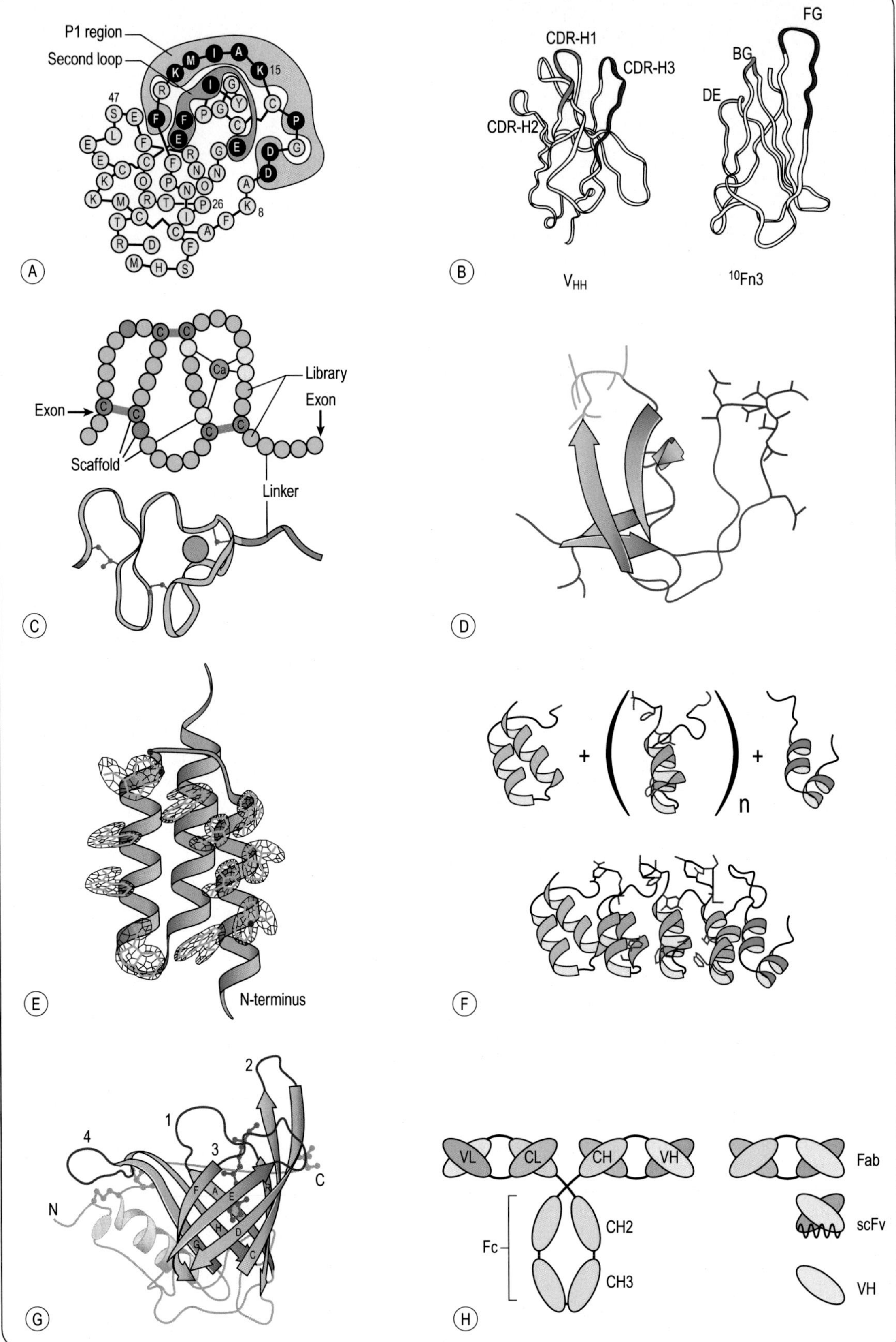
P1 region
Second loop
A
CDR-H1
CDR-H3
CDR-H2
FG
BG
DE
B
V_{HH}
^{10}Fn3
Library
Exon
Exon
Scaffold
Linker
C
D
N-terminus
E
n
F
2
1
4
3
C
N
G
VL
CL
CH
VH
Fab
Fc
CH2
CH3
scFv
VH
H

- Creating a library of protein mutants by introducing diversity at a contiguous patch of the surface of the protein (e.g. loops)
- Using a genotype-phenotype display system (e.g. phage display) to select a range of binders to a therapeutic target of interest
- Screening the binders obtained by the selection procedure for the desired biological activity, e.g. by enzyme-linked immunosorbent assay (ELISA).

Mutations introduced in the protein scaffold to produce diversity may compromise the three-dimensional structure, stability and solubility of the protein scaffold, thus making the isolation of protein binders based on folding frameworks other than the immunoglobulin fold difficult. Nevertheless, more than 50 scaffolds have been described for the generation of new protein binders (reviewed in Binz et al., 2005; Gebauer and Skerra, 2009). Being mainly a topic of academic interest at first, nowadays the development and use of non-antibody classes of proteins is being pursued by small- and medium-sized biotechnology companies (Hey et al., 2005). The common basis for the successful development of well-designed protein drugs lies in the availability of both a well-behaving protein scaffold and an efficient selection or screening technology in order to find suitable candidate proteins in the large repertoire created by mutagenesis. The next sections will introduce selected classes of protein scaffolds (see also Figure 13.1) that have been successfully used and commercialized by small- and medium-sized companies. The first scaffold derived drug has been recently approved by the FDA for treatment of hereditary angioedema (see kunitz type domains), others are being investigated in clinical trials. Therefore, we will learn more in the near future about this interesting field of antibody alternatives.

Kunitz type domains

Proteases have important biological functions, they have been identified as key regulators of cellular processes such as ovulation, fertilization, wound healing, angiogenesis, apoptosis, peptide hormone release, coagulation and complement activation (Nixon and Wood, 2006). Because unregulated proteolysis in any of these processes will have undesirable effects, effective control of protease activity is critical. Indeed, unregulated activity has been implicated in the pathogenesis of many diseases (e.g. cancer, inflammatory diseases, chronic obstructive pulmonary disease (COPD), chronic pancreatitis, muscular dystrophy and Alzheimer's disease (Naruse et al., 1999; Egeblad and Werb, 2002; Nunan and Small, 2002; Shapiro, 2002; Laval and Bushby, 2004; Parks et al., 2004), making proteases important target proteins. It is notable, that there are only a few marketed drugs (such as HIV protease inhibitors, angiotensin-converting enzyme inhibitors, the proteasome inhibitor bortezomib and the renin inhibitor aliskiren), since a key challenge in the discovery of new inhibitors is the ability to identify drugs which are both potent and specific. Structural similarities within the active site of most proteolytic enzyme families often result in a simultaneous inhibition of several family members, which

Fig. 13.1 Schematic representation of representative scaffolds. A, Kunitz type domain (LAC–D1) (Ley et al., 1996). Varied positions are depicted in black, the P1 and second loop positions are enclosed. B, Structural comparison of a llama V_{HH} domain and the wild-type human ^{10}Fn3 domain (Xu et al., 2002). Despite the lack of significant sequence identity, both domains fold into similar beta sheet sandwiches. The CDRs of the V_{HH} domain and the residues randomized in the ^{10}Fn3 domain are shown in color. C, Fixed and variable positions of the A-domain library, as well as the disulfide topology, are indicated (Silverman et al., 2005). Each circle represents an amino acid position. Calcium-coordinating scaffold residues are yellow, structural scaffold residues are blue, cysteine residues are red and variable positions are green. A ribbon diagram of a prototypical A-domain structure is included (Protein Data Bank entry 1AJJ). D, Fyn SH3 wt protein structure (Protein Data Bank entry 1M27) The RT-Src loop is in red, and the *n*-Src loop is in green. E, Electron density for all 13 mutated residues in the affibody (Hogbom et al., 2003). For clarity, only the electron density around the side chains is displayed. F, Schematic representation of the library generation of designed ankyrin repeat proteins (Binz et al., 2004). (upper part) Combinatorial libraries of ankyrin repeat proteins were designed by assembling an N-terminal capping ankyrin (green), varying numbers of the designed ankyrin repeat module (blue) and a C-terminal capping ankyrin (cyan); side chains of the randomized residues are shown in red. (lower part) Ribbon representation of the selected MBP binding ankyrin repeat protein (colours as above) This binder was isolated from a library of N-terminal capping ankyrin repeat, three designed ankyrin repeat modules and a C-terminal capping ankyrin repeat. G, General structure of human retinol-binding protein, a prototypic lipocalin (Schlehuber and Skerra, 2005). Ribbon diagram of the crystal structure of RBP with the bound ligand retinol (magenta, ball and stick representation). The eight antiparallel strands of the conserved β-barrel structure are shown in blue with labels A to H, and the four loops, which are highly variable among the lipocalin family, are colored red and numbered. The typical α-helix that is attached to the central β-barrel in all lipocalins, the loops at the closed end the N- and C-terminal peptide segments are shown in grey. The three disulfide bonds of RBP are depicted in yellow. H, Schematic representation of full-sized antibodies, multidomain and single-domain antigen-binding fragments (Saerens et al., 2008). Classical IgG consists of two light chains and two heavy chains. The light chain is composed of one variable (VL) and one constant (CL) domain, whereas the heavy chain has one variable (VH) and three constant domains (CH1, CH2, and CH3). The smaller antigen-binding antibody fragments are shown, that is, Fab, scFv, and the single-domain antibody (sdAb) fragment, VH.

can lead to an unacceptable toxicity profile. One solution to this problem represents the use of endogenous, engineered protease inhibitors that make more contacts with the target protease and therefore allow for tighter control over specificity. One type of endogenous inhibitors include the kunitz domain inhibitors, e.g. bovine pancreatic trypsin inhibitor (BPTI) (Ascenzi et al., 2003).

In 1992, Ladner and co-workers produced a small library of mutants of kunitz domain BPTI, displayed on phage and screened for the ability to bind to elastase (Roberts et al., 1992), a serine protease that is believed to play a causative role in a variety of lung diseases, including COPD and cystic fibrosis (Hautamaki et al., 1997). Isolates that were able to bind to elastase were expressed, purified and tested for inhibition of elastase. The P-loop (see Figure 13.1A), the region that was varied in the library, of the best inhibitor (K_i ~1 pM) was transferred to a human kunitz domain without subsequent loss of potency (Ley et al., 1997). The resulting engineered molecule, depelestat (Dyax/Debiopharm SA), inhibited human neutrophile elastase (HNE) activity in the sputum of cystic fibrosis patients, was demonstrated to be safe in an aerolized format in monkeys and no adverse effects were reported in Phase I clinical trials (Delacourt et al., 2002; Grimbert et al., 2003; Nixon and Wood, 2006). Pharmacodynamic reports of a Phase IIa clinical trial have been shown to inhibit completely sputum HNE in 52.6% of the patients and to decrease interleukin-8 levels, a biomarker of inflammation, in the sputum of treated patients (Saudubray et al., 2003).

In 1996, another human kunitz domain, the lipoprotein-associated coagulation inhibitor (LACI-D1), was used as a scaffold for the successful isolation of a very specific and potent inhibitor of human kallikrein (Markland et al., 1996). Kallikrein is believed to be an important mediator of hereditary angioedema (HAE), a rare disorder with attacks of oedema in the hands, face, feet, abdomen and/or throat. This condition is caused by a genetic deficiency of C1 esterase inhibitor (C1-Inh), which is an endogenous inhibitor of plasma kallikrein. In Europe, HAE is treated with plasma-derived C1-Inh which attenuates attacks and may prove life-saving, but C1-Inh is expensive and requires the use of pooled blood product (Nixon and Wood, 2006). After an iterative selection and screening approach chosen by the authors (Markland et al., 1996), the plasma kallikrein inhibitor DX-88 (Dyax Corp/Genzyme Corp) was isolated and proved to be a potent inhibitor (K_i = 40 pM) with high selectivity (Table 1 in Williams and Baird, 2003). The use of DX-88 in a C1-Inh deficient mouse model demonstrated that DX-88 is effective in preventing changes in vascular permeability (Han et al., 2002). In December 2009, DX-88 (ecallantide) was approved by FDA for the treatment of HAE.

With the first approved drug kunitz type domains represent the most advanced scaffold in this field. The strategy of taking a human protease inhibitor as a scaffold and improving it by protein engineering works well for certain therapeutic applications. At the same time, kunitz type domains have the limitation of binding only to proteases, and thus, at present, they do not represent a universal source for the generation of binding proteins to a variety of targets.

Tenth type III domain of fibronectin (Adnectins)

The tenth type III domain of human fibronectin (^{10}Fn3) is a 94 aminoacid residue structural protein with an immunoglobulin-like fold that is used as an antibody-mimic scaffold. High thermal stability (T_M = 90°C) and solubility (>15 mg/mL), high expression yields in *Escherichia coli* and the lack of cysteines in its structure are attractive properties that make the ^{10}Fn3 a good scaffold candidate (Xu et al., 2002). Three of the solvent exposed loops in ^{10}Fn3, named BC, DE and FG are structurally analogous to the V_H complementary-determining regions (CDR) (Figure 13.1B).

The first report on the use of the ^{10}Fn3 domain as a protein with artificial binding sites was published in 1998 (Koide and Koide, 1998). In that study, a library of 10^8 distinct ^{10}Fn3 mutants was made by deleting three residues in the FG loop and by randomizing five residues in the BC loop and four residues in the FG loop. The library, displayed on phage, was used in affinity selection experiments with immobilised ubiquitin as model target protein. After five rounds of panning, clones were randomly picked for sequencing. A clone designated as Ubi4-Fn3 dominated the population of selected protein mutants and was subjected to further analysis. Ubi4-Fn3 was demonstrated to bind in phage enzyme-linked immunosorbent assay (ELISA) experiments. However, when expressed as a single domain protein in *E. coli*, Ubi4-Fn3 exhibited low solubility at neutral pH, unspecific binding to the dextran matrices of the size-exclusion chromatography column and the dextran coated biosensor chips used for the subsequent characterization of Ubi-Fn3. More importantly, the affinity was relatively low; the IC_{50} determined by competition ELISA was 5 μM.

In order to select ^{10}Fn3 domains binding to a target of interest with improved properties than Ubi4-Fn3, an alternative library design in combination with a fully in vitro selection system (mRNA display (Wilson et al., 2001)) was used for the isolation of ^{10}Fn3 variants binding to tumour necrosis factor-α (TNF-α) (Xu et al., 2002). Clones from the ninth and tenth round of selection were cloned in *E. coli*, sequenced and expressed. Affinity constants were determined by incubating the in vitro translated ^{35}S-methionine labelled proteins with biotinylated TNF-α at different concentrations. The solution containing the ^{10}Fn3 mutants bound to TNF-α were aspirated by vacuum onto a membrane coated with streptavidin, therefore capturing protein complexes on the membrane. Binding was analysed by measuring the radioactivity on the membrane, the K_D for selected mutants were found in the range of 1-24 nM. Further affinity maturation procedures revealed K_D values around 100 pM, the best being 20 pM, and analytical gel filtration showed that the apparent molecular weight of purified, soluble wild-type (wt) and mutant domains was consistent with the variants being monomeric. The reported affinities, especially for TNF-α, are very high. However, these values should be evaluated critically because first, the capture step of the biotinylated TNF-α-Fn3 protein complexes was performed in a solid phase format, and second, TNF-α is homotrimeric protein, so avidity effects may contribute to the high apparent affinity observed.

Other ^{10}Fn3 variants were shown to recognize αvβ3-integrin expressed on cell surface and inhibiting αvβ-dependent cell adhesion (Richards et al., 2003) and to bind to vascular endothelial growth factor receptor 2 (VEGF-R2) inhibiting the activation by VEGF-A, -C and –D (Parker et al., 2005; Getmanova et al., 2006). Indeed, the test case of ^{10}Fn3 for the in vivo behaviour in human patients is the VEGF-R2 binding CT-322 (K_D = 11 nM), currently in clinical development by Bristol Myers Squibb in cancer patients (Choy et al., 2002; Molckovsky and Siu, 2008). The CT-322 ^{10}Fn3 domain is coupled via a C-terminal cysteine to a 40-kDa polyethylene glycol (PEG) to increase the size of the molecule above the threshold for kidney-mediated clearance. In a Phase I study in patients with solid tumours, CT-322 administered intravenously at 1 mg/kg showed a terminal half-life of 68.7 hours, based on the first dose of a weekly dosing regimen (Molckovsky and Siu, 2008). The half-life in humans is substantially shorter than that of IgG (7–26 days), as expected for a molecule lacking FcRn binding, and also shorter than the 14-day half-life reported for Cimzia, a pegylated Fab that binds to TNF-α (Choy et al., 2002). Still, the pharmacokinetics of CT-322 supported weekly intravenous dosing, and a biomarker for VEGF-R2 blockade showed sustained elevation over several repeated weekly doses. Immunogenicity was also assessed in this Phase I trial showing that 31 out of 39 patients developed antibodies to CT-322 (Beyond Antibodies Conference, 2009, San Diego) but these did not lead to a clinical significant immunogenicity (Bloom and Calabro, 2009). As for other biologics, immunogenicity should be monitored carefully for this scaffold, especially for the generation of cross-reactive antibodies binding not only to the injected mutant, but also to the endogenous fibronectin domain. In the near future we will learn more about this scaffold, since patients are currently being enrolled in a Phase II trial in glioblastoma multiforme, in which CT-322 will be tested alone or in combination with irinotecan (Campto, Pfizer), a cytostatic agent inhibiting DNA-topoisomerase I. The technology of using the ^{10}Fn3 domain was commercialized by Adnexus, which was acquired by Bristol Myers Squibb for $430 million in 2007, proving the interest and significant potential of antibody alternatives in the field of pharmaceutical biotechnology.

A-domains (Avimers)

A family of A-domains (Huang et al., 1999; North and Blacklow, 1999) has been described to be suitable as a scaffold for the generation of new binding proteins (Silverman et al., 2005). A-domains occur as strings of multiple domains in several cell-surface receptors (Figure 13.1C). Domains of this family bind over 100 different known targets, including small molecules, proteins and viruses (Krieger and Herz, 1994; Gliemann, 1998). Such a target is typically contacted by multiple A-domains with each domain binding independently to a unique epitope, thereby binding with high avidity. Each of the 217 human A-domains comprises approximately 35 amino acids and the domains are separated by linkers that average five amino acids in length. Native A-domains fold quickly and efficiently to a uniform, stable structure mediated by calcium binding and disulfide formation. A conserved scaffold motif of only 12 amino acids is required for this common structure (Koduri and Blacklow, 2001). Stemmer and co-workers have designed a phage display library of A-domains, consisting of a conserved consensus sequence in the scaffold motif and variable amino acids at different positions (Silverman et al., 2005). Like other directed evolution technologies, the process the authors developed to isolate binding proteins, included multiple recursive cycles, each consisting of library generation and screening in functional assays. However, rather than mutagenizing the protein between cycles (e.g. for affinity maturation purposes), they added a new domain library adjacent to the domain(s) selected in previous rounds.

The result of this process is a single protein chain containing multiple domains, each of which having a separate binding function. The A-domains are therefore called 'avimers', from avidity multimers. A heterotetramer consisting of three IL-6 binding A-domains and an IgG binding domain (named C326) showed a remarkable affinity (picomolar range) to its target and exhibited sub-picomolar IC_{50}s in cell-proliferation assays (Silverman et al., 2005). Moreover, C326 completely abrogated acute-phase protein induction by human IL-6 in mice in a dose-dependent manner, suggesting that C326 inhibited IL-6 functions in vivo. The technology of using the modular platform of A-domains was commercialized by Avidia Inc. that was acquired by Amgen for $290 million in 2006. A placebo-controlled Phase I study of C326 was registered in the United States in September 2006, with patients suffering from Crohn's disease. Since then, to our knowledge, new results have not been published in the public domain. Recent data (Beyond Antibodies Conference, 2009, San Diego) indicate that Amgen is further engineering avimers for the neutralization of IL-6 mediated effects.

SH3 domain of Fyn kinase (Fynomers)

Fyn kinase is a 59 kDa member of the Src family of tyrosine kinases (Cooke and Perlmutter, 1989; Resh, 1998). As a result of alternative splicing, the Fyn protein is expressed as two isoforms, differing in approximately 50 amino acids in a region between their SH2 and kinase domain. One form is found in thymocytes, splenocytes and some hematolymphoid cell lines (FynT), while the second form accumulates principally in the brain (Cooke and Perlmutter, 1989). Its biological functions are diverse and related to Fyn's ability to associate and to phosphorylate a variety of intracellular signaling molecules. One of the best known functions of Fyn kinase is the phosphorylation of SLAM (signalling lymphocyte activation molecule) in T cells, inducing a signalling complex modulating interferon-γ expression (Li, 2005). The interaction between Fyn and SLAM occurs via the SH3 domain of Fyn and the adaptor protein SAP (SLAM associated protein), forming a ternary complex. Interestingly, Fyn SH3 associates with SAP through a surface–surface interaction that does not involve the canonical PXXP recognition motif of SH3 domains (Chan et al., 2003). The Fyn SH3 domain comprises 63 residues (amino acids 83–145 of the sequence reported by Kawakami et al., 1986; Semba et al., 1986) and shows the typical SH3 topology of two perpendicular β-sheets and a single turn of 3_{10} helix (Figure 13.1D). Interacting regions of the Fyn SH3 domain include the RT-loop, n-src loop and single residues of the β3- and β4 strands (Chan et al., 2003). With its biophysical properties and its primary structure, Fyn SH3 perfectly matches important criteria for a scaffold to be used as alternative to antibodies: (i) it is expressed in bacteria at high level in soluble, monomeric form (Morton et al., 1996), (ii) it is stable (T_M: 70.5° C) (Filimonov et al., 1999), (iii) it does not contain any cysteine residues, (iv) it is from human origin and (v) its amino acid sequence is conserved in mouse, rat, monkey (gibbon) and man. As mentioned above, its binding mode to SAP has been resolved and indicates that this particular domain does not necessarily need a PXXP core binding motif (Chan et al., 2003), which is an important prerequisite to be well suited for the isolation of binders against a variety of different target epitopes. Recently, we presented the design, construction, and characterization of a human Fyn SH3 phage library containing more than 1 billion individual clones, where both loops of the Fyn SH3 domain (the RT- and n-Src-loop) were randomized (Grabulovski et al., 2007). Using phage display technology, the isolation and in vitro characterization of Fyn SH3 proteins (termed Fynomers) binding to the extra-domain B (EDB) of fibronectin (Castellani et al., 1994; Kaspar et al., 2006), a marker of angiogenesis, was described. Fibronectin is a large glycoprotein that is present in large amounts in plasma and body tissues. EDB is a 91-amino acid type III homology domain that becomes inserted into the fibronectin molecule by a mechanism of alternative splicing at the level of the primary transcript (Zardi et al., 1987). The Fynomer clone termed D3 exhibited low nM affinities to EDB (Grabulovski et al., 2007). Furthermore, genetically fused homodimers of D3 were cloned, expressed and analysed for their capability to target tumoural neo-vasculature in vivo. In addition, we could demonstrate that neither Fyn SH3 WT nor the D3 mutant was immunogenic in mice after repeated intravenous injections (Grabulovski et al., 2007).

In another study, Bertschinger et al. successfully used Covalent DNA Display technology (Bertschinger and Neri, 2004) to isolate Fynomers binding to mouse serum albumin (Bertschinger et al., 2007). More recently, we have shown the construction of a novel, large Fyn SH3 library comprising more than 8×10^{10} individual clone members (Advancing Protein Therapeutics Conference, 2010, Frankfurt, Germany). In addition, a large collection of formats (homo-dimers, homo-trimers, bispecific dimers, bivalent and tetravalent Fc fusions) and subnanomolar Fynomer derivatives binding to human IL-17A have been presented. Overall, the single-pot Fyn SH3 library may provide useful reagents for many biochemical and biomedical applications as an alternative to more conventional IgG-based immunochemical technologies.

Affibodies: Z-domain of staphylococcal protein A

The immunoglobulin binding domain of staphylococcal protein A (SPA) is widely used as an immunochemical ligand for the purification or detection of antibodies and serves as affinity tag in fusion proteins (Uhlen et al., 1992). The IgG binding domain of SPA consists of five highly homologous three-helix bundle domains of approximately 58 amino acid residues each. Because SPA is known as a non-cysteine containing, highly soluble, proteolytically and thermally stable protein, an engineered version of one of the SPA domains, the so-called Z-domain (Nilsson et al., 1987), was chosen as a scaffold for the development of novel affinity proteins designated as 'affibodies' (Figure 13.1E). Utilizing structural data available for the complex between a native SPA domain and the Fc fragment of human IgG1, 13 positions distributed across two helices, located at the surface of the domain and involved in the Fc interaction, were chosen for random mutagenesis, and subsequently, for the creation of phage libraries (Nord et al., 1995). In 1997, from two medium-sized libraries comprising about 4×10^7 individual clones, binding proteins against three model target proteins (*Taq* DNA polymerase, human insulin, and a human apolipoprotein A-1 variant) were isolated, with binding affinities in the micromolar range (Nord et al., 1997). In the meantime, affibodies have been isolated against a variety of protein targets (e.g. human factor VIII (Nord et al., 2001), human immunoglobulin A (Ronnmark et al., 2002) and CD28 (Sandstrom et al., 2003)). In a more recent paper (Wikman et al., 2004), an affibody ligand binding to human epidermal growth factor receptor 2 (Her2) was isolated with a dissociation constant (K_D) of 50 nmol/L. Dimerization of this affibody molecule resulted in improved target binding affinity ($K_D = 3$ nmol/L), and radioiodination of the dimer allowed selective targeting and imaging of Her2-expressing xenografts in vivo (Steffen et al., 2006). Further affinity maturation strategies led to an affibody molecule with a dissociation constant in the range of 20 pmol/L and to better tumour targeting and imaging results in the same tumour mouse model (Orlova et al., 2006). A fully synthetic affibody molecules has also been described, site-specifically and homogenously conjugated with a DOTA (1,4,7,10-tetra-azacyclododecane-N,N′,N″,N‴-tetraacetic acid) chelator, produced in a single chemical process by peptide synthesis (Orlova et al., 2007).

Importantly, the first clinical investigation of ^{68}Ga- and ^{111}In-labelled anti Her2 affibody molecule (ABY-002) in three patients with metastatic breast cancer showed that Her2-specific affibody molecules have the potential to visualize Her2-expressing metastatic lesions (Löfblom et al., 2010). High contrast SPECT or PET images were obtained already 2–3 h after injection. Over-expression of Her2 in two metastases was confirmed on biopsy tissue samples using the HercepTest™ indicating that ABY-002 specifically targets Her2 also in humans. Further clinical studies are warranted to assess the sensitivity and specificity of radiolabelled Her2-targeting affibody molecules (Löfblom et al., 2010). For therapeutic applications, concerns about the immunogenic potential of this class of proteins should be seriously considered, owing to its bacterial origin.

Ankyrin repeat proteins (DARPins)

Ankyrin repeat (AR) proteins, first isolated in mammalian erythrocytes, are involved in the targeting, mechanical stabilization and orientation of membrane proteins to specialized compartments within the plasma membrane and endoplasmic reticulum. Natural ankyrin repeat proteins consist of many 33-amino-acid modules, each comprising a β-turn and two anti-parallel α-helices (Sedgwick and Smerdon, 1999). In most known complexes, the β-turn and the first α-helix mediate the interactions with the target, and different numbers of adjacent repeats are involved in binding. The reported target binding affinities of natural AR proteins are in the low nanomolar range (Suzuki et al., 1998). Ankyrin repeat proteins were built and diversified to create a library from which ankyrin variants were selected binding to maltose-binding-protein and two eukaryotic kinases (Binz et al., 2004; Amstutz et al., 2005; Zahnd et al., 2006). In the approach chosen by the authors, a consensus ankyrin repeat module consisting of six diversified potential interaction residues and 27 framework residues was designed based on sequence alignments and structural analyses (Figure 13.1F). Varying numbers of this repeat module were cloned between capping repeats, which are special terminal repeats of ankyrin domains shielding the hydrophobic core. Two libraries were created with two and three, respectively, randomized ankyrin repeats in between an N-terminal and a C-terminal cap.

Using a library with more than 10^{10} individual members in combination with the ribosome display selection methodology, binding variants (termed DARPins) were selected by performing four or five rounds of selection. Dissociation constants were determined by surface plasmon resonance and found to be in the range of 2–20 nM against these model target proteins. More recently, a so-called SRP phage display methodology was employed for efficient filamentous phage display of DARPins. Using a phage DARPin library with more than 10^{10} individual members resulted in isolation of well-behaved and highly specific DARPins against a broad range of target proteins (such as the Fc domain of human IgG, TNFalpha, ErbB1 (EGFR), ErbB2 (Her2) and ErbB4 (Her4)) having affinities as low as 100 pM directly from this library, without affinity maturation (Steiner et al., 2008).

In April 2010, the first cohorts of patients were enrolled in two separate Phase I trials with the first DARPin (MP0112) neutralizing VEGF for a single intravitreal injection in wet age-related macular degeneration (wet AMD) and diabetic macular edema (DME) (www.molecularpartners.ch). The trials are investigating the safety and tolerability of MP0112, but the studies will also allow a preliminary assessment of efficacy and the duration of action of MP0112. The DARPin was engineered to have a long ocular half-life, but fast systemic clearance. In general, as the DARPins were newly designed and are not found in nature in this format, their immunogenic potential should be investigated in detail, especially after repeated systemic administration.

Lipocalins

The lipocalins represent a family of functionally diverse, small proteins that comprise 160–180 amino acid residues and have weak sequence homology, but high similarity at the tertiary structural level (Skerra, 2000). Members of this family have important biological functions in a variety of organisms, from bacteria to humans. The majority of lipocalins are responsible for the storage and transport of compounds that have low solubility or are chemically sensitive, such as vitamins, steroids and metabolic products (Flower, 1995). An example of human lipocalin is the retinol binding protein (RBP), of which the three-dimensional-structure has been elucidated by X-ray cristallography (Cowan et al., 1990). RBP transports the poorly soluble and oxidation-prone vitamin A from the liver, where it is stored as a fatty acid ester, to several target tissues. Despite their extremely poor sequence homology, the lipocalins share a structurally conserved β-barrel as their central folding motif, which consists of eight antiparallel β-strands that are arranged in a cylindrical manner (Figure 13.1G). The binding specificity for low-molecular-weight compounds is well-characterized for many lipocalins: some bind their ligands with high specificity, whereas others form complexes with a considerable range of lipophilic molecules (Schlehuber and Skerra, 2005). Typically, the ligand affinities of lipocalins are moderate with dissociation constants of approximately 1 μM, which is consistent with their presumed function as a physiological buffer for the bound substance; however, there are notable exceptions, e.g. the tick histamine-binding protein (HBP)-2 with a K_D of 1.7 nM (Paesen et al., 1999). The insect bilin binding protein (BBP) from *Pieris brassicae* served as a model lipocalin in initial studies to create artificial binding sites for several ligands. Sixteen amino acid positions located within the four loops at the open end of the β-barrel and adjoining regions of the β-strands were subjected to targeted random mutagenesis (Beste et al., 1999). The resulting molecular random library with about 4×10^8 members was subjected to selection towards several low-molecular-weight compounds using phage display. BBP variants, so-called 'anticalins', that specifically recognize fluorescein, digoxigenin, phthalic acid esters and doxorubicin were obtained, with affinities in the nM range (Beste et al., 1999; Schlehuber et al., 2000; Mercader and Skerra, 2002). In order to extend the concept of anticalins, several human lipocalins were subjected to random mutagenesis generating libraries that enable recognition of macromolecular protein targets. Because proteins have larger molecular dimensions than small compounds, they cannot penetrate into the ligand-binding pocket of lipocalins. Consequently, side chains of lipocalins at more exposed positions, close to the tips of the four loops at the open end of the β-barrel, were subjected to random mutagenesis. Following this strategy, a panel of anticalins based on human lipocalins with specificities for several therapeutic targets such as cytotoxic T-lymphocyte-associated antigen (CTLA-4), c-met, IL-4Ra, VEGF and other undisclosed targets were isolated (www.pieris-ag.com). The VEGF binding anticalin (PRS-050) is about to enter clinical trials and we will learn more about this scaffold in the near future.

Single domain antibodies

Although not belonging to the strict definition of antibody alternative protein 'frameworks', single domain antibody fragments are included as well in this chapter since they share a lot of common properties with the 'classical' scaffolds (e.g. small domains with high expression yields in bacteria). Moreover, they represent a valuable source for the generation of new binding proteins.

In a seminal early publication (Ward et al., 1989), mouse single variable domains (V_H) were shown to be functional, and it was proposed that they could potentially target cryptic epitopes normally hidden for whole antibodies and even for smaller fragments thereof. However, they were described to be poorly soluble and often prone to aggregation, because of their exposed hydrophobic surface normally 'capped' by the V_L domain. Interest was recently revived when it was discovered that at least two types of organisms, the camelids and cartilaginous fish have evolved high-affinity V-like single domains, mounted on an Fc-equivalent constant domain framework as an integral and crucial component of their immune system (De Genst et al., 2004; Dooley and Flajnik, 2005).

Unlike mouse V_H domains (Ward et al., 1989), camelid VhH (termed nanobodies) and shark V-NAR domains are in general soluble and can be produced as stable in vitro reagents. However, for in vivo administration, humanization (or deimmunization) may be crucial to reduce immunogenicity. Human single domain antibodies (dAbs) (Figure 13.1H) would be even more preferable, and the problems of poor stability and solubility have been solved for some human V domains by the identification and design of mutations that minimize the hydrophobic V_H/V_L interface (Dottorini et al., 2004; Jespers et al., 2004a). Moreover, in a publication of Jespers and co-workers (2004b), aggregation-resistant domain antibodies could be directly selected on phage by heat denaturation. Starting from a DP47d domain antibody (a typical human V_H dAb), which unfolds irreversibly and forms aggregates if heated above 55 °C, a repertoire containing approximately 1 billion different mutants was cloned by diversification of the CDR loops. The library was multivalently displayed on phage and after three rounds of heat denaturation followed by selection on protein A (a ligand common to folded dAbs), 179 out of 200 colonies secreted dAb phage that retained more than 80% of protein A-binding activity after heating (in contrast to the starting protein DP47d, which loses binding by a factor of 560 after heating). Twenty clones were sequenced and revealed many unique dAb sequences with a large variability in the CDR length and sequences, which shows that mutations located only in the CDR loops of the dAbs are sufficient to confer resistance to aggregation. Interestingly, the T_M of the mutants was not higher than the one of the parental clone DP47d, which shows that the selected dAbs are not heat stable, but can fold reversibly.

Most data in the public domain describe serum albumin-binding domain antibodies (AlbudAbs) fusions, which extend the serum half-life of otherwise short-lived proteins, such as the interleukin-1 receptor antagonist IL-1ra (Holt et al., 2008) and interferon (IFN)-α2b (Walker et al., 2010). In the latter study, IFN-α2b was fused to both human serum albumin (termed HSA-IFN-α2b) and to an AlbuDab (termed IFN-α2b-DOM7h-14). The fusion proteins were subjected to a pharmacokinetic (PK) analysis in rats following intravenous dosing. The in vivo half-life of both fusion proteins was significantly increased in comparison with the IFN-α standard (22.6 and 14.2 h for

IFN-α2b-DOM7h-14 and HSA-IFN-α2b, respectively compared with 1.2 h for IFN-α standard). The $t_{1/2}$ of IFN-α2b-DOM7h-14, interestingly, is approximately 1.5 times longer than that of HSA-IFN-α2b. Moreover, similar AUC values were obtained for IFN-α2b-DOM7h-14 and HSA-IFN-α2b, 737.5 and 689.2 h mg/mL, respectively, which in both cases represents a significant increase over the value of 18.8 h mg/mL observed with the IFN-α standard. A further study was carried out to determine PKs following subcutaneous administration in rats. As with the i.v. study the in vivo half-life of both fusion proteins was increased in comparison with IFN-α standard. Interestingly, the antiviral efficacy of the AlbuDab fusion IFN-α2b-DOM7h-14 was 5.8 fold greater in comparison with albumin fusion HSA-IFN-α2b, as determined by an in vitro antiviral assay with A549 human lung carcinoma cells, indicating that in this particular case fusion of IFN-α to the Albudab represents an attractive avenue to prolong its half-life.

Today, the single domain antibody technology is commercialized by Glaxo Smith Kline, which acquired Domantis Ltd. in December 2006 for £230 million, and certainly reflects the interest of big pharmaceutical companies in single domain protein scaffolds.

Other domains

The preceding sections introduced important domain scaffolds that have been commercialized and for which published data are available. A recent review by Gebauer and Skerra (2009) listed more than 50 scaffolds that have been described for the generation of new binding proteins. The majority of them have been used for research purposes only (e.g. probing the specificity determinants of WW-domains to their ligands (Dalby et al., 2000), elucidating target recognition rules of SH3 domains (Hiipakka et al., 1999; Panni et al., 2002) or identifying signal transduction pathways with the staphylococcal nuclease as scaffold (Norman et al., 1999)). Other domains have been commercialized by companies for in vitro applications (e.g. PDZ domains for the generation of high-affinity detection reagents (Biotech Studio; Ferrer et al., 2005) or for intracellular signalling interference applications (thioredoxin, Aptanomics; Kunz et al., 2006)). Antibody fragments of the constant domain have also been used as scaffolds, e.g. the CH2 domain of human IgG1 has been used as a library scaffold, and isolated CH2 domains with specific binding affinity to a HIV-1 gp120-CD4 complex have been described (Xiao et al., 2009). There, the new binding site is formed by engineered sequences in the BC and FG loops of the CH2 domain located at the N-terminal tip of the domain. Another approach was chosen by Wozniak-Knopp and co-workers (2010), where the whole Fc fragment of IgG1 was used as an alternative small-size antibody format. With the exception of the antigen binding site, the full Fc of an IgG1 has all the properties of a complete antibody, i.e. the ability to elicit effector functions via binding to Fc-gamma receptors and to the complement activator C1q, as well as the long half-life of antibodies mediated through binding to FcRn. Using their CH3 library and yeast display selection technologies these authors described recently the isolation of a Her2 binding Fc mutant with low nM affinities (Wozniak-Knopp et al., 2010).

A few other scaffolds have also been commercialized by small- and medium-sized companies; however, no refereed publications are available (ubiquitin by Scil Proteins, C-type lectin domain by Anaphore, and a not disclosed scaffold by Amunix; information obtained from the corresponding websites).

CONCLUDING REMARKS

Overall, the engineering and practical uses of binding proteins derived from non-Ig scaffolds are established and these will push biological chemistry toward both basic research and applied science. Although some rational justification may be given for the choice of almost any scaffold described so far, the true potential of the various protein scaffolds for human therapy, including in vivo diagnostics, and considering the different approaches to the implementation of effector functions, will only become clear once a number of additional Phase I/II trials have been completed in the near future.

REFERENCES

Amstutz P, Binz HK, Parizek P, et al. Intracellular kinase inhibitors selected from combinatorial libraries of designed ankyrin repeat proteins. Journal of Biological Chemistry 2005;280:24715–22.

Ascenzi P, Bocedi A, Bolognesi M, et al. The bovine basic pancreatic trypsin inhibitor (Kunitz inhibitor): a milestone protein. Current Protein & Peptide Science 2003;4: 231–51.

Bertschinger J, Neri D. Covalent DNA display as a novel tool for directed evolution of proteins in vitro. Protein Engineering, Design & Selection 2004;17:699–707.

Bertschinger J, Grabulovski D, Neri D. Selection of single domain binding proteins by covalent DNA display. Protein Engineering, Design & Selection 2007;20:57–68.

Beste G, Schmidt FS, Stibora T, et al. Small antibody-like proteins with prescribed ligand specificities derived from the lipocalin fold. Proceeding of the National Academy of Sciences of USA 1999;96:1898–903.

Binz K, Pluckthun A. Engineered proteins as specific binding reagents.

Current Opinion in Biotechnology 2005;16:459–69.

Binz HK, Amstutz P, Kohl A, et al. High-affinity binders selected from designed ankyrin repeat protein libraries. Nature Biotechnology 2004;22:575–82.

Binz HK, Amstutz P, Plückthun A. Engineering novel binding proteins from nonimmunoglobulin domains. Nature Biotechnology 2005;23:1257–68.

Bloom L, Calabro V. FN3: a new protein scaffold reaches the clinic. Drug Discovery Today 2009;14:949–55.

Castellani P, Viale G, Dorcaratto A, et al. The fibronectin isoform containing the ED-B oncofetal domain: a marker of angiogenesis. International Journal of Cancer 1994;59:612–18.

Chan B, Lanyi A, Song HK, et al. SAP couples Fyn to SLAM immune receptors. Nature Cell Biology 2003;5:155–60.

Choy EH, Hazleman B, Smith M, et al. Efficacy of a novel PEGylated humanized anti-TNF fragment (CDP870) in patients with rheumatoid arthritis: a phase II double-blinded, randomized, dose-escalating trial. Rheumatology (Oxford) 2002;41:1133–7.

Cooke MP, Perlmutter RM. Expression of a novel form of the fyn proto-oncogene in hematopoietic cells. New Biology 1989;1:66–74.

Cowan SW, Newcomer ME, Jones TA. Crystallographic refinement of human serum retinol binding protein at 2A resolution. Proteins 1990;8:44–61.

Dalby PA, Hoess RH, DeGrado WF. Evolution of binding affinity in a WW domain probed by phage display. Protein Science 2000;9:2366–76.

De Genst E, Handelberg F, Van Meirhaeghe A, et al. Chemical basis for the affinity maturation of a camel single domain antibody. Journal of Biological Chemistry 2004;279:53593–601.

Delacourt, C, Hérigault S, Delclaux C, et al. Protection against acute lung injury by intravenous or intratracheal pretreatment with EPI-HNE-4, a new potent neutrophil elastase inhibitor. American Journal of Respiratory Cell Molecular Biology 2002;26:290–7.

Dooley H, Flajnik MF. Shark immunity bites back: affinity maturation and memory response in the nurse shark, Ginglymostoma cirratum. European Journal of Immunology 2005;35:936–45.

Dottorini T, Vaughan CK, Walsh MA, et al. Crystal structure of a human VH: requirements for maintaining a monomeric fragment. Biochemistry 2004;43:622–8.

Dyax Corp. (Ley AC, L. R, Guterman SK, Roberts Bruce L, Markland W, Ken RB) Engineered human-derived kunitz domains that inhibit human neutrophil elastase. US056633143 patent. 1997.

Egeblad M, Werb Z. New functions for the matrix metalloproteinases in cancer progression. Nat Review. Cancer 2002;2:161–74.

Ferrer M, Maiolo J, Kratz P, et al. Directed evolution of PDZ variants to generate high-affinity detection reagents. Protein Engineering, Design & Selection 2005;18:165–73.

Filimonov VV, Azuaga AI, Viguera AR, et al. A thermodynamic analysis of a family of small globular proteins: SH3 domains. Biophysical Chemistry 1999;77:195–208.

Flower DR. Multiple molecular recognition properties of the lipocalin protein family. Journal of Molecular Recognition 1995;8:185–95.

Gebauer M, Skerra A. Engineered protein scaffolds as next-generation antibody therapeutics. Current Opinion in Chemical Biology 2009;13:245–55.

Getmanova EV, Chen Y, Bloom L, et al. Antagonists to human and mouse vascular endothelial growth factor receptor 2 generated by directed protein evolution in vitro. Chemical Biology 2006;13:549–56.

Gliemann J. Receptors of the low density lipoprotein (LDL) receptor family in man. Multiple functions of the large family members via interaction with complex ligands. Biological Chemistry 1998;379: 951–64.

Grabulovski D, Kaspar M, Neri D. A novel, non-immunogenic Fyn SH3-derived binding protein with tumor vascular targeting properties. Journal of Biological Chemistry 2007;282:3196–204.

Grimbert D, Vecellio L, Delépine P, et al. Characteristics of EPI-hNE4 aerosol: a new elastase inhibitor for treatment of cystic fibrosis. Journal of Aerosol Medicine 2003;16:121–9.

Han ED, MacFarlane RC, Mulligan AN, et al. Increased vascular permeability in C1 inhibitor-deficient mice mediated by the bradykinin type 2 receptor. Journal of Clinical Investment 2002;109:1057–63.

Hautamaki RD, Kobayashi DK, Senior RM, et al. Requirement for macrophage elastase for cigarette smoke-induced emphysema in mice. Science 1997;277:2002–4.

Hey T, Fiedler E, Rudolph R, et al. Artificial, non-antibody binding proteins for pharmaceutical and industrial applications. Trends in Biotechnology 2005;23:514–22.

Hiipakka M, Poikonen K, Saksela K. SH3 domains with high affinity and engineered ligand specificities targeted to HIV-1 Nef. Journal of Molecular Biology 1999;293: 1097–106.

Hogbom, M, Eklund M, Nygren PA, et al. Structural basis for recognition by an in vitro evolved affibody. Proceeding of the National Academy of Sciences of USA 2003;100:3191–6.

Holliger P, Hudson PJ. Engineered antibody fragments and the rise of single domains. Nature Biotechnology 2005;23:1126–36.

Holt LJ, Basran A, Jones K, et al. Anti-serum albumin domain antibodies for extending the half-lives of short lived drugs. Protein Engineering, Design & Selection 2008;21:283–8.

Huang, W, Dolmer K, Gettins PG. NMR solution structure of complement-like repeat CR8 from the low density lipoprotein receptor-related protein. Journal of Biological Chemistry 1999;274:14130–6.

Jespers L, Schon O, Famm K, et al. Aggregation-resistant domain antibodies selected on phage by heat denaturation. Nature Biotechnology 2004a;22:1161–5.

Jespers L, Schon O, James LC, et al. Crystal structure of HEL4, a soluble, refoldable human V(H) single domain with a germ-line scaffold. Journal of Molecular Biology 2004b;337:893–903.

Kaspar M, Zardi L, Neri D. Fibronectin as target for tumor therapy. International Journal of Cancer 2006;118:1331–9.

Kawakami T, Pennington CY, Robbins KC. Isolation and oncogenic potential of a novel human src-like gene. Molecular Cell Biology 1986;6:4195–201.

Koduri V, Blacklow SC. Folding determinants of LDL receptor type A modules. Biochemistry 2001;40:12801–7.

Koide A, Koide S. The fibronectin type III domain as a scaffold for novel binding proteins. Journal of Molecular Biology 1998;284: 1141–51.

Krieger M, Herz J. Structures and functions of multiligand lipoprotein receptors: macrophage scavenger receptors and LDL receptor-related protein (LRP). Annual Reviews in Biochemstry 1994;63:601–37.

Kunz C, Borghouts C, Buerger C, et al. Peptide aptamers with binding specificity for the intracellular domain of the ErbB2 receptor interfere with AKT signaling and sensitize breast cancer cells to Taxol. Molecular Cancer Researchearch 2006;4:983–98.

Laval SH, Bushby KM. Limb-girdle muscular dystrophies – from genetics to molecular pathology. Neuropathology and Applied Neurobiology 2004;30:91–105.

Ley AC, LR, Guterman SK, Roberts Bruce L, et al. *US056633143 patent* 1997.

Ley AC, Markland W, Ladner RC. Obtaining a family of high-affinity, high-specificity protein inhibitors of plasmin and plasma kallikrein. Molecular Divers 1996;2:119–24.

Li SS. Specificity and versatility of SH3 and other proline-recognition domains: structural basis and implications for cellular signal transduction. Biochemical Journal 2005;390:641–53.

Löfblom J, Feldwisch J, Tolmachev V, et al. Affibody molecules: engineered proteins for therapeutic, diagnostic and biotechnological applications. FEBS Letters. Epub ahead of print 11 April 2010.

Markland W, Ley AC, Ladner RC. Iterative optimization of high-affinity protease inhibitors using phage display. 2. Plasma kallikrein and thrombin. Biochemistry 1996;35:8058–67.

Mercader JV, Skerra A. Generation of anticalins with specificity for a nonsymmetric phthalic acid ester. Annals of Biochemstry 2002;308:269–77.

Molckovsky A, Siu LL. First-in-class, first-in-human phase I results of targeted agents: highlights of the 2008 American Society of Clinical Oncology meeting. Journal of Hematology and Oncology 2008;1:20.

Morton CJ, Pugh DJ, Brown EL, et al. Solution structure and peptide binding of the SH3 domain from human Fyn. Structure 1996;4: 705–14.

Naruse S, Kitagawa M, Ishiguro H. Molecular understanding of chronic pancreatitis: a perspective on the future. Molecular Medicine Today 1999;5:493–9.

Nilsson B, Moks T, Jansson B, et al. A synthetic IgG-binding domain based on staphylococcal protein A. Protein Engineering 1987;1:107–13.

Nixon AE, Wood CR. Engineered protein inhibitors of proteases. Current Opinion in Drug Discovery and Development 2006;9:261–8.

Nord K, Nilsson J, Nilsson B, et al. A combinatorial library of an alpha-helical bacterial receptor domain. Protein Engineering 1995;8:601–8.

Nord K, Gunneriusson E, Ringdahl J, et al. Binding proteins selected from combinatorial libraries of an alpha-helical bacterial receptor domain. Nature Biotechnology 1997;15:772–7.

Nord K, Nord O, Uhlén M, et al. Recombinant human factor VIII-specific affinity ligands selected from phage-displayed combinatorial libraries of protein A. European Journal of Biochemistry 2001;268:4269–77.

Norman TC, Smith DL, Sorger PK, et al. Genetic selection of peptide inhibitors of biological pathways. Science 1999;285:591–5.

North CL, Blacklow SC. Structural independence of ligand-binding modules five and six of the LDL receptor. Biochemistry 1999;38:3926–35.

Nunan J, Small DH. Proteolytic processing of the amyloid-beta protein precursor of Alzheimer's disease. Essays in Biochemistry 2002;38:37–49.

Nygren PA, Uhlen M. Scaffolds for engineering novel binding sites in proteins. Current Opinion in Structural Biology 1997;7:463–9.

Orlova A, Magnusson M, Eriksson TL, et al. Tumor imaging using a picomolar affinity HER2 binding affibody molecule. Cancer Research 2006;66:4339–48.

Orlova A, Tolmachev V, Pehrson R, et al. Synthetic affibody molecules: a novel class of affinity ligands for molecular imaging of HER2-expressing malignant tumors. Cancer Research 2007;67: 2178–86.

Paesen GC, Adams PL, Harlos K, et al. Tick histamine-binding proteins: isolation, cloning, and three-dimensional structure. Molecular Cell 1999;3:661–71.

Panni S, Dente L, Cesareni G. In vitro evolution of recognition specificity mediated by SH3 domains reveals target recognition rules. Journal of Biological Chemistry 2002;277: 21666–74.

Parker MH, Chen Y, Danehy F, et al. Antibody mimics based on human fibronectin type three domain engineered for thermostability and high-affinity binding to vascular endothelial growth factor receptor two. Protein Engineering, Design & Selection 2005;18:435–44.

Parks WC, Wilson CL, López-Boado YS. Matrix metalloproteinases as modulators of inflammation and innate immunity. Nature Review. Immunology 2004;4:617–29.

Reichert JM. Editorial for PEDS special issue on antibodies. Protein Engineering, Design & Selection 2010;23:153–4.

Resh MD. Fyn, a Src family tyrosine kinase. International Journal of Biochemistry and Cell Biology 1998;30:1159–62.

Richards J, Miller M, Abend J, et al. Engineered fibronectin type III domain with a RGDWXE sequence binds with enhanced affinity and specificity to human alphavbeta3 integrin. Journal of Molecular Biology 2003;326:1475–88.

Roberts BL, Markland W, Ley AC, et al. Directed evolution of a protein: selection of potent neutrophil elastase inhibitors displayed on M13 fusion phage. Proceeding of the National Academy of Sciences of USA 1992;89:2429–33.

Ronnmark J, Grönlund H, Uhlén M, et al. Human immunoglobulin A (IgA)-specific ligands from combinatorial engineering of protein A. European Journal of Biochemistry 2002;269:2647–55.

Saerens D, Ghassabeh GH, Muyldermans S. Single-domain antibodies as building blocks for novel therapeutics. Current Opinion in Pharmacology 2008;8:600–8.

Sandstrom K, Xu Z, Forsberg G, et al. Inhibition of the CD28–CD80 co-stimulation signal by a CD28-binding affibody ligand developed by combinatorial protein engineering. Protein Engineering 2003;16:691–7.

Saudubray F, Labbé A, Durieu I. Phase IIa clinical study of a new human neutrophil elastase inhibitor (HNE), EPI-HNE4 (DX-890), with repeated administration by inhalation in adult cystic fibrosis patients. Journal of Cystic Fibrosis 2003;2:A85.

Schlehuber S, Beste G, Skerra A. A novel type of receptor protein, based on the lipocalin scaffold, with specificity for digoxigenin. Journal of Molecular Biology 2000;297:1105–20.

Schlehuber S, Skerra A. Lipocalins in drug discovery: from natural ligand-binding proteins to anticalins. Drug Discovery Today 2005;10:23–33.

Sedgwick SG, Smerdon SJ. The ankyrin repeat: a diversity of interactions on a common structural framework. Trends in Biochemical Science 1999;24:311–16.

Semba K, Nishizawa M, Miyajima N, et al. yes-related protooncogene, syn, belongs to the protein-tyrosine kinase family. Proceeding of the National Academy of Sciences of USA 1986;83:5459–63.

Shapiro SD. Proteinases in chronic obstructive pulmonary disease. Biochemical Society Transactions 2002;30:98–102.

Silverman J, Liu Q, Bakker A, et al. Multivalent avimer proteins evolved by exon shuffling of a family of human receptor domains. Nature Biotechnology 2005;23:1556–61.

Skerra A. Lipocalins as a scaffold. Biochimica et Biophysica Acta 2000;1482:337–50.

Smith G. Patch engineering: a general approach for creating proteins that have new binding activities. Trends in Biochemical Science 1998;23: 457–60.

Steffen AC, Orlova A, Wikman M, et al. Affibody-mediated tumour targeting of HER-2 expressing xenografts in mice. European Journal of Nuclear Medicine and Molecular Imaging 2006;33:631–8.

Steiner D, Forrer P, Plückthun A. Efficient selection of DARPins with sub-nanomolar affinities using SRP phage display. Journal of Molecular Biology 2008;382:1211–27.

Suzuki F, Goto M, Sawa C, et al. Functional interactions of transcription factor human GA-binding protein subunits. Journal of Biological Chemistry 1998;273:29302–8.

Tomlinson IM. Next-generation protein drugs. Nature Biotechnology 2004;22:521–2.

Uhlen M, Forsberg G, Moks T, et al. Fusion proteins in biotechnology. Current Opinion in Biotechnology 1992;3:363–9.

Walker A, Dunlevy G, Rycroft D, et al. Anti-serum albumin domain antibodies in the development of highly potent, efficacious and long-acting interferon. Protein Engineering, Design & Selection 2010;23:271–8.

Ward ES, Güssow D, Griffiths AD, et al. Binding activities of a repertoire of single immunoglobulin variable domains secreted from Escherichia coli. Nature 1989;341:544–6.

Wikman M, Steffen AC, Gunneriusson E, et al. Selection and characterization of HER2/neu-binding affibody ligands. Protein Engineering, Design & Selection 2004;17:455–62.

Williams A, Baird LG. DX-88 and HAE: a developmental perspective. Transfusion and Apheresis Science 2003;29:255–8.

Wilson DS, Keefe AD, Szostak JW. The use of mRNA display to select high-affinity protein-binding peptides. Proceedings of the National Academy of Sciences of USA 2001;98:3750–5.

Wozniak-Knopp G, Bartl S, Bauer A, et al. Introducing antigen-binding sites in structural loops of immunoglobulin constant domains: Fc fragments with engineered HER2/neu-binding sites and antibody properties. Protein Engineering, Design & Selection 2010;23:289–97.

Xiao X, Feng Y, Vu BK, et al. A large library based on a novel (CH2) scaffold: identification of HIV-1 inhibitors. Biochemical and Biophysical Research Communications 2009;387: 387–92.

Xu L, Aha P, Gu K, et al. Directed evolution of high-affinity antibody mimics using mRNA display. Chemical Biology 2002;9:933–42.

Zahnd C, Pecorari F, Straumann N, et al. Selection and characterization of Her2 binding-designed ankyrin repeat proteins. Journal of Biological Chemistry 2006;281:35167–75.

Zardi L, Carnemolla B, Siri A, et al. Transformed human cells produce a new fibronectin isoform by preferential alternative splicing of a previously unobserved exon. The EMBO Journal 1987;6:2337–42.

Section 3

Drug development

Chapter **14**

Drug development: introduction

H P Rang, R G Hill

INTRODUCTION

Drug development comprises all the activities involved in transforming a compound from drug candidate (the end-product of the discovery phase) to a product approved for marketing by the appropriate regulatory authorities. Efficiency in drug development is critical for commercial success, for two main reasons:

- Development accounts for about two-thirds of the total R&D costs. The cost per project is very much greater in the development phase, and increases sharply as the project moves into the later phases of clinical development. Keeping these costs under control is a major concern for management. Failure of a compound late in development represents a lot of money wasted.
- Speed in development is an important factor in determining sales revenue, as time spent in development detracts from the period of patent protection once the drug goes to market. As soon as the patent expires, generic competition sharply reduces sales revenue.

Despite a high level of awareness in the pharmaceutical industry of the need to reduce the money and time spent on development, both have actually increased significantly over the last two decades (see Chapter 22). This is mainly due to external factors, particularly the increased stringency applied by regulatory authorities in assessing the safety and efficacy of new compounds (see Chapter 20). The development burden is, therefore, tending to increase, thereby increasing the need for companies to improve their performance in this area in order to remain profitable and competitive.

THE NATURE OF DRUG DEVELOPMENT

Drug discovery, as described in Section 2, is invariably an exploration of the unknown, and successful projects may end up with compounds quite different from what had originally been sought: there is a large component of 'unplannability'. In contrast, drug development has a very clear-cut goal: to produce the drug in a marketable form, and to gain regulatory permission to market it for use in the target indication(s) as quickly as possible. The work required to do this falls into three main parts, respectively *technical, investigative* and *managerial*:

- Technical development – solving technical problems relating to the synthesis and formulation of the drug substance, aimed mainly at ensuring the *quality* of the end-product:
  - Main functions involved: chemical development, pharmaceutical development.
- Investigative studies – establishing the safety and efficacy of the product, including assessment of whether it is pharmacokinetically suitable for clinical use in man:
  - Main functions involved: safety pharmacology, toxicology, pharmacokinetics, clinical development.
- Managerial functions:
  - Coordination – managing quality control, logistics, communication and decision making in a large multidisciplinary project to ensure high-quality data and to avoid unnecessary delays:
  - Main function involved: project management

- Documentation and liaison with regulatory authorities – collating and presenting data of the type, quality and format needed to secure regulatory approval
- Main function involved: regulatory affairs.

An important distinction between the technical and investigative aspects of development is that, in tackling technical problems, it is assumed that a solution does exist, and so the team's task is to find and optimize it as quickly as possible, whereas in assessing safety and efficacy it cannot be assumed that the compound reaches the required standards – rather, the object is to discover this as quickly and cheaply as possible. In other words, technical development is essentially an exercise in problem solving, whereas clinical and toxicological development is a continuing investigation of the properties of the compound. Although technical problems, such as an unacceptably complex and poor-yielding synthesis route, or difficulty in developing a satisfactory formulation, can result in abandonment of the project, this is relatively uncommon. Failure on account of the drug's biological properties, such as toxicity, poor efficacy or unsatisfactory pharmacokinetics, is, however, very common, and largely accounts for the fact that only some 10% of compounds entering Phase I clinical trials are eventually marketed. An important aspect of the management of drug-development projects, therefore, is to establish firm 'no-go' criteria, and to test the compound against them as early as possible.

Development proceeds along much more clearly defined lines than discovery, and is consequently more 'plannable', particularly the non-clinical studies, where standard experimental protocols exist for most of the work that needs to be carried out. This applies also in Phase I clinical studies. Delays can nevertheless occur if unexpected findings emerge, for example poor oral absorption in humans, or species-specific toxic effects, which require additional work to be carried out before clinical trials can proceed. If the drug has a completely novel mechanism of action this often prolongs the technical phase whilst off-target effects are explored (sometimes at the insistence of the regulatory authority).

Beyond Phase I, the route to be followed is generally much less well charted, and success depends to a much greater extent on strategic decisions by the project team as to which clinical indications should be investigated (see Chapter 17). They will need to assess, for example, whether recruiting patients to the trial will be easy or difficult, what exclusion criteria should apply, what clinical outcome measures should be used, and how long the treatment and assessment periods will need to be. To achieve registration as quickly as possible, it may, for example, be expedient to select a relatively low-market, but quick-to-test, clinical indication for the initial trials, and to run these trials in parallel with more prolonged trials in the major indication. Careful attention needs to be given to the patient group selected for the trial, so as to maximize the chance of success in obtaining a clear-cut result. Experience shows that inconclusive clinical trials resulting from poor decisions of this sort are a common cause of failure or delay in drug development. Where the indication allows this an adaptive trial design may allow a more efficient evaluation of the drug (see Chapter 17).

COMPONENTS OF DRUG DEVELOPMENT

Figure 14.1 summarizes the main activities involved in developing a typical synthetic compound. It shows the main tasks that have to be completed before the compound can be submitted for regulatory approval, but needs to be translated into an operational plan (Figure 14.2) that will allow the project to proceed as quickly and efficiently as possible. It is obvious that certain tasks have to be completed in a particular order. For example, a supply of pure compound, prepared in an acceptable formulation, has to be available before Phase I clinical studies can begin. Animal toxicity data must also be available before the compound can be given to humans. Deciding on the dosage schedule to be used in efficacy trials requires knowledge of the pharmacokinetics and metabolism of the compound in humans. Because the data generated will be included in the final registration proposal, it is essential that each part of the work should be formally reported and 'signed off' by the group responsible and archived for future reference. A typical development project is likely to involve several hundred individuals, expert in different disciplines and working on different aspects of the project, and coordinating their work is a complex and demanding task. For this reason, most companies assign specialist project managers to this task. Their role is to design a project plan, based on input from the experts involved, to monitor progress and to adapt the plan accordingly. As well as being good organizers, project managers need to be excellent communicators, diplomatic, and with a good understanding of the scientific and technological aspects of the project. Figure 14.2 is a much-simplified outline of a project plan of the development of a typical orally active drug. Each 'task', represented by an arrow, starts and ends at a circular symbol (representing an 'event'), and decision points are marked by diamond symbols. This type of graphical format, which is widely used as a project management tool and implemented in many commercially available software packages, is known as a PERT (project evaluation and review technique) chart. By assigning times – shortest possible, maximum, and expected – to each task, the timing of the whole project can be assessed and the *critical path* – i.e. the sequence of tasks that need to be completed on time in order to avoid an overall delay – defined. In Figure 14.2 the process has been reduced to a

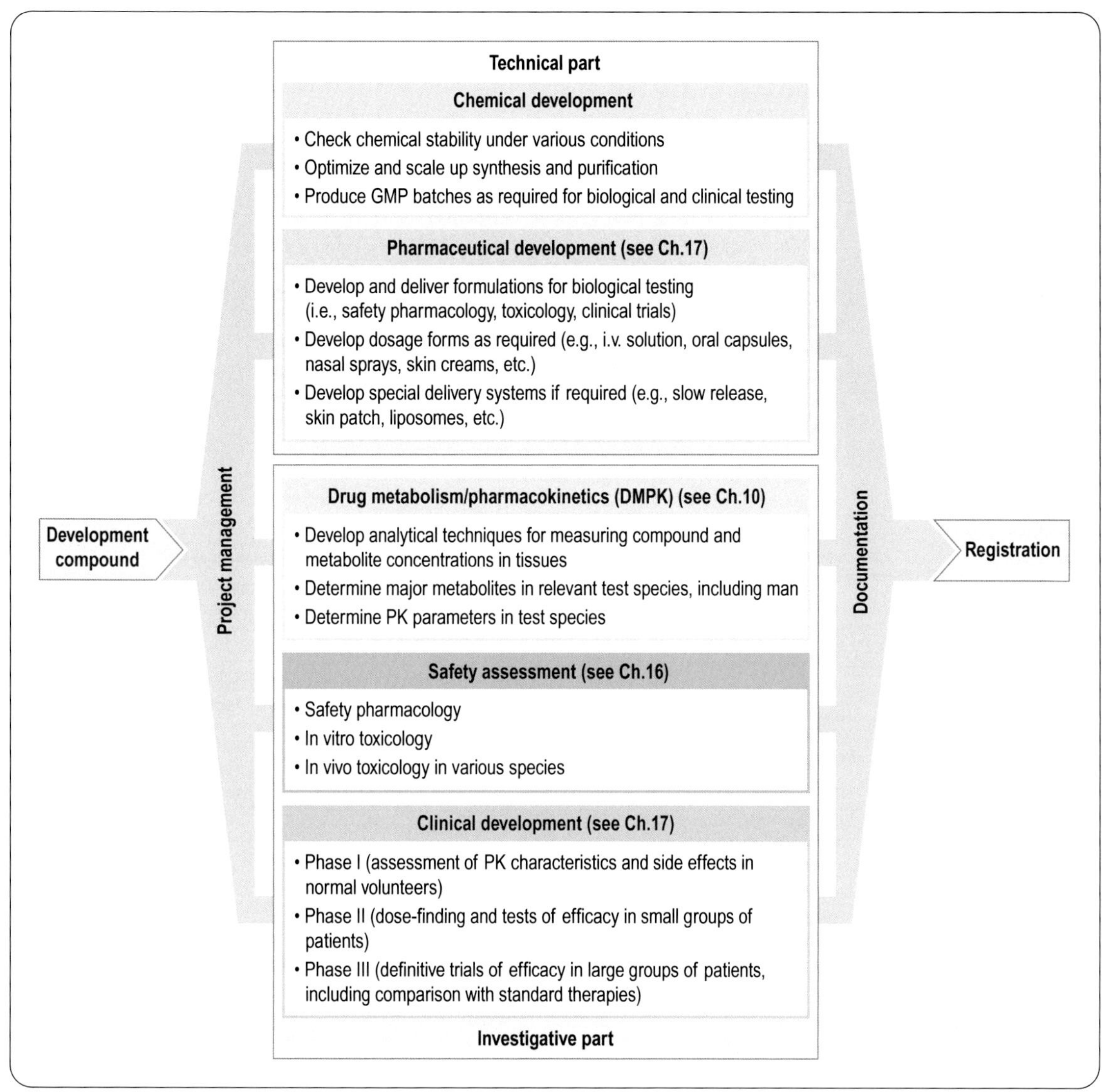

Fig. 14.1 The main technical and investigative components of a typical drug development project.

bare minimum to allow representation on a single page; in practice, each of the 'tasks' shown (e.g. develop formulations, perform Phase I studies, etc.) needs to be further subdivided into a series of subtasks and timings to enable the project to be planned and monitored at the operational level. The complete diagram for a typical drug development project will be of such size and complexity as to frighten all but the most hardened project management professionals. Software tools, fortunately, are available which allow the project to be viewed in different ways, such as Gantt charts, which are barcharts set against a calendar timescale, showing the expected start and completion dates for each task, many of which will be running simultaneously on any given date[1].

In this section of the book we outline the main technical and experimental parts of the work that goes into drug development, namely toxicology, pharmaceutical development and clinical studies. Chapter 19 discusses the principles underlying the patenting of drugs. Chapter 20

[1]In Robert Burns' words 'The best-laid plans of mice and men gang aft agley'. Drug development is no exception to this principle – managers prefer the euphemism 'slippage'.

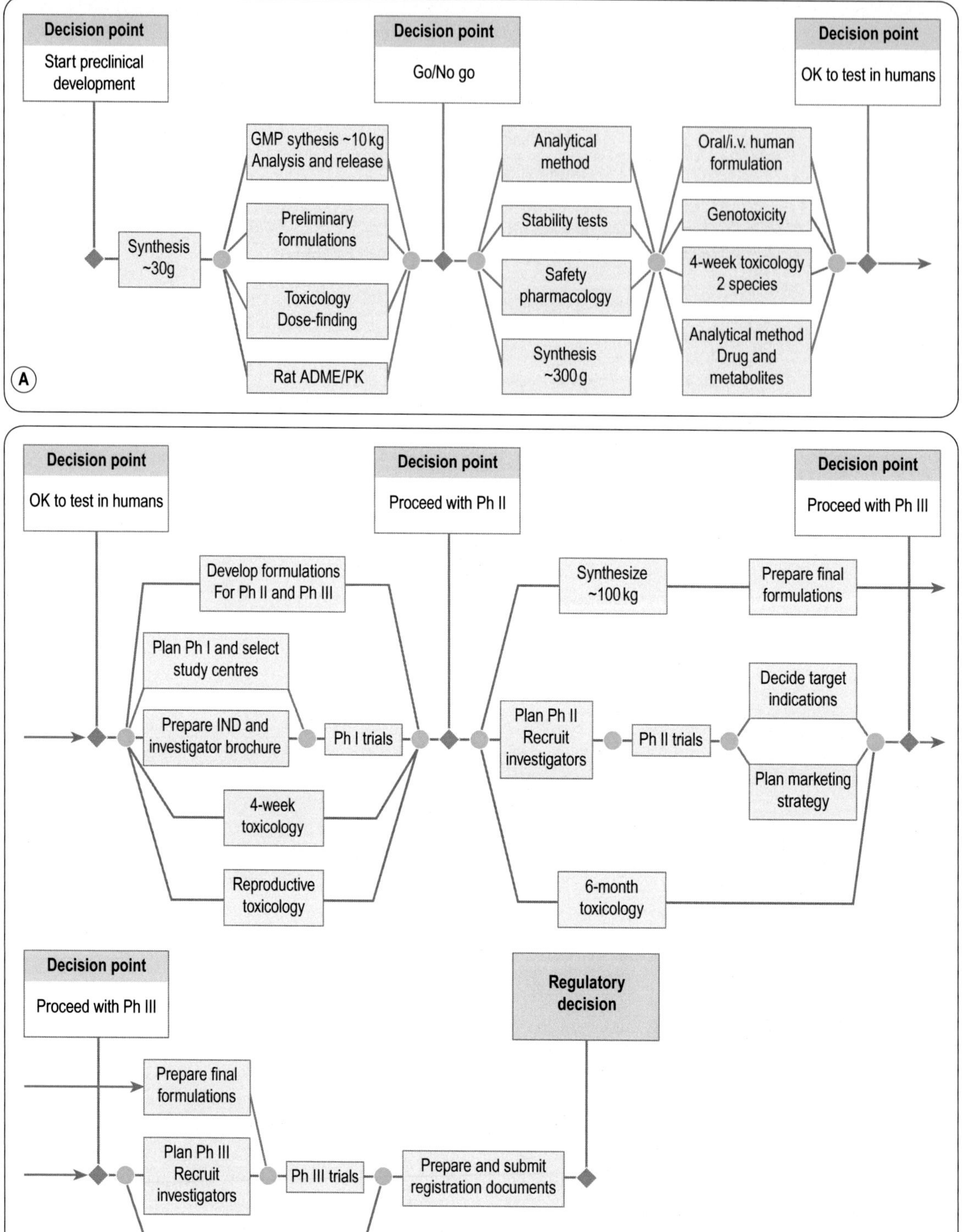

Fig. 14.2 Simplified flowchart showing the main activities involved in drug development. The nodes indicated by circles represent the start and finish points of each activity, and the diagram indicates which activities need to be completed before the next can begin. By assigning timescales to each activity, the planned overall development time can be determined and critical path activities identified. (A) Preclinical development. (B) Clinical development.

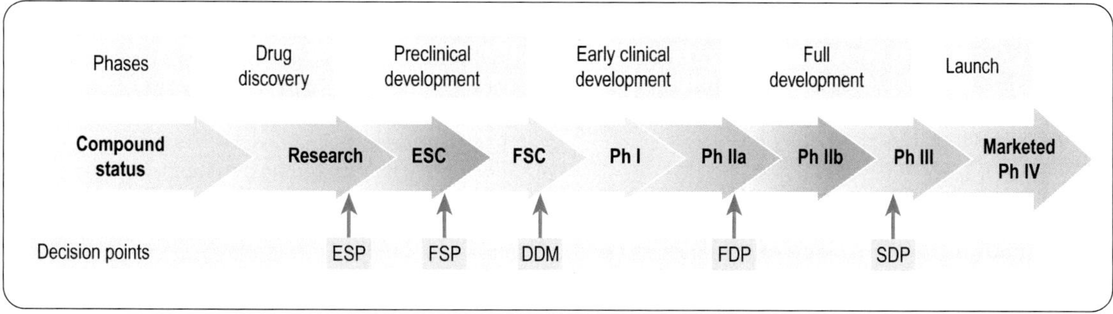

Fig. 14.3 Strategic decision points in drug development. ESP, early selection point; FSP, final selection point; DDM, decision to develop in man; FDP, full development decision point; SDP, submission decision point.

describes how regulatory bodies go about evaluating new compounds for registration, and Chapter 21 presents an introduction to the principles of pharmaceutical marketing. Chemical development, covering the specialized technical aspects of producing the drug substance economically and safely on a large scale, as well as the control measures needed to ensure consistent high quality of the final product, is beyond the scope of this book (see Gadamasetti, 2007; Repic, 1998 for a full account of this subject).

THE INTERFACE BETWEEN DISCOVERY AND DEVELOPMENT

For the purposes of this book, drug development is presented as an operation separate from discovery and following on from it, but the distinction is actually not clear-cut. Increasingly, as has been stressed in Chapters 9 and 10, activities previously undertaken during development are taking place earlier, as an integral part of the discovery process. The emphasis on the 'druggability' of leads (Chapter 9) reflects a concern for focusing on structures that are least likely to have unsatisfactory pharmacokinetic, toxicological or stability problems. Whereas in vitro tests of absorption and metabolism were traditionally performed on individual compounds during the development phase, they are now being incorporated into medium-throughput screens in the discovery phase (Chapter 10), as are in vitro toxicity tests. Formulation work also often begins during the discovery phase, particularly if the characteristics of the lead compounds suggest that specialized formulations are likely to be required for use in pharmacological profiling of compounds in vivo. Furthermore, the selection of a single compound for full development will sometimes be deferred until data from Phase I trials on several candidates have been obtained. Thus, the preliminary work needed before Phase I, and the Phase I trials themselves, will need to be performed on a group of candidate compounds. This is clearly more expensive than choosing the development compound before Phase I, but may be justified as a strategy for reducing the risk of failure at a later (and more expensive) stage.

DECISION POINTS

The decision to advance a drug candidate into early development is the first of several key strategic decision points in the history of the drug development project. The timing, nomenclature and decision-making process vary from company to company, and Figure 14.3 shows a typical scheme, developed by Novartis:

- The early selection point (ESP) is the decision to take the drug candidate molecule into early (preclinical) development. The proposal will normally be framed by the drug discovery team and evaluated by a research committee, which determines whether the criteria to justify further development have been met. After this checkpoint, responsibility normally passes to a multidisciplinary team with representatives from research, various development functions, patents, regulatory affairs and marketing, under the direction of a professional project manager. In a large multinational company the team will have international representation, and the development plan will be organized to meet global development standards as far as possible.
- The decision to develop in man (DDM) controls entry of the compound into Phase I, based on the additional information obtained during the preclinical development phase (i.e. preliminary toxicology, safety pharmacology, pharmacokinetics, etc.). An important task once this decision point is passed is normally the production of a sufficient quantity (usually 2–5 kg) of clinical-grade material.

Passing this decision point takes the project into Phase I and Phase IIa clinical studies, described in more detail in Chapter 17, which are designed to reveal whether the drug has an acceptable pharmacokinetic and side-effect profile in normal volunteers (Phase I), and whether it shows evidence of clinical efficacy in patients (Phase IIa). For drugs acting by novel mechanisms, Phase IIa provides the all-important first 'proof of concept', on which the decision whether or not to proceed with the serious business of full development largely rests[2].

- The full development decision point (FDP) is reached after the Phase I and Phase IIa ('proof-of-concept') studies have been completed, this being the first point at which evidence of clinical efficacy in man is obtained. It is at this point that the project becomes seriously expensive in terms of money and manpower, and has to be evaluated strictly in competition with other projects. Evaluation of the likely commercial returns as well as the chances of successful registration and the time and cost of the 'pivotal' Phase III studies, are, therefore, important considerations at this point.
- The submission decision point (SDP) is the final decision to apply for registration, based on a check that the amount and quality of the data submitted are sufficient to ensure a smooth passage through the regulatory process. Hold-ups in registration can carry serious penalties in terms of the cost and time required to perform additional clinical studies, as well as loss of confidence among financial analysts, who will have been primed to expect a new product to bring in revenues according to the plan as originally envisaged.

A couple of aphorisms are often applied to drug development, namely:

- In research, surprise = discovery; in development, surprise = disaster
- It is as valuable to stop a project as to carry one forward.

Like most aphorisms they contain a grain of truth, but only a small one. With regard to the first, equating surprise with disaster applies, if at all, only to the technical parts of development, not to the investigational parts, which are, as discussed above, a continuation of research into the properties of the drug. Surprises in this arena can be good or bad for the outcome of the project. Finding, to the company's surprise, that sildenafil (Viagra) improved the sex life of trial subjects, set the development project off in a completely new, and very successful, direction.

The value attached to stopping projects reflects the frustration – commonly felt in large research organizations – that projects that have little chance of ending in success tend to carry on, swallowing resources, through sheer inertia, sustained mainly by the reluctance of individuals to abandon work to which they may have devoted many years of effort. In practice, of course, the value of stopping a project depends only on the possibility of redeploying the resources to something more useful, i.e. on the 'opportunity cost'. If the resources used cannot be redeployed, or if no better project can be identified, there is no value in stopping the project. What is certain is that it is only by carrying projects forward that success can be achieved. Despite the aphorism, it is no surprise that managers who regularly lead projects into oblivion achieve much less favourable recognition than those who bring them to fruition!

THE NEED FOR IMPROVEMENT

As emphasized elsewhere in this book, innovative new drugs are not being registered as fast as the spectacular developments in biomedical science in the last decades of the 20th century had led the world to expect. The rate of new drug approvals in recent years has shown a disheartening decline and there is little sign of the anticipated surge (see Chapter 22), despite a steadily rising R&D spend. This worrying problem was analysed in a 2004 report by the FDA, which lays the blame firmly on the failure of the development process to keep up with advances in biomedicine. The report comments: 'the applied sciences needed for medical product development have not kept pace with the tremendous advances in the basic sciences'. The report outlines a historical success rate (i.e. chance of reaching the market) for new compounds entering Phase I clinical trials of 14% and comments that this figure did not improve between 1985 and 2000. Furthermore, a recent analysis cited in this report shows that the cost of development, per compound registered, almost doubled in 2000–2002 compared with 1995–2000, whereas the cost of discovery changed very little. In their view, too little effort is being made to develop an improved 'product development toolkit' that places more reliance on early laboratory data, and relies less on animal models and clinical testing in assessing safety and efficacy. The FDA and other regulatory bodies hold a large amount of data

[2]The division of Phase II clinical trials, which are exploratory tests involving relatively small numbers of patients (100–300), and lack the statistical power of the later 'pivotal' Phase III trials, into two stages (a and b) is a fairly recent idea, now widely adopted. Phase IIa is essentially a quick look to see whether the drug administered in a dose selected on the basis of pharmacokinetic, pharmacodynamic and toxicological data has any worthwhile therapeutic effect. Phase IIb, also on small numbers, is aimed at refining the dosage schedule to optimize the therapeutic benefit, and to determine the dosage to be tested in the large-scale, definitive Phase II trials. It marks the beginning of full development, following the key decision (FDP) whether to proceed or stop. For the discovery team, the outcome of Phase IIa largely determines whether they throw their hats in the air or retire to lick their wounds.

which could be used to analyse in a much more systematic way than has so far been done by the predictive value of particular laboratory tests in relation to clinical outcome. New screening technologies and computer modelling approaches need to be brought into the same frame. Currently, extrapolation from laboratory and animal data to the clinical situation relies largely on biological intuition – it is assumed, for example, that a compound that does not cause hepatotoxicity in animals is unlikely to do so in man – but there may well be cheaper and quicker tests that would be at least as predictive. There are many other examples, in the FDA's view, where new technologies offer the possibility of replacing or improving existing procedures, with substantial savings of money and time. The task is beyond the capabilities of any one pharmaceutical company, but needs collaboration and funding at the national or international level. The FDA has continued to issue reports aimed at improving the regulatory process and reducing delays in approval of important new drugs (see CDER 2011; FDA, 2010).

The remaining chapters in this section give a simple overview of the main activities involved in drug development. Griffin and O'Grady (2002) describe the drug development process in more detail.

REFERENCES

CDER. Identifying CDER's science and research needs – report July 2011, 2011. p. 24

FDA Report. Innovation stagnation: challenge and opportunity on the critical path to new medical products. 2004. www.fda.gov/oc/initiatives/criticalpath/whitepaper.html

FDA Report. Advancing regulatory science for public health. 2010. www.fda.gov/scienceresearch/specialtopics/regulatoryscience/ucm228131.htm

Gadamasetti K, editor. Process chemistry in the pharmaceutical industry, vol. 2. Chichester: CRC Press/Taylor and Francis; 2007. p. 520.

Griffin JP, O'Grady JO. The textbook of pharmaceutical medicine, 4th ed. London: BMJ Books; 2002.

Repic O. 1998 Principles of process research and chemical development in the pharmaceutical industry. New York: John Wiley.

Chapter 15

Assessing drug safety

H P Rang, R G Hill

INTRODUCTION

Since the thalidomide disaster, ensuring that new medicines are safe when used therapeutically has been one of the main responsibilities of regulatory agencies. Of course, there is no such thing as 100% safety, much as the public would like reassurance of this. Any medical intervention – or for that matter, any human activity – carries risks as well as benefits, and the aim of drug safety assessment is to ensure, as far as possible, that the risks are commensurate with the benefits.

Safety is addressed at all stages in the life history of a drug, from the earliest stages of design, through preclinical investigations (discussed in this chapter) and preregistration clinical trials (Chapter 17), to the entire post-marketing history of the drug. The ultimate test comes only after the drug has been marketed and used in a clinical setting in many thousands of patients, during the period of Phase IV clinical trials (post-marketing surveillance). It is unfortunately not uncommon for drugs to be withdrawn for safety reasons after being in clinical use for some time (for example *practolol*, because of a rare but dangerous oculomucocutaneous reaction, *troglitazone* because of liver damage, *cerivastatin* because of skeletal muscle damage, *terfenadine* because of drug interactions, *rofecoxib* because of increased risk of heart attacks), reflecting the fact that safety assessment is fallible. It always will be fallible, because there are no bounds to what may emerge as harmful effects. Can we be *sure* that drug X will not cause kidney damage in a particular inbred tribe in a remote part of the world? The answer is, of course, 'no', any more than we could have been sure that various antipsychotic drugs – now withdrawn – would not cause sudden cardiac deaths through a hitherto unsuspected mechanism, hERG channel block (see later). What is not hypothesized cannot be tested. For this reason, the problem of safety assessment is fundamentally different from that of efficacy assessment, where we can define exactly what we are looking for.

Here we focus on non-clinical safety assessment – often called preclinical, even though much of the work is done in parallel with clinical development. We describe the various types of in vitro and in vivo tests that are used to predict adverse and toxic effects in humans, and which form an important part of the data submitted to the regulatory authorites when approval is sought (a) for the new compound to be administered to humans for the first time (IND approval in the USA; see Chapter 20), and (b) for permission to market the drug (NDA approval in the USA, MAA approval in Europe; see Chapter 20).

The programme of preclinical safety assessment for a new synthetic compound can be divided into the following main chronological phases, linked to the clinical trials programme (Figure 15.1):

- *Exploratory toxicology*, aimed at giving a rough quantitative estimate of the toxicity of the compound when given acutely or repeatedly over a short period (normally 2 weeks), and providing an indication of the main organs and physiological systems involved. These studies provide information for the guidance of the project team in making further plans, but are not normally part of the regulatory package that has to be approved before the drug can be given to humans, so they do not need to be perfomed under good laboratory practice (GLP) conditions.
- *Regulatory toxicology*. These studies are performed to GLP standards and comprise (a) those that are required by regulatory authorities, or by ethics committees, before the compound can be given for the first time to humans; (b) studies required to

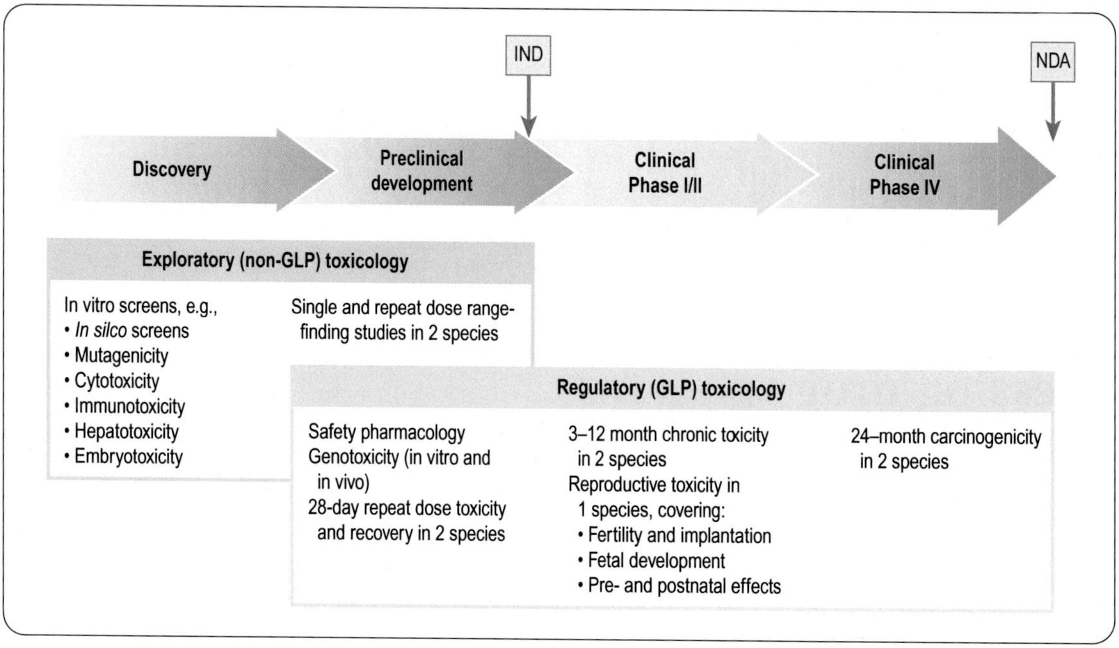

IND

NDA

Discovery

Preclinical development

Clinical Phase I/II

Clinical Phase IV

Exploratory (non-GLP) toxicology

In vitro screens, e.g.,
- *In silco* screens
- Mutagenicity
- Cytotoxicity
- Immunotoxicity
- Hepatotoxicity
- Embryotoxicity

Single and repeat dose range-finding studies in 2 species

Regulatory (GLP) toxicology

Safety pharmacology
Genotoxicity (in vitro and in vivo)
28-day repeat dose toxicity and recovery in 2 species

3–12 month chronic toxicity in 2 species
Reproductive toxicity in 1 species, covering:
- Fertility and implantation
- Fetal development
- Pre- and postnatal effects

24–month carcinogenicity in 2 species

Fig. 15.1 Timing of the main safety assessment studies during drug discovery and development.

support an application for marketing approval, which are normally performed in parallel with clinical trials. Full reports of all studies of this kind are included in documentation submitted to the regulatory authorities.

Regulatory toxicology studies in group (a) include 28-day repeated-dose toxicology studies in two species (including one non-rodent, usually dog but sometimes monkey especially if the drug is a biological), in vitro and in vivo genoxocity tests, safety pharmacology and reproductive toxicity assessment. In vitro genotoxicity tests, which are cheap and quick to perform, will often have been performed much earlier in the compound selection phase of the project, as may safety pharmacology studies.

The nature of the tests in group (b) depends greatly on the nature and intended use of the drug, but they will include chronic 3–12-month toxicological studies in two or more species, long-term (18–24 months) carcinogenicity tests and reproductive toxicology, and often interaction studies involving other drugs that are likely to be used for the same indications.

The basic procedures for safety assessment of a single new synthetic compound are fairly standard, although the regulatory authorities have avoided applying a defined checklist of tests and criteria required for regulatory approval. Instead they issue guidance notes (available on relevant websites – USA: www.fda.gov/cder/; EU: www.emea.eu.int; international harmonization guidelines: www.ich.org), but the onus is on the pharmaceutical company to anticipate and exclude any unwanted effects based on the specific chemistry, pharmacology and intended therapeutic use of the compound in question. The regulatory authorities will often ask companies developing second or third entrants in a new class to perform tests based on findings from the class leading compound.

There are many types of new drug applications that do not fall into the standard category of synthetic small molecules, where the safety assessment standards are different. These include most biopharmaceuticals (see Chapter 12), as well as vaccines, cell and gene therapy products (see below). Drug combinations, and non-standard delivery systems and routes of administration are also examples of special cases where safety assessment requirements differ from those used for conventional drugs. These special cases are not discussed in detail here; Gad (2002) gives a comprehensive account.

TYPES OF ADVERSE DRUG EFFECT

Adverse reactions in man are of four general types:

- Exaggerated pharmacological effects – sometimes referred to as *hyperpharmacology* or *mechanism-related effects* – are dose related and in general predictable on the basis of the principal pharmacological effect of the drug. Examples include hypoglycaemia caused by antidiabetic drugs, hypokalaemia induced by diuretics, immunosuppression in response to steroids, etc.

- Pharmacological effects associated with targets other than the principal one – covered by the general term *side effects* or *off-target effects*. Examples include hypotension produced by various antipsychotic drugs which block adrenoceptors as well as dopamine receptors (their principal target), and cardiac arrythmias associated with hERG-channel inhibition (see below). Many drugs inhibit one or more forms of cytochrome P450, and hence affect the metabolism of other drugs. Provided the pharmacological profile of the compound is known in sufficient detail, effects of this kind are also predictable (see also Chapter 10).
- Dose-related *toxic effects* that are unrelated to the intended pharmacological effects of the drug. Commonly such effects, which include toxic effects on liver, kidney, endocrine glands, immune cells and other systems, are produced not by the parent drug, but by chemically reactive metabolites. Examples include the gum hyperplasia produced by the antiepileptic drug phenytoin, hearing loss caused by aminoglycoside antibiotics, and peripheral neuropathy caused by thalidomide[1]. Genotoxicity and reproductive toxicity (see below) also fall into this category. Such adverse effects are not, in general, predictable from the pharmacological profile of the compound. It is well known that certain chemical structures are associated with toxicity, and so these will generally be eliminated early in the lead identification stage, sometimes in silico before any actual compounds are synthesized. The main function of toxicological studies in drug development is to detect dose-related toxic effects of an unpredictable nature.
- Rare, and sometimes serious, adverse effects, known as *idiosyncratic reactions*, that occur in certain individuals and are not dose related. Many examples have come to light among drugs that have entered clinical use, e.g. aplastic anaemia produced by *chloramphenicol*, anaphylactic responses to *penicillin*, oculomucocutaneous syndrome with *practolol*, bone marrow depression with *clozapine*. Toxicological tests in animals rarely reveal such effects, and because they may occur in only one in several thousand humans they are likely to remain undetected in clinical trials, coming to light only after the drug has been registered and given to thousands of patients. (The reaction to clozapine is an exception. It affects about 1% of patients and was detected in early clinical trials. The bone marrow effect, though potentially life-threatening, is reversible, and clozapine was successfully registered, with a condition that patients receiving it must be regularly monitored.)

Safety pharmacology testing and *dose range-finding studies* are designed to detect pharmacological adverse effects; *chronic toxicology testing* is designed to detect dose-related toxic effects, as well as the long-term consequences of pharmacological side effects; idiosyncratic reactions may be revealed in Phase III clinical trials, but are likely to remain undetected until the compound enters clinical use.

SAFETY PHARMACOLOGY

The pharmacological studies described in Chapter 11 are exploratory (i.e. surveying the effects of the compound with respect to selectivity against a wide range of possible targets) or hypothesis driven (checking whether the expected effects of the drug, based on its target selectivity, are actually produced). In contrast, safety pharmacology comprises a series of protocol-driven studies, aimed specifically at detecting possible undesirable or dangerous effects of exposure to the drug in therapeutic doses (see ICH Guideline S7A). The emphasis is on acute effects produced by single-dose administration, as distinct from toxicology studies, which focus mainly on the effects of chronic exposure. Safety pharmacology evaluation forms an important part of the dossier submitted to the regulatory authorities.

ICH Guideline S7A defines a *core battery* of safety pharmacology tests, and a series of *follow-up* and *supplementary tests* (Table 15.1). The core battery is normally performed on all compounds intended for systemic use. Where they are not appropriate (e.g. for preparations given topically) their omission has to be justified on the basis of information about the extent of systemic exposure that may occur when the drug is given by the intended route. Follow-up studies are required if the core battery of tests reveals effects whose mechanism needs to be determined. Supplementary tests need to be performed if the known chemistry or pharmacology of the compound gives any reason to expect that it may produce side effects (e.g. a compound with a thiazide-like structure should be tested for possible inhibition of insulin secretion, this being a known side effect of thiazide diuretics; similarly, an opioid needs to be tested for dependence liability and effects on gastrointestinal motility). Where there is a likelihood of significant drug interactions, this may also need to be tested as part of the supplementary programme.

The core battery of tests listed in Table 15.1 focuses on acute effects on cardiovascular, respiratory and nervous systems, based on standard physiological measurements.

[1]This notorious drug is undergoing a therapeutic revival in the treatment of myeloma, a serious type of bone marrow cancer, progressive muscle weakness and sensory loss due to peripheral neuropathy being the most common and troublesome side effects.

Table 15.1 Safety pharmacology

Type	Physiological system	Tests
Core battery	Central nervous system	Observations on conscious animals
		Motor activity
		Behavioural changes
		Coordination
		Reflex responses
		Body temperature
	Cardiovascular system	Measurements on anaesthetized animals
		Blood pressure
		Heart rate
		ECG changes
		Tests for delayed ventricular repolarization (see text)
	Respiratory system	Measurements on anaesthetized or conscious animals
		Respiratory rate
		Tidal volume
		Arterial oxygen saturation
Follow-up tests (examples)	Central nervous system	Tests on learning and memory
		More complex test for changes in behaviour and motor function
		Tests for visual and auditory function
	Cardiovascular system	Cardiac output
		Ventricular contractility
		Vascular resistance
		Regional blood flow
	Respiratory system	Airways resistance and compliance
		Pulmonary arterial pressure
		Blood gases
Supplementary tests (examples)	Renal function	Urine volume, osmolality pH
		Proteinuria
		Blood urea/creatinine
		Fluid/electrolyte balance
		Urine cytology
	Autonomic nervous system	Cardiovascular, gastrointestinal and respiratory system responses to agonists and stimulation of autonomic nerves
	Gastrointestinal system	Gastric secretion

Table 15.1 ***Continued***

Type	Physiological system	Tests
		Gastric pH
		Intestinal motility
		Gastrointestinal transit time
	Other systems (e.g. endocrine, blood coagulation, skeletal muscle function, etc.)	Tests designed to detect likely acute effects

The follow-up and supplementary tests are less clearly defined, and the list given in Table 15.1 is neither prescriptive nor complete. It is the responsibility of the team to decide what tests are relevant and how the studies should be performed, and to justify these decisions in the submission to the regulatory authority.

Tests for QT interval prolongation

The ability of a number of therapeutically used drugs to cause a potentially fatal ventricular arrhythmia (*'torsade de pointes'*) has been a cause of major concern to clinicians and regulatory authorities (see Committee for Proprietary Medicinal Products, 1997; Haverkamp et al., 2000). The arrhythmia is associated with prolongation of the ventricular action potential (delayed ventricular repolarization), reflected in ECG recordings as prolongation of the QT interval. Drugs known to possess this serious risk, many of which have been withdrawn, include several *tricyclic antidepressants*, some antipsychotic drugs (e.g. *thioridazine, droperidol*), antidysrhythmic drugs (e.g. *amiodarone, quinidine, disopyramide*), antihistamines (*terfenadine, astemizole*) and certain antimalarial drugs (e.g. *halofantrine*). The main mechanism responsible appears to be inhibition of a potassium channel, termed the hERG channel, which plays a major role in terminating the ventricular action potential (Netzer et al., 2001).

Screening tests have shown that QT interval prolongation is a common property of 'drug-like' small molecules, and the patterns of structure–activity relationships have revealed particular chemical classes associated with this effect. Ideally, these are taken into account and avoided at an early stage in drug design, but the need remains for functional testing of all candidate drug molecules as a prelude to tests in humans.

Proposed standard tests for QT interval prolongation have been formulated as ICH Guideline S7B. They comprise (a) testing for inhibition of hERG channel currents in cell lines engineered to express the hERG gene; (b) measurements of action potential duration in myocardial cells from different parts of the heart in different species; and (c) measurements of QT interval in ECG recordings in conscious animals. These studies are usually carried out on ferrets or guinea pigs, as well as larger mammalian species, such as dog, rabbit, pig or monkey, in which hERG-like channels control ventricular repolarization, rather than in rat and mouse. In vivo tests for proarrhythmic effects in various species are being developed (De Clerck et al., 2002), but have not yet been evaluated for regulatory purposes.

Because of the importance of drug-induced QT prolongation in man, and the fact that many diverse groups of drugs appear to have this property, there is a need for high-throughput screening for hERG channel inhibition to be incorporated early in a drug discovery project. The above methods are not suitable for high-throughput screening, but alternative methods, such as inhibition of binding of labelled *dofetilide* (a potent hERG-channel blocker), or fluorimetric membrane potential assays on cell lines expressing these channels, can be used in high-throughput formats, as increasingly can automated patch clamp studies (see Chapter 8). It is important to note that binding and fluorescence assays are not seen as adequately predictive and cannot replace the patch clamp studies under the guidelines (ICH 7B). These assays are now becoming widely used as part of screening before selecting a clinical candidate molecule, though there is still a need to confirm presence or absence of QT prolongation in functional in vivo tests before advancing a compound into clinical development.

EXPLORATORY (DOSE RANGE-FINDING) TOXICOLOGY STUDIES

The first stage of toxicological evaluation usually takes the form of a *dose range-finding study* in a rodent and/or a non-rodent species. The species commonly used in toxicology are mice, rats, guinea pigs, hamsters, rabbits, dogs, minipigs and non-human primates. Usually two species (rat and mouse) are tested initially, but others may be used if there are reasons for thinking that the drug may exert species-specific effects. A single dose is given to each test animal, preferably by the intended route of administration in the clinic, and in a formulation shown by previous pharmacokinetic studies to produce satisfactory absorption and duration of action (see also Chapter 10). Generally, widely spaced doses (e.g. 10, 100, 1000 mg/kg) will be tested first, on groups of three to four rodents, and the animals will be observed over 14 days for obvious signs of toxicity. Alternatively, a *dose escalation* protocol may be used, in which each animal is treated with increasing doses of the drug at intervals (e.g. every 2 days) until signs of toxicity appear, or until a dose of 2000 mg/kg is reached. With either protocol, the animals are killed at the end of the experiment and autopsied to determine if any target organs are grossly affected. The results of such dose range-finding studies provide a rough estimate of the *no toxic effect level* (NTEL, see Toxicity measures, below) in the species tested, and the nature of the gross effects seen is often a useful pointer to the main target tissues and organs.

The dose range-finding study will normally be followed by a more detailed single-dose toxicological study in two or more species, the doses tested being chosen to span the estimated NTEL. Usually four or five doses will be tested, ranging from a dose in the expected therapeutic range to doses well above the estimated NTEL. A typical protocol for such an acute toxicity study is shown in Figure 15.2. The data collected consist of regular systematic assessment of the animals for a range of clinical signs on the basis of a standardized checklist, together with gross autopsy findings of animals dying during a 2-week observation period, or killed at the end. The main signs that are monitored are shown in Table 15.2.

Single-dose studies are followed by a multiple dose-ranging study in which the drug is given daily or twice daily, normally for 2 weeks, with the same observation and autopsy procedure as in the single-dose study, in order to give preliminary information about the toxicity after chronic treatment.

The results of these preliminary in vivo toxicity studies will help in the planning and design of the next steps of the development programme; they will also help to decide whether or not it is worthwhile to continue the research effort on a given chemical class.

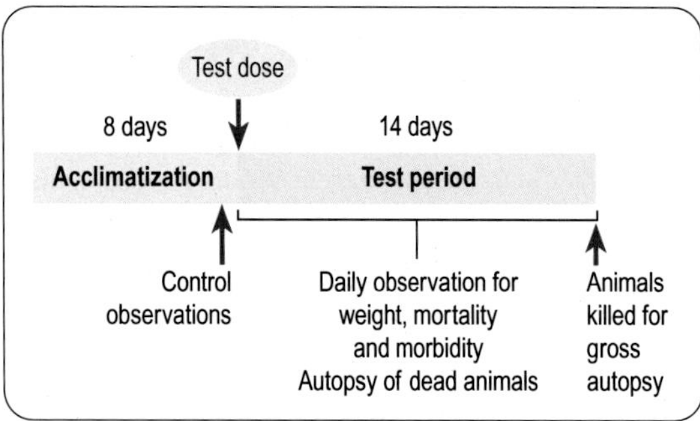

Fig. 15.2 Typical protocal for single-dose toxicity study.

As mentioned above, these toxicology studies are preliminary, and usually they are not sufficient for supporting the first human evaluation of the medicine. Very often, they are not conducted under good laboratory practice (GLP) conditions, nor are they conducted with test material which has been produced according to good manufacturing practice (GMP).

Subsequent work is guided by regulatory requirements elaborated by the International Conference of Harmonization or by national regulatory authorities. Their published guidelines specify/recommend the type of toxicological evaluation needed to support applications for carrying out studies in humans. These documents provide guidance, for example, on the duration of administration, on the design of the toxicological study, including the number of animals to be studied, and stipulate that the work must be carried out under GLP conditions and that the test material must be of GMP standard. The test substance for the toxicology evaluation has to be identical in terms of quality and characteristics to the substance given to humans.

GENOTOXICITY

Foreign substances can affect gene function in various ways, the two most important types of mechanism in relation to toxicology being:

- *Mutagenicity*, i.e. chemical alteration of DNA sufficient to cause abnormal gene expression in the affected cell and its offspring. Most commonly, the mutation arises as a result of covalent modification of individual bases (point mutations). The result may be the production of an abnormal protein if the mutation occurs in the coding region of the gene, or altered expression levels of a normal protein if the mutation affects control sequences. Such mutations occur continuously in everyday life, and are counteracted more or less effectively by a variety of DNA repair mechanisms. They are important particularly because certain mutations can interfere with mechanisms controlling cell division, and thereby lead to malignancy or, in the immature organism, to adverse effects on growth and development. In practice, most carcinogens are mutagens, though by no means all mutagens are carcinogens. Evidence of mutagenicity therefore sounds a warning of possible carcinogenicity, which must be tested by thorough in vivo tests.
- *Chromosomal damage*, for example chromosome breakage (clastogenesis), chromosome fusion, translocation of stretches of DNA within or between chromosomes, replication or deletion of chromosomes, etc. Such changes result from alterations in DNA, more extensive than point mutations and less well understood mechanistically;

Table 15.2 Clinical observations in acute toxicity tests

System	Observation	Signs of toxicity
Nervous system	Behaviour	Sedation
		Restlessness
		Aggression
	Motor function	Twitch
		Tremor
		Ataxia
		Catatonia
		Convulsions
		Muscle rigidity or flaccidity
	Sensory function	Excessive or diminished response to stimuli
Respiratory	Respiration	Increased or decreased respiratory rate
		Intermittent respiration
		Dyspnoea
Cardiovascular	Cardiac palpation	Increase or decrease in rate or force
	?Electrocardiography	Disturbances of rhythm.
		Altered ECG pattern (e.g. QT prolongation)
Gastrointestinal	Faeces	Diarrhoea or constipation
		Abnormal form or colour
		Bleeding
	Abdomen	Spasm or tenderness
Genitourinary	Genitalia	Swelling, inflammation, discharge, bleeding
Skin and fur		Discoloration
		Lesions
		Piloerection
Mouth		Discharge
		Congestion
		Bleeding
Eye	Pupil size	Mydriasis or miosis
	Eyelids	Ptosis, exophthalmos
	Movements	Nystagmus
	Cornea	Opacity
General signs	Body weight	Weight loss
	Body temperature	Increase or decrease

they have a similar propensity to cause cancerous changes and to affect growth and development.

The most important end results of genotoxicity – carcinogenesis and impairment of fetal development (teratogenicity) – can only be detected by long-term animal studies. There is, therefore, every reason to pre-screen compounds by in vitro methods, and such studies are routinely carried out before human studies begin. Because in many cases the genotoxicity is due to reactive metabolites rather than to the parent molecule, the in vitro tests generally include assays carried out in the presence of liver microsomes or other liver-derived preparations, so that metabolites are generated. Often, liver microsomes from rats treated with inducing agents (e.g. a mixture of chlorinated biphenyls known as Arochlor 1254) are used, in order to enhance drug metabolizing activity.

Selection and interpretation of tests

Many in vitro and in vivo test systems for mutagenicity have been described, based on bacteria, yeast, insect and mammalian cells (see Gad, 2002 for details). The ICH Guidelines S2A and S2B, stipulate a preliminary battery of three tests:

- *Ames test: a test of mutagenicity in bacteria*. The basis of the assay is that mutagenic substances increase the rate at which a histidine-dependent strain of *Salmonella typhimurium* reverts to a wild type that can grow in the absence of histidine. An increase in the number of colonies surviving in the absence of histidine therefore denotes significant mutagenic activity. Several histidine-dependent strains of the organism which differ in their susceptibility to particular types of mutagen are normally tested in parallel. Positive controls with known mutagens that act directly or only after metabolic activation are routinely included when such tests are performed.
- *An in vitro test for chromosomal abnormalities in mammalian cells or an in vitro mouse lymphoma* tk *cell assay*. To test chromosomal damage Chinese hamster ovary (CHO) cells are grown in culture in the presence of the test substance, with or without liver microsomes. Cell division is arrested in metaphase, and chromosomes are observed microscopically to detect structural aberrations, such as gaps, duplications, fusions or alterations in chromosome number. The mouse lymphoma cell test for mutagenicity involves a heterozygous (*tk* +/–) cell line that can be killed by the cytotoxic agent BrDU. Mutation to the *tk* –/–) form causes the cells to become resistant to BrDU, and so counts of surviving cells in cutures treated with the test compound provide an index of mutagenicity. The mouse lymphoma cell mutation assay is more sensitive than the chromosomal assay, but can give positive results with non-carcinogenic substances. These tests are not possible with compounds that are inherently toxic to mammalian cells.
- *An in vivo test for chromosomal damage in rodent haemopoietic cells*. The mouse micronucleus test is commonly used. Animals are treated with the test compound for 2 days, after which immature erythrocytes in bone marrow are examined for micronuclei, representing fragments of damaged chromosomes.

If these three tests prove negative, no further tests of genotoxicity are generally needed before the compound can be tested in humans. If one or more is positive, further in vitro and in vivo genotoxicity testing will usually be carried out to assess more accurately the magnitude of the risk. In a few cases, where the medical need is great and the life expectancy of the patient population is very limited, development of compounds that are clearly genotoxic – and, by inference, possibly carcinogenic – may still be justified, but in most cases genotoxic compounds will be abandoned without further ado. An updated version of the guideline is open for consultation at the time of writing.

Whereas early toxicological evaluation encompasses acute and subacute types of study, the full safety assessement is based on subchronic and chronic studies. The focus is more on the harmful effects of long-term exposure to 'low' doses of the agent. The chronic toxic effects can be very different from the acute toxic effects, and could accumulate over time. Three main categories of toxicological study are required according to the regulatory guidelines, namely chronic toxicity special tests and toxicokinetic analysis.

CHRONIC TOXICOLOGY STUDIES

The object of these studies is to look for toxicities that appear after repetitive dosing of the compound, when a steady state is achieved, i.e. when the rate of drug administration equals the rate of elimination. In long-term toxicity studies three or more dose levels are tested, in addition to a vehicle control. The doses will include one that is clearly toxic, one in the therapeutic range, and at least one in between. Ideally, the in-between doses will exceed the expected clinical dose by a factor of 10 for rodents and 5 for non-rodents, yet lack overt toxicity, this being the 'window' normally required by regulatory authorities. At least one recovery group is usually included, i.e. animals treated with the drug at a toxic level and then allowed to recover for 2–4 weeks so that the reversibility of the changes observed can be assessed. The aim of these studies is to determine (a) the cumulative biological effects produced by the compound, and (b) at what exposure level (see below) they appear. The initial repeated-dose studies, by revealing the overall pattern of toxic effects produced, also give pointers to particular aspects (e.g. liver toxicity, bone marrow depression) that may need to be addressed later in more detailed toxicological investigations.

The standard procedures discussed here are appropriate for the majority of conventional synthetic compounds intended for systemic use. Where drugs are intended only for topical use (skin creams, eye drops, aerosols, etc.) the test procedures are modified accordingly. Special considerations apply also to biopharmaceutical preparations, and these are discussed briefly below.

Experimental design

Chronic toxicity testing must be performed under GLP conditions, with the formulation and route of administration to be used in humans. Tests are normally carried out on one rodent (usually rat) and one non-rodent species (usually dog), but additional species (such as monkey or pig) may be tested if there are special reasons for suspecting that their responses may predict effects in man more accurately than those of dogs. Pharmacokinetic measurements are included, so that extrapolation to humans can be done on the basis of the concentration of the drug in blood and tissues, allowing for differences in pharmacokinetics between laboratory animals and humans (see Chapter 10). Separate male and female test groups are used. The recommended number of animals per test group (see Gad, 2002) is shown in Table 15.3. There are strong reasons for minimizing the number of animals used in such studies, and the figures given take this into account, representing the minimum shown by experience to be needed for statistically reliable conclusions to be drawn. An average study will require 200 or more rats and about 60 dogs, dosed with compound and observed regularly, including blood and urine sampling, for several months before being killed and autopsied, with tissue samples being collected for histological examination. It is a massive and costly experiment requiring large amounts of compound prepared to GMP standards, the conduct and results of which will receive detailed scrutiny by regulatory authorities, and so careful planning and scrupulous execution are essential.

Regulatory authorities stipulate the duration of repeat-dose toxicity testing required before the start of clinical testing, the ICH recommendations being summarized in Table 20.1. These requirements can be relaxed for drugs aimed at life-threatening diseases, the spur for this change in attitude coming from the urgent need for anti-HIV drugs during the 1980s. In such special cases chronic toxicity testing is still required, but approval for clinical trials – and indeed for marketing – may be granted before they have been completed.

Evaluation of toxic effects

During the course of the experiment all animals are inspected regularly for mortality and gross morbidity, severely affected animals being killed, and all dead animals subjected to autopsy. Specific signs (e.g. diarrhoea, salivation, respiratory changes, etc.) are assessed against a detailed checklist and specific examinations (e.g. blood pressure, heart rate and ECG, ocular changes, neurological and behavioural changes, etc.) are also conducted regularly. Food intake and body weight changes are monitored, and blood and urine samples collected at intervals for biochemical and haematological analysis.

At the end of the experiment all animals are killed and examined by autopsy for gross changes, samples of all major tissues being prepared for histological examination. Tissues from the high-dose group are examined histologically and any tissues showing pathological changes are also examined in the low-dose groups to enable a dose threshold to be estimated. The reversibility of the adverse effects can be evaluated in these studies by studying animals retained after the end of the dosing period.

As part of the general toxicology screening described above, specific evaluation of possible *immunotoxicity* is required by the regulatory authorities, the main concern being immunosuppression. If effects on blood, spleen or thymus cells are observed in the 1-month repeated-dose studies, additional tests are required to evaluate the strength of cellular and humoral responses in immunized animals. A battery of suitable tests is included in the FDA Guidance note (2002).

Table 15.3 Recommended numbers of animals for chronic toxicity studies (Gad, 2002)

Study duration	Rats (per sex)	Dogs (per sex)	Primates (per sex)
4 weeks	5–10	3–4	3
3 months	20	6	5
6 months	30	8	5
12 months	50	10	10
2-year (carcinogenicity)	50–80		

The large body of data collected during a typical toxicology study should allow conclusions to be drawn about the main physiological systems and target organs that underlie the toxicity of the compound, and also about the dose levels at which critical effects are produced. In practice, the analysis and interpretation are not always straightforward, for a variety of reasons, including:

- Incorrect choice of doses
- Variability within the groups of animals
- Spontaneous occurrence of 'toxic' effects in control or vehicle-treated animals
- Missing data, owing to operator error, equipment failure, unexpected death of animals, etc.
- Problems of statistical analysis (qualitative data, multiple comparisons, etc.).

Overall, it is estimated that correctly performed chronic toxicity tests in animals successfully predict 70% of toxic reactions in humans (Olson et al., 2000); skin reactions in humans are the least well predicted.

Biopharmaceuticals

Biopharmaceuticals now constitute more than 25% of new drugs being approved. For the most part they are proteins made by recombinant DNA technology, or monoclonal antibodies produced in cell culture. As a rule, proteins tend to be less toxic than synthetic compounds, mainly because they are normally metabolized to smaller peptides and amino acids, rather than to the reactive compounds formed from many synthetic small molecule compounds, which are the cause of most types of drug toxicity, especially genotoxicity. Biopharmaceuticals are, therefore, generally less toxic than synthetic compounds. Their unwanted effects are associated mainly with 'hyperpharmacology' (see above), lack of pharmacological specificity or immunogenicity. Many protein therapeutics are highly species specific and this often means that safety studies have to be performed in monkeys or that a rodent-selective analogue has to be made. This applies to biological mediators, such as hormones, growth factors, cytokines, etc., as well as to monoclonal antibodies. The presence of impurities in biopharmaceutical preparations has an important bearing on safety assessment, as unwanted proteins or other cell constituents are often present as contaminants, and may vary from batch to batch. Quality control presents more problems than with conventional chemical products, and is particularly critical for biopharmaceuticals.

The safety assessment of new biopharmaceuticals is discussed in ICH Guidance Note S6 and the Addendum issued in June 2011. The main aspects that differ from the guidelines relating to conventional drugs are: (1) careful attention to choice of appropriate species; (2) no need for routine genotoxicity and carcinogenicity testing (though carcinogenicity testing may be required in the case of mediators, such as growth factors, which may regulate cell proliferation); and (3) specific tests for immunogenicity, expressed as sensitization, or the development of neutralizing antibodies.

Newer types of biopharmaceuticals, such as DNA-, RNA- and cell-based therapies (see Chapter 3), pose special questions in relation to safety assessment (see FDA Guidance Note, 1998). Particular concerns arise from the use of genetically engineered viral vectors in gene therapy, which can induce immune responses and in some cases retain potential infectivity. The possibility that genetically engineered foreign cells might undergo malignant transformation is a further worrisome risk. These specialized topics are not discussed further here.

SPECIAL TESTS

In addition to the the general toxicological risks addressed by the testing programme discussed above, the risks of carcinogenicity and effects on reproduction (particularly on fertility and on pre- and postnatal development) may be of particular concern, requiring special tests to be performed.

Carcinogenicity testing

Carcinogenicity testing is normally required before a compound can be marketed – though not before the start of clinical trials – if the drug is likely to be used in treatment continuously for 6 months or more, or intermittently for long periods. It is also required if there are special causes for concern, for example if:

- the compound belongs to a known class of carcinogens, or has chemical features associated with carcinogenicity; nowadays such compounds will normally have been eliminated at the lead identification stage (see Chapter 9)
- chronic toxicity studies show evidence of precancerous changes
- the compound or its metabolites are retained in tissues for long periods.

If a compound proves positive in tests of mutagenicity (see above), it must be *assumed* to be carcinogenic and its use restricted accordingly, so no purpose is served by in vivo carcinogenicity testing. Only in very exceptional cases will such a compound be chosen for development.

ICH Guidelines S1A, S1B and S1C on carcinogenicity testing stipulate one long-term test in a rodent species (usually rat), plus one other in vivo test, which may be either (a) a short-term test designed to show high sensitivity to carcinogens (e.g. transgenic mouse models) or to detect early events associated with tumour initiation or promotion; or (b) a long-term carcinogenicity test in a second rodent species (normally mouse). If positive results emerge in either study, the onus is on the pharmaceutical company to provide evidence that carcinogenicity will not be a significant risk to humans in a therapeutic setting. Until recently, the normal requirement was for long-term studies in two rodent species, but advances in the understanding of tumour biology and the availability of new models that allow quicker evaluation have brought about a change in the attitude of regulatory authorities such that only one long-term study is required, together with data from a well-validated short-term study.

Long-term rat carcinogenicity studies normally last for 2 years and are run in parallel with Phase III clinical trials. (Oral contraceptives require a 3-year test for carcinogenicity in beagles.)

Three or four dose levels are tested, plus controls. Typically, the lowest dose tested is close to the maximum recommended human dose, and the highest is the maximum tolerated dose (MTD) in rats (i.e. the largest dose that causes no obvious side effects or toxicity in the chronic toxicity tests). Between 50 and 80 animals of each sex are used in each experimental group (see Table 15.3), and so the complete study will require about 600–800 animals. Premature deaths are inevitable in such a large group and can easily ruin the study, so that housing the animals under standard disease-free conditions is essential. At the end of the experiment, samples of about 50 different tissues are prepared for histological examination, and rated for benign and malignant tumour formation by experienced pathologists. Carcinogenicity testing is therefore one of the most expensive and time-consuming components of the toxicological evaluation of a new compound. New guidelines for dose selection were adopted from 2008 which allow a more rational approach to the selection of the high dose on the basis of a 25-fold higher exposure of the rodent than that seen in human subjects on the basis of AUC measurements in plasma rather than MTD (Van der Laan, 2008).

Several transgenic mouse models have been developed which provide data more quickly (usually about 6 months) than the normal 2-year carcinogenicity study (Gad, 2002). These include animals in which human proto-oncogenes, such as hRas, are expressed, or the tumour suppressor gene P53 is inactivated. These mice show a very high incidence of spontaneous tumours after about 1 year, but at 6 months spontaneous tumours are rare. Known carcinogens cause tumours to develop in these animals within 6 months.

Advances in this area are occurring rapidly, and as they do so the methodology for carcinogenicity testing is expected to become more sophisticated and faster than the conventional long-term studies used hitherto (www.alttox.org/ttrc/toxicity-tests/carcinogenicity/).

Reproductive/developmental toxicology studies

Two incidents led to greatly increased concern about the effects of drugs on the fetus. The first was the thalidomide disaster of the 1960s. The second was the high incidence of cervical and vaginal cancers in young women whose mothers had been treated with diethylstilbestrol (DES) in early pregnancy with the aim of preventing early abortion. DES was used in this way between 1940 and 1970, and the cancer incidence was reported in 1971. These events led to the introduction of stringent tests for teratogenicity as a prerequisite for the approval of new drugs, and from this flowed concern for other aspects of reproductive toxicology which now must be fully evaluated before a drug is marketed. Current requirements are summarized in ICH Guideline S5A.

Drugs can affect reproductive performance in three main ways:

- Fertility (both sexes, fertilization and implantation), addressed by *Segment 1* studies
- Embryonic and fetal development or teratology, addressed by *Segment 2* studies
- Peri- and postnatal development, addressed by *Segment 3* studies.

It is usually acceptable for Phase I human studies on male volunteers to begin before any reproductive toxicology data are available, so long as the drug shows no evidence of testicular damage in 2- or 4-week repeated-dose studies. The requirement for reproductive toxicology data as a prelude to clinical trials differs from country to country, but, as a general rule, clinical trials involving women of childbearing age should be preceded by relevant reproductive toxicology testing. In all but exceptional cases, such as drugs intended for treating life-threatening diseases, or for use only in the elderly, registration will require comprehensive data from relevant toxicology studies so that the reproductive risk can be assessed.

Segment 1 tests of fertility and implantation involve treating both males (for 28 days) and females (for 14 days) with the drug prior to mating, then measuring sperm count and sperm viability, numbers of implantation sites and live and dead embryos on day 6 of gestation. For drugs that either by design or by accident reduce fertility, tests for reversibility on stopping treatment are necessary.

Segment 2 tests of effects on embryonic and fetal development are usually carried out on two or three species (rat, mouse, rabbit), the drug being given to the female during the initial gestation period (day 6 to day 16 after mating in the rat). Animals are killed just before parturition, and the embryos are counted and assessed for structural abnormalities. In vitro tests involving embryos maintained in culture are also possible. The main stages of early embryogenesis can be observed in this way, and the effects of drugs added to the medium can be monitored. Such in vitro tests are routinely performed in some laboratories, but are currently not recognized by regulatory authorities as a reliable measure of possible teratogenicity.

Segment 3 tests on pre- and perinatal development entail dosing female rats with the drug throughout gestation and lactation. The offspring are observed for motility, reflex responses, etc., both during and after the weaning period, and at intervals some are killed for observations of structural abnormalities. Some are normally allowed to mature and are mated, to check for possible second-generation effects. Mature offspring are also tested for effects on learning and memory.

Reproductive and developmental toxicology is a complex field in which standards in relation to pharmaceuticals have not yet been clearly defined. The experimental studies are demanding, and the results may be complicated by species differences, individual variability and 'spontaneous' events in control animals.

It is obvious that any drug given in sufficient doses to cause overt maternal toxicity is very likely to impair fetal development. Non-specific effects, most commonly a reduction in birthweight, are commonly found in animal studies, but provided the margin of safety is sufficient – say 10-fold – between the expected therapeutic dose and that affecting the fetus, this will not be a bar to developing the compound. The main aim of reproductive toxicology is to assess the risk of specific effects occurring within the therapeutic dose range in humans. Many familiar drugs and chemicals are teratogenic in certain species at high doses. They include *penicillin, sulfonamides, tolbutamide, diphenylhydantoin, valproate, imipramine, acetazolamide, ACE inhibitors* and *angiotensin antagonists*, as well as many *anticancer drugs* and also *caffeine, cannabis* and *ethanol*. Many of these are known or suspected teratogens in humans, and their use in pregnancy is to be avoided. A classification of drugs based on their safety during pregnancy has been developed by the FDA (A, B, C, D or X). Category A is for drugs considered safe in human pregnancy, that is, adequate and well-controlled studies in pregnant women have failed to demonstrate a risk to the fetus in any trimester of pregnancy. Few drugs belong to this category. Category X is reserved for drugs (e.g. *isotretinoin, warfarin*) that have been proved to cause fetal abnormalities in man, and are therefore contraindicated in pregnancy. Category B covers drugs with no evidence of risk in humans; category C covers drugs in which a risk cannot be ruled out; and category D covers drugs with positive evidence of risk. Requirements for the reproductive safety testing of biologicals are laid out in the Addendum to S6 (2011) and there are specific considerations, e.g. the inability of some high-molecular-weight proteins to cross the placenta which do not apply to small molecules.

Other studies

The focus of this chapter is on the core battery of tests routinely used in assessing drug safety at the preclinical level. In practice, depending on the results obtained from these tests, and on the particular therapeutic application and route of administration intended for the drug, it is nearly always necessary to go further with experimental toxicology studies in specific areas. It must be remembered that the regulatory authorities put the onus firmly on the pharmaceutical company to present a dossier of data that covers all likely concerns about safety. Thus, where toxic effects are observed in animals, evidence must be presented to show either that these are seen only at exposure levels well outside the therapeutic range, or that they involve mechanisms that will not apply in humans. If the compound is observed to cause changes in circulating immune cells, or in lymphoid tissues, further tests for immunosuppression will be needed, as well as studies to determine the mechanism. Potential toxicological problems, not necessarily revealed in basic toxicology testing, must also be anticipated. Thus, if the compound is potentially immunogenic (i.e. it is a peptide or protein, or belongs to a known class of haptens), tests for sensitization will be required. For drugs that are intended for topical administration, local tissue reactions, including allergic sensitization, need to be investigated. For some classes of drugs skin photosensitization will need to be tested.

Interaction toxicology studies may be needed if the patients targeted for the treatment are likely to be taking another medicine whose efficacy or toxicity might be affected by the new therapeutic agent.

In summary, it is essential to plan the toxicology testing programme for each development compound on a case-by-case basis. Although the regulatory authorities stipulate the core battery of tests that need to be performed on every compound, it is up to the development team to anticipate other safety issues that are likely to be of concern, and to address them appropriately with experimental studies. In planning the safety assessment programme for a new drug, companies are strongly advised to consult the regulatory authorities, who are very open to discussion at the planning stage and can advise on a case-by-case basis.

TOXICOKINETICS

Toxicokinetics is defined in ICH Guideline S3A as 'the generation of pharmacokinetic data, either as an integral component in the conduct of non-clinical toxicity studies, or in specially designed supportive studies, in order to assess systemic exposure'. In essence, this means pharmacokinetics applied to toxicological studies, and the methodology and principles are no different from those of conventional absorption, distribution, metabolism and excretion (ADME) studies. But whereas ADME studies address mainly drug and metabolite *concentrations* in different body compartments as a function of dose and time, toxicokinetics focuses on *exposure*. Although exposure is not precisely defined, the underlying idea is that toxic effects often appear to be a function of both local concentration and time, a low concentration persisting for a long time being as likely to evoke a reaction as a higher but more transient concentration. Depending on the context, exposure can be represented as peak plasma or tissue concentration, or more often as average concentrations over a fixed period. As with conventional pharmacokinetic measurement, attention must be paid to plasma and tissue binding of the drug and its metabolites, as bound material, which may comprise 98% or more of the measured concentration, will generally be pharmacologically and toxicologically inert. The principles of toxicokinetics as applied to preclinical studies are discussed in detail by Baldrick (2003).

Despite the difficulties of measuring and interpreting exposure, toxicokinetic measurements are an essential part of all in vivo toxicological studies. Interspecies comparisons and extrapolation of animal data to humans are best done on the basis of measured plasma and tissue concentrations, rather than administered dose, and regulatory authorities require this information to be provided.

As mentioned earlier, the choice of dose for toxicity tests is important, and dose-limiting toxicity should ideally be reached in toxicology studies. This is the reason why the doses administered in these studies are always high, unless a maximum limit based on technical feasibility has been reached.

TOXICITY MEASURES

Lethal dose (expressed as LD_{50}, the estimated dose required to kill 50% of a group of experimental animals) has been largely abandoned as a useful measure of toxicity, and no longer needs to be measured for new compounds. Measures commonly used are:

- *no toxic effect level* (NTEL), which is the largest dose in the most sensitive species in a toxicology study of a given duration which produced no observed toxic effect
- *no observed adverse effect level* (NOAEL), which is the largest dose causing neither observed tissue toxicity nor undesirable physiological effects, such as sedation, seizures or weight loss
- *maximum tolerated dose* (MTD), which usually applies to long-term studies and represents the largest dose tested that caused no obvious signs of ill-health
- *no observed effect level* (NOEL), which represents the threshold for producing any observed pharmacological or toxic effect.

The estimated NTEL in the most sensitive species is normally used to determine the starting dose used in the first human trials. The safety factor applied may vary from 100 to 1000, depending on the information available, the type and severity of toxicities observed in animals, and whether these anticipated toxicities can be monitored by non-invasive techniques in man.

VARIABILITY IN RESPONSES

The response to a given dose of a drug is likely to vary when it is given to different individuals or even to the same individual on different occasions. Factors such as age, sex, disease state, degree of nutrition/malnutrition, co-administration of other drugs and genetic variations may influence drug response and toxicity. As elderly people have reduced renal and hepatic function they may metabolize and excrete drugs more slowly, and, therefore, may require lower doses of medication than younger people. In addition, because of multiple illnesses elderly people often may be less able than younger adults to tolerate minor side effects. Likewise, children cannot be regarded as undersized adults, and drug dosages relative to body weight may be quite different. Drug distribution is also different between premature infants and children. The dosages of drugs for children are usually calculated on the basis of weight (mg/kg) or on the basis of body surface area (mg/m^2). These important aspects of drug safety cannot be reliably assessed from preclinical data, but the major variability factors need to be identified and addressed as part of the clinical trials programme.

CONCLUSIONS AND FUTURE TRENDS

No drug is completely non-toxic or safe[2]. Adverse effects can range from minor reactions such as dizziness or skin reactions, to serious and even fatal effects such as anaphylactic reactions. The aims of preclinical toxicology are (a) to reduce to a minimum the risk to the healthy volunteers and the patients to whom the drug will be given in clinical trials; and (b) to ensure that the risk in patients treated with the drug once it is on the market is commensurate with the benefits. The latter is also a major concern during clinical development, and beyond in Phase IV.

It is important to understand the margin of safety that exists between the dose needed for the desired effect and the dose that produces unwanted and possibly dangerous side effects. But the extrapolation from animal toxicology to safety in man is difficult because of the differences between species in terms of physiology, pathology and drug metabolism.

Data from preclinical toxicity studies may be sufficiently discouraging that the project is stopped at that stage. If the project goes ahead, the preclinical toxicology data provide a basis for determining starting doses and dosing regimens

[2]Nor, of course, are any other everyday technologies, such as ladders, kitchen knives, pots of paint or trains. None the less, public opinion seems particularly sensitive to iatrogenic medical risks and is inclined to demand what is impossible, namely 'proof that this drug/vaccine/procedure is 100% safe'.

for the initial clinical trials, and for identifying likely target organs and surrogate markers of potential toxicity in humans. Two particular trends in preclinical toxicology are noteworthy:

- Regulatory requirements tend to become increasingly stringent and toxicology testing more complex as new mechanisms of potential toxicity emerge. This has been one cause, over the years, of the steady increase in the cost and duration of drug development (see Chapter 22). Only in the last 5–10 years have serious efforts been made to counter this trend, driven by the realization that innovation and therapeutic advances are being seriously slowed down, to the detriment, rather than the benefit, of human healthcare. The urgent need for effective drugs against AIDS was the main impetus for this change.
- In an effort to reduce the time and cost of testing, and to eliminate development compounds as early as possible, early screening methods are being increasingly developed and applied during the drug discovery phase of the project, with the aim of reducing the probability of later failure. One such approach is the use of cDNA microarray methods (see Chapter 7) to monitor changes in gene expression resulting from the application of the test compound to tissues or cells in culture. Over- or underexpression of certain genes is frequently associated with the occurrence of specific toxic effects, such as liver damage (Nuwaysir et al., 1999; Pennie, 2000), so that detecting such a change produced by a novel compound makes it likely that the compound will prove toxic, thereby ruling it out as a potential development candidate. Such high-throughput genomics-based approaches enable large databases of gene expression information to be built up, covering a diverse range of chemical structures. The expectation is that the structure–activity patterns thus revealed will enable the prediction in silico of the likely toxicity of a wide range of hypothetical compounds, enabling exclusion criteria to be applied very early in the discovery process. This field of endeavour, dubbed 'toxicogenomics', is expected by many to revolutionize pharmaceutical toxicology (Castle et al., 2002).

At present, extensive toxicity testing in vivo is required by regulatory authorities, and data from in vitro studies carry little weight. There is no likelihood that this will change in the near future (Snodin, 2002). What is clearly changing is the increasing use of in vitro toxicology screens early in the course of a drug discovery programme to reduce the risk of toxicological failures later (see Chapter 10). New guidelines have recently (2009) been introduced to avoid delays in the evaluation of anticancer drugs (S9 ICH). The main impact of new technologies will therefore be – if the prophets are correct – to reduce the attrition rate in development, not necessarily to make drug development faster or cheaper.

REFERENCES

Baldrick P. Toxicokinetics in preclinical evaluation. Drug Discovery Today 2003;8:127–33.

Castle AL, Carver MP, Mendrick DL. Toxicogenomics: a new revolution in drug safety. Drug Discovery Today 2002;7:728–36.

Committee for Proprietary Medicinal Products. Points to consider for the assessment of the potential QT prolongation by non-cardiovascular medicinal products. Publication CPMP 986/96. London: Human Medicines Evaluation Unit; 1997.

De Clerck, F, Van de Water A, D'Aubiol J, et al. In vivo measurement of QT prolongation, dispersion and arrhythmogenesis: application to the preclinical cardiovascular safety pharmacology of a new chemical entity. Fundamental and Clinical Pharmacology 2002; 16:125–40.

FDA Guidance Note. Cell therapy and gene therapy products. 1998. http://www.fda.gov/cber/gdlns/somgene.pdf.

FDA Guidance Note. Immunotoxicology evaluation of investigational new drugs. 2002. www.fda.gov/guidance/index.htm.

Gad SC. Drug safety evaluation. New York: Wiley Interscience; 2002.

Haverkamp W, Breitlandt G, Comm AJ, et al. The potential for QT prolongation and proarrhythmias by non-anti-arrhythmic drugs: clinical and regulatory implications. European Heart Journal 2000;21:1232–7.

ICH Guideline S1A: Guideline on the need for carcinogenicity studies of pharmaceuticals. www.ich.org.

ICH Guideline S1B: Testing for carcinogenicity of pharmaceuticals. www.ich.org.

ICH Guideline S1C: Dose selection for carcinogenicity studies of pharmaceuticals and S1C(R): Addendum: addition of a limit dose and related notes. www.ich.org.

ICH Guideline S2A: Genotoxicity: guidance on specific aspects of regulatory tests for pharmaceuticals. www.ich.org.

ICH Guideline S2B: Genotoxicity: a standard battery for genotoxicity testing for pharmaceuticals. www.ich.org.

ICH Guideline S3A: Note for guidance on toxicokinetics: the assessment of systemic exposure in toxicity studies. www.ich.org.

ICH Guideline S5A: Detection of toxicity to reproduction for medicinal products. www.ich.org.

ICH Guideline S6: Preclinical safety evaluation of biotechnology-derived pharmaceuticals. www.ich.org.

ICH Guideline 6 – Addendum 2011 www.ich.org.

ICH Guideline S7A: Safety pharmacology studies for human pharmaceuticals. www.ich.org.

ICH Guideline S7B: Safety pharmacology studies for assessing the potential for delayed ventricular repolarization (QT interval prolongation) by human pharmaceuticals. www.ich.org.

ICH Guideline S9: Non clinical evaluation for anticancer pharmaceuticals. www.ich.org.

Netzer R, Ebneth E, Bischoff U, et al. Screening lead compounds for QT interval prolongation. Drug Discovery Today 2001;6:78–84.

Nuwaysir EF, Bittner M, Trent J, et al. Microassays and toxicology; the advent of toxicogenomics. Molecular Carcinogenesis 1999;24:152–9.

Olson H, Betton G, Robinson D, et al. Concordance of the toxicity of pharmaceuticals in humans and animals. Regulatory Toxicology and Pharmacology 2000;32: 56–67.

Pennie WD. Use of cDNA microassays to probe and understand the toxicological consequences of altered gene expression. Toxicology Letters 2000;112:473–7.

Snodin DJ. An EU perspective on the use of in vitro methods in regulatory pharmaceutical toxicology. Toxicology Letters 2002;127: 161–8.

Van der Laan JW. Dose selection for carcinogenicity studies of pharmaceuticals. 2008. www.ich.org.

Chapter 16

Pharmaceutical development

T Lundqvist, S Bredenberg

INTRODUCTION

Active pharmaceutical ingredients (API) in pharmaceutical products must be formulated to dosage forms suitable for handling, distribution and adminstration to patients. Common dosage forms are tablets and capsules, liquids for injection, patches for transdermal administration and semisolids for dermal application. Development and documentation of dosage forms is complex involving several stages and areas of expertise. In the preformulation phase the chemical and physicochemical properties of the drug substance are characterized. This information serves together with information about the disease, intended doses and preferred route of administration as the starting point for the formulation development. Stability of the drug substance is a cornerstone in the preformulation phase. Analytical pharmaceutical chemistry is crucial for successful formulation development. Impurities and degradation products must be identified and quantified. Uniformity of content in unit dosage forms is vital to assure that the patient is treated with correct doses.

This chapter describes the main steps involved in pharmaceutical development and is illustrated with examples of the most common formulations, tablets and capsules, since development of these dosage forms contains most of the steps involved in formulation development *per se*. Development of solutions for injection/infusion or other sterile dosage forms are not specifically discussed in this chapter.

PREFORMULATION STUDIES

As a starting point to developing dosage forms, various physical and chemical properties of the drug substance need to be documented. These investigations are termed *preformulation studies*. Most synthetic drugs are either weak bases (~75%) or weak acids (~20%), and will generally need to be formulated as salts. Salts of a range of acceptable conjugate acids or bases therefore need to be prepared and tested. Intravenous formulations of relatively insoluble compounds may need to include non-aqueous solvents or emulsifying agents, and the compatibility of the test substance with these additives, as well as with the commonly used excipients that are included in tablets or capsules, will need to be assessed.

The main components of preformulation studies are:

- Development of a suitable spectroscopic assay method for determining concentration and purity
- Determination of solubility and dissolution rates of parent compound and salts in water and other solvents
- Chemical stability of parent compound and salts in solution and solid state
- Determination of pK_a and pH dependence of solubility and chemical stability
- Determination of lipophilicity (i.e. oil:water partition coefficient, expressed as K_d)
- Determination of particle morphology, melting point and suitability for milling
- Characterizations of importance for the dosage forms of choice, e.g. bulk density, powder flow, angle of repose and compression properties.

Theoretical treatments of these molecular properties, and laboratory methods for measuring them, which are beyond the scope of this book, are described in textbooks such as Burger and Abraham (2003), Aulton (2007) and Allen (2008). Here we consider some issues that commonly arise in drug development.

Solubility and dissolution rate

The question of solubility, already emphasized in Chapters 9 and 10, is particularly important in relation to the development of pharmaceutical formulation. It is measured by standard laboratory procedures and involves determining the concentration of the compound in solution after equilibration – usually after several hours of stirring – with the pure solid. In general, compounds whose aqueous solubility exceeds 10 mg/mL present no problems with formulation (Kaplan, 1972). Compounds with lower solubility are likely to require conversion to salts, or the addition of non-aqueous solvents, in order to achieve satisfactory oral absorption. Because the extreme pH values needed to induce ionization of very weak acids or bases are likely to cause tissue damage, the inclusion of a miscible solvent of relatively low polarity, such as 20% propylene glycol or some other biocompatible solubilizing agent (see below), will often be required for preparing injectable formulations. Complications may arise with oral formulations if the solubility is highly dependent on pH, because of the large pH difference between the stomach and the small intestine. Gastric pH can range from near neutrality in the absence of any food stimulus to acid secretion, to pH 1–2, whereas the intestinal pH is around 8. Basic substances that dissolve readily in the stomach can therefore precipitate in the intestine and fail to be absorbed. Compounds that can exist in more than one crystal form can also show complex behaviours. The different lattice energies of molecules in the different crystal forms mean that the intrinsic solubility of the compound is also different. Different crystal forms may correspond to different hydration states of the compound, so that a solution prepared from the unhydrated solid may gradually precipitate as hydrated crystals. Selecting the best salt form to avoid complications of this sort is an important aspect of preformulation studies.

Compounds that have low intrinsic solubility in aqueous media can often be brought into solution by the addition of a water-miscible *solubilizing agent,* such as polysorbates, ethanol or polyethylene glycol (PEG). Preformulation studies may, therefore, include the investigation of various solubilizing agents, such as methylcellulose or cyclodextrin, which are known to be relatively free of adverse effects in man.

As well as intrinsic solubility, *dissolution rate* is important in determining the rate of absorption of an oral drug. The process of dissolution involves two steps: (a) the transfer of molecules from the solid to the immediately adjacent layer of fluid, known as the *boundary layer;* and (b) escape from the boundary layer into the main reservoir of fluid, which is known as the *bulk phase* and is assumed to be well stirred so that its concentration is uniform. Step (a) is invariably much faster than step (b), so the boundary layer quickly reaches saturation. The overall rate of dissolution is limited by step (b), and depends on the intrinsic solubility of the compound, the diffusion coefficient of the solute, the surface area of the boundary layer, and the geometry of the path leading from the boundary layer to the bulk phase.

In practice, dissolution rates depend mainly on:

- Intrinsic solubility (since this determines the boundary layer concentration)
- Molecular weight (which determines diffusion coefficient)
- Particle size and dispersion of the solute (which determine the surface area of the boundary layer and the length of the diffusion path).

In pharmaceutical development, dissolution rates are often manipulated intentionally by including different polymers, such as methylcellulose into tablets or capsules, to produce 'slow-release' formulations of drugs such as *diclofenac,* allowing once-daily dosage despite the drug's short plasma half-life.

Stability

For routine use, a drug product is expected to have a shelf-life, representing less than 5% decomposition and no significant physical change under normal storage conditions, of at least 3 years.

During the preformulation studies stability tests are often carried out for 1–4 weeks. The chemical stability of the solid is measured at temperatures ranging from 4 to 75°C, and moisture uptake at different relative humidities is also assessed.

Measurements of stability in solution at pH values ranging from 1 to 11 at room temperature and at 37°C will be performed, including formulations with solubilizing agents where appropriate. Sensitivity to UV and visible light, and to exposure to oxygen, is also measured.

The rate of degradation in short-term studies under these harsh conditions is used to give a preliminary estimate of the likely rate of degradation under normal storage conditions. Sensitivity to low pH means that degradation is likely to occur in the stomach, requiring measures to prevent release of the compound until it reaches the intestine.

These preformulation stability tests serve mainly to warn that further development of the compound may be difficult or even impossible. Definitive tests of the long-term (3 years or more) stability of the formulated preparation will be required at a later stage of development for regulatory purposes.

Particle size and morphology

Ideally, for incorporation into a tablet or capsule the drug substance needs to exist in small, uniformly sized particles, forming a smoothly flowing powder which can be uniformly blended with the excipient material. Rarely, the compound will emerge from the chemistry laboratory as non-hygroscopic crystals, and the melting point will be sufficiently high that it can be reduced to a uniform fine powder by mechanical milling. More often it will take the form of an amorphous, somewhat waxy solid, and additional work will be needed later in development to produce it in a form suitable for incorporation into tablets or capsules.

Preformulation studies are designed to reveal how far the available material falls short of this ideal. Various laboratory methods are available for analysing particle size and morphology, but in the preformulation stage simple microscopic observation is the usual method.

Particles larger than a few micrometres, particularly if the particle size is very variable, are difficult to handle and mix uniformly. Hygroscopic materials and polymorphic crystal forms are a disadvantage, as already mentioned. These issues are unlikely to matter greatly in the early stages of development, as Phase I studies can usually be carried out with liquid formulations if necessary, but can be a major hurdle later, so the main aim of the preformulation studies is to give a warning of likely problems to come.

ROUTES OF ADMINISTRATION AND DOSAGE FORMS

With the knowledge of the characteristics of the drug substance from preformulation studies, the administration route has to be selected and the substance to be included into a dosage form which is effective and convenient for the patient. The preferred dosage form for therapeutic agents is almost always an oral tablet or capsule, either taken as needed to control symptoms, or taken regularly once or several times a day. However, there are many alternatives, and Table 16.1 lists some of the main ones. An important consideration is whether it is desirable to achieve *systemic exposure* (i.e. distribution of the drug to all organs via the bloodstream) or *selective local exposure* (e.g. to the lungs, skin or rectum) by applying the drug topically. In most cases systemic exposure will be required, and an oral capsule or tablet will be the desired final dosage form. Even so, an intravenous formulation will normally be required for use in safety pharmacology, toxicology and pharmacokinetic studies in man.

Table 16.1 The main routes of administration and dosage forms

Exposure required	Routes of administration	Dosage forms	
Systemic	Oral	Tablet, capsule, solution, suspension, emulsion	Liquid forms are particularly suitable for children, and for patients unable to swallow tablets. Unsuitable for foul-tasting medicines
	Parenteral		
	Injection (intravenous, subcutaneous, intramuscular) Needle-free injection	Solution, emulsion, suspension, implant	Examples: cytotoxic drugs liable to damage GI tract, drugs needed for unconscious patients, drugs unstable in GI tract (e.g. peptide hormones)
	Percutaneous	Skin patches	
	Inhalation	Gas, vapour	Applicable mainly to anaesthetic agents
	Intranasal	Aerosol	Used for some hormone preparations that are not absorbed orally, e.g. vasopressin analogues, gonadotropin-releasing hormone
Topical	Skin	Ointment, cream, gel, aerosol	
	Respiratory tract	Aerosol, inhaled powder	
	Rectum, vagina	Suppository	
	Eye	Solution, ointment	

The main routes of administration for drugs acting systemically, apart from oral and injectable formulations, are *transdermal, intranasal and oromucosal. Rectal, vaginal* and *pulmonary* routes are also used in some cases, though these are used mainly for drugs that act locally.

Transdermal administration of drugs formulated as small adhesive skin patches has considerable market appeal, even though such preparations are much more expensive than conventional formulations. To be administered in this way, drugs must be highly potent, lipid soluble and of low molecular weight. Examples of commercially available patch formulations include *nitroglycerin, scopolamine, fentanyl, nicotine, testosterone, estradiol* and *ketoprofen*, and several others in development. The main limitation is the low permeability of the skin to most drugs and the small area covered, which mean that dosage is limited to a few milligrams per day, so only very potent drugs can be given systemically via this route of administration. Variations in skin thickness affect the rate of penetration, and the occurrence of local skin reactions is also a problem with some drugs. Various penetration enhancers, mainly surfactant compounds of the sort discussed above, are used to improve transdermal absorption. The transfer rate can be greatly enhanced by applying a small and painless electric current (about 0.5 mA/cm^2), and this is effective in achieving transfer of peptides (e.g. *calcitonin)* and even *insulin* through the skin. It also offers promise as a route of administration of oligonucleotides in gene therapy applications (see Chapter 12). These procedures are used for administration of nucleotides and in gene therapy and are being used experimentally in the clinic, but are not yet available as commercial products for routine clinical use. Ultrasonic irradiation is also under investigation as a means of facilitating transdermal delivery. These procedures would also allow the administration to be controlled according to need. Intranasal drug administration (Illium, 2002, 2003) is another route that has been used successfully for a few drugs. The nasal epithelium is much more permeable than skin and allows the transfer of peptide drugs as well as low-molecular-weight substances. Commercially available preparations have been developed for peptide hormones, such as *vasopressin analogues, calcitonin, buserelin* and others, as well as for conventional drugs such as *triptans, opioids*, etc. The main disadvantages are that substances are quickly cleared from the nasal epithelium by ciliary action, as well as being metabolized, and the epithelial permeability is not sufficient to allow most proteins to be given in this way. Ciliary clearance can be reduced by the use of gel formulations, and surfactant permeability enhancers can be used to improve the penetration of larger molecules. The possibility of administering insulin, growth factors or vaccines by this route is the subject of active research efforts. Some studies have suggested (see Illium, 2003) that substances absorbed through the nasal epithelium reach the brain more rapidly than if they are given intravenously, possibly bypassing the blood–brain barrier by reaching the CNS directly via the nerves to the olfactory bulb.

Oromucosal delivery (Madhav et al., 2009) and especially utilizing the buccal and sublingual mucosa as the absorption site is a drug delivery route which promotes rapid absorption and almost immediate pharmacological effect. The sublingual mucosa, especially, is highly vascularized and this route bypasses the gastrointestinal tract and, thus, the first-pass metabolism. However, not all drugs can be efficiently absorbed through the oral mucosa because of physicochemical properties or enzymatic breakdown of the drug and the amount of drug that could be absorbed is limited to a few milligrams. The drug has to be soluble, stable and able to easily permeate the mucosal barrier at the administration site. Also some formulation aspects have to be taken into consideration, using a tablet formulation for a rapid onset of effect a prerequisite is a fast disintegration and dissolution in the oral cavity resulting in an optimal exposure of active substance to the small volume of dissolving fluids. Swallowing of the drug could be a potential problem, but can be minimized by using technologies using mucoadhesive components (Bredenberg et al., 2003; Brown and Hamed, 2007). An optimized formulation and using this administration route has the potential for very fast absorption (Kroboth et al., 1995) and obtaining peak blood levels within 10 to 15 minutes. It is thereby potentially a more comfortable and convenient alternative to the intravenous route of administration.

FORMULATION

Formulation of an active substance into a dosage form, where there are no special requirements for modified release, involves a good deal of engineering. As already mentioned, the 'ideal' drug substance, intended for use as an oral preparation, has the following characteristics:

- Water solubility
- Chemical stability (including stability at low pH)
- Permeability across the gastrointestinal epithelium
- Good access to site of action (e.g. blood–brain barrier penetration, if intended to work in the brain)
- Resistance to first-pass metabolism.

If these conditions are met the formulation of oral formulations presents no special problems, but they rarely are, and it falls to the pharmaceutical development group to develop formulations that successfully overcome the shortcomings of the compound. Firstly, the drug substance must be dried and converted to a powder form that can be precisely dispensed. Further, depending on the dosage form and the desired properties, other substances called excipients, have to be included.

As mentioned above, tablets and capsules are the most common dosage form (probably due to a combination of convenience for the patient and a cost-effective manufacturing process, at least for conventional tablets). Even for a tablet without special requirements for its drug release profile a range of excipients are needed, e.g. the tablet should be sufficiently strong to withstand handling but also has to disintegrate after intake in order to release the drug.

Inert diluents or fillers, such as lactose or starch, are added to produce tablets of a manageable size (generally 50–500 mg). The filler should have good compactability and flow properties, be non-hygroscopic and have acceptable taste. Binders, such as cellulose and other polymeric materials, may be needed to assist compaction into a solid tablet that will not crumble. A binder could be added both in dry form and in the granulation liquid depending on the manufacturing process. Disintegrating agents, such as starch and cellulose, ensure that the tablet disintegrates rapidly in the gastrointestinal tract. For a very fast disintegration, so-called super disintegrants acting to produce extensive swelling could be used. Slippery, non-adherent materials, such as magnesium stearate, may be needed to ensure that the powder runs smoothly in the tablet machine, by reduction of friction between particles and between particles and parts of the machine in contact. The tablet may need to be coated with cellulose or sugar to disguise its taste.

Capsule formulations are often used for initial clinical trials, as they are generally simpler to develop than compressed tablets, but are less suitable for controlled-release formulations (see below). A two-piece gelatin capsule can be used to contain drugs also in semisolid or liquid form. Other advantages are that capsules are easy to swallow and provide effective taste-masking. Drug dissolution rate could, with a fast dissolving capsule, be increased compared to a conventional tablet resulting in improved drug absorption, especially for poorly soluble substances.

The choice of excipients and the manufacturing process is very much dependent on the characteristics of drug substance and the desired properties of the dosage form. Drug release profile is just one aspect, while the homogeneity or uniformity of content is another. If the drug substance is very potent and cohesive then mixing a small amount of drug with a high amount of filler could lead to a product with low homogeneity. This problem is most severe if the drug particles are micronized to improve the dissolution rate. Then it is important to also choose the most appropriate manufacturing process, such as dry mixing with larger filler paticles, so-called ordered or interactive mixing, wet granulation or drug coating of placebo tablets. Different processes used in drug development and manufacturing are described in textbooks such as Aulton (2007).

As mentioned in the preformulation section the shelf-life of the drug product should preferably be at least 3 years. The presence of moisture is the main contributor to the degradation of the drug substance. Tablets normally have a longer shelf-life than other formulations such as oral and parental liquids since they are a dry dosage form. However, it is important to choose excipients which are not hygroscopic since small amounts of moisture could decrease the stability of the drug. Therefore, selection of the packing material is also an important aspect to take into consideration: for example, moisture-sensitive freeze-dried tablets are often packed in almost impenetrable aluminium blisters.

In reality, formulation development has to take into account not only the properties of the drug substance, but also the desired delivery system and the form of the final product. In developing a new nitrate preparation for treating angina, for example, the preferred delivery system might be a skin patch to be packaged in a foil sachet, or a nasal spray to be packaged as a push-button aerosol can. Although a simple oral preparation may be feasible, the medical need and patient convenience might require the development of different dosage forms, and the development plan would have to be directed towards this more demanding task.

PRINCIPLES OF DRUG DELIVERY SYSTEMS

In recent years, drug delivery systems have become progressively more sophisticated, for three main reasons. First, biopharmaceuticals represent an increasing proportion of new drugs. They are very unlikely to conform to the 'ideal' profile summarized above, and so ingenuity in formulation is often needed to turn them into viable products. Second, there is increasing emphasis on selective targeting of drugs to sites of disease via the use of specialized delivery systems. This is particularly relevant for anticancer drugs. Third, controllable delivery systems are being developed for specific indications. The use of electrophoresis to provide a steady flux of drug through the skin (see below) appears promising and has been applied, for example, to the treatment of pain using fentanyl as the active drug. A further step is to incorporate sensors (e.g. for blood glucose concentration) into devices that control the delivery of insulin, in order to provide feedback control of blood glucose.

Polymers and surfactants

Combining the drug substance with different polymers and surfactants permits it to adopt states that are intermediate between the pure solid and a free aqueous solution. Polymers in colloidal, gel or solid form can be used to entrap drug molecules, and have many applications in drug formulations (Torchilin, 2001; Dimitriu, 2002; Kim et al., 2009; Savic et al., 2010):

- Polymers and surfactants in liquid form give rise to micelles or emulsions, which can greatly enhance the solubility of drug molecules while at the same time protecting them from chemical degradation, and sometimes improving permeation through tissue barriers, such as the gastrointestinal epithelium and the blood–brain barrier.
- Polymers that form soft hydrated gels are used mainly in topical dermatological preparations.
- Solid gel formulations can be used as implantable depot preparations which can be inserted under the skin to give sustained release of the drug (see below). Skin patches can be made from sheet of such a flexible polymer, loaded with the drug substance.
- Polymers are commonly used in tablets and capsules for several purposes, either to facilitate the manufacturing process or for a specific drug release profile, e.g. binders, disintegrants, film coating agents.

The range of polymers available for drug formulation is vast. A few important examples are shown in Figure 16.1. By combining hydrophilic and hydrophobic domains in a single polymer, as in 'Pluronic', micelle formation is encouraged (see below). The inclusion of acidic or basic side chains, as in polyaspartate or polylysine, enables the polymer to bind oppositely charged drug molecules, thereby increasing their effective solubility.

Micelles

Micelles (Figure 16.2) consist of aggregates of a few hundred *amphiphilic* molecules that contain distinct hydrophilic and hydrophobic regions. In an aqueous medium, the molecules cluster with the hydrophilic regions facing the surrounding water and the hydrophobic regions forming an inner core. Micelles typically have diameters of 10–80 nm, small enough not to sediment under gravity, and to pass through most filters. Micelle-forming substances have limited aqueous solubility, and

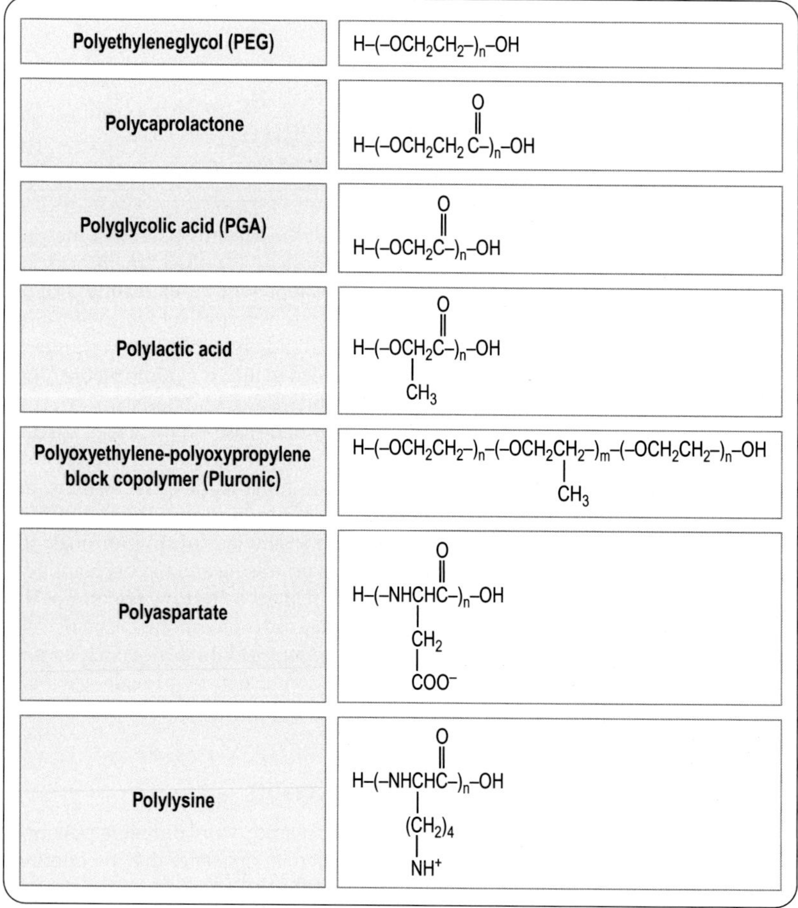

Fig. 16.1 Amphiphilic polymer.

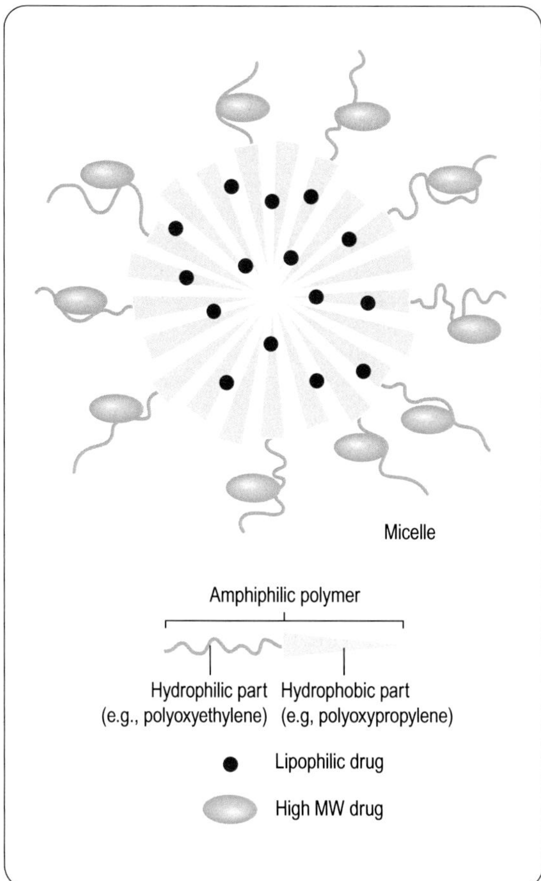

Fig. 16.2 Structures of some common pharmaceutical polymers.

when the free aqueous concentration reaches a certain point – the *critical micelle concentration* – typically in the millimolar range, micelles begin to form; further addition of the substance increases their abundance. With some compounds, as the density of micelles increases a gel is formed, consisting of a loosely packed array of micelles interspersed with water molecules. Lipophilic drug molecules often dissolve readily in the inner core allowing concentrations to be achieved that greatly exceed the aqueous solubility limit of the drug. Amphiphilic substances also tend to associate with micelles, as do high-molecular-weight substances such as peptides and proteins, which have affinity for surfaces, on account of the large surface area which micelles present.

Micelle formation is a natural property of bile acids, which are secreted into the duodenum under physiological conditions and which play an important role in fat absorption by the intestine. Micellar drug formulations are thus an extension of a normal physiological process. Micellar absorption by the gastrointestinal tract is directed mainly to the lymphatic system rather than the vascular system. Thus, unlike substances absorbed directly from aqueous solution, micelle-associated compounds tend to bypass the hepatic portal circulation, and thereby escape first-pass metabolism.

Micelle formation is a general property of amphiphilic molecules, and many chemical forms have been developed for pharmaceutical use (Pillai and Panchagnula, 2001; Torchilin, 2001). Some examples are shown in Figure 16.2, and additional information on the many types of polymers used in pharmaceutical formulation is given by Kumar and Kumar (2001), as well as in many textbooks (e.g. Ansel et al., 1999; Dimitriu 2002; Aulton, 2007). A particularly versatile group is that of *copolymers*, containing more than one type of polymer unit, one of which, typically, is hydrophilic (e.g. polyethylene glycol), whereas the other is hydrophobic (e.g. polypropylene glycol). Alternating blocks of these two units form a copolymer (known commercially as Pluronic, see Figure 16.2) which is commonly used in drug formulations. Copolymers of this sort at low concentrations form a liquid micellar suspension, but at higher concentrations the micelles may aggregate in an ordered array to form a water-containing gel. Such gel formulations are commonly used to prepare controlled-release preparations (see below). The polymer components may include anionic or cationic groups, which have the effect of altering their affinity for charged drug molecules, and also of altering their pharmacokinetic behaviour.

Micelles and other drug vehicles, such as cyclodextrins and liposomes (see below), have a considerable – and generally beneficial – effect on the pharmacokinetic properties of the drug. Often, but not invariably, absorption from gastrointestinal tract is improved, though the reasons for this are not well understood. Preferential uptake into lymphatics, as mentioned above, reduces the extent of first-pass metabolism. Circulating micelles protect the drug from metabolic degradation, so the plasma half-life is generally prolonged. Micelles are too large to cross 'tight' capillary endothelium, so transfer across the blood–brain barrier is not increased. They are able to cross the fenestrated capillaries that occur in most tissues, but the rate of permeation is less than that of the uncomplexed drug. Malignant tumours and inflamed tissues generally have rather leaky capillaries with large fenestrations, so that transfer of micellar drug complexes into such tissues is more rapid than into normal tissues. This mechanism results in a degree of selectivity in the distribution of the drug to diseased tissues, a phenomenon known as *passive targeting* (see below).

Liposomes

Liposomes were first discovered in 1965 and proposed as drug carriers soon afterwards (see Samad et al., 2007 for a

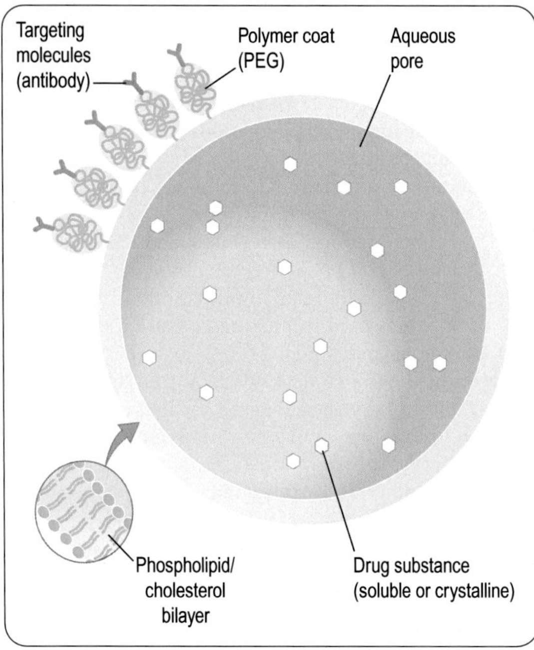

Fig. 16.3 Structure of drug delivery liposome.

recent short review). They are microscopic vesicles formed when an aqueous suspension of phospholipid is exposed to ultrasonic agitation. Depending on the conditions, large multilayered vesicles 1–5 μm in diameter, or small single-layered vesicles 0.02–0.1 μm in diameter, may be formed. The vesicles are bounded by a phospholipid bilayer, which is impermeable to non-lipophilic compounds. They can act as drug carriers in various ways (Figure 16.3):

- Non-lipophilic drugs are carried in solution in the aqueous core, by adding them to the aqueous medium in which the liposomes are produced. Techniques for introducing drug molecules into preformed liposomes have also been described.
- Lipophilic drugs occupy the phospholipid membrane phase.
- Some peptides and proteins, as well as amphiphilic drugs, can be sequestered at the lipid–water interface.

The main purpose of using liposomes is to improve the pharmacokinetic behaviour of drugs. Drugs contained in liposomes are inaccessible to metabolizing enzymes and transport systems, and their effective biological half-life is determined by the rate of clearance of the liposomes. These drug-containing vesicles are easy and cheap to manufacture, and in most cases are stable as aqueous suspensions. Simple phospholipid-based liposomes are unsatisfactory as drug carriers for several reasons: they are relatively permeable to drug molecules and tend to disintegrate in the circulation, and so fail to retain the drug satisfactorily; and their circulating half-life is short, because they are rapidly taken up by tissue macrophages, mainly in liver and spleen, so these tissues receive most of the drug as a brief bolus. The biological characteristics of liposomes, however, can be improved by chemical modifications of various kinds:

- The inclusion of cholesterol, and other alterations of the phospholipid composition, improves the stability of liposomes and renders them less permeable to drug molecules.
- Attaching other substances to their surface. Such substances include polyethylene glycol (PEG; see Figure 16.3), charged compounds, or antibodies directed at antigens expressed by tissues in which the drug is intended to act.

Altering the size, lipid composition and charge on the vesicle surface affects the rate at which circulating liposomes are taken up by tissue macrophages. Liposomes are not generally suitable for oral administration, as they are destroyed by enzymes and bile acids in the small intestine. Nor do they cross the blood–brain barrier, so they cannot be used to improve the access of drugs to the brain. Despite an extensive literature acclaiming liposomes as the answer to almost every imaginable formulation problem, the application of liposome technology in commercial products is so far limited to a very few examples, in the field of anticancer and antifungal drugs. Liposome technology has received much attention in the design of drug delivery systems (e.g. Harrington et al., 2002; Sapra and Allen, 2003; Gabizon et al., 2006), though the developments mostly are at the experimental stage and remain to show added value in clinical applications. Recent reviews providing information on trends and expectations in this field include Barratt (2003), Sapra and Allen (2003), Goyal et al. (2005) and Samad et al. (2007).

Nanontechnology more then nanoparticles

Nanotechnology, using materials in the nanometre scale, is a new rapidly growing scientific field. The first approved products using formulations based on nanoparticles were liposomes, polymer protein conjugates polymeric substances or suspensions (EMEA, 2006). Medical applications of nanontechnology (nanomedicine) has also been suggested to have the potential to create new 'intelligent materials' in nano scale to be used as diagnostic materials, in stents with and without drugs. In drug development the technology has been suggested to have a great potential for targeted drug delivery in the treatment of cancer and organ-specific drug delivery, e.g. to CNS (Singh and Lillard, 2009). However, the safety issue of delivering such small particles is currently also under discussion and evaluation (e.g. EMEA 2006; De Jong and Borm, 2008). Several new drug-delivery technologies using a number of materials

Table 16.2 Drug delivery applications of nanotechnology

Drug delivery system	Application
Liposomes	Targeting drug/ oligonucleotide/gene delivery
Micelles	Targeting drug/ oligonucleotide/gene delivery
Nanoemulsions and nanogels	CNS disorders, targeted across blood–brain barrier
Nanoparticles, e.g. metallic, mesoporous silica, solid lipids	Carrier, site-specific delivery and contrast agents in cancer therapy Oligonucleotides
Nanoprobes	Biomarkers

such as polymers, metals and ceramics are under development where surfaces or pores in nanoscale are loaded with pharmaceutical substances. The drug release is rate determined or programmed using nanotechnology and conventional pharmaceutical formulation principles in combination. Besides the size other physicochemical properties, such as surface properties, particle morphology and structure, and drug release are of importance for understanding and interpreting in vivo results (Putheti et al., 2008). Table 16.2 exemplifies drug delivery applications of nanotechnology.

Modified-release drug formulations

The most common challenge in drug formulation is to shorten the time to onset of action or prolong the duration of action of a drug. In either situation the rate of absorption must be determined by the rate of release of the active substance from the dosage form. The most common method is to delay the rate of release of the drug substance from the dosage form causing it to be absorbed gradually. Ideally, the rate of absorption should reach a steady level that is maintained for hours or days, depending on the application, until the reservoir is used up. This is known as *sustained release*. It is widely used to produce once-daily oral preparations, or long-lasting depot injections (e.g. contraceptives, hormone replacements, antipsychotic drugs) where the drug effect is required to last for weeks or months.

Other types of modified release include *delayed release*, used mainly for oral drugs that are unstable at the low pH of the stomach, and *controlled release*, produced by specialized devices that allow the rate of release to be adjusted according to need. Some of the approaches used to develop controlled-release formulations are discussed briefly below.

There are many different ways of producing sustained-release oral preparations, some of which are shown in Figure 16.4. They rely mainly on the use of impermeable coatings that are slowly eroded as the pill passes through the gut, or water-absorbing polymer gels which slowly become hydrated. Injectable implants operate in the same way over a longer period, and have the advantage that they can be removed if necessary. Depot injections of drugs dissolved in oil can also be used to provide long-lasting sustained release, but these generally produce a less constant rate of administration and cannot be removed.

Controlled release represents a stage beyond sustained release and involves coupling a sensing mechanism, responding to changes in temperature or pH, for example, to the drug release mechanism. Examples of the many kinds of device that could meet this need include temperature-sensitive liposomes, which disintegrate when the temperature is increased to, say, 40 °C, and temperature-sensitive polymers which aggregate into a gel when the temperature is increased. The idea is that local heating of a tumour will cause the drug to be released at that site. Another example is the pH-sensitive system, which can be used to delay the release of acid-sensitive drugs (particularly peptides) until they have passed beyond the stomach. Drug delivery can also, in principle, be targeted to regions of low pH, such as inflamed or hypoxic tissues, by the use of pH-sensitive polymers. A particularly ingenious approach is to incorporate insulin into pH-sensitive gels loaded with glucose oxidase (known to specialists in this field as *GOD-gels*). If the ambient glucose concentration increases, enzymic oxidation causes a fall in pH and the release of insulin. (For more details of 'responsive' polymers and their application in controlled drug delivery, see Soppimath et al. (2002), Gupta et al. (2002) and Kim et al. (2009).)

Delivery and formulation of biopharmaceuticals

In contrast to traditional small drug molecules biopharmaceutical drugs are protein-based, built up of amino acid chains, and structurally complex with many functional groups. Examples are: human insulin in diabetes therapy, different vaccines and interferons in, e.g., lung cancer, leukaemia and hepatitis therapy (see Chapter 12). Since these molecules are large, the diffusional transport across epithelial barriers in the gastrointestional tract is slow, and enzymes present there result in fast degradation of the molecules; a majority of the biotech drugs are, therefore, delivered via the parenteral route. Despite that, the market for biotech products is growing and they accounted for one-fifth of all blockbuster drugs in the US market in 2008 (Malik, 2008).

Formulation of proteins and peptides are a real challenge since they are usually more unstable compared to

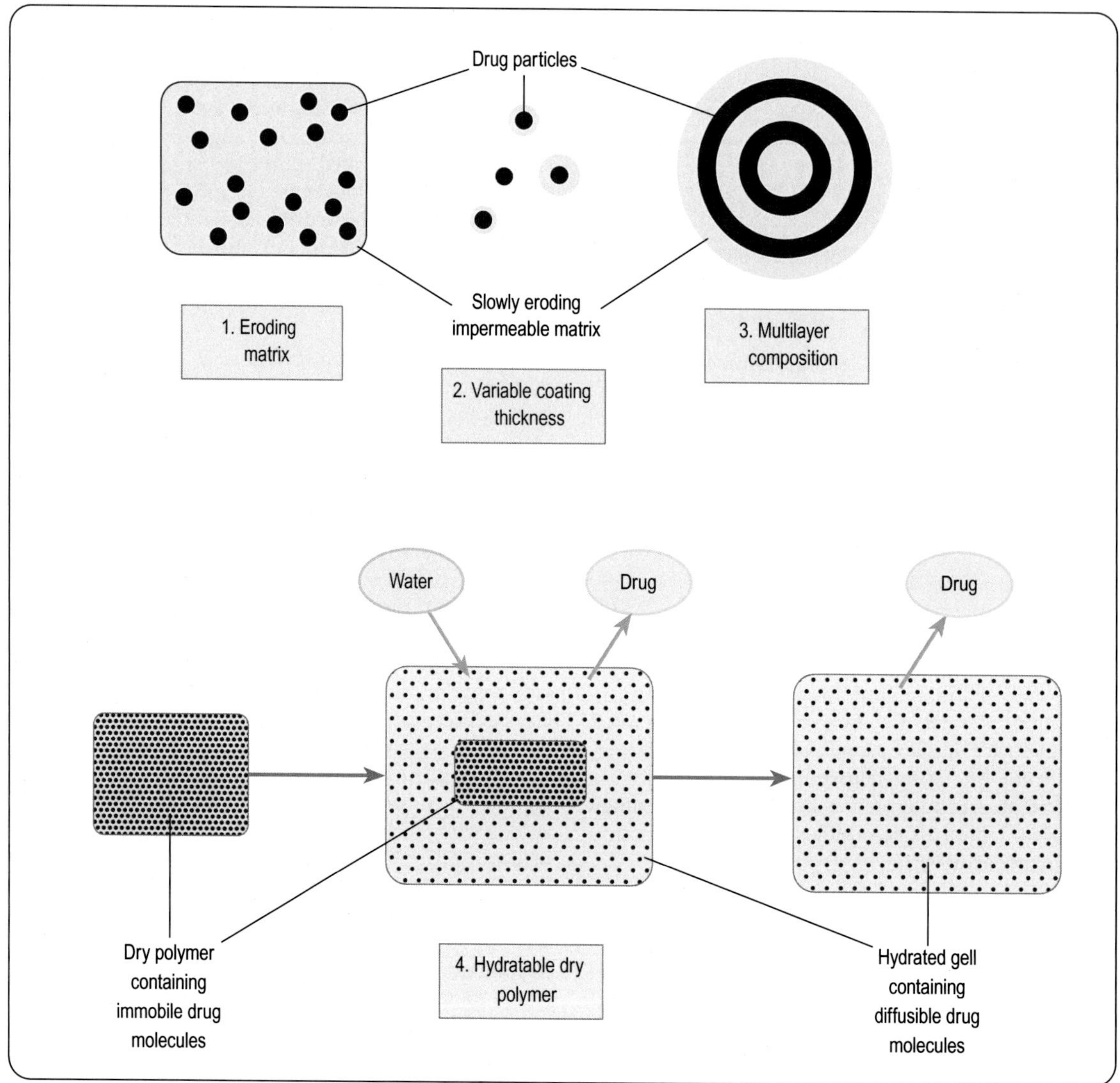

Fig. 16.4 Types of sustained-release preparation.

small molecules and the formulation strategy needs a high focus on stabilization. The structures are often both chemically and physically unstable. These molecules are often designed for specific mechanisms of action; loss of activity can arise with, for example, increased temperature or a change in pH and, therefore, heating should obviously be avoided and the right pH conditions need to be selected. Biopharmaceuticals also have fast degradation in aqueous solutions and, therefore, freeze-drying is a common technique to transfer them into a dry state for longer shelf-life. However, it is important to select the right temperature and pressure to avoid damage of the molecule during the process. Further instability problems that could arise with biopharmaceuticals are protein aggregation and oxidation. Liposomes, micelles and the addition of polymers and surfactants, as described above, are used to overcome these stability problems with biopharmaceuticals.

Drug delivery to the central nervous system

Brain capillaries, unlike those in most parts of the body, are non-fenestrated, so that drug molecules must traverse the endothelial cells, rather than passing between them, to move from circulating blood to the extracellular space of the brain (see Chapter 10). Three main routes of access are important (Scherrmann, 2002):

- Lipophilic compounds of low molecular weight cross the membrane of endothelial cells very easily, and

comprise the great majority of CNS-acting drugs. Peptides, proteins, non-lipophilic or ionized drugs are, for the most part, unable to cross the endothelial cell membrane.
- The endothelial cells also possess various active transport mechanisms that can allow certain non-lipophilic compounds to enter the brain. Examples include *levodopa*, used for treating Parkinson's disease, *baclofen*, a GABA analogue used to treat spasticity, and the cytotoxic drug *melphalan*, all of which are transported across the blood–brain barrier by the amino acid transporter. Attempts have been made to couple other drugs with amino acids or sugars which are carried via this transport system. Despite being successful in animal models, however, such compounds have not been developed for clinical use. Active transport out of the brain also occurs with many compounds, including drugs such as *penicillins*, which are able to enter passively.
- Molecules can be carried as endocytotic vesicles across the endothelial cells. This type of transcytosis occurs with molecules that are bound to receptors or other proteins on the endothelial cell surface. An approach that has been tested extensively, though not yet applied for clinical use, is to couple active peptides and proteins to the monoclonal antibody OX26, which recognizes the endothelial transferrin receptor. Binding to this receptor stimulates transcytosis, carrying the antibody and its cargo across the blood–brain barrier. Transcytosis can also be stimulated by the non-specific binding of small cationic peptides to the acidic glycoprotein components of the endothelial cell surface. Conjugates of various cytotoxic and antimicrobial drugs to such peptides show improved brain penetration in animal models, and may prove to be applicable clinically.

Recent approaches for improving drug delivery to the brain are described in more detail by Denora et al. (2009), Patel et al. (2009) and Pardridge (2010).

Enabling impermeant drugs to reach the brain represents a major challenge for formulation chemists, and there are actually very few examples where it has been overcome. Most often, the drug molecule has to be redesigned to increase its lipophilicity. Formation of a lipid-soluble prodrug is one strategy, but is rarely effective in this context because conversion to the active, non-lipophilic compound is likely to take place in the circulation before the drug reaches the brain.

SUMMARY

Pharmaceutical development comprises all the activities needed to turn a therapeutic drug substance into a marketable product that will perform reliably when used in real life. Preformulation studies consist of a series of chemical and physicochemical investigations on the drug substance which indicate the kinds of formulation that are likely to be satisfactory. In some cases problems (for example, poor solubility or chemical instability) will emerge at this stage, requiring modification of the drug molecule before development can proceed – in other words, back to the drawing board. Therefore it is important to run preformulation activities in parallel with early drug development of new chemical entitites.

The process of formulation will depend greatly not only on information from preformulation activites, but also on the medical condition and on the intended route of administration of the drug. In most cases, where the intention is to produce a tablet or capsule for oral use, an intravenous formulation will also be developed for use in clinical trials, and the oral form used in initial efficacy trials (clinical Phase II) may not be the same as the intended marketed form.

Even in cases where no problems are encountered, formulation studies require considerable time and resources. The end result has to be a product that can be manufactured on a large scale and meet strict quality-control standards, and can be stored in thousands of homes under varying conditions of temperature and humidity without significant deterioration.

Very often pharmaceutical development is called on to improve the characteristics of the drug substance, for example by improving its solubility using amorphous substances or new salts, disguising its taste, increasing its plasma half-life or reducing unwanted effects, and work of this kind increases the value of a substance clinically and commercially. Increasing use is being made of colloidal systems, such as micelles, polymers and liposomes as vehicles for drug molecules. Such formulations have a considerable effect on the drug's pharmacokinetic properties, and can also be used to achieve a degree of targeting of the drug to the tissues on which it is required to act. Drug targeting based on these and other principles, e.g. antibodies, are currently the subject of much experimental work. The principles have only proved applicable so far to a few anticancer and antifungal drugs, but many more applications are expected in the foreseeable future.

Overall, work on more sophisticated formulations, new routes of administration and new delivery systems, e.g. based on nanotechnology for currently used drugs and biopharmaceuticals, is thought likely to contribute as much to improved therapeutics as the discovery of new drugs, and is seen by the pharmaceutical industry as an important parallel approach to drug discovery, particularly at times – like the present – when drug discovery runs into a phase of disappointingly low productivity.

REFERENCES

Allen LV. The art, science and technology of pharmaceutical compounding. 3rd ed. Washington DC: American Pharmaceutical Association; 2008.

Ansel HC, Allen LV, Popovich NG. Pharmaceutical dosage forms and drug delivery systems. 7th ed. Baltimore: Lippincott Williams & Wilkins; 1999.

Aulton ME, editor. Aulton's pharmaceutics. The design and manufacture of medicines. 3rd ed. Edinburgh: Churchill Livingstone; 2007.

Barratt G. Colloidal drug carriers: achievements and perspectives. Cellular and Molecular Life Sciences 2003;60:21–37.

Bredenberg S, Duberg M, Lennernäs B, et al. In vitro and pharmacokinetic evaluation of a new sublingual tablet system for rapid oromucosal absorption using fentanyl citrate as the active substance. European Journal of Pharmaceutical Sciences 2003;20:327–34.

Brown BA-S, Hamed E. oraVescent® Technology offers greater oral transmucosal delivery. Drug Delivery Technology 2007;7:42–5.

Burger A, Abraham D, editors. Burger's medicinal chemistry and drug discovery. New York: John Wiley and Sons; 2003.

Denora N, Trapani A, Laquintana V, et al. Recent advances in medicinal chemistry and pharmaceutical technology – strategies for drug delivery to the brain. Current Topics in Medicinal Chemistry 2009;9:182–96.

De Jong WH, Borm PJA. Drug delivery and nanoparticles: applications and hazards. International Journal of Nanomedicine 2008;3:133–49.

Dimitriu S, editor. Polymeric biomaterials. New York: Marcel Dekker; 2002.

EMEA (European Medicines Agency) (2006) Reflection paper on nanotechnology-based medicinal products for human use. EMEA/CHMP/79769/2006.

Gabizon AA, Shmeeda H, Zalipsky S. Pros and cons of the liposome platform in cancer drug targeting. Journal of Liposome Research 2006;16:175–83.

Goyal P, Goyal K, Vijaya Kumar SG, et al. Liposomal drug delivery systems – clinical applications. Acta Pharmaceutica 2005;5:1–25.

Gupta P, Vermani K, Garg S. Hydrogels: from controlled release to pH-responsive drug delivery. Drug Discovery Today 2002;7:569–79.

Harrington KJ, Syrigos KN, Vile RG. Liposomally targeted cytotoxic drugs for the treatment of cancer. Journal of Pharmaceutics and Pharmacology 2002;54:1573–600.

Illium L. Nasal drug delivery: new developments and strategies. Drug Discovery Today 2002;7:1184–9.

Illium L. Nasal drug delivery – possibilities, problems and solutions. Journal of Controlled Release 2003;87:187–98.

Kaplan SA. Relationships between aqueous solubility of drugs and their bioavailability. Drug Metabolism Reviews 1972;1:15–32.

Kim S, Kim J-H, Jeon O, et al. Engineered polymers for advanced drug delivery. European Journal of Pharmaceutics and Biopharmaceutics 2009;71:420–30.

Kroboth PD, McAuley JW, Kroboth FJ, et al. Triazolam pharmacokinetics after intravenous, oral, and sublingual administration. Journal of Clinical Psychopharmacology 1995;15:259–62.

Kumar RMNV, Kumar H. Polymeric controlled drug-delivery systems: perspective issues and opportunities. Drug Development and Industrial Pharmacy 2001;27:1–30.

Madhav NVS, Shakya AK, Shakya P, et al. Orotransmucosal drug delivery systems: a review. Journal of Controlled Release 2009;140:2–11.

Malik NN. Drug discovery: past, present and future. Drug Discovery Today 2008;13:909–12.

Pardridge WM. Biopharmaceutical drug targeting to the brain. Journal of Drug Targeting 2010;18:157–67.

Patel MM, Goyal BR, Bhadada SV, et al. Getting into the brain: approaches to enhance brain drug delivery. CNS Drugs 2009;23:35–58.

Pillai O, Panchagnula R. Polymers in drug delivery. Current Opinion in Chemical Biology 2001;5:447–51.

Putheti RR, Okigbo RN, Sai advanapu M, et al. Nanotechnology importance in the pharmaceutical industry. African Journal of Pure and Applied Chemistry 2008;2:27–31.

Samad A, Sultana Y, Aqil M. Liposomal drug delivery systems: an update review. Current Drug Delivery 2007;4:297–305.

Sapra P, Allen TM. Ligand-targeted liposomal anticancer drugs. Progress in Lipid Research 2003;42:439–62.

Savic S, Tamburic S, Savic MM. From conventional towards new – natural surfactants in drug delivery systems design: current status and perspectives. Expert Opinion in Drug Delivery 2010;7:353–69.

Scherrmann JM. Drug delivery to brain via the blood–brain barrier. Vascular Pharmacology 2002;38:349–54.

Singh R, Lillard Jr JW. Nanoparticle-based targeted drug delivery. Experimental and Molecular Pathology 2009;86:215–23.

Soppimath KS, Aminabhavi TM, Dave AM, et al. Stimulus-responsive 'smart' hydrogels as novel drug delivery systems. Drug Development and Industrial Pharmacy 2002;28:957–74.

Torchilin V. Structure and design of polymeric surfactant-based drug delivery. Journal of Controlled Release 2001;73:137–72.

Chapter 17

Clinical development: present and future

C Keywood

INTRODUCTION

Clinical development is the art of turning science into medicine. It is the point at which all the data from basic science, preclinical pharmacology and safety are put into medical practice to see whether scientific theory can translate into a valuable new medicine for patients. The fundamental purpose of the clinical development programme is to provide the clinical information to support the product labelling, which ultimately tells the healthcare professional and patient how to use the drug effectively and safely.

The segments of product label coming from clinical trials are the pharmacokinetics, the dosing regimen in the main population and in special populations, e.g. the elderly or those with hepatic and renal impairment, the clinical pharmacology/mechanism of action in man, drug interactions, contraindications, warnings, precautions, efficacy in the indication, safety and side effects. All this information has to be generated from a development programme designed to investigate these specific properties.

Clinical development has to satisfy the demands of regulators who will grant product approval, government organizations responsible for reimbursement in countries where healthcare is state subsidized, managed care organizations in the USA and also the marketing team who will sell the product. The needs are sometimes conflicting and a challenge of clinical development is to design a trials programme that not only demonstrates that the new drug is effective and safe, but also balances the various desires and requirements of the different parties, for the product profile.

Bringing new drugs to the market is not only complex but also costly, time and resource consuming. Taking into account failure of drugs in development to make it to market, Di Masi (2003) estimated the costs to be around US$802 million and Adams and Brantner (2006) made an estimate of US$868 million but within a range of $500 million to $2 billion, depending on the indication pursued and the company performing the development. Of this total amount the clinical development accounts for just over half, i.e. about US$480 million.

In spite of heavy investment in research and development, new product approvals have been decreasing in the last 10 years (Woodcock and Woosley, 2008). Pipelines of large pharmaceutical companies have been declining and the productivity of large pharmaceutical companies in new drug development has been diminishing in an environment of increasing costs of clinical development and increasing risk aversion of companies, regulators and the general public. New strategies are needed to overcome this problem, both in the way companies source and develop new drugs and also in the way regulators approach the evaluation of efficacy and safety of new medicines.

This new environment is leading to an evolution in clinical development strategy, with the type of indications being pursued and in the sourcing and development of new compounds. There is a move away from blockbuster medicines, i.e. 'one size fits all' in major indications, towards more specialized unmet medical needs and patient-tailored therapies, i.e. personalized medicine. The success of the human genome project was supposed to have heralded a new era for patient-specific drug development. However, for now, the art of medicine appears to continue to outwit the theory of basic science and drug development based purely upon genomic approaches has yet to live up to its promises.

There is an increasing trend for large pharmaceutical companies to collaborate with small pharmaceutical companies and biotech companies in order to enhance discovery pipelines and drug development productivity. Large companies have a great deal of resources to put behind development programmes but internal competition for resources, risk aversion and political pressures within these organizations can mean they are less flexible and creative in clinical development. Small pharmaceutical companies can provide the flexibility, innovation and creativity to complement the large pharmaceutical company development activities and there is an increasing trend for new drug development to be performed in partnership.

In the United Sates the Food and Drug Administration (FDA) published a white paper in 2004 (FDA, 2004a) that identified that the current methods of drug development were partly behind the decline of new drug applications and has set up the Critical Path Initiative (FDA, 2004b) in order to address some of the problems of low productivity and high late-stage attrition rates, the idea being to encourage novel approaches to clinical development in trial design and measuring outcomes. The Innovative Medicines Initiative (EFPIA, 2008), underway in Europe, is also looking to encourage public and private collaboration with small and large enterprises and academia, to share knowledge, enhance the drug discovery and development process, reduce late-stage attrition and, ultimately, bring good medicines to patients in a cost- and time-effective manner.

These factors are changing the way clinical development is being performed and will be performed in the future. In this chapter the conventional path of clinical development will be explained along with the new strategies for merging phases and using adaptive trial design to enhance the development of new medicines.

CLINICAL DEVELOPMENT PHASES

The conventional path of clinical development involves four phases:

- Phase I, pharmacokinetics, safety and tolerability and clinical pharmacology
- Phase IIa, exploratory efficacy
- Phase IIb, efficacy and dose range finding
- Phase III, pivotal efficacy and safety and larger population
- Phase IV, post-marketing safety and efficacy evaluation.

A summary of these phases is given in Table 17.1.

Traditionally these phases have been conducted in a step-wise manner with decisions to proceed to the next stage being made once the preceding stage was completed. However, more recently, the margins between phases are becoming less distinct as more seamless drug development programmes are being performed and adaptive trial designs adopted. Therefore, it may be more appropriate to describe the phases as: clinical pharmacology, including first in man – Phase I; exploratory, proof of concept – Phase IIa; confirmatory efficacy and dose range finding – Phase IIb; confirmatory, large scale efficacy and safety – Phase III; marketing authorization application, license extension and post-marketing surveillance – Phase IIIb/IV.

Phase I – Clinical pharmacology

Phase I is somewhat of a misnomer for, although the first studies in man are performed as part of Phase I, many of the other components of Phase I, for example drug–drug interactions, special populations and human radiolabelled studies, are conducted in parallel with later phase studies. Hence it is probably more appropriate to call these 'clinical pharmacology studies'.

A typical Phase I programme may contain around 20 clinical pharmacology studies. The main objectives of the programme are to define the pharmacokinetics, metabolism and safety of the intended formulation given alone and with other drugs that have potential to interact either kinetically or dynamically with the new drug. How the drug is handled by certain populations, such as the elderly, ethnic groups or those with hepatic or renal impairment, is also studied. All of this information goes into the prescribing information to guide the safe and effective use and dosing of the drug. Some efficacy information can also be gathered in human pharmacological models in order to assist dose selection for trials in patients. The principal components are as follows:

- First in man single ascending dose pharmacokinetics and safety
- Multiple ascending repeat dose pharmacokinetics and safety
- Pharmacodynamic studies
- Bioavailability absolute and bioequivalence of new formulations
- Absorption distribution metabolism excretion in man (radiolabelled studies)
- Drug–drug interaction studies
- Safety pharmacology, e.g. thorough QT studies and abuse liability studies
- Elderly pharmacokinetics and safety
- Ethnic groups pharmacokinetics and safety
- Hepatic and renal impairment, pharmacokinetics and safety.

Clinical pharmacology studies and in particular 'first in man' studies are conducted by specialist medical staff, trained in clinical pharmacology, in specialized units either within or close to a major hospital. The units are specifically equipped for the preparation and correct administration of the test drugs (and in some cases manufacture of the drug product), collection and storage of biological samples and management of subject safety, including full resuscitation facilities. The subjects selected

Table 17.1 Phases of clinical development

Clinical phase	General aim	Subjects/design	Data collected	Approx number of subjects	Approx cost ($ 000)	Approx time required
Ia	Exploratory; safety, tolerability and PK to support patient studies	Healthy subjects. Escalating single-dose, placebo-controlled, randomized, double-blind	Adverse events PK parameters PD measures (sometimes)	40–60	200–400	6 months
Ib	Exploratory; safety, tolerability and PK to support patient studies	Healthy subjects. Escalating repeat-dose, placebo-controlled, randomized double-blind	Adverse events PK parameters PD measures (sometimes)	30–50	200–400	6 months
IIa	Exploratory; preliminary safety and efficacy to support go/no-go decision	Patients; intended clinical dose and regimen based on Ph I results Usually placebo-controlled randomized double-blind, but sometimes open label	Adverse events PK parameters Preliminary evidence of efficacy. 'Proof of concept'	50–200	500–1000	9 months–2 years
IIb	Confirmatory; dose selection to support registration	Patients in one or more indications Selected dose levels/regimens compared to placebo and/or standard treatment, randomized double-blind	Statistically rigorous analysis of dose–response relationships Confirmation of clinical dose and regimen for optimum efficacy, safety and tolerability	200–500	2000–5000+	2–3 years
III	Confirmatory; efficacy and safety data to support registration; may include pharmacoeconomic evaluation	Patients in target indication(s) but including different groups (age, ethnicity, etc.). Selected dose level compared with placebo and/or standard treatment(s) randomized double-blind	Statistically rigorous measurements demonstrating safety and efficacy in comparison with placebo or existing therapies May include pharmacoeconomic analysis	500–1000+	2000–10 000+	2–5+ years
IV	Obligatory post-marketing surveillance to reveal unexpected adverse effects or toxicity	Treated patients	Adverse events	10 000+	10 000+	2–4+ years

for studies are usually enrolled from the unit's subject volunteer panel. Typically a clinical pharmacology unit will advertise for subjects to join their database. People who are interested in taking part in trials are then carefully screened for their physical health, their ability to comprehend the requirements of taking part in the studies and their motivation to comply with the constraints of the studies, to check whether they are suitable to join the volunteer panel. In some countries (e.g. France), the subjects have to be registered on a national database to make sure they comply with laws governing participation in clinical trials. For most large professional units, the database will comprise a variety of healthy subjects including young men and women (18–45 years), older healthy subjects (over 55 years), subjects of non-Caucasian origin (e.g. Japanese) and subjects with genetic polymorphisms for CYP metabolism. As the subjects gain no medical benefit from taking part in the studies and have to undergo procedures which can be mildly unpleasant or inconvenient, they are paid for taking part. However, the amount they can be paid is restricted to be commensurate with the inconvenience and discomfort of the study and is not so high as to be an inducement to take part. The subjects' reimbursement is reviewed and has to be approved by the ethics committee, before the study can go ahead. The number of studies that subjects can take part in annually is also restricted. Most protocols demand that a subject cannot be exposed to another investigational drug within 90 days of taking part in a study and so that limits how many studies in which a given subject can participate, in any one year.

First in man, single ascending dose, pharmacokinetics and safety

First dose in man (FDIM), also known as single ascending dose (SAD), is a red-letter day for the drug development team, when single doses of the drug are given to small cohorts of subjects in a sequential manner until the maximum tolerated dose is achieved.

Objectives

The objectives of the SAD study are to evaluate the safety (physiological effects on body systems), tolerability (occurrence of side effects) and pharmacokinetics of different doses of the test drug, and to identify the maximum tolerated dose (MTD). That is the dose at which either the occurrence of intolerable side effects and/or unacceptable safety findings are encountered. The MTD is important to identify for estimation of the therapeutic window, which is the dose range within which the drug is effective but safe and well tolerated. In some cases it is not possible to achieve the MTD, perhaps if the drug is very well tolerated, or has poor bioavailability, in which case the maximum feasible dose can be used to estimate the therapeutic window.

Subjects

In most cases the subjects in first in man studies will be conducted in healthy young men usually aged 18–45 years. The idea behind this is to have a fairly homogeneous population in which to study the effects of the new drug and so limit variability, and also to have a population who will be more able to withstand any unexpected toxicity caused by the test drug. Healthy subjects are those who have no underlying diseases that could interfere with the conduct of the study or confound the interpretation of the safety or pharmacokinetic data. Criteria for inclusion into the study based upon medical history, physical examination, use of concomitant medications, alcohol, cigarettes and recreational drugs, as well as the results of blood testing 12-lead ECG, blood pressure heart rate are laid out in the study protocol. Male subjects are generally preferred, because at this early stage of development, reproductive toxicology testing in animals will not have been completed and the risk to the fetus of female subjects who might be pregnant or become pregnant shortly before or after the study, has not been characterized. Once the segment 2 reproductive toxicology has been completed (see Chapter 15), female subjects of non-childbearing potential, i.e. post-menopausal, surgically sterilized, sexually abstinent or using effective methods of contraception, may be included in European studies. In the USA, female subjects may be included prior to reproductive toxicology data being available if they are of non-childbearing potential. In some cases it is not appropriate to use healthy young men, for example, studies of female hormone products or products for oncology, and in these cases the subjects will be selected from the appropriate population.

Design

The classical design of the SAD study is a double-blind, placebo-controlled sequential cohort design; where the first cohort takes the lowest dose and then the dose is escalated through subsequent cohorts, provided the tolerability and safety in the preceding cohort are acceptable. The size of each group is usually six to eight subjects, with two of the subjects being randomized to placebo. The use of placebo and the double-blinding, where neither the investigator nor the subject knows the treatment being taken, allows for a more objective evaluation of the safety and tolerability of the test drug.

The choice of doses to be administered in the SAD trials should be based on the highest dose at which no adverse effects were seen in the most sensitive species tested in toxicology studies (the *no observed adverse effect level*, or NOAEL; see Chapter 15) and on the nature of the toxicity observed. The starting dose should be at least 10-fold lower than the NOAEL, but specific guidelines exist for the accurate determination of the starting dose on a case-by-case basis (FDA; http:www.fda.gov/cber/gdlns/dose.htm).

The dose escalation plan will depend on the characteristics of the drug and its metabolites, and especially on the nature of any toxicity seen in preclinical toxicology testing at doses above the NOAEL. It will also be influenced by the relationship between dose, systemic exposure as determined by its pharmacokinetic (PK) profile in animals, and the pharmacodynamic (PD) effects observed in preclinical pharmacology studies. Each dose escalation step will be dependent on satisfactory safety data from the previous dose level, according to the clinical judgment of the investigator.

Usually the drug is administered only once to each subject so that each dose group comprises separate subjects. This has the advantage of maximizing the population exposed to the test drug. Sometimes, however, it may be appropriate for each subject to receive two or three of the planned doses at successive visits, with the proviso that each dose is administered only after the response to the preceding dose in the series has been evaluated. In this way the required number of subjects is reduced, but each has to attend more than once.

Typical dose escalation schedules from a starting dose of X are:

- Dose escalation schedule 1: X, 2X, 4X, 8X, 16X, 32X
- Dose escalation schedule 2: X, 2X, 4X, 6X, 8X, 10X.

The dose escalation schedule is guided primarily by safety considerations. Dose escalation schedule 1, where the dose is increased exponentially, would be appropriate for a drug that has shown low toxicity in animal testing. Schedule 2, where the dose increments are constant, is more conservative and might be more appropriate for a drug which has a toxicology profile that calls for a more cautious approach to dose escalation in man. There are many other possible dose escalation patterns, and each is considered on its own merits. The ideal is to exceed the dose predicted to effective from preclinical pharmacology studies, by a good margin. A drug for which the MTD is close to the dose predicted for therapeutic effect is less likely to be successful than one that has a wide therapeutic margin.

As it is common for the PK profiles of orally administered drugs to be affected by the presence or absence of food in the stomach at the time of dosing, the food effect is usually investigated at the end of the SAD study. A dose level that is safe and well tolerated (e.g. one-quarter of the MTD) will be given to healthy subjects on two occasions once in the fed state (following a standard high-fat breakfast) and once fasted (overnight fast). The order of fed and fasted administration is randomized among the subjects and the two dose periods are separated by an appropriate washout period, so that the results of the second period are not affected by the drug administration on the first period. The results of the fed/fasted comparison will form the basis of the dosing instructions for all future studies with the drug.

Outcome measures

In the SAD study the principal outcome measures are safety, tolerability and pharmacokinetics.

Throughout the study, for an appropriate period after each dose, the subjects are intensively monitored for signs and/or symptoms of toxicity (adverse events). The safety parameters measured include, blood pressure, heart rate and rhythm, 12-lead ECG (intervals and morphology), body temperature, haematology, liver function and renal function, as well as observation for any other unwanted effects. Tolerability is evaluated by the documentation of adverse events which are collected throughout the study and then categorized by severity, duration, outcome and causality. If an adverse event meets certain specific criteria (for instance if it is life-threatening or necessitates hospitalization) it is classified as a *serious adverse event* (SAE) and must be reported without delay to the ethics committee, and usually also to the regulatory authority.

Whereas assessment of safety and tolerability is the primary objective, pharmacokinetic evaluation is the secondary objective of a SAD study. Blood samples will normally be taken before dosing and at specified intervals after dosing to measure the amount of drug in the blood or plasma at various time points after each dose. A typical sampling schedule is shown in Figure 17.1A. In addition, urine and/or faeces may be collected to measure the excretion of the drug via the kidneys and/or liver (in bile). The results enable the rate of absorption, metabolism and excretion of the drug to be explored, and the PK parameters to be estimated (see also Chapter 10).

The plasma or serum PK parameters usually derived are:

- C_{max}: peak drug and/or metabolite(s) concentration
- T_{max}: time to peak drug and/or metabolite(s) concentration
- $AUC_{0-\infty}$: area under the concentration–time curve of the drug and/or metabolite(s), extrapolated to infinity
- AUC_{0-T}: area under the concentration–time curve of the drug and/or metabolite(s), calculated to a specific time point T
- $t_{1/2}$: time taken for levels of drug and/or metabolite(s) to decrease by half (a measure of the rate of elimination of the drug from plasma).

Other PK parameters may also be determined, including:

- V_D: volume of distribution of drug and/or metabolite(s)
- *Cl*: clearance of drug and/or metabolite, i.e. the volume of plasma/serum cleared of drug and/or metabolite(s) per unit time, e.g. mL/min, L/h
- *MRT*: mean residence time, i.e. the average time a drug molecule remains in the body after rapid i.v. injection.

Specialist pharmacokineticists perform the calculation of these parameters.

Single-dose study

Time	0	15 min	30 min	1h	1½h	2h	4h	6h	8h	12h	24h	48h
Dose	↑											
Blood sample	●	●	●	●	●	●	●	●	●	●	●	●

(A)

Repeat-dose study

Day 1	0	15 min	30 min	1h	1½h	2h	4h	6h	8h	12h
	↑									
	●	●	●	●	●	●	●	●	●	●

Days 2–7	0	15 min	30 min	1h	1½h	2h	4h	6h	8h	12h
	↑									↑
	●									●

Day 8	0	15 min	30 min	1h	1½h	2h	4h	6h	8h	12h	24h	48h
	↑											
	●	●	●	●	●	●	●	●	●	●	●	●

(B)

Fig. 17.1A, B A, A typical sampling schedule. B, A typical Phase MAD blood sampling schedule.

A comparison of the PK parameters at each dose level, e.g. AUC_{∞}, C_{max}, will indicate whether they increase proportionately (linear kinetics) or disproportionately (non-linear kinetics) with increasing dose. This information will influence the selection of dose levels, regimen and duration of dosing for the multiple, ascending repeat-dose study (MAD). The single-dose PK data can also be used to predict the drug/metabolite(s) concentrations expected on repeated dosing, based on the assumption that the kinetics do not change with time.

Multiple ascending repeat-dose studies

After review of the safety data and the single-dose PK profile, two or three safe and well-tolerated dose levels are chosen and the multiple ascending (repeated-dose) study (MAD) is designed. Its purpose is to test safety, tolerability and PK when the drug is given repeatedly.

Design

A typical MAD study design will be double-blind, placebo-controlled with two or three cohorts of eight (six active two placebo) to 12 (eight active four placebo) subjects taking successively higher doses for several days. As for the SAD, the decision to escalate to the next dose level is based upon the safety and tolerability of the preceding dose level. The dose regimen in the MAD study is based upon the PK characteristics seen in the SAD and designed to give the PK profile necessary to allow the drug to exert its therapeutic effect and to achieve 'steady state' in which the drug's input rate is balanced by its rate of elimination. The duration of the dosing is based upon the desire to achieve steady state but also to collect sufficient safety information to support use in Phase II studies. For indications where chronic dosing is required a duration of around 7–10 days is usual in MAD studies.

Outcome measures

Safety assessment is necessary under these conditions, as steady-state blood levels are usually higher than blood levels following a single administration. It is also important to know whether the PK of the drug and/or metabolite(s) changes on repeated dosing. For instance, saturation of elimination pathways (e.g. metabolizing enzyme systems) could cause the drug to accumulate to toxic levels in the body, or alternatively stimulation (induction) of drug-metabolizing enzyme systems could cause the levels of drug and/or metabolite(s) to decrease to subtherapeutic levels. A comparison of the predicted and observed plasma–serum concentration time curves will provide evidence of any such non-linear or time-dependent kinetics for the drug and/or metabolite(s).

The general requirements and procedures for MAD studies are the same as those for Phase I SAD. A typical Phase MAD blood sampling schedule is shown in Figure 17.1B. Blood samples for PK profiling will generally be taken on the first and last days of dosing, with additional single samples taken immediately before the first morning dose each day, to measure the levels of drug remaining in the blood immediately before the next dose is administered, i.e. the trough level.

The results of the Phase I SAD and MAD studies together support the decision as to whether to administer the drug to patients and, if so, at what dose and regimen and for how long.

Pharmacodynamic studies

Pharmacodynamic (PD) assessments may be included in the MAD studies, or specific PD studies can be performed separately. Usually prior to Phase IIa, the objective of these studies is to establish whether the drug has some pharmacological effect in man that may be relevant to its therapeutic effect, and to determine at what doses and plasma concentrations the effects are seen, with a view to optimizing dose selection for Phase IIa. Such studies are termed PK/PD studies.

This approach must still be treated with some caution, as the physiology in patients may differ from that in healthy subjects, and clinical efficacy may therefore not be reliably predicted from Phase I results. It is not uncommon for drugs that are highly effective in patients suffering from a certain condition to have little or no effect on the same body system in healthy subjects. This is particularly true of drugs acting on psychiatric diseases as these conditions are very difficult to emulate in healthy subjects. The ideal PD assessments in Phase I are those that have biological or surrogate markers that are measurable in healthy subjects and are relevant to drug's mechanism of action and/or therapeutic effect. For example, the ability of a β-adrenoceptor antagonist to inhibit exercise-induced tachycardia, or the effect of a proton pump inhibitor on acid gastric secretion are relevant effects that can easily be measured objectively in volunteers. However, such markers are not always available (e.g. in the case of many psychiatric diseases) or may be misleading (pain is a good example because the endpoints are subjective rather than objective), and the interpretation of such data is usually approached with care. Nonetheless, Phase I PK/PD studies can be very useful to confirm that a new drug is actually having the pharmacological effect in man that was predicted from animal studies. As well as studying pharmacodynamics in healthy subjects, patients with a mild form of disease can be studied. An example is asthma, where a new drug could be studied for a short period of time in mild asthmatics to observe a pharmacological response, without necessarily intending to provide a long-term therapeutic benefit. Such subjects are known as patient volunteers and, like healthy subjects, as they are not entering the study to seek a cure for their disease, they can receive some financial compensation for their time and inconvenience.

Drug–drug interaction studies

The objective of drug–drug interaction studies (DDI) is to determine whether the test drug's efficacy, safety or pharmacokinetics will be altered if it is given with other drugs that the target patient population may also be taking. The timing of drug interaction studies depends partly on the importance of understanding interactions prior to treating patients. Some DDIs may need to be performed prior to Phase IIa if the patient population in the study cannot be excluded from taking concomitant medications that might interact with the test drug. Otherwise DDIs can be conducted later in the development programme when more is known about the target treatment population and the efficacy and safety of the new drug. The choice of which DDI studies to perform is based on the following: the metabolism of the new drug (for example if it inhibits, induces or is metabolized by certain cytochrome p450 enzymes – see Chapter 10); the pharmacodynamic action of the drug; and which drugs the target population may be taking concomitantly. Drug interactions can occur on a metabolic level, so that the exposure to a certain dose may be changed by a drug interaction or on a pharmacodynamic level so that pharmacological effects may be increased or diminished by the interacting drug. It is important to known whether co-administration of the relevant drugs leads to a change in exposure or a change in pharmacodynamic effect of either the test drug or the interacting drug.

In a typical DDI study, subjects are dosed with the interacting drug until steady state is achieved and then a single dose of the test drug is given and the PK, safety, and sometimes PD effects are evaluated. The information from the DDI studies gives guidance as to whether any dose alterations are necessary when the new drug is co-administered with a drug with which it interacts and the information is included on the product label.

Absolute bioavailability and bioequivalence of new formulations

Absolute bioavailability studies are performed to compare the exposure of an intravenous preparation of the study drug which has 100% bioavailability, with the formulation intended for clinical use which is to be given by another route, e.g. oral or subcutaneous. The absolute bioavailability information is needed for the product label, but also assists further formulation development as modifications to the formulation can be made in order to optimize exposure to the drug. The studies are conducted in healthy subjects in a crossover fashion where each subject receives an intravenous dose and then one or more doses of the study drug given by its intended clinical route of administration. Standard pharmacokinetic parameters are measured and the absolute bioavailability calculated by comparing the pharmacokinetics of the intravenous and non-intravenous doses.

In the initial clinical pharmacology trials and in the exploratory efficacy studies it is not usual to use a formulation that would be the final commercial formulation. Development of a commercial formulation is performed in parallel with the early phase studies and the data from those studies guides the formulation development activity. Once a commercial type formulation or formulations has been identified, the safety and pharmacokinetics are compared with the prototype formulation in comparative bioavailability studies. As for absolute bioavailability, the studies are conducted in healthy subjects in a crossover fashion. If there is no more than 5% difference in exposure (AUC) between two formulations, they are considered to be bioequivalent. Dosing information obtained from exploratory efficacy studies using a prototype formulation which is bioequivalent to the commercial type formulation, can, therefore, be applied directly to confirmatory efficacy dose range finding studies. If the formulations are not bioequivalent, further multiple dose pharmacokinetics and pharmacodynamic studies may be needed to determined dosing regimens for the dose range finding studies. Depending on the intricacy of the formulation development, comparative bioavailability studies may need to be performed on more than one occasion.

Absorption distribution metabolism excretion (ADME) in man (radiolabelled studies)

The objective of the human ADME is to identify precisely the handling of the drug by the body and to look for and quantify metabolites that might also have effects on its efficacy and safety. The study involves giving a small number (usually four to six) of male subjects a dose of radiolabelled compound and then sampling blood urine and faeces over a period commensurate with its elimination half-life. Unless information about metabolite presence and activity is needed more urgently, the study is usually performed in late Phase II or early in Phase III.

Other safety pharmacology studies

The clinical pharmacology programme also contains studies to examine safety aspects, notably the ability of the new compound to cause QT prolongation, which may carry a risk of a potentially fatal ventricular arrhythmia, called torsade de pointes, or for some central nervous system drugs, abuse liability studies are needed. There are specific study designs to look for whether a drug has potential for abuse. Other studies such as effect on reaction time or driving ability may also be needed, particularly for central nervous system compounds.

The need for thorough QT studies has become a general requirement for all NCEs in the past few years, whether or not the compound demonstrates any potential to cause cardiac conduction abnormalities in vitro or in non-clinical studies. The studies are usually conducted in mid-stage of development when efficacy has been shown, the likely therapeutic dose is known and prior to large scale confirmatory studies. They are conducted in healthy male and female subjects with no evidence of heart disease or concomitant medication that could affect cardiac conduction. The study typically comprises four arms in a crossover, that is the test drug at the intended clinical dose, the test drug dosed at or near the MTD, an active comparator known to cause QTc prolongation, e.g. moxifloxacin and placebo. Drug dosing on each treatment day is followed by the collection of multiple ECGs at multiple time points, especially around C_{max}, that are read by hand by a blinded central observer. As the studies require approximately 50 subjects and hundreds of ECGs to be read they are laborious and expensive. The Guidance ICH E14 from 2005 sets out the conduct and interpretation of thorough QT studies. However, the true predictiveness of these studies for *torsade de pointes* remains to be proven and it is likely that a number of useful drugs may be halted in development due to an observation of prolongation of QTc that may not represent a risk of dangerous arrhythmia to patients.

Special populations

In order to provide accurate dosing information in the product label, to cover administration to different patient types in the target population, the pharmacokinetics and safety are studied in patient subgroups. These include elderly subjects, specific ethnic groups, subjects belonging to a defined genetic subgroup for metabolism (fast or slow metabolizers) and also subjects with hepatic impairment and subjects with renal impairment. These studies are usually conducted once the clinically effective dose is fairly certain, as they are performed with the intended clinical dose. As many news drugs will be given to patients over 65 years old, elderly subjects are required in order to assess safety and kinetics in a group of healthy subjects more representative of the target patient population. Specific ethnic groups, on the other hand, will be required when a drug being developed in Caucasian populations is also being submitted for approval in a different population (e.g. Japanese). In this case, it is to determine whether significant differences exist in the pharmacokinetics and pharmacodynamics of the two ethnic groups, and whether different dosage regimens will be necessary. Specific genetic metabolic subtypes might be selected in order to ensure that where slow metabolizer subtypes exist this does not cause accumulation of the drug and related toxicity in those individuals. Finally, as most drugs are eliminated via the kidney and/or the liver, alteration of the function of these organs could change the kinetics and safety when the drug is given to patients with hepatic or renal impairment; hence these studies are performed to make dosing recommendations for those patients.

Phase IIa – Exploratory efficacy

Objectives

The exploratory efficacy studies have different objectives depending on whether the drug in development has a novel mechanism of action, i.e. is a first in class drug, or if it has a known mechanism and others in the class are already available for patient use in the indication, i.e. a 'follow-on drug'. In the case of the former, The 'proof of concept' (PoC) studies in Phase IIa will be the first time the drug is tested in patients and this is when scientific theory is tested in clinical reality. It is interesting for the non-clinical and the clinical teams to see how translational the animal models turn out to be in patients. As it is the first time the drug is given to patients, safety evaluation is the key objective. The design of PoC for novel mechanisms is crucial to ensure that meaningful clinical effect can be identified, if it exists and likewise if there is no clinical effect this also needs to be identified, so that a decision about the future of the drug in the indication can be determined.

In the case of a follow-on drug with a known mechanism of action, the PoC studies will be more orientated towards establishing points of differentiation with drugs on the market that have the same mechanism of action. The existing product may have weaknesses of efficacy, side effects or pharmacokinetics which the follower drug can improve upon. An example of this is the class of oral triptans for acute treatment of migraine, where speed of onset of action and duration of action, manifest by a lower headache recurrence rate, were differentiators of interest compared to the market leader sumatriptan. Follow-on compounds in the class concentrated on having either a more rapid onset of action or a long half-life leading to lower headache recurrence. The design of studies for follow on compounds will be orientated towards drawing out these differentiating features rather than answering the question 'does it work or not?'

Design consideration for first in class compounds – large pharma vs small pharma

Phase IIa PoC studies are small in size and designed carefully to answer the questions about whether the drug has any meaningful therapeutic activity in the case of first in class compounds, or whether it has any useful differentiating features in the case of follow-on compounds. As the studies are not fully statistically powered to demonstrate treatment differences it is important to determine *a priori* what are the criteria for success or failure in the study. This requires objectivity and an experienced development team.

The objectives of a large pharmaceutical company in conducting PoC with a novel mechanism of action may be different to those of a small pharmaceutical company. For the large company, the most important aspect will be to show as soon as possible that they have a novel mechanism of action that is safe and well tolerated and works in man, to feedback to the discovery teams working on the back-up programme. To that end they may choose a drug which is good enough for exploratory clinical trials, but may have features that are not optimal for a final commercial medicinal product, for example a short half-life or poor solubility. However, once PoC has been demonstrated with the novel mechanism of action they can accelerate development of back-up molecules, which have better properties to become medicinal products. On the other hand if the PoC fails, then this line of research can be abandoned.

For a small company with more limited resources and fewer pipeline programmes, the Phase IIa PoC studies may be make or break for the entire company. Start-up companies funded by venture capital may only have one lead product going into Phase IIa, no products on the market and other compounds in their pipeline may well be a long way from the clinic. In that case a great deal of the company's fortune rides on the drug being tested in Phase IIa becoming a medicinal product. The small company may well have done their best to select a molecule with good drug-like properties which they believe could make it to the market, prior to entering into man. The objectives of Phase IIa for this type of company are to demonstrate convincing therapeutic effect with acceptable safety so that the compound can be advanced further into development. It is not generally the intention to go back to other molecules that might look a bit better, as in the case of large companies, unless there is a major problem with the lead compound. Whatever the size of the company, the basic tenet of Phase IIa is to gain robust data upon which to base decisions about the future of the drug. Given that the PoC studies are fundamental to the go/no-go decision for an entire development project in both large and small companies, the design of the studies is crucial.

Design

In most cases, a double-blind placebo-controlled study is an ideal approach as this allows for a more objective measure of efficacy and safety. However, there are notable exceptions, for example in oncology, where a comparison with, or add-on to a standard therapy is usually needed as it would be unethical to withhold known effective treatments from patients with cancer. It is possible to perform open-label small 'look see' studies in Phase IIa using historical comparison with efficacy of other drugs used in the indication, but this is not an ideal strategy as there is a substantial risk of bias if there is no control arm. The dosing regimen will have been determined from the Phase I studies and also from supporting non-clinical pharmacology data. There are numerous possibilities for choosing the dose, but the principal objective is to be as sure as possible that the dose or doses chosen for the study have a high likelihood of showing an effect if there is one and that the doses have acceptable safety and tolerability. A maximum tolerated dose approach is often used, especially for drugs with good safety and tolerability. Doses can be selected to achieve plasma concentrations that have been shown to be effective in animal studies or which are likely to give a particular receptor occupancy if PET studies have been performed previously. The number of dose groups in Phase IIa studies is usually limited to one or two active groups and a placebo group. The treatment groups may be parallel or the study can be done as a crossover, which is when the patient is randomized to receive each of the treatments in a random order, separated by a suitable washout period. The advantage of a crossover is that the patient acts as his/her own control and the number of patients can be reduced. The disadvantage is that there can be an order effect where the previous treatment affects the outcome of the subsequent treatment. Also crossovers are generally more suitable for indications where the outcome variables are rapidly measurable, e.g. pain, or have objective endpoints, e.g. blood pressure. Crossovers are less suitable for indications where the efficacy measurement is highly dependent on patient reported outcomes, e.g. anxiety, because they are more prone to bias from order effects. As the patients have to have more than one treatment the crossover study may also take longer to complete than a parallel group. However, if patient recruitment for a particular indication is difficult (for example rarer diseases or highly competitive therapeutic trial areas) a study with a larger parallel group population may take longer to complete. As they are exploratory, Phase IIa studies lend themselves to adaptive trial designs where the dosing may be adjusted during the study according to the response of the study population. Adaptive trial designs are discussed in more detail below.

In Phase IIa, as clinical data are required rapidly, the preclinical programme may well be lean, and focused on getting only the data needed to support initial study in humans, therefore the formulation development is likely to be incomplete. If the compound is highly soluble, an intravenous or simple oral formulation (solution or simple tablet) can be used in early Phase I and Phase IIa. Information from these studies, in particular the PK-PD data, will help with the development of a commercial type formulation, to be used in confirmatory efficacy studies. If the compound is poorly soluble more formulation development will have taken place prior to entry into man. Nevertheless, in Phase IIa it is not usual to use a final commercial type formulation as the results of the initial clinical studies do influence the final formulation development.

The duration of Phase IIa studies for novel drugs is influenced by the indication, but is usually shorter than for larger scale later phase studies, for two reasons. Firstly it is important to gain information on clinical effect as soon as possible so that decisions on compound development can be made. Secondly, the toxicology programme to support the shorter studies, e.g. up to 1 month in duration, will also be shorter. Clinical trials of 3 and 6 months dosing duration require toxicology studies in two species of corresponding duration to support the human dosing. To make this type of investment in a toxicology programme for a novel mechanism of action drug before its clinical effects are known, is not always desirable, particularly for smaller companies. For follow-on compounds, however, studies of more than 1 month in duration might be needed in Phase IIa for indications in which clinical differentiation will only become apparent after longer-term administration, for example in Parkinson's disease or psychiatric indications.

Patients to be studied

The PoC is usually the first time that the drug will be used in patients with the relevant disease; therefore, careful patient selection is vital to the success of a PoC study, especially those of novel compounds. It important to be clear about what question is being asked in the study and what patient group should be targeted so that question can be answered. Typically in the exploratory phase, as the population is small, a more homogeneous patient group is selected to reduce variability that might dilute the possibility of seeing a result. The inclusion and exclusion criteria at this stage may be more restrictive than at later stages of development. In the exploratory efficacy phase less is known about the safety of the drug in diverse clinical situations and the drug–drug interactions will not have been fully explored. A subgroup of patients within a disease entity who are considered most likely to show a benefit can be studied at this early stage. For example, to evaluate the benefit of reflux inhibition with a novel drug in patients with gastroesophageal reflux disease (GORD), patients with non-erosive reflux disease and classical symptoms of heartburn and regurgitation would be selected, in order to increase the likelihood of seeing a response to the drug. Once convincing efficacy and satisfactory safety/tolerability have been demonstrated, subsequent studies can include patients with more severe disease, or more diverse symptoms. In the case of GORD this could extend to patients with erosive oesophagitis and symptoms other than heartburn and regurgitation that are thought to be due to GORD.

Outcome measures

Thorough safety and adverse event monitoring is performed in these initial patient studies, with close attention paid to looking for untoward effects in patients that might not have been seen in healthy subjects. With regards to efficacy, as the PoC studies have a relatively small population and short duration, it is necessary to have robust outcome measures. In the exploratory phase it can be tempting to try and answer a lot of questions in one clinical trial. This is not a good idea because putting too much into the trial increases the complexity of its execution and can confound the interpretation of the data. It is by far better to have one clear principal objective and, at most, two smaller less important objectives. The ease of having robust measurable endpoints depends a lot on the indication. Those indications with objective measures, e.g. hypertension and diabetes, are straightforward to demonstrate in terms of proof of concept. However, for licensing in such indications it is not sufficient to show that the drug lowers blood pressure or glucose alone, it has to be shown that the drug improves patient outcome in reducing mortality or cardiovascular morbidity, which presents a substantial challenge in late phase development. In the middle are pain-type indications, as pain is rapidly treatable. However, as one is relying on the patient to report the severity of pain, the outcome can be subject to bias and a high placebo response. For other indications where long-term treatment is needed to evaluate the full benefit, a good surrogate marker can be used in the PoC. One example would be in the case of the treatment of rheumatoid arthritis where measuring inflammatory mediators in the blood can indicate evidence of meaningful pharmacological effect. Another example comes from a study of the prevention of vasospasm post subarachnoid haemorrhage, with an endothelin antagonist. Ultimately it needs to be known if treatment with the drug improves patient outcome, i.e. mortality and morbidity, but in the PoC trial the occurrence of vasospasm was measured with angiography, transcranial Doppler and the presence of infarcts on CT scanning, to see if the drug was able to prevent physiological vasospasm and its anatomical sequelae.

Pharmacokinetic samples may also be taken in the Phase IIa studies to examine the PK-PD response and also to see if the pharmacokinetics in patients are different from healthy subjects; migraine patients, for example, have gastric stasis during an attack and this can alter the absorption of orally administered drugs. Phase IIa may be the first time that the PK–PD relationship is studied and the information can be used to guide the dose selection for Phase IIb.

In summary, the characteristics of Phase IIa PoC studies are short, focused, using carefully selected patient populations and robust endpoints to enable go/no-go decisions for new drugs in development.

Phase IIb to III dose range finding and confirmatory efficacy studies

Objectives

The purpose of this phase of development is to confirm the initial efficacy seen in the Phase IIa PoC studies and to provide the pivotal data which will support the application for market approval, as such extensive, comprehensive data from well-designed and adequately powered studies are required. The data from the confirmatory studies will be used to make the claims in the product label upon which the drug can be promoted. Therefore, during this part of the development, the clinical team needs to liaise closely with Regulatory and Marketing so that the trials can be designed to fulfil the desired product label. Usually the first step is a Phase IIb dose range finding study to confirm the preliminary safety and efficacy data and to explore the dose–response relationship in detail, to select the dose that has the optimal efficacy and safety profile to be used for large-scale Phase III efficacy and long-term safety studies. The eventual marketing strategy is a major guiding factor for the design of the Phase III programme, especially for follow-on drugs where product differentiation to existing treatments, whether it be on efficacy, safety or cost effectiveness, is crucial to its success.

Design

The standard design of Phase IIb dose-finding studies is parallel-group randomized double-blind and, placebo-controlled and/or active comparator controlled. The placebo group in theory allows for a comparison of active intervention with 'no treatment' and, therefore, should provide a clear view of the efficacy benefits and safety of the test drug. However, it is well documented that patients in clinical trials do have a response to placebo (Beecher, 1955). Strictly speaking, taking placebo does not mean that the patient has no treatment. The very act of taking part in a clinical trial and receiving extra medical attention can contribute to an improvement to a patient's underlying condition. This is particularly true for psychiatric conditions or those exacerbated by stress or anxiety. Trials in psychiatry and those which rely heavily on patient reported outcomes have notoriously high placebo response rates. Occasionally the enthusiasm of the investigating physician for the new treatment can colour their view of the efficacy, which can also contribute to high placebo response rates. In some medical conditions, for example oncology or other serious conditions for which effective treatment exists, it is not appropriate for patients to receive placebo. In this case the new drug can be tested either against a gold standard, single active comparator or against a standard-care treatment regimen. In the latter case the test drug might also be added to standard care in one group while the other group just receives standard care alone.

Another way to minimize placebo response in the active treatment phase, is to have a single blind, placebo run-in period, where all patients take placebo but only the investigator knows that they are on placebo. At the end of the period, those who continue to fulfil the predefined eligibility criteria can be randomized to the double-blind phase. For pivotal efficacy Phase IIb or III studies in Europe, it is a requirement to have at least one study with an active comparator arm. The choice of comparator will depend on marketing considerations and what the potential advantages the new drug can offer, whether it be in terms of safety, tolerability, efficacy or cost effectiveness. Active comparator studies may be designed to show superiority, equivalence or non-inferiority compared to the gold standard treatment. The choice will depend upon the efficacy and the safety of the drug. For example, if the drug is thought to have similar efficacy but a superior safety profile to the existing treatment an equivalence or non-inferiority design may be chosen for the primary efficacy, because the main objective is to demonstrate the better safety and tolerability. The treatment selected for comparison has to be justified to the regulatory authorities when submitting the trial application and can be discussed with them in advance, for example at an end of Phase II meeting. The only exception to this is for indications where no treatment is currently licensed. An example of this is levodopa-induced dyskinesia in Parkinson's disease. Even so, the non-use of an active comparator needs to be justified in the clinical trial application.

These trials form the basis of the marketing authorization application and so they have to have a sufficient sample size to demonstrate efficacy with confidence. Also sufficient safety data to support exposure to the target patient population needs to be generated. Statistical calculations are made to ensure enough patients are enrolled to have robust efficacy results that will support the desired claims on the product label. In the case of a parallel group, multiple, dose-range finding Phase IIb study, although the power of the study might be lower than required for a Phase III pivotal efficacy study (e.g. 85% rather than 90%), sample size calculations have to take into account adjustment for comparisons of the multiple dose arms. Typically the studies will have several hundred patients or in the case of some cardiovascular intervention (e.g. hypertension) studies, a few thousand patients may be required. The dosing duration must be sufficient not only to demonstrate efficacy but also to establish safety. For indications where long-term chronic use is intended, even if it is intermittent dosing, the safety database should contain information on dosing for at least 12 months in an adequate number of patients. These data are often generated by enrolling patients from the Phase IIb and III studies into a long-term, open-label, extension study at the intended clinical dose.

The dose range for Phase IIb will be selected based upon the efficacy and safety data from the Phase I and Phase IIa studies. If the Phase IIb study is successful it will have identified the dose level and dosing regimen which gives the optimal balance between efficacy, safety and tolerability. This dosing regimen is subject to confirmation in Phase III.

Patients and study setting

For the later phases of development it is important to study the drug in a more 'real-life' setting, because the safety and efficacy data from these studies has to support the use in the patient population in the target market. Therefore, the trial eligibility criteria are expanded in Phases IIb and III to enroll patients that are more representative of the final target population. By this stage more safety and drug interaction data are available, so reducing the restrictions on patient recruitment can be done with more confidence. The countries, study sites and doctors selected for the late phase studies will generally be more diverse than in Phase IIa and influenced by marketing as well as regulatory needs. It is perfectly possible to apply for a product licence in a country or region without conducting pivotal efficacy trials there, because the trials are conducted according to ICH GCP so the trials should be acceptable as long as the data generated cover any intrinsic (genetic) or extrinsic (e.g. diet, medical practice) differences that exist in that region. However, for the major territories of USA, Europe and Japan it is usual to conduct at least one study in that region and, for Japan, bridging studies may be needed to demonstrate that the properties of the drug demonstrated in a 'European type' population are applicable to Japanese patients.

Outcome measures

In the large-scale confirmatory studies the surrogate endpoints of Phase IIa give way to demonstrating clinically meaningful benefit. This means that simply demonstrating a reduction in blood pressure, or preventing cerebral vasospasm or reflux events from occurring, to name but a few examples, has to be shown to provide a benefit on disease-free survival or a benefit to the patient's ability to function in their daily life. It also has to be shown in many cases that the new medicine will be cost effective. This means that the outcome measures in Phase IIb and III are more orientated towards patient and physician reported outcomes. For example, in oncology tumour markers used in Phase IIa will give way to demonstrating survival over a predefined period of time. In hypertension, the measurement of blood pressure may need to be accompanied by data on the incidence of cardiovascular morbidity and mortality, and in neurology and psychiatry there are a host of validated questionnaires to demonstrate meaningful clinical benefit. In addition, in many cases pharmacoeconomic data needs to be collected, if not to justify marketing authorization, then to justify the pricing of the drug to reimbursement committees and managed care plans in the various countries where the drug is to be sold. As these reported outcomes have various factors that can influence them the sample size needed to show a positive effect is generally much larger than when objectively measured surrogate markers are used. For many indications where treatments exist there are outcome measures that are recognized by the regulatory authorities as being the gold standard efficacy measure for the particular indication. These measures are not always appropriate for drugs with novel mechanism of action or for a subset of patients within an indication. It is possible to stray from the path of the standard efficacy measure and use outcomes more adapted to the clinical scenario, but it requires good justification and careful negotiation with the relevant competent authorities.

Phase IIIb and IV studies

The data included in the submission package from the Phase I to III studies is very comprehensive; however, it is not possible to guarantee that all adverse effects that could be observed when the drug is on the market, have been identified in the pre-marketing studies; especially for those events that occur with an incidence of less than 1 in 10 000. Indeed there are many cases of drugs being withdrawn from the market for safety reasons, or having significant labelling amendments applied to them, once more information has become available. Regulatory authorities recognize that to ask companies to collect tens of thousands of patients' safety data in the initial submission package would be costly, time consuming, and could cause unnecessary delay, or even prevent the marketing of useful new medicines. Therefore, in order to protect patient safety once the drug is on the market, the authorities request that the companies perform post-marketing safety surveillance, through specific studies designed to evaluate safety of the marketed drug and by means of filing Periodic Safety Update Reports (PSURS). The data for these reports are collected by the company's pharmacovigilance group, whose members are specially trained in drug safety surveillance. The reports are required to be filed at regular intervals and include data from ongoing trials and spontaneous adverse event reports, which can arise from a variety of sources, e.g. doctors, patients, clinical trials, journal articles, etc.

Clinical trials collecting additional data can be started while the initial marketing authorization submission is being reviewed. Authorities will sometimes accept dossiers for review with limited duration safety data if the company continues the collection of data during the review period and has sufficient patient exposure by the time the authority comes to make their decision. Studies conducted in this peri-approval period are known as Phase IIIb studies. If a company wishes to expand the indication, they may also conduct additional pivotal efficacy studies in the peri-approval period or shortly after product launch and these studies also fall into the category of Phase IIIb.

The Phase IV studies, which take place once the product is on the market, may take the form of collecting safety data as required by authorities, but they may also be used to collect additional simple efficacy data which are used to support the marketing effort. Phase IV studies are generally large in scale, conducted at widespread sites but usually of simple design, and are orientated towards looking at how the drug is used in everyday practice within the confines of the existing product licence. As for any clinical trial, Phase IIIb and IV studies are subject to the conditions of ICH GCP.

Bridging studies

Data generated in the USA and/or Europe and used to support marketing approval of the drug in Japan present more problems, owing to the more significant intrinsic (e.g. genetic) differences between Caucasian and Japanese populations. An example is the greater frequency of polymorphisms in the cytochrome P450 enzyme CYP2A6 (Oscarson, 2001) seen in Chinese and Japanese populations, and the related differences in nicotine metabolism. It is therefore usually necessary for a study to be carried out to 'bridge' Caucasian data into Japan, i.e. to test the validity of Caucasian data in a Japanese population. This is done by studying the drug's pharmacokinetics, and usually its pharmacodynamic properties, in both populations and analysing the results to determine whether they are comparable.

In considering the issue of extrapolating drug safety and efficacy data from one population to the other, the objective is to do this safely while not repeating clinical trials unnecessarily. Specific ICH guidelines exist for the extrapolation of data from one ethnic group to another (ICH, E5 latest update 2006). There are several strategies and approaches for exploring ethnic differences in drug response, but none is appropriate for all circumstances and each situation must be carefully evaluated, with a detailed understanding of the requirements of the target regulatory authority and its acceptance of foreign data.

Patient recruitment in efficacy studies

In exploratory efficacy studies, as the efficacy and safety in the patient population are yet to be determined, it is desirable to have a relatively homogeneous population in order to minimize variability which might confound the results. The entry criteria for patients in exploratory studies will therefore be more stringent than in the later phases where it is then desirable to study patients who are more representative of the population, which will use the drug once it is on the market. Patients can be recruited from the patient pool known to the clinic if they are regular outpatients or if they have already participated in a clinical trial in the indication. In some studies the patients may already be in the hospital (e.g. in studies of interventions in acute medical emergencies, such as myocardial infarction, stroke, or inflammatory bowel disease). Patients may be referred to the investigator from other clinics, or it is possible to source patients externally by means of advertising. There are various possibilities for advertising. Media such as radio and television are popular in the USA but less so in Europe, partly because the cost is not always commensurate with the return. Publicity in local papers and posters and fliers in hospital or general practice clinics are often effective, as are advertisements on a hospital website. The appropriateness of external advertising will depend on the indication. For common, straightforward ailments, such as migraine or allergies, external advertising can be a good way to recruit patients, but for more complex indications, for example in neurology or oncology, it may not be appropriate. The disadvantage of advertising is that the patient coming in 'off the street', is not already known to the investigator and so a thorough check of the patient's medical history and trial eligibility, including likelihood of good compliance, needs to be made. All advertising materials, including the scripts for radio and television advertisements, have to be reviewed and approved by ethics committees before they can be used. Patients who take part in the efficacy trials may anticipate deriving some clinical benefit; therefore, they are not volunteers as such, and cannot be paid for their participation, as is the case for subjects in Phase I studies. However, the patients can receive a modest sum to cover out-of-pocket costs for transport and subsistence associated with the study clinic visits, the amount of which has to be approved by the ethics committee.

CLINICAL TRIALS IN CHILDREN

As part of the overall clinical development plan it is now a requirement in the EU and USA to include a paediatric drug development plan. The objective is to have thorough testing of the safety, pharmacokinetics and efficacy of drugs that may also be used in children, so that correct dosing information, using an appropriate formulation, can be given for this population. In the past, companies tended to shy away from testing their drugs in children due to ethical concerns and also because the paediatric market was not seen to be particularly commercially attractive. Adult drugs were used off-label in children, often by extrapolating the adult dose to the weight of the child with no proper guidance in the product label for paediatric use. However, there are many medical conditions that occur in children as well as in adults. Examples of drugs commonly used by children as well as adults include anti-epileptics, asthma drugs, anti-inflammatory and anti-infectives. The therapeutic margin of some of these compounds can be quite narrow and so precise information about safety and dosing in children is very important. Differences in metabolism exist between adults and children and at different times in childhood, e.g. during adolescence, that may alter the kinetics or safety of the adult medicine. Also formulations used by adults many not be suitable for use in children. The purpose of the plan, therefore, is to ensure that companies will develop medicines that can also safely and effectively treat important conditions in children. The draft plan is usually requested by the end of Phase II. The timing of the start of the paediatric trials is usually within a year after the product licence for the adult use has been granted. However, this can be varied according to the indication or need. Exemptions to paediatric development can be obtained if the disease does not exist in children, for example Parkinson's disease or Alzheimer's disease, or in certain age categories, e.g. migraine, which does not really occur in children less than 6 years old.

REGULATORY AND ETHICAL ENVIRONMENT

In most parts of the world, clinical trials are a legal requirement before a new drug can be sold or any claims made for its therapeutic benefit or safety. All clinical trials, including Phase I studies, are subject to international, national and, sometimes, also local regulation. International regulatory requirements for human administration of a new active substance (NAS) are set out in a series of guidelines published by the International Committee on Harmonization (ICH; see Chapter 20). This committee was formed to harmonize the regulation of clinical trials in the three major pharmaceutical development regions (European Union, USA and Japan), with the aim of avoiding duplication of clinical research programmes when applying for approval in all three ICH regions. National and local regulations still exist and may vary from country to country within these regions, but ICH guidelines still apply and usually have the force of law. Clinical development of new drugs for registration in any of these regions must comply, and be seen to comply, with ICH guidelines if the data are to be accepted for registration purposes in the ICH regions, irrespective of where in the world they were generated. This means it is not possible to sidestep the requirements of the ICH guidelines by developing drugs outside the ICH regions in a manner that would not comply with them. As the EU, USA and Japan represent the three biggest world markets for new drugs, there is little incentive for non-compliance.

All human studies are performed according to strict ethical requirements. The Declaration of Helsinki (World Medical Association, 2008) and ICH Guidance E6 (CPMP/ICH/135/95) 2002 set the rules for all clinical development. In one sentence, the message comes through: 'It is the duty of the physician in medical research to protect the life, health, privacy, and dignity of the human subject'. The major points of the Declaration of Helsinki and ICH E6 Good Clinical Practice are summarized below:

- The risks and potential benefits must be assessed before trials are initiated, and the benefits must outweigh the risks.
- The interests of the individual study subjects must take precedence over those of science or society.
- All trial subjects must freely give their informed consent prior to participation.
- Trials must be scientifically sound and clearly described in a trial protocol.
- The trial must be carried out according to the protocol, which must be reviewed and approved by a properly constituted ethics committee.
- Only properly qualified physicians may provide medical care to trial subjects, and all other staff involved in clinical trials must be appropriately educated, qualified and experienced for the tasks they carry out.
- Human administration must be supported by the results of adequate preclinical testing in compliance with ICH guidelines for the administration of drugs to man.
- Data from clinical trials must be recorded, handled and stored in a way that allows accurate reporting, interpretation and verification.
- Trial subjects' privacy and confidentiality must be respected and assured.
- The material to be administered must be of acceptable quality and purity, as defined by the relevant ICH guidelines. This means both the drug substance and the formulated drug product must be manufactured in compliance with ICH Guidelines (2000) for good manufacturing practice (GMP) and used in accordance with the trial protocol.
- The trial must be registered in a publicly available database prior to the first subject being recruited.

Ethical procedures

The safety of subjects is always the paramount consideration in clinical trials. There are two main bodies responsible for evaluating proposals for trials: the national drug regulatory authority in the country where the trial will take place, and the local ethics committee (EC) or, in the USA, the institutional review board (IRB) of the clinic in which the study will be performed. All clinical trials must be approved by a properly convened and correctly functioning EC or IRB before they can be initiated. Ethics committees are composed of independent experts and lay members, who review the proposed study (protocol, investigator's brochure, insurance arrangements, patient information sheet, informed consent documentation and any other patient facing materials, e.g. electronic or paper diaries, questionnaires, etc.) and decide whether it is justified on ethical grounds. They evaluate the study in terms of the risk to the subjects, the appropriateness of any remuneration offered to both subjects and the clinical investigator, the design of the study and its ability to fulfil its primary objective(s), the qualifications, experience and clinical trial performance of the clinical investigator, the text of any advertising used to recruit subjects, etc., and approve or reject the proposed trial on the basis of these ethical considerations. If it is approved, the EC/IRB remains involved with the trial until it is completed: for example, it must be informed of any serious adverse events (see below) that occur, and of any other major issues that cause concern during the study. Changes to an approved protocol may not normally be implemented without the EC/IRB approval.

In the case of regulatory authorities the degree of involvement varies from country to country (see Chapter 20), some reviewing all of the available data on the drug and some only requiring notification that EC/IRB approval has been given and that the trial will take place.

Clinical trial operations and quality assurance

As described above, all clinical trials have to be conducted to ICH Good Clinical Practice (GCP) by investigators and staff properly trained in the conduct of clinical trials. The sponsor has a duty to ensure that the trials are being conducted according to GCP both at the investigational site and within the sponsor's organization. The constraints of ICH and their local rules place a large organizational and administrative burden on the trial centres, which need to be selected with care, based on inspection of their facilities and an assessment of the investigator's and site staff's qualifications, experience and availability to carry out the study to the standard required.

The sponsor has specific responsibilities to train those involved in the trial in the requirements of the study protocol and ICH GCP standards, and then to monitor the project on site to ensure compliance monitor the performance of the sites during the study. Study staff training and monitoring may be performed by the sponsor company or delegated to a subcontractor, i.e. a clinical research organization (CRO), in which case the Sponsor has to oversee the activities of the CRO to ensure and be seen to ensure, that they are compliant with GCP. The study monitoring is performed by specially trained clinical monitors who visit the sites regularly throughout the trial and, using specific written procedures, verify the study data, check that the study is being conducted in accordance with the protocol and that there are no breaches of GCP. To further ensure compliance, additional quality assurance (QA) is carried out in the form of an independent audit. Study sites will be selected for auditing. The clinical monitor is instrumental in identifying the sites for auditing. Typically those sites who are high recruiters or who have had particular problems with the study are selected. In addition, if the monitor suspects any irregularity in the data, or even fraud, a site may undergo a 'for cause' audit. Auditors are responsible for thoroughly inspecting the data and documentation files to validate the site and the data it produces in terms of ICH compliance.

Finally, the regulatory authority itself may choose to inspect one or more clinical sites and/or the files of the sponsoring company or its CRO, as a final check on data quality. Issues arising at this late stage cast suspicion on the whole dossier and can delay or prevent the granting of marketing approval. A detailed overview of the regulatory requirements for product development and licensing are given in Chapter 20.

Issues of confidentiality and disclosure

Since 2008 it has become a requirement for all clinical trials to be registered on a publicly accessible database before the first patient is enrolled. In the USA and Europe clinical trials can be registered on http//www.clinicaltrials.gov or http//pharmacos.eudra.org which provide details of the purpose and plan of the trial, the clinical centres and investigators involved, and the stage the trial has reached. For every trial a registration number (International Standardized Randomized Controlled Trial Number, ISRCTN) is assigned, allowing public access to information on all prospective studies involving experimental and registered compounds. Its main aim is to avoid unnecessary repetition of clinical trials. These databases do not, however, include the *results* of completed trials, which frequently remain unpublished.

Regulatory authorities (see Chapter 20) require detailed results of all clinical trials approved by them – including trials of marketed compounds – to be reported to them, but this information is not, in general, publicly accessible, except to the extent that the Summary Basis of Approval (USA) or Centralized Evaluation Report (EU) that is published when a drug is approved, includes a summary of the clinical trials results on which the approval was based. Clinical trial sponsors are under an obligation to report to the regulatory authority any safety issues that come to light, and in the case of marketed drugs the regulatory authority may respond by altering the terms of the marketing approval (for example by including a warning in the package insert, or, in an extreme case, by withdrawing the approval altogether). Publication of trial results in the open literature is not obligatory. Trial sponsors often choose to publish their data in refereed journals, although they are not obliged to do so, and both they and journal editors tend to give preference to positive rather than negative findings (Hopewell et al., 2009). Publication bias inevitably means that good news receives more publicity than does bad news. The most recent Declaration of Helsinki, from 2008, states that authors should publish trial results or make them publicly available whether they are positive, negative or inconclusive. GlaxoSmithKline, has a publicly available database of trial results summaries for its marketed drugs and www.clinicalstudyresults.org also contains study results for marketed compounds. For drugs that fail in development there is no obligation to put the results into a public database, nevertheless, there is increasing pressure for companies to publish data about their drugs in development whether positive or negative. Such transparency could help drug development in general as much can be learned from the development programmes of drugs that do not make it to market.

SEAMLESS DRUG DEVELOPMENT WITH ADAPTIVE CLINICAL TRIAL DESIGN: THE FUTURE OF CLINICAL DEVELOPMENT?

The disadvantage of the conventional step-wise approach to clinical development where drugs move to the next Phase once the preceding Phase is finished is that it is time-consuming, costly and drugs may fail in late Phase development. It is estimated currently that approximately 40% of drugs entering Phase III do not make it through registration (Di Masi et al., 2010). The success rate is somewhat dependent on the indication, with GI, CNS and cardiovascular drugs having the lowest overall success rates (Di Masi et al., 2010). This is a great waste of resources for the pharmaceutical industry and a missed opportunity for medical practice. Late-stage attrition rates may be reduced by adopting a more seamless approach to the clinical development programme using adaptive clinical trial designs so that ineffective drugs can be identified earlier and their development terminated and those drugs with promising efficacy can be accelerated through development, with a higher likelihood of successful registration.

There are a number of ways in which the development stages can be merged or overlapped. Broadly speaking the development path is looking to have initial safety testing with exploratory efficacy leading to a go/no-go decision and then confirmatory efficacy and safety, leading up to filing the registration dossier. It is becoming more common for initial Phase I protocols to contain more than one stage. For example, within the same protocol it is possible to do a single ascending dose study, a food effect crossover at a dose determined from the SAD, and then, based upon these results, go into the multiple ascending dose study, which itself might contain pharmacodynamic evaluations relevant to the desired indication. Using this combined approach saves time in making repeated applications to regulators and ethics committees. Provided the decision points to proceed to the next stage within the study are clear and subjects' safety is maintained throughout, combination Phase I protocols can be approved at a single regulatory and ethical review. If efficacy in an indication can be shown with a single dose, an initial proof of concept study in patients could commence after the SAD and be conducted in parallel with the MAD, thereby overlapping Phase IIa with Phase I. This always assumes that safety and tolerability in the SAD were acceptable. A good example of this is acute treatment of migraine, where efficacy can be shown with a single dose of study medication to treat a single attack of migraine. For indications where repeat dosing and/or steady state plasma levels are considered necessary to see a treatment effect one can consider performing the MAD study in patients, again assuming that the level of tolerability is acceptable for proceding straight to patients after the SAD. Most likely a relevant surrogate marker of efficacy will be required as the full effect on symptom control or control of the disease may not be evident until after several weeks' treatment. An example of this could be treatment of gastro-esophageal reflux with a reflux inhibitor. The effect of a study drug on the occurrence of reflux events and transient lower oesophageal sphincter relaxations, following a challenge meal, can be monitored with oesophageal impedance-pH monitoring and manometry respectively, on a single day at steady state. Clinical symptoms could be monitored as a secondary objective because a significant effect on clinical symptom control would not necessarily be anticipated with such a short duration study. In the case of oncology studies it is routine to look for clinical effects in patients using surrogate markers in clinical pharmacology studies, as it is not possible to test most anticancer drugs in healthy subjects.

Once a go/no-go decision has been achieved in the exploratory phase, dose range finding Phase IIb studies can be combined with Phase III to achieve the objective of finding the optimal dose and having adequate, well-controlled, pivotal efficacy and safety data. An example of this approach is to have a parallel group, dose range finding study that has sufficient sample size and power so that it can be considered pivotal. Patients on the optimal dose can then continue either into an open-label safety phase or generate further efficacy and safety data in a double-blind controlled study extension Adaptive trial designs are useful in this regard, because the optimal dose could be selected from several dose arms on an interim measure, and then the study continued with the optimal dose to achieve full power (Orloff et al., 2009). Using the seamless Phase II to Phase III design, the second pivotal efficacy study can be started with the optimal dose as soon as it has been identified and the start of this study would overlap with the end of, or continuation of the dose range finding study. As the sample size for this type of study is likely to be larger than a conventional stand-alone Phase IIb dose range finding study, there needs to be sufficient confidence that the results of exploratory studies will be replicated in the larger scale trials at the doses chosen.

Adaptive design trials are those where an interim adaptation of treatment or endpoint during the study is decided before the study is started. The *a priori* protocol design incorporates the changes within it. The FDA's draft guidance from February 2010 (FDA, 2010) defines adaptive trial design studies as 'a prospectively planned opportunity for modification of one or more specific aspects of the study design and hypotheses based on analysis of the data (usually interim data) from subjects in the study'.

The purpose is to make studies more efficient, either by having a shorter duration, fewer patients, more appropriate patients, increasing the likelihood of identifying drug activity if it exists, or making the study more informative, for example in understanding better the dose response, the patients, or part of the indication most likely to benefit.

The adaptations may include the following:

- Change of sample size to either increase or decrease it according to results of an interim analysis
- Reallocate treatment distribution; dose groups may be added or dropped according to predefined criteria for doing so
- Changing the treatment duration
- Refining the study entry criteria: certain patient types may be dropped if they appear to have no benefit, alternatively the population can be enriched with patient types who appear to be deriving benefit.

The types of adaptations used may differ according to whether the trial is in the exploratory or confirmatory phase (Orloff et al., 2009). For example, surrogate endpoints such as biomarkers may be used to evaluate patient progress in an exploratory study, whereas clinical outcome measures would be needed in a confirmatory study. In an exploratory study it may be possible to use a single (patient) blind approach to reallocate treatments. An example of this was a study of migraine. The investigator knew the treatment allocation but the patients did not. The first patient at each site was allocated to start on a mid-range dose of the treatment. If the patient had a headache response, the next patient was allocated the next dose down, if not, the next patient was allocated the next dose up. The doses were changed up or down by the investigator according to each patient's response. The results of this study turned out to closely predict the dose that was chosen as the optimal effective dose by a subsequent, conventional, parallel, dose-range finding study.

It is crucial that making the adaptations while the study is ongoing does not compromise the integrity or outcome of the study. The FDA draft Guidance 2010 (FDA, 2010) lays out the major design and performance considerations to be taken into account for adaptive clinical trials. The study needs to be carefully designed and the protocol clearly written to incorporate any interim analyses, the conduct of which must be performed in such a way as to not compromise the study blinding, or influence interpretation of the data. Close liaison with statisticians, who will have to model the effects of proposed adaptations on statistical outcomes, will be required when designing the study. Likewise the regulatory affairs group needs to be involved to help craft a protocol that will be acceptable and justify the use of the adaptive design to competent authorities. This means that the study design and protocol writing stage may take longer than a conventional study, but the reward should come in the form of a study that may be shorter to perform and have a higher chance of a successful outcome.

Adaptive clinical trials lend themselves better to some indications than others. The ideal scenario is to have an indication where the effect of treatment is rapidly evident and objectively measurable. For example, as blood glucose and blood pressure are objective and respond rapidly to effective intervention, Phase IIa studies in diabetes or hypertension could use adaptive design to good advantage, to rapidly identify doses and the target patient population. Acute treatment of migraine is a good example of an indication where adaptive design could be used throughout the development. Migraine attacks occur frequently in the study population and the gold standard efficacy parameter 'pain free at 2 hours post dose' is easily identifiable, even though it relies on the patient to report it. Indications where drug benefit takes months or years to become apparent and rely heavily on patient reported outcome are more challenging. This includes studies in oncology, neurology and psychiatry. Nevertheless, in the exploratory phase it may well be possible to perform an adaptive design using surrogate markers, to improve the dose and patient selection for confirmatory efficacy in these indications.

To summarize, the schematic in Figure 17.2A shows the stages and timelines of a conventional clinical development path and Figure 17.2B shows how a new form of clinical development might look, using seamless development with adaptive clinical trial design.

CONCLUSIONS

Clinical development is the cornerstone of bringing new medicines to the market. It is a complex, highly regulated,

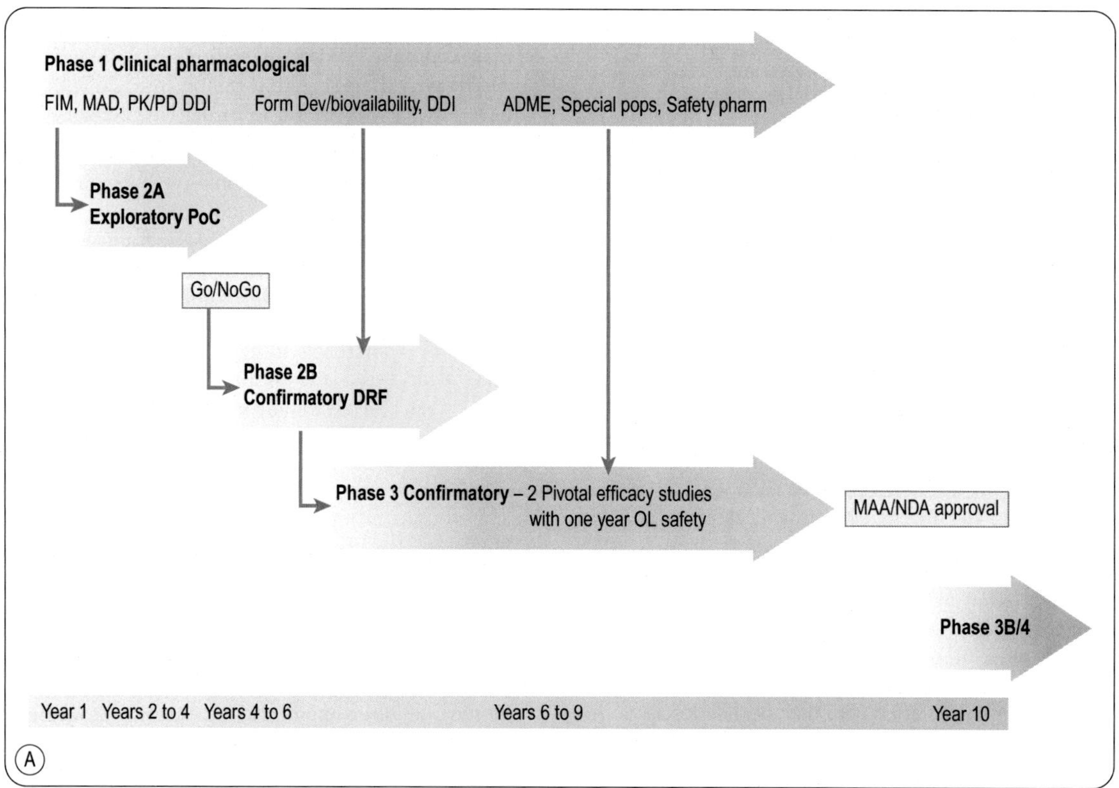

Fig. 17.2 A, Conventional path of clinical development.

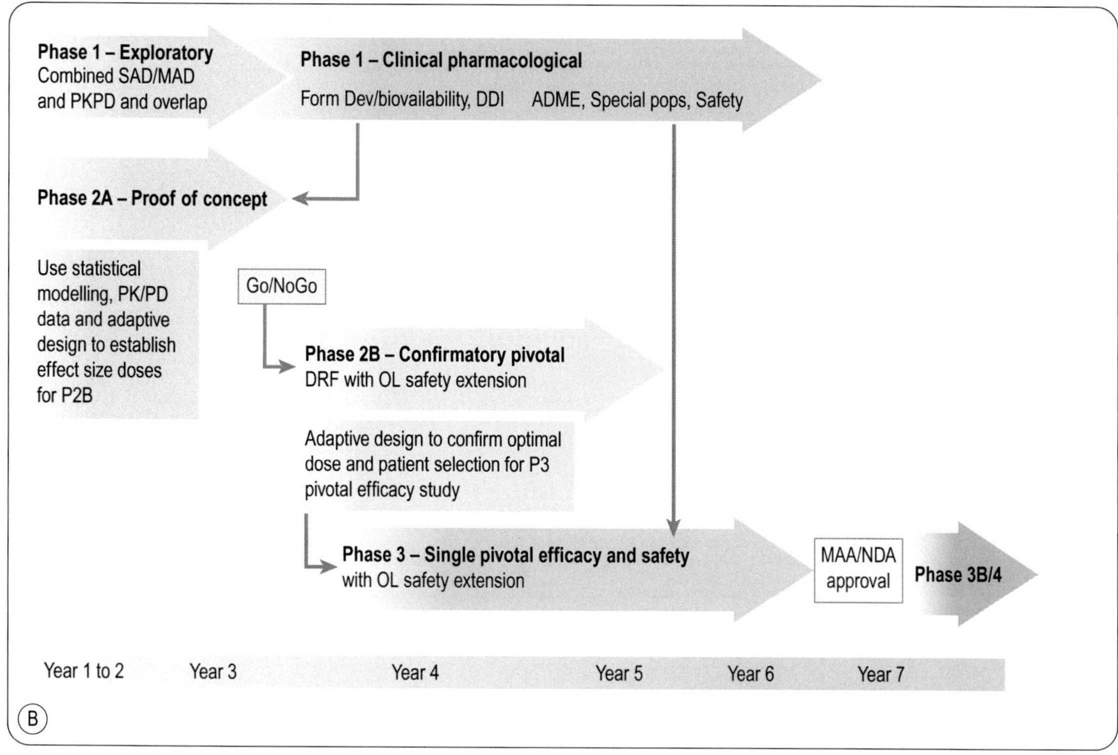

Fig. 17.2 ***Continued*** B, Seamless development with adaptive trial designs.

time-consuming and very costly part of the overall drug development process, with a substantial risk of failure. The traditional path of clinical development hitherto has served the pharmaceutical industry reasonably well and has enabled high-quality innovative medicines to be delivered to patients. However, the current process has a high attrition rate which is wasteful of financial, medical and patient resources. New initiatives are being launched at the input end to improve the sourcing of the drug development pipeline through public and private partnership, partnership with academia and partnership between small and large pharmaceutical companies and at the output end, by modifying the traditional clinical development pathway. It is hoped that adopting these new initiatives will enable companies to bring new medicines to the market and to patients more effectively and rapidly.

REFERENCES

Adams CP, Brantner VV. Estimating the cost of new drug development: is it really 802 million dollars? Health Affairs 2006;25:420–8.

Beecher HK. The powerful placebo. Journal of the American Medical Association 1955;159:1602–6.

Di Masi JA, Hansen RW, Grabowski HG. The price of innovation: new estimates of drug development costs. Journal of Health Economics 2003;22:151–85.

Di Masi JA, Feldman L, Seckler A, et al. Trends in risks associated with new drug development: success rates for investigational drugs. Clinical Pharmacology and Therapeutics 2010;87:272–7.

EFPIA. The Innovative Medicines Initiative. www.imi-europe.org; 2008.

FDA. US Food and Drug Administration 2004. Innovation or stagnation: challenge and opportunity on the critical path to new medicinal products. www.fda.gov/oc/initiatives/criticalpath/whitepaper.html; 2004a.

FDA. US Food and Drug Administration 2004. Innovation or stagnation: critical path opportunities report and list. www.fda.gov/oc/initiatives/criticalpath/reports/opp_report.pdf; 2004b.

FDA (2010) FDA Guidance for industry: adaptive design clinical trials for drugs and biologics. Feb 2010.

Hopewell S, Loudon K, Clarke MJ, et al. Publication bias in clinical trials due to statistical significance or direction of trial results. Cochrane Database Systematic Review 2009;1:MR000006.

Orloff J, Douglas F, Pinheiro J, et al. The future of drug development: advancing clinical trial design. Nature Reviews Drug Discovery 2009;8:949–57.

Oscarson M. Nicotine metabolism by the polymorphic cytochrome P450 2a6 (cyp2a6) enzyme: implications for interindividual differences in nicotine metabolism. Drug Metabolism and Disposition 2001;29:91–5.

Woodcock J, Woosley R. The FDA critical path initiative and its influence on new drug development. Annual Review of Medicine 2008;59:1–12.

World Medical Association. Declaration of Helsinki. Ethical principles for medical research involving human subjects. 59th WMA General Assembly, Seoul, October 2008. www.wma.net/en/30publications/10policies/b3/index.html; 2008.

Chapter 18

Clinical imaging in drug development

P M Matthews

INTRODUCTION

Preclinical and clinical imaging has already made a significant contribution to drug development. Almost 30% of new molecular entities approved for neuropsychiatric indications by the FDA between 1995 and 2004 were developed with contributions from imaging (Zhang and Raichle, 2010) and there will be a growing need in drug development for information provided by imaging. New ways of thinking about clinical development are putting a premium on integration of early biology and clinical development in the context of 'experimental medicine'.

Therapeutics development increasingly involves research that is hypothesis led, performed across levels of biological complexity (e.g. cells to the whole human), or inspired by concepts translated across species (e.g. mouse to man). Similar non-invasive imaging methods can be applied in both clinical and preclinical applications. Regulatory authorities also are putting an increasing emphasis on the need to have a deeper understanding of pharmacology and the biology of disease in approvals for new chemical entities, as well as the potential for delivering individualized therapies. The Critical Path Initiative (CPI) (www.fda.gov/ScienceResearch/SpecialTopics/CriticalPathInitiative/default.htm) sets out a strategy for transforming the way FDA-regulated products – drugs, biological products, medical devices and veterinary drugs – are developed and manufactured. Central to this is developing better evaluation methods (including specifically better imaging methods, as well as advancing genetics and bioinformatics – see also Chapter 7) and applying these to the acceleration of development of personalized medicine.

A useful way of considering how imaging tools can contribute to clinical drug development is through their roles in addressing major questions in new drug development:

1. *Target validation:* does the chosen therapeutic target potentially play a central role in determining the disease or symptom of interest?
2. *Biodistribution:* does the molecule reach the tissue of interest in potentially pharmacologically active concentrations?
3. *Target interactions:* does the molecule interact with the target of interest? What is the relationship between administered dose and interaction with the target?
4. *Pharmacodynamics:* what are the effects of the drug and how long do they last?
5. *Patient stratification and personalized medicine:* how can the most responsive patient population be identified for more efficient clinical trials? How can a medicine be given in the clinic to patients who will experience the greatest benefit?

This chapter will provide a brief overview of clinical imaging applications in drug development. Preclinical imaging is a larger topic, beyond the scope of this review, although reference will be made to some aspects of imaging for direct translation of pharmacological hypotheses from preclinical to clinical applications. Preclinical studies also enable the validation of innovative imaging methods that can be applied to clinical development applications.

IMAGING METHODS

Positron emission tomography (PET)

PET imaging relies on the design and manufacture of radiolabelled ligands which can bind selectively to a target of interest with minimal non-specific binding. These ligands are most typically labelled with positron-emitting

Table 18.1 Some examples of PET radioisotopes useful in drug development applications

Radioisotope	Half-life (min)
^{15}O	2.1
^{11}C	20.4
^{68}Ga	68
^{18}F	109

radioisotopes that decay with a relatively short half-life (Table 18.1). The short half-life allows high enough doses to be administered for a strong imaging signal without substantially increasing long-term health risks associated with the ionizing radiation.

PET imaging is based on the principle that emitted positrons collide with local electrons to produce pairs of photons that travel at 180° to each other and can be detected as coincident events by γ-detectors surrounding the subject. The relative positions of detection of coincident events and their precise timing enable localization of the original annihilation events for reconstruction of the spatial distribution of the radiolabelled ligand. By following the time course of the emissions (and appropriate instrument corrections) across different tissues, the rates of delivery of the radiotracer and the amount retained can be modelled.

Only microdoses of radioligands or other radiolabelled molecules need to be used; PET is exquisitely sensitive and even nanomoles of labelled material (e.g. with ^{11}C-labelling) can be detected. However, spatial resolution is limited intrinsically by the distance over which the annihilation event occurs (and, in practice, is typically ~4 mm). The PET data can be co-registered with structural data from computed tomography (CT) or MRI images to localize the signal anatomically.

Magnetic resonance imaging (MRI)

MRI imaging conventionally relies on the interaction of the weak magnetic dipole of the hydrogen nucleus with a strong applied magnetic field varying in a well-defined way across the body. Energy in the radiofrequency range modulates this with a specific frequency that depends on the precise magnetic field at each point in the body. As most hydrogen atoms in the body are in water (or fat), the frequencies of the mix of signals detected can be used to reconstruct tissue morphology as an image. Additional information comes from the intensity and duration of the signal detected. These are determined by the concentration of hydrogen atoms (e.g. how much water or fat) and their local environment, respectively.

The effect of the environment of the hydrogen atoms is expressed as two parameters: the T_1 and T_2 relaxation times. Changes in the way in which the radiofrequency is applied and the signal received by the scanner, mix the relative contributions of T_1 and T_2 parameters to signal in different ways. This allows image contrast (grey scale variation) between different tissues (e.g. grey matter and white matter in the brain) or regions of a heterogenous tissue to be generated. Images thus allow tissue size and shape to be measured and are sensitive to the state of tissue (e.g. changing with evolution of the pathology of stroke in the brain).

The signal of blood relative to tissue can be enhanced on a T_1-weighted imaged by intravenous injection of a gadolinium chelate 'contrast agent' that alters local relaxation properties of water in the blood. Quantitative assessments of signal change after the injection of contrast agent provides one way by which MRI can measure blood volume and flow. Leak of plasma across the vascular endothelium (e.g. with a damaged blood–brain barrier or with tumour neovascularization) can be detected as abnormal, sustained tissue signal enhancement after this contrast administration.

MRI images usually measure volumes between 1 and 5 mm^3. Morphological measures can be conducted with high precision because of the high soft tissue contrast. Moreover, the method is non-ionizing and without known health risks.

Functional magnetic resonance imaging (fMRI)

fMRI is based on indirect measures of neuronal response by being sensitive to changes in relative blood oxygenation (Jezzard, 2001). Increased neuronal activity is associated with a local haemodynamic response involving both increased cerebral blood flow and blood volume. This *neurovascular coupling* appears to be a consequence predominantly of presynaptic neurotransmitter release and thus reflects local signalling.

The most commonly used fMRI (or pHMRI) imaging method applies blood oxygen level dependent contrast (BOLD). MRI is sensitive to changes in blood oxygenation because deoxyhaemoglobin is paramagnetic and, therefore, locally distorts the static magnetic field used for MR imaging. In the MRI magnet, the magnetic field is made highly homogeneous, but the presence of deoxyhaemoglobin leads to small magnetic field *inhomogeneities* around blood vessels, the magnitude of which increases with the amount of paramagnetic deoxyhaemoglobin. A relationship between neuronal activation and blood oxygenation is observed because blood flow increases with higher neuronal activity and this increase in blood flow is larger than is needed simply for increased oxygen delivery with greater tissue demands: the local oxygen extraction fraction decreases with synaptic signalling. The signal, therefore, is not a measure of blood flow directly. Note also that these signal changes are small (typically, 0.5–5% at 3T).

A typical experiment would involve acquisition of a series of brain images during infusion of a drug or over the course of a changing cognitive state (e.g. performing a visually presented working memory task vs. attending to a simple matched visual stimulus). Regions of significant signal change with drug infusion or between cognitive states then are defined by statistical analysis of the time series of signal change. Quantitative measurement of this change allows measures relevant to drug action on the brain to be defined.

HUMAN TARGET VALIDATION

Confidence in progression of drug development from target validation in preclinical models (e.g. by demonstration of a phenotype plausibly related to the human disease with knockout of the gene of interest) is often limited. The approach arguably is particularly problematic for chronic diseases, for diseases that are determined by the interaction of multiple biological factors and the environment and particularly for those with uniquely human phenotypes (e.g. most neurological or psychiatric disorders). This has brought an increasing interest in validation of new therapeutic targets using experimental medicine and human disease 'models'. Imaging supports this by providing a range of methods for directly assessing molecular interactions, biochemistry and physiology in humans non-invasively. To date, most applications have been to targets for neuropsychiatric diseases.

Human models can support target validation for symptom management. For example, sleep deprivation has been used as a model for mild cognitive impairment. FMRI can be applied as a probe for physiological changes specific to sleep deprivation-associated cognitive impairment to enable assessment of any responses to a test agent interacting with the target of interest (Chuah and Chee, 2008). In this instance, the ability of fMRI to report quantitatively on physiological modulation in specific functional anatomical regions relevant both to diseases of cognitive impairment and the model (e.g. the hippocampus) adds specificity to associated behavioural measures. Modulation of impaired hippocampal activation during memory tasks after sleep deprivation by a molecule interacting with a novel target provides compelling evidence supporting validation of the target for symptomatic treatment of disorders of memory.

An alternative concept for target validation in humans involves testing for modulation of disease-related brain systems by allelic variation at candidate target loci. This approach employs structural MRI or fMRI outcomes as *endophenotypes* (heritable quantitative traits). For example, indirect evidence has suggested that glycogen synthase kinase-3beta (GSK3β) and canonical Wnt pathway function contribute to the molecular pathology of major depressive disorder (MDD). Brain structural changes also have been associated with MDD. To test the hypothesis that GSK3β is relevant to the disease, variations in brain grey volume were associated with GSK3β polymorphisms in a mixed population of healthy controls and MDD patients to demonstrate an interaction between genetic variation and MDD (Inkster et al., 2009). Supporting evidence for a functional association also can come from similar analyses linking brain structural variation to genetic polymorphisms related to genes encoding multiple proteins contributing to the same signalling pathway (Inkster et al., 2010).

Functional imaging methods can be used in similar ways. Patients with a history of affective disorders carrying the S allele of the common 5-HTTLPR polymorphism in the serotonin transporter gene (SLC6A4) have an exaggerated fMRI response (in the amygdala) to environmental threat relative to L allele homozygotes (Hariri et al., 2002). Other work has supported hypotheses regarding genetic variation associated with other disorders. For example, polymorphisms linked to the genes DISC1, GRM3 and COMT all have been related to imaging endophenotypes for schizophrenia and associated with altered hippocampal structure and function (Callicott et al., 2005), glutamatergic fronto-hippocampal function (Egan et al., 2004) and prefrontal dopamine responsiveness (Egan et al., 2004), respectively.

Application of functional MRI approaches that define neurobiological bases for general cognitive processes (such as in the context of psychiatric disease, motivation or reward) facilitate understanding of the general importance of targets relevant to more than one disease. For example, fMRI approaches have contributed to the current appreciation for neural mechanisms common to addictive behaviours across a wide range of substance abuse states. Studies of cue-elicited craving have defined similar activities of the mesolimbic reward circuit in a range of addictions (e.g. nicotine (David et al., 2005)). Combination of fMRI with PET receptor mapping on the same subjects has the potential to relate systems-level dysfunction directly with the molecular targets of drug therapies to further speed target validation in appropriate circumstances.

With the potential to define the relationship between in vivo molecular pathology and disease expression, the relevance of a target can be inferred more confidently in some instances than is possible based on post-mortem studies only. For example, central to current therapeutic hypotheses for schizophrenia is targeting of dopamine receptor signalling. PET imaging with a receptor-specific radiotracer allows the receptor densities and distributions to be mapped in vivo in patient and healthy control populations. Using this approach, D_2/D_3 binding potential values have been shown to be abnormal in schizophrenics in both striatal and extrastrial regions and to vary with age (Kegeles et al., 2010).

A limitation of the PET measure, however, is that it does not distinguish between effects of abnormal receptor availability or dopamine release (and neurotransmitter occupancy of the receptor that reduces the free receptor available for binding to the radiotracer). To more specifically test the therapeutic hypothesis that dopamine receptor antagonism is relevant to schizophrenia, dynamic changes in receptor binding potential can be studied before and after an intervention modulating dopamine release. For example, dopamine depletion leads to a larger increase in PET D_2 receptor availability in patients with schizophrenia than in healthy controls, suggesting a higher synaptic dopamine concentration in the patients (Kegeles et al., 2010).

The relevance of a target to symptoms or behaviours can be validated in a similar fashion. For example, because dopamine is known to be an important mediator of the reinforcing effects of cocaine, it was hypothesized that alterations in dopamine function are involved in cocaine dependence. To validate dopamine receptor modulation as a therapeutic target for the treatment of drug dependence, pre- and postsynaptic dopamine function were characterized by assessing the receptor-specific binding of a PET radiotracer in recently detoxified cocaine-dependent subjects and related directly to drug-seeking behaviour in the same group of subjects (Martinez et al., 2007).

BIODISTRIBUTION

Microdialysis can provide accurate measurements of the free concentration of a drug in the brain or other organ or direct assays of tissue uptake can be performed on biopsies or performed *post mortem*. However, because of its relative inaccessibility, whether a drug intended for a CNS target crosses the blood–brain barrier in sufficient amounts to be pharmacologically active can be very difficult to answer early in new drug development using conventional approaches to Phase I and IIa studies (see also Chapter 10). Confidence in extrapolation of measures directly from rodents to humans is limited (Figure 18.1). Recognized species differences in blood–brain barrier penetration are related to species-specific patterns of expression of transport enzymes, for example. PET provides the most general method for assessing distribution of a drug molecule. Imaging biodistribution can answer the question: does a molecule reach the tissue of interest in concentrations high enough to be potentially pharmacologically active?

The principles for a PET biodistribution study are straightforward. The time course of data from the blood and tissue allow the clearance from plasma to tissue (a function of the blood flow and the tissue extraction of the molecule from the blood) to be estimated. If the tissue uptake is low, then separate estimates of the blood volume and allowance in the kinetics for the amount of the labelled molecule in the blood at any point are needed. An important caution, however, is that it is only the

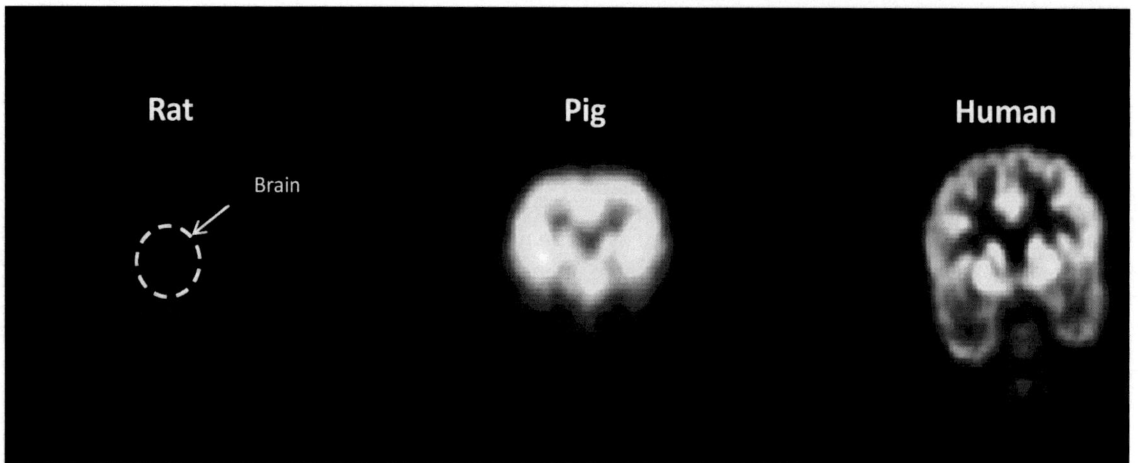

Fig. 18.1 Species differences in blood–brain barrier penetration. A novel CNS active molecule was labelled with ^{11}C for PET biodistribution studies in a rodent, pig and human. The studies illustrate how poorly predictive rodent studies can be regarding distribution into the human brain. The small rodent brain lies at the arrowhead. A detected signal scale (standardized uptake value or SUV) is shown to the right.

Images courtesy of the GSK Clinical Imaging Centre, London.

distribution of the positron-emitting isotope 'label' that is being measured with PET. Information also is needed regarding the concentration and the nature of any metabolites carrying the isotope that are generated during the imaging period and appropriate corrections made to the uptake model.

Molecules in the tissue will distribute to varying extents into tissue 'free' and 'bound' compartments. Binding can be either specific (e.g. binding to a receptor) or non-specific, reflecting, for example, lipophilic interactions or the action of non-specific uptake mechanisms. In the general case, a non-linear relationship between the relative tissue distribution of a molecule and the amount that is specifically bound is expected. To define this, a kinetic analysis of the tissue compartment signal change over time is needed, ideally with respect to another compartment in which there is similar non-specific, but no specific, binding (a 'reference' region).

Moreover, if the plasma free concentration of the labelled molecule is measured and it is assumed that the molecule distributes passively, measures over the time course to a steady-state distribution allow an estimation of the tissue free concentration (Slifstein and Laruelle, 2001). Defining the volume of distribution of a molecule along with measurement of the plasma free concentration allows the occupancy of a receptor (OR) to be estimated if the assumption that the in vitro and in vivo K_D are equivalent, where:

$$OR = C_{\text{free plasma}}/(C_{\text{free plasma}} + K_D)$$

The passive distribution assumption can be tested with separate, invasive preclinical experiments (ideally in a non-human primate for brain studies) exploring the relationship between plasma concentration of the molecule and the concentration in the tissue of interest as demonstrated by microdialysis.

The passive distribution model does not hold in situations in which there is high expression of active transporters for the molecule of interest, such as P-glycoprotein, at the blood–brain barrier. Evidence for transporters can be derived from demonstration of exclusion of tracer doses of the radiolabelled molecule but increasing tissue uptake with increasing plasma concentrations of the unlabelled molecule or after a transporter inhibitor is administered (Loscher and Potschka, 2005).

Reaching the tissue of interest in amounts sufficient to have a pharmacological effect is such a fundamental requirement for drug action that, if there is uncertainty, biodistribution data should be acquired at the earliest stages of new drug development. Relative biodistribution can be a factor contributing to selection of the lead molecule for development at candidate selection. Non-human primate or other preclinical studies can be performed efficiently prior to filing for registration of a labelled drug molecule as an investigational medicinal product (IMP). However, as the labelled drug molecule is used in microdoses only, toxicity testing for IMP filing can be limited to studies in a single species, allowing even human volunteer studies to progress early in a drug development programme.

While the greatest application of biodistribution studies thus far has been in the development of CNS drugs, biodistribution studies should also play an important role in optimizing anticancer drugs, as up-regulation of pumps that may exclude drugs from tumours is well described. When a pump mechanism is suspected, then the dependence of distribution on the dose of the unlabelled molecule can be explored. This approach was used to characterize the brain and tumour distribution of temozolomide, an alkylating agent used in the treatment of brain tumours. Normal brain and brain tumour temozolomide concentration profiles were estimated for different temozolomide dosing regimens. A relatively impaired plasma–tissue barrier in the tumour (presumed to be related to both breakdown of the blood–brain barrier and tumour angiogenesis) was demonstrated for the drug (Rosso et al., 2009).

There is a potential for integration of PET with conventional drug metabolism and pharmacokinetic (DMPK) radiotracer studies of new molecules, although it is not an approach that has been used widely. Subjects can be administered simultaneously both ^{11}C and ^{14}C-labelled molecules. The radiation burden added by the ^{14}C molecule at radiotracer doses is small. The long half-life of ^{14}C (5700 years) means that there is no time pressure on sample handling for the additional analyses! This potentially allows the ^{14}C to be used to provide more detailed information on PK behaviour, which can improve modelling in the PET experiment. An alternative would be to use ^{13}C label with GC-MS, allowing additional information on molecule absorption, distribution, metabolism and excretion (ADME) to be obtained. The value of the information can be enhanced by performing the study after administering varying pharmacological doses of the unlabelled 'cold' drug. However, the cost of this combined approach is high, limiting its use to specialized applications.

A creative extension of the traditional biodistribution experiment was demonstrated in use of the differential distribution of alternatively labelled molecules to provide information on drug metabolism directly from the PET experiment. The approach demands sophisticated radiochemistry, but provides an elegant reminder that what is measured by PET is the distribution of the label, not the molecule specifically. Temozolomide undergoes decarboxylation and ring opening in the 3–4 position to produce the highly reactive methyldiazonium ion that alkylates DNA. To evaluate this directly in humans, a dual radiolabelling strategy was employed in which [^{11}C]temozolomide was radiolabelled separately both in the 3-N-methyl and 4-carbonyl positions. ^{11}C in the C-4 position of [4-^{11}C-carbonyl]temozolomide will be converted to

$[^{11}C]CO_2$ and an inactive metabolite. Paired studies were performed with both forms of $[^{11}C]$temozolomide in 6 patients with gliomas. A third PET scan was performed with ^{11}C-radiolabelled bicarbonate to provide data allowing quantitative modelling of the labelled CO_2 release from the independently performed temozolomide experiment. Data were obtained on activities of $[^{11}C]$temozolomide and $[^{11}C]$metabolites in plasma collected during scanning and $[^{11}C]CO_2$ was measured in the expired air. Greater amounts of $[^{11}C]CO_2$ in the plasma and exhaled air and lower tumour $[^{11}C]$temozolomide signal with the $[4\text{-}^{11}C$-carbonyl]temozolomide relative to that labelled in the 3-N-methyl position confirmed ring-opening as a mechanism for metabolic activation of temozolomide (Saleem et al., 2003).

Monoclonal antibodies and other biopharmaceuticals are becoming an increasingly important part of new therapeutics development. An increasing range of methods are available for labelling such large molecules with positron emitting isotopes in well-defined ways (van Dongen and Vosjan, 2010). Because of the much longer distribution times for these large molecules, long-lived position emitters such as ^{89}zirconium, ^{64}copper or ^{124}iodine have been used. Considerable information potentially is available, but the slow approaches to steady-state and the distinct range of non-specific interactions and metabolism of these large molecules makes the conduct and interpretation of these studies more challenging than for small molecules. While promising, this area still is in an early stage of development. There are special challenges in defining a meaningful distribution for radiotracers with very high affinities (especially if the binding site availability [B_{avail}] also is high), as the distribution may reflect delivery (blood flow) more than the distribution of specific binding sites.

TARGET INTERACTION

Does a potential drug interact with the intended target to an extent that could be pharmacologically active? What is the relationship between plasma concentrations (and, thus, administered dose) and the extent of target interaction?

Direct demonstration of interaction of a molecule with the tissue target confirms distribution into the tissue. Target interaction studies also allow estimation of relevant tissue binding of a molecule without making assumptions regarding correspondences between in vivo and in vitro measures or between human and preclinical in vivo receptor affinities.

Target interaction studies are more informative if there is a strong hypothesis concerning the degree of target interaction needed for a pharmacological effect. In such cases, data relating plasma concentration to target occupancy can guide dose selection directly. For example, for inhibitors of G-protein coupled receptors, preclinical (and clinical) studies suggest that free concentrations sufficient to provide at least 70% receptor occupancy are needed. By demonstrating the relationship between plasma concentration and target interaction, doses sufficient to achieve this degree of interaction can be defined. If this information is available before dose ranging studies, the range of doses that need to be explored is reduced, allowing the number of volunteers exposed to the experimental molecule (and cost) to be minimized at this early stage.

Target interaction studies demand availability of a radioligand that has good affinity and relative specificity for the target (Cunningham, 2005). The selected radioligand with relative target selectivity then can be used for imaging the extent of target available before and after a pharmacological dose of the molecule of interest. The ratio of the specifically bound radioligand to its free concentration (estimated from the plasma free concentration) in the tissue is termed the 'binding potential' (BP). The estimated BP at equilibrium is the ratio of the target availability (B_{avail}) relative to the radioligand dissociation constant from the receptor (B_{avail}/K_D). With prior administration of the unlabelled (drug) molecule that binds to the same target, the measured BP varies with the local concentration and the affinity of the unlabelled molecule. Over a range of doses of the unlabelled molecule, the variation in radioligand BP thus allows binding affinity of the unlabelled molecule to be estimated. As a rule of thumb, the radiotracer BP before any drug administration should be greater than about 0.5 for sufficient signal to detect binding changes.

Estimates of in vivo BP for alternative candidate molecules for a target can provide particularly important information if there are dose limiting toxicities (Figure 18.2). In such cases, the BP measures and simultaneous measures of plasma concentration allow estimation of the pharmacologically active dose range, the upper limit of which can be related directly to the minimum dose at which adverse events are expected.

PET studies are expensive and theoretically confer some additional long-term health risks for volunteers arising from the additional radiation exposure. It therefore is important to optimize the efficiency of study designs to use the smallest number of subjects and the optimal selection of doses for defining the in vivo binding affinity. In contrast to the approach with a fixed dose design, adaptive designs use information gained from each experiment to improve the selection of the subsequent dose (see also Chapter 17). Adaptive designs are well suited to PET measurements of this type, as outcomes data can be provided soon after completion of a study of any one subject to contribute to dose selection for the next. The less prior knowledge concerning dosing that is available, the greater the potential efficiency gains with adaptive designs (Zamuner et al., 2010) .

Is there 'added value' from human in vivo target interaction studies in drug development? In some cases, human

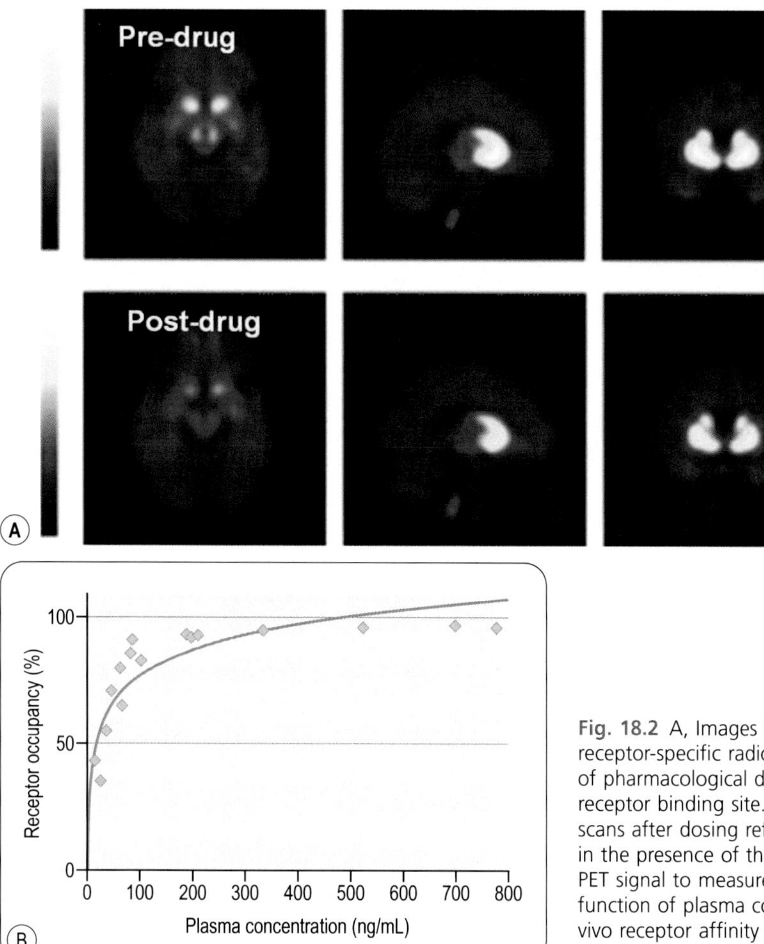

Fig. 18.2 A, Images illustrating the specific binding of a receptor-specific radioligand before and after administration of pharmacological doses of a drug targeting the same receptor binding site. The reduced specific signal on the PET scans after dosing reflects decreased receptor site availability in the presence of the drug. B, Quantitative modelling of the PET signal to measure specific binding of the radioligand as a function of plasma concentration for the drug allows the in vivo receptor affinity of the drug to be estimated.
Images courtesy of the GSK Clinical Imaging Centre, London.

in vivo binding potentials can be very different from those measured in vitro or in preclinical models. A histamine H_3 subtype antagonist, for example, was shown to have an in vivo binding potential in humans substantially greater than that estimated on the basis of preclinical studies. This observation had a substantial impact on the related drug-development programme, as it gave a rationale and confidence for a major reduction in dosing and subsequent evaluation of doses that were well tolerated by patients. The study also highlighted unexpectedly slow receptor 'off' rates for the molecule, leading to a re-estimation of the optimal dosing frequency. In general, tissue PK or target interactions and plasma PK are not the same except for the limiting case of molecules with fast equilibrium binding properties that diffuse passively between the plasma and relevant tissue compartments.

Non-human primate or preclinical studies of other species can be used to estimate relevant plasma concentration-time-target interaction relationships prior to obtaining approval of IMP approval for a molecule. Potentially important information for prioritization of candidate molecules prior to selection for clinical development can be obtained in this way. Data from preclinical (especially non-human primate) studies also can establish 'priors' that will reduce the number of volunteers needed for estimation of the human in vivo BP.

An interesting variant of this application is to the 'reverse engineering' of empirically established treatments to better define factors that may be driving therapeutic efficacy. A recent example was to better understand differences in dopamine receptor subtype interactions between atypical and typical antipsychotics. PET imaging was used in baboons with [^{11}C]PHNO to determine the binding of clozapine and haloperidol to dopaminergic D_2 and D_3 receptor subtypes. Scans were acquired following single doses of antipsychotic drugs and compared with baseline scans. The percent changes in binding (ΔBP(ND)) following challenges with antipsychotic drugs were measured. A regression model, based on published values of regional D_2 and D_3 fractions of [^{11}C]PHNO BP(ND) in six brain regions then was used to infer the specific occupancy separately on the D_2 and D_3 receptors (Girgis et al., 2011).

Target interaction studies typically have been conducted with single dose studies for experimental convenience. A follow-up study, informed by the prior data, then is possible after repeat dosing to confirm dose–occupancy relationships with more chronic drug administration. However, if it is known (or can reasonably be assumed) that repeat dosing does not induce changes in receptor expression or availability, a consistent relationship between plasma concentration and target occupancy can be assumed and repeat-dose brain target occupancy can be estimated based on the basis of the combined occupancy data obtained after administration of a single dose and plasma pharmacokinetic (PK) data. The principles behind this kind of analysis were illustrated with a study of single and repeat dose target interactions for the antidepressant duloxetine. Integrated plasma concentration-time-target occupancy models were fitted to the single dose data to characterize the model parameters and then applied to an estimated repeat dose duloxetine plasma time course to predict the 5-HTT occupancy after repeat dosing (Abanades et al., 2011).

PHARMACODYNAMICS

Imaging methods can provide information on in vivo tissue structure, physiology or biochemistry. Based on questions derived from the pharmacological hypotheses for the study, these approaches thus can be used to provide pharmacodynamic information for proof of principle or molecule differentiation. The full range of imaging methods has been – or could be – applied with the common objective of answering the question: does a molecule exert a pharmacological effect on the biological system of therapeutic interest? The potential range of applications is illustrated by some general principles and specific examples (Box 18.1).

Pharmacological studies of diseases of the brain have been a particularly important area for the development of new imaging pharmacodynamic markers, in part simply because the privileged localization of the brain limits access to tissue and the informativeness of circulating biomarkers. MRI fundamentally changed how clinical trials in multiple sclerosis (MS) were performed. An initial therapeutic goal was to limit new inflammatory lesions, which are sensitively marked by gadolinium-enhancement of T_1-weighted images in the hyperacute stage and hyperintensity on T_2-weighted images in the acute and chronic stages. The observation that the frequency of new gadolinium enhancement is as much as 10-fold the rate of disease relapse (Arnold and Matthews, 2002) and validation of the correlation between changes in these imaging markers and changes in relapse rate with treatments (Sormani et al., 2009) have given confidence that early phase trials with MRI endpoints for anti-inflammatory therapies can be reliably informative, demand smaller numbers of patients for meaningful endpoints and can be completed more quickly than trials with clinical outcome measures. An additional advantage of the close MRI monitoring is that *adverse* consequences of immune modulation also can be identified early. In such cases, the costs and complexity of serial MRI scans for the evaluation of the frequency of new enhancing lesions or the volume of T_2 hyperintense lesions is well offset by the gains in trial efficiency and informativeness. Additional endpoints are now in various stages of validation, allowing specific neuropathological changes to be

Box 18.1 **Selected applications of imaging in drug development**

Marketed drugs

- Differentiation between available treatments
- Earlier detection of disease or associated pathology:
  - Improved disease classification/diagnosis
  - Diagnosis of pre-symptomatic or minimally symptomatic disease
  - Improved identification of chronic disease exacerbation/recurrence
  - Patient stratification based on disease sub-phenotype or early treatment response

Late phase development

- Surrogate markers of response more sensitive than clinical measures
- Stratification of patients based on potential for treatment efficacy
- Pharmacological differentiation of asset from marketed drugs or new competitor compounds

Early phase development

- Biodistribution studies confirming molecule reaches the target tissue and does not accumulate in non-target sites of potential toxicity
- Target PK (dose-target occupancy) measurements guiding dose selection
- Pharmacodynamic biomarkers for proof of pharmacology, stronger 'reasons to believe' or contributing key rationale for proof of concept
- Translational preclinical imaging to identify or validate new imaging biomarkers or provide early differentiation between candidates based on target PK or PD responses

Safety and toxicity

- Imaging biomarkers as non-invasive, in vivo surrogates for direct, ex vivo studies of tissues and their translation from preclinical to clinical studies monitored to report on drug actions for remyelination, axonal loss or neurodegeneration, for example.

Alzheimer's disease (AD) has been a major recent area of new research for evaluation of imaging markers in therapeutics development because of the slow rate of progression of the disease and thus long periods over which clinical measures need to be followed for meaningful outcomes. The most striking neuropathological feature of AD is the progressive brain atrophy related to neuronal dystrophy (retraction of the extensive ramification of neurites extending from the neuronal cell body) and death. This is reflected in shrinking of the cortex (and other grey matter), which leads to generalized brain atrophy. Measurement of the rate of brain atrophy provides a pharmacodynamic index related to neurodegeneration (assuming that changes in water content or the relative size of associated cell compartments, such as glia, are not significant). Robust, automated brain MRI measures of volume and volume change provide reproducible indices of the progression of disease (Smith et al., 2009). Recent interest has focused on development of similarly robust approaches for the measurement of regional brain volumes defining atrophy specifically of the hippocampus, for example, which begins in the earliest stages of the disease and progresses faster than that for the whole brain.

Pharmacodynamic biomarkers ideally should be tailored very specifically to the drug development question. For example, a number of preclinical and pilot clinical studies had suggested that peroxisome proliferator activated receptor gamma (PPAR-γ) -gamma agonism could reverse bioenergetic defects related to abnormal insulin signalling and reduced glucose uptake in AD that might be contributing to neurodegeneration. The brain has a high metabolic rate and glucose is the preferred substrate. A reduced rate of glucose utilization, particularly in the hippocampus and temporal-parietal cortex, is an early discriminant of people at risk of developing AD. The cerebral glucose metabolic rate slows progressively over time with development of the disease. Changes are also disproportionate to decreases in volume, suggesting that they represent neuronal dysfunction prior to the neuronal dystrophy or loss assessed by structural measures. Together, this prior knowledge allowed a precise pharmacodynamic hypothesis to be generated a proof of principle study of the efficacy of the PPAR-gamma agonist rosiglitazone in AD: does treatment enhance uptake of the glucose analogue [^{18}F]-fluoro-dexoyglucose (FDG) as measured by PET and is this associated with slowing of the progressive reduction in FDG uptake expected with the natural history of the disease? A novel multi-centre FDG PET trial with 80 subjects demonstrated a trend for an improvement in FDG uptake over the first month of treatment, but provided no evidence for slowing of the progression of neurodegeneration (Tzimopoulou et al., 2010; Fig. 18.3). These data were

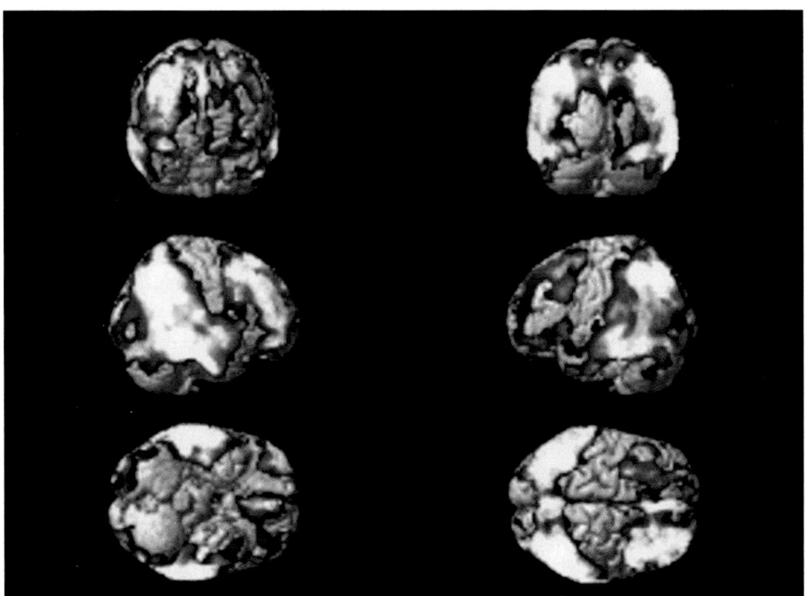

Fig. 18.3 FDG PET as an imaging biomarker for the progression of neuropathology in Alzheimer's disease. Rendering of the location of voxels with significant decreases in glucose metabolism (red) over a 12-month period are overlaid on the surface of a reference brain (grey). Changes in the rate of decrease of brain glucose metabolism can be used as a pharmacodynamic marker for therapies intended to slow neurodegeneration (Tzimopoulou et al., 2010).
Images courtesy of the GSK Clinical Imaging Centre, London.

consistent with clinical results from two large phase III trials (involving many hundreds of patients) that had been conducted in parallel. The experience highlights how directly well-selected imaging pharmacodynamic markers can be related to underlying pharmacological hypotheses. It also suggests the potential cost and trial efficiency gains that could come with optimal staging of imaging studies able to address key pharmacodynamic questions like this in a clinical development plan.

This is further illustrated by a recent study of treatment effects on brain amyloid deposition in AD. Genetic findings in families with familial disease have suggested that excessive or abnormal amyloid protein may be a cause of neurodegeneration in AD. This has led a number of pharmaceutical companies to develop anti-amyloid antibodies intended to provide a 'peripheral sink' binding amyloid and lowering the free plasma and brain amyloid concentrations. Brain amyloid deposits can be assessed by PET measures of brain binding of the radiotracer [^{11}C]-Pittsburgh compound B (PIB), which shows a relative affinity for the beta sheet structure of the deposits. In a recent Phase IIa study, time- and dose-dependent reductions in brain PIB binding were reported with use of the amyloid binding antibody bapineuzumab (Rinne et al., 2010). Imaging in this case is molecularly specific and provides a pharmacodynamic marker. PIB PET does not report directly on the free amyloid peptide or amyloid oligomers, however, and would not necessarily provide a useful pharmacodynamic marker for a treatment addressing another, independent mechanism of genesis, expression or progression of AD. Pharmacodynamic markers – whether imaging or other kinds of biomarkers – need to be tailored to meet the demands of the specific treatment question.

Similar considerations hold for the development of therapeutics in oncology. A growing 'toolkit' of imaging markers for activity of biological processes commonly altered by many therapies is becoming available. For example, quantitative FDG PET provides a marker for the elevated glucose metabolism in tumours as a concern of the upregulation of glycolysis (the 'Warburg' effect). Changes in FDG uptake can reflect specific effects on insulin signalling and glucose uptake (e.g. of use with Akt or PI3 kinase specific inhibitors), as well as non-specific effects on glycolytic enzyme expression or cell viability. Relative cell turnover rates can be probed through assessment of the activity of the thymidine salvage pathway with [^{18}F] fluoro-L-thymidine (FLT). Dynamic contrast enhanced (DCE) MRI uses the time course of signal change in a tumour after injection of a bolus of gadiolinium contrast into the circulation to model tissue blood volume, perfusion and the contrast agent permeability, which is increased with tumour neoangiogenesis. Pharmacodynamic effects of angiogenesis inhibitors should be reflected in these parameters.

Less specific markers also can be useful. X-ray computed tomography (CT) estimates of tumour size changes are at the basis of the current, widely accepted RECIST criteria for assessment of longitudinal changes with treatment. Several MRI markers of tumour volume, tissue microstructure or metabolism promise additional approaches (Workman et al., 2006). PET radiotracers are being developed to image hypoxic, apoptotic or dying cells or other parameters relevant to potential tissue responses.

fMRI is an emerging imaging pharmacodynamic marker for drugs that have actions – direct or indirect – on brain activity, for example, for measurement of brain activity while the symptom of interest is experienced, or during performance of tasks that engage cognitive processes putatively related to the symptom. The method is of particular interest as a way of providing an objective, neurophysiological measure of brain events related to subjective experiences such as pain. This could be of special value in patients who are unwilling or – as for those with AD – unable to report accurately. An advantage of fMRI is that similar imaging approaches can be adapted to address a broad range of pharmacodynamic questions simply by applying them in the context of different behavioural task challenges.

An emerging alternative to task-related fMRI is the use of resting state fMRI, which probes a class of functional interactions between brain regions (Zhang and Raichle, 2010). There is a continued background activity in the brain, the modulation of which is measured with task-constrained fMRI. A component of this background activity can be monitored as fMRI signal fluctuations at rest that occur at low frequencies (0.01–0.05 Hz) and show with coherent changes between widely separated brain regions. These consistent spatiotemporal coherence patterns define common activity networks that correspond functional anatomically with those engaged by task-constrained activations (Smith et al., 2009). These and related coherence measures can define drug effects (Cole et al., 2010).

Pharmacodynamic measures can be integrated with those for biodistribution to define PK-pharmacodynamic relationships directly. This innovative strategy was applied to the characterization of a novel antisense oligonucleotide strategy for tumour treatment. The antisense oligonucleotide was labelled with ^{11}C and a PET biodistribution study performed to demonstrate its accumulation within the tumour tissue, while biochemical studies performed on samples obtained from biopsies of the same tumours were used to relate these measures to direct tests of the pharmacodynamic hypothesis (Talbot et al., 2010).

PATIENT STRATIFICATION AND PERSONALIZED MEDICINE

A critical issue in early drug development is to establish an appropriate level of confidence in the potential of a new molecule to become a therapy. One way in which this can be facilitated is by better controlling for intrinsic variations in therapeutic responses between individuals. As well demonstrated in oncology, stratification of patients based on specific disease characteristics can allow for more powerful trial designs. Consider, hypothetically, the difference in outcomes of trials first for a population in which a new molecule has a 50% treatment effect in 20% of patients (leading to a *10%* net treatment effect) and then in a stratified population enriched so that 70% are responders (net *35%* treatment effect). If able to predict potential responders, imaging could suggest ways of best selecting optimal patient groups for applications of new molecules. Of course, developing such a strategy is predicated on having an understanding of pharmacology sufficient to make useful guesses regarding the selection of stratification criteria.

Imaging-based stratification is already applied in clinical practice to better ensure efficacy and limit adverse outcomes, e.g. to limit surgical treatments to patients with localized neoplastic disease, or tissue plasminogen activator (tPA) therapy to patients presenting within a few hours after ischaemic stroke. Enrichment of clinical trials based on imaging indices also is well established in specific areas, e.g. enrichment of MS trial populations for active inflammatory disease by screening for gadolinium-enhancing lesions at trial entry.

There are obvious cautions to the use of enrichment or stratification methods. First, they can increase trial cost or complexity to an undesirable extent. Individual scans and the additional demands for image data management, quality control and expert support in analysis add to trial cost. The demands of research imaging in busy clinical settings can limit times for scheduling subjects in a trial, introducing constraints that make trial execution more difficult. Information sheets for volunteers and consent forms inevitably become more difficult to understand as imaging procedures and their safety concerns are explained, potentially reducing recruitment. Specialized types of imaging (e.g. PET scanning with advanced radiotracers) may be able to be performed at a very limited number of sites. A consequence can be less efficient trial design and execution. These consequences need to be factored into decisions to use imaging for stratification. Optimally efficient statistical methods able to evaluate likelihoods of causality to derive maximum utility from the data and an understanding of the clinical relevance of strategies add value. In addition, for situations where imaging metrics derived from imaging that is part of routine clinical care can be used for stratification, immediate gains may be expected.

However, the gains can be lower than might initially be expected. There are a number of reasons for this. One is that use of quantitative imaging methods demands explicit consideration of ways of controlling for inter-session or inter-site variance in measurements with a care that generally has not been needed for good diagnostic imaging. A recent report also has highlighted the possibility that a stratified population behaves differently from the general population, so that gains from the investment in stratification are reduced. In this example, modelling showed that an increase in outcome variance in a subgroup of mild cognitive impairment (MCI) patients selected according to proposed criteria significantly offset the gains expected from the population as a whole (Schneider et al., 2010).

Towards personalized medicine

Personalized medicine (PM) is an extension of the concept of stratification of patients in trials to their stratification in medical care delivery. The President's Council of Advisors on Science and Technology (PCAST), in their September 2008 report entitled 'Priorities for Personalized Medicine', define *'personalized medicine'* as *'the tailoring of medical treatment to the individual characteristics of each patient. The intent is for treatments to be concentrated on those who will benefit, sparing expense and side effects for those who will not.'*

The underlying concepts are not novel. Healthcare delivery has long relied on physiological or pathological indices, as well as their clinical assessments to optimize (personalize) the diagnosis and treatment of patients. Current efforts in PM are evaluating the use of new biomarkers (including imaging based measures) together with an understanding of both pharmacology and disease to make more rational treatment choices for individual patients. Potential applications of this approach in an imaging context would include:

- Selection of patients for a treatment based on imaging
- Dose adjustment based on imaging measures
- Identification of risks or early markers of adverse events with use of the drug based on imaging
- Using imaging to monitor treatment responses
- Selection of pre-symptomatic people with developing pathology for treatment based on imaging criteria.

PM approaches ultimately will demand a common vision from the pharmaceutical industry and regulatory agencies, and likely will be most powerfully applied when a PM strategy can be incorporated into new drug development. Treatments ultimately approved for use with imaging support will need to be able to include sufficient information in the drug label to ensure that the correct patients can be selected for treatment in routine practice. This will demand that measures are both available and able to be appropriately standardized. Instrument manufacturers and relevant professional bodies are already implementing approaches to facilitate this.

IMAGING AS A SURROGATE MARKER

Enthusiasts of imaging in drug development often explain the benefits of any imaging approach through its potential to become a surrogate marker for clinical treatment responses in pivotal trials. However, the instances in which this will be possible are likely to be rather limited.

The Food, Drug and Cosmetics Act is interpreted by the FDA as demanding evidence that the drug confers a clinical benefit. This establishes a clear need to acquire data for efficacy, as the usual, most meaningful clinical measures which, in general, are not expressed simply as imaging outcomes. While this does not mean that key questions cannot be addressed with primary imaging endpoints in early phase development or that imaging data may not become a general part of regulatory packages to support the therapeutic rationale, it does not suggest that primary outcomes for late phase studies will often be able to be framed as an imaging measure.

There are circumstances in which registration based on imaging markers could be possible. For example, especially if the relationship between amyloid and Alzheimer's disease becomes firmly established, therapies to lower brain amyloid might be approved on the basis of PET molecular imaging markers of brain amyloid.

This and other special situations in which imaging may provide a primary outcome measure may be considered within the provisions of subpart H, 21 CFR 314.50 of the Accelerated Approval Provision, which allows approval on the basis of a surrogate marker *likely* to predict clinical benefit. However, a central tenet of this regulation is that it is applied in a situation in which there is an 'inability' to assess a clinical outcome with a feasible trial. Applications to the evaluation of treatments for rare diseases with known pathophysiological mechanisms, for which there are well established imaging markers, may be the most obvious areas for immediate application, e.g. in rare storage disorders such as adrenomyeloneuropathy.

Even in such situations, for the first agent in a new therapeutic class, the use of imaging markers is unlikely to meet generally acceptable criteria as a measure of efficacy. The most obvious example of how such an approach would be developed would be to follow imaging observational studies of the disease and validation of the biomarker against usual measures of progression or even against a 'gold standard' intervention. However, a simple correlation between the natural history of progression and a measure will not establish predictive *likelihood* in the context of a new treatment. Even validation against a 'gold standard' treatment does not establish the general relationship because of the potential for multiple mechanisms or therapeutic effects other than those originally postulated.

IMAGING IN THE REAL WORLD – CHALLENGES TO IMPLEMENTATION

As with any aspect of trial conduct, conceptually elegant, robust implementation of clinical imaging in the context of a new drug trial brings substantial challenges. While imaging markers can have a high statistical power in some pharmacological applications, the measures are quantitative, continuous and often dependent on multiple factors. Controlling for variance in data between sites or even between examinations at a single site can be demanding. Reasonable prior estimates of the expected treatment effect size and the reproducibility of measures is needed to estimate the potential study power. Progression of overpowered studies incorporating complex and expensive outcomes will be not be sustainable.

In general, studies with designs based on reproducibility of measures within a single site can substantially underestimate true variance. For example, structural measures based on MRI are dependent on the homogeneity and linearity of the MR gradients, which can vary between instruments and installations of even the same instruments. Fortunately, considerable effort has been expended in standardizing measurements (Boellaard et al., 2008; Friedman and Glover, 2006; Stocker et al., 2005). In analogous ways, the sensitivity of PET scanners varies. In both cases, calibrations with standard phantoms used across sites can be used to minimize variances. Even so, instrument or site bias in measurements can be introduced in many ways, e.g. differences in radiofrequency coil coupling for MRI, detection mode for PET scanners or injection timing for radiopharmaceuticals or contrast agents. Analysis of results allowing for confounding of site-to-site variation helps to ensure that site bias can be recognized and optimally accounted for.

More fundamentally, introduction of more sophisticated imaging endpoints can limit the availability sites. Training on specialized techniques may not be accessible widely, e.g. cardiac MRI demands cardiologist and radiographer training and ongoing experience to maintain skills if it is to be performed well. Some methods may be implemented only at institutions with relevant research interests. PET methods relying on molecular probes other than the few that are obtainable commercially are only available at a limited number of sites and shorter-lived isotopes (e.g., for [^{11}C] PET radiotracers) can only be used where there are radiopharmaceutical manufacturing facilities and a cyclotron are accessible on site.

The outcomes from many methods depend on precisely how they are implemented. Consensus criteria have been developed to minimize site variation in DCE-MRI measures, for example (Leach et al., 2003). Analytical techniques can be designed that are relatively robust to many aspects of patient or site variability. The issues have been discussed before in different contexts, e.g. for precision in the assessment of brain atrophy rates or dynamic changes in FDG measures of brain glucose utilization in AD (Smith et al., 2002; Tzimopoulou et al., 2010).

Imaging approaches are variably complex (or can confer additional health risks) for patients or volunteers. These factors limit volunteer interest and complicate recruitment. MRI studies can be as short as 7–10 min (e.g. a whole body scan for fat-water assessment) or less, but multi-sequence studies demand cooperation for periods of 30–60 min in what to the volunteers may be the alien environment of the high field magnet bore and with the sometimes distressing noise from the MR gradients. Prior familiarization of subjects with both the magnet and the noise, and attentive support from staff, can reduce complaints of claustrophobia and increase tolerance of more extended procedures. Contrast or radiopharmaceutical injections demand placement of intravenous catheters, so are not strictly non-invasive. While intravenous catheters are generally well tolerated, the intra-arterial (typically placed in the radial artery) cannulation needed for serial blood sampling to allow accurate estimation of the input function for fully quantitative PET can be uncomfortable. Finally, all of the imaging methods using ionizing radiation carry some estimated additional health risks for subjects. It is important, therefore, to minimize demands on volunteers to those strictly needed to answer the question(s) of interest and to ensure that the procedures and risks are explained well, that procedures are optimized to give subjects the best experience possible, and that they are conducted by highly trained staff to minimize risk or discomfort.

Some kinds of clinical studies for drug development already are incorporating imaging routinely to provide data for development decisions because of the demands of usual clinical care delivery or the need for imaging-based safety readouts. For these, the extra care in site setup and data analysis needed for quantitative imaging endpoints may add minimally to either trial cost or complexity. However, in other instances, imaging endpoints typically add substantially to cost and trial complexity and can make recruitment more difficult. Feasibility of the design of any imaging supported clinical trial needs to be carefully explored with potential trial sites. Sometimes, relatively small issues – such as the extra time needed in the clinical centre for a full imaging examination – add so much to the burden of the trial for patients communicating into a research centre, that recruitment within desired time frames is not possible. It is important, therefore, that the value of the imaging outcome is high, commensurate with these direct and indirect costs. In the planning stage, designs and development plans that do not rely on imaging need to be considered to balance the information available with respect to both ease of implementation by the sites and participation by volunteers.

Imaging supported clinical drug development is still an immature field and experience is limited. Validation of methods in the context of novel targets or classes of therapeutic molecules is even more limited. Potential applications need to be anticipated sufficiently and investments made well in advance of need if imaging is to be applied most powerfully in these contexts. This is most easily illustrated by considering molecular imaging markers. Biodistribution studies demand the site-specific labelling and quantitative modelling of the distribution of signal in the tissues of interest. Implementation demands evaluation of labelling feasibility under the constraints of automated or semi-automated radiochemical methods, tailored for the appropriate half-life and the development and validation of the specific radiopharmaceutical and metabolite quantitative analysis methods for the radiotracer of interest. While timelines are highly variable and depend on both the molecule and on particular capabilities of the imaging centre, typical estimates from our site with recent molecules suggest that even an optimal progression timeline demands at least 3–4 months for feasibility to be established, and 3 months for validation of a novel-labelled molecule. Thus, the decision to incorporate a PET biodistribution study needs to be made well in advance of the need for information. Fortunately, as a microdosing experiment, this planning can be done and implementation completed as one of the earliest experiments in the sequence of clinical development studies.

Target occupancy studies are more demanding, especially if a radioligand suitable for use as a reporter for the target needs to be developed. Radioligand development is as challenging as the first stages of any drug development programme, as affinity and specificity need to be balanced for the molecule. Candidate radioligands show high attrition along the course of development and validation. Limiting non-specific binding is a particular challenge. In general, useful radioligands should be lipophilic enough to diffuse well between tissue compartments without being so lipophilic that they accumulate in fatty tissues to a substantial extent. However, recent advances in a design based biomathematical modelling approaches (Guo et al., 2009) and the great potential for radioligand development to benefit from medicinal chemistry experience in the syntheses of related drug candidates suggest that there are substantial opportunities for more efficient development in the future.

Pharmacological fMRI offers the advantages of a potentially general marker for brain pharmacodynamic studies and has been used for a broad range of applications in healthy volunteers and patients. However, major challenges to the meaningful quantitative interpretations of pHMRI measures remain. First, the relationship of blood flow changes with altered presynaptic activity depends on the physiological (and, potentially, pharmacological) context. Even the direction of changes in relative activation in pathological states may be difficult to interpret precisely. For example, reduced activation in the aging brain may reflect either brain functional impairment or improved efficiency. Experimental designs need to accommodate this, for example by studying dose–response relations and behavioural correlates in individual studies. Additionally, BOLD signal changes arising from any direct (or indirect, e.g. with changes in ventilation rate (Wise et al., 2004)) need to be controlled. Nonetheless, experience has shown that fMRI provides pharmacologically discriminative measures (Matthews, 2009) and that studies can be implemented across multiple sites and the resulting data meaningfully integrated (Bosnell et al., 2008).

Future methodological developments promise to make fMRI even more informative. Computational advances already allow robust analyses in real time. In the context of pHMRI, this could enable improved quality control during an examination or more precise tailoring of the protocol to the question being asked about an individual patient. Some limitations to interpretation of the BOLD response can also be addressed with use of complementary forms of MRI contrast or through the integration of BOLD MRI and other measures in simultaneous data acquisition. For example, direct measures of brain blood flow can be made using non-invasive 'arterial spin labelling' (ASL) MRI methods which have greater stability over time for better assessment of slow (of the order of a minute or more) changes in brain responses now can be implemented robustly (Xie et al., 2010). With care for safety issues and correction of the artefacts induced by the shifting magnetic field gradients used for MRI, high-quality EEG now can be obtained simultaneously during an fMRI examination (Lemieux, 2004), allowing simultaneous pHMRI and pharmaco-EEG studies. Variance in measures can be reduced by correcting for variations in pCO_2 across the ventilatory cycle (Wise et al., 2004). In the near future, advances in positron detection methods should support commercial availability of combined human PET/MRI scanners that will allow integrated experiments examining target occupancy and pharmacodynamics (Herzog et al., 2010).

SUMMARY

Clinical imaging has an important role in drug development. The utility already has been well demonstrated in several applications reviewed here. It can facilitate more seamless transitions from preclinical to clinical development. Imaging also will facilitate answering critical questions earlier in development and directly with human studies, adding to confidence in decision-making. While implementation of imaging-supported protocols can add to trial complexity and cost per patient, where imaging has greater sensitivity, the gains can translate into smaller numbers of subjects in trials. This would have a particularly large impact on the potential to pursue studies for rare diseases for which it may be possible to recruit only small numbers of subjects or for highly stratified populations amongst even prevalent diseases for which PM is sought.

There now is an opportunity to substantially extend the range of situations in which, and the extent to which, imaging is used in clinical drug development. However, optimal use will demand the development of preclinical and clinical imaging strategies to support molecule development from the earliest stages of programme planning to ensure that methods are validated and ready to be implemented as critical decision points in projects are being approached. Wider use in development should catalyse new applications for imaging-based PM to better ensure that the right medicine is used by the right patient.

ACKNOWLEDGMENTS

The author would like to thank his colleagues in the GSK Clinical Imaging Centre for their substantial contributions to the ideas that have developed into this chapter. He also wishes to thank Mrs Rachel Green for careful editorial assistance.

REFERENCES

Abanades S, van der Aart J, Barletta JA, et al. Prediction of repeat-dose occupancy from single-dose data: characterisation of the relationship between plasma pharmacokinetics and brain target occupancy. Journal of Cerebral Blood Flow and Metabolism 2011;31:944–52, Epub Oct 13 2010.

Arnold DL, Matthews PM. MRI in the diagnosis and management of multiple sclerosis. Neurology 2002;58:S23–31.

Boellaard R, Oyen WJ, Hoekstra CJ, et al. The Netherlands protocol for standardisation and quantification of FDG whole body PET studies in multi-centre trials. European Journal of Nuclear Medicine and Molecular Imaging 2008;35:2320–33.

Bosnell R, Wegner C, Kincses ZT, et al. Reproducibility of fMRI in the clinical setting: implications for trial designs. Neuroimage 2008;42:603–10.

Callicott JH, Straub RE, Pezawas L, et al. Variation in DISC1 affects hippocampal structure and function and increases risk for schizophrenia. Proceedings of the National Academy of Sciences of the USA 2005;102:8627–32.

Chuah LY, Chee MW. Cholinergic augmentation modulates visual task performance in sleep-deprived young adults. Journal of Neuroscience 2008;28:11369–77.

Cole DM, Beckmann CF, Long CJ, et al. Nicotine replacement in abstinent smokers improves cognitive withdrawal symptoms with modulation of resting brain network dynamics. Neuroimage 2010;52:590–9.

Cunningham VJ, Parker CA, Rabiner EA, et al. PET studies in drug development: methodological considerations. Drug Discovery Today: Technologies 2005;2:311–5.

David SP, Munafo MR, Johansen-Berg H, et al. Ventral striatum/nucleus accumbens activation to smoking-related pictorial cues in smokers and nonsmokers: a functional magnetic resonance imaging study. Biology and Psychiatry 2005;58:488–94.

Egan MF, Straub RE, Goldberg TE, et al. Variation in GRM3 affects cognition, prefrontal glutamate, and risk for schizophrenia. Proceedings of the National Academy of Sciences of the USA 2004;101:12604–9.

Friedman L, Glover GH. Report on a multicenter fMRI quality assurance protocol. Journal of Magnetic Resonance Imaging 2006;23: 827–39.

Girgis R, Xu X, Miyake N, et al. In vivo binding of antipsychotics to D(3) and D(2) receptors: a PET study in baboons with [(11)C]-(+)-PHNO. Neuropsychopharmacology 2011;36:887–95, Epub Dec 22 2010.

Guo Q, Brady M, Gunn RN. A biomathematical modeling approach to central nervous system radioligand discovery and development. Journal of Nuclear Medicine 2009;50:1715–23.

Hariri AR, Mattay VS, Tessitore A, et al. Serotonin transporter genetic variation and the response of the human amygdala. Science 2002;297:400–3.

Herzog H, Pietrzyk U, Shah NJ, et al. The current state, challenges and perspectives of MR-PET. Neuroimage 2010;49:2072–82.

Inkster B, Nichols TE, Saemann PG, et al. Association of GSK3beta polymorphisms with brain structural changes in major depressive disorder. Archives of General Psychiatry 2009;66:721–8.

Inkster B, Nichols TE, Saemann PG, et al. Pathway-based approaches to imaging genetics association studies: Wnt signaling, GSK3beta substrates and major depression. Neuroimage 2010;53:908–17.

Jezzard P, Matthews PM, Smith S. Functional magnetic resonance imaging: methods for neuroscience. Oxford: Oxford University Press; 2001.

Kegeles LS, Abi-Dargham A, Frankle WG, et al. Increased synaptic dopamine function in associative regions of the striatum in schizophrenia. Archives of General Psychiatry 2010;67:231–9.

Leach MO, Brindle KM, Evelhoch JL, et al. Assessment of antiangiogenic and antivascular therapeutics using MRI: recommendations for appropriate methodology for clinical trials. British Journal of Radiology 2003;1(76 Spec No):S87–91.

Lemieux L. Electroencephalography-correlated functional MR imaging studies of epileptic activity. Neuroimaging Clinics of North America 2004;14:487–506.

Loscher W, Potschka H. Role of drug efflux transporters in the brain for drug disposition and treatment of brain diseases. Progress in Neurobiology 2005;76:22–76.

Martinez D, Narendran R, Foltin RW, et al. Amphetamine-induced dopamine release: markedly blunted in cocaine dependence and predictive of the choice to self-administer cocaine. American Journal of Psychiatry 2007;164:622–9.

Matthews PM, Filippi M. Pharmacological applications of fMRI. In: fMRI Techniques and Protocols. Heidelberg and New York: Springer-Verlag; 2009.

Rinne JO, Brooks DJ, Rossor MN, et al. 11C-PiB PET assessment of change in fibrillar amyloid-beta load in patients with Alzheimer's disease treated with bapineuzumab: a phase 2, double-blind, placebo-controlled, ascending-dose study. Lancet Neurology 2010;9:363–72.

Rosso L, Brock CS, Gallo JM, et al. A new model for prediction of drug distribution in tumor and normal tissues: pharmacokinetics of temozolomide in glioma patients. Cancer Research 2009;69:120–7.

Saleem A, Brown GD, Brady F, et al. Metabolic activation of temozolomide measured in vivo using positron emission tomography. Cancer Research 2003;63:2409–15.

Schneider LS, Kennedy RE, Cutter GR. Requiring an amyloid-beta1-42 biomarker for prodromal Alzheimer's disease or mild cognitive impairment does not lead to more efficient clinical trials. Alzheimers and Dementia 2010;6:367–77.

Slifstein M, Laruelle M. Models and methods for derivation of in vivo neuroreceptor parameters with PET and SPECT reversible radiotracers. Nuclear Medicine and Biology 2001;28:595–608.

Smith SM, Zhang Y, Jenkinson M, et al. Accurate, robust, and automated longitudinal and cross-sectional brain change analysis. Neuroimage 2002;17:479–89.

Smith SM, Fox PT, Miller KL, et al. Correspondence of the brain's functional architecture during activation and rest. Proceedings of the National Academy of Sciences of the USA 2009;106:13040–5.

Sormani MP, Bonzano L, Roccatagliata L, et al. Magnetic resonance imaging as a potential surrogate for relapses in multiple sclerosis: a meta-analytic approach. Annals in Neurology 2009;65:268–75.

Stocker T, Schneider F, Klein M, et al. Automated quality assurance routines for fMRI data applied to a multicenter study. Human Brain Mapping 2005;25:237–46.

Talbot DC, Ranson M, Davies J, et al. Tumor survivin is downregulated by the antisense oligonucleotide LY2181308: a proof-of-concept, first-in-human dose study. Clinical Cancer Research 2010;16:6150–8.

Tzimopoulou S, Cunningham VJ, Nichols TE, et al. A multi-center randomized proof-of-concept clinical trial applying [(1)F]FDG-PET for evaluation of metabolic therapy with rosiglitazone XR in mild to moderate Alzheimer's disease. Journal of Alzheimer's Disease 2010;22:1241–56.

van Dongen GA, Vosjan MJ. Immuno-positron emission tomography: shedding light on clinical antibody therapy. Cancer Biotherapy and Radiopharmaceuticals 2010;25:375–85.

Wise RG, Ide K, Poulin MJ, et al. Resting fluctuations in arterial carbon dioxide induce significant low frequency variations in BOLD signal. Neuroimage 2004;21:1652–64.

Workman P, Aboagye EO, Chung YL, et al. Minimally invasive pharmacokinetic and pharmacodynamic technologies in hypothesis-testing clinical trials of innovative therapies. Journal of the National Cancer Institute 2006;98:580–98.

Xie J, Clare S, Gallichan D, et al. Real-time adaptive sequential design for optimal acquisition of arterial spin labeling MRI data. Magnetic Resonance in Medicine 2010;64:203–10.

Zamuner S, Di Iorio VL, Nyberg J, et al. Adaptive-optimal design in PET occupancy studies. Clinical Pharmacology and Therapeutics 2010;87:563–71.

Zhang D, Raichle ME. Disease and the brain's dark energy. Nature Reviews. Neurology 2010;6:15–28.

Chapter 19

Intellectual property in drug discovery and development

P Grubb

As is clear from the rest of this book, it costs a great deal of effort and money to discover and develop a new drug. No one would make such an investment if the results could simply be copied by an imitator who had invested nothing. The best way to protect the investment is by obtaining a patent for the drug. In this chapter we will look at what patents are, what kinds of inventions can be patented, and how a patent may be obtained and enforced.

Patents are not the only form of intellectual property (IP), but they are by far the most important for the pharmaceutical industry. Many patents that are filed and granted prove to be worth nothing, but a patent protecting a blockbuster drug against generic competition may be worth millions of dollars for each day that it is in force. An unexpected loss of patent protection may have a much larger effect upon the market value of the company holding the patent. In August 2000, when a US patent covering Prozac was held invalid by the Court of Appeal for the Federal Circuit, thereby reducing by about 3 years the expected term of exclusivity for this drug, 29% of the value of Eli Lilly stock was lost in 1 day – over $35 billion. This is serious money by any standards.

WHAT IS A PATENT?

A patent is the grant by a nation state of the exclusive right to commercialize an invention in that state for a limited time. During that time (the 'term' of the patent, usually 20 years from the filing date) the patent owner can go to the courts and enforce his or her rights by suing an infringer. An owner who wins the infringement suit can get damages or other compensation, and more importantly can obtain a court order (an injunction) to stop any further infringement. Note that although the state grants the patent right, the state does not check whether the right is being infringed – the patent owner must do that.

It is important to realize that the rights given by a patent do not include the right to practise the invention, but only to exclude others from doing so. Many inventors and business managers think that having a patent gives them freedom to operate, but this is not so. The patentee's freedom to use the invention may be limited by laws or regulations having nothing to do with patents, or by the existence of other patents. For example, owning a US patent for a new drug does not give the right to market that drug in the USA without permission from the FDA (see Chapter 20).

What is less obvious is that having a patent does not give the right to infringe an earlier existing patent. To take a simple example, if A has a patent for a process using an acid catalyst, and B later finds that nitric acid (not disclosed in A's patent) gives surprisingly good results, B may be able to get a patent for the process using nitric acid as catalyst. However, because this falls under the broad description of acid catalysis covered in A's patent, B is not free to use his invention without the permission of A. On the other hand, A cannot use nitric acid without a licence from B, and in this situation, cross-licensing may allow both parties to use the improved invention.

Patents are important to industry because they give the innovator a period during which imitations can be excluded and the investment in R&D can be recovered. They are of particular importance to the pharmaceutical industry because once the chemical structure of a drug is published it is usually rather easy to copy the product, and because the manufacturing cost of a pharmaceutical is only a small part of the selling price, an imitator who has no R&D costs to recover can sell the product cheaply and still make a profit.

THE PATENT SPECIFICATION

A patent (which strictly speaking is just a one-page certificate of grant) is in most countries published with a printed *patent specification*, which typically will be 10–100 pages long, or even more. The patent specification consists of three parts, the bibliographic details and abstract, the description, and the claims. Each part has a different purpose.

Bibliographic details

The title page usually sets out the bibliographic details, giving information such as the names of the inventors, the owner or assignee of the patent, the title, the dates of priority, filing, publication and grant, and the name of the attorney, if any, who acted for the patentee. It may also give the international search classification, and a list of prior published documents considered by the Patent Office when examining the application. Generally it will also have an abstract summarizing the invention; this is meant as a tool for searching purposes and is not used in determining the scope of protection given by the patent.

Description

The longest part of the specification is the description, the purpose of which is to give enough information about the invention to enable a reader who is technically qualified in the relevant field to reproduce it. This ensures that when the patent is no longer in force the invention will be fully in the public domain and able to be used by anyone having the necessary skills. The description will usually start with a brief account of the background to the invention, followed by a summary of the invention, then present full details, with actual examples where appropriate. There may also be figures (drawings, structural formulae, graphs, photographs, etc.) and if DNA or amino acid sequences are disclosed there will be sequence identifiers in standard form.

Claims

At the end of the specification come one or more claims, which have the legal purpose of setting out exactly what is covered by the scope of the exclusionary right. Readers who see that what they wish to do clearly falls within the claims of someone else's patent are put upon notice that if they go ahead they may be sued for infringement, and will have to stop their activities unless they can prove that the patent is invalid. Unfortunately the reverse situation is not so clear. In many countries, particularly the USA, even an activity that does not fall within the literal wording of a patent claim may nevertheless be held to infringe by 'equivalence'. The consequence is that before doing anything in the USA that is even close to the claims of a granted US patent, you must make sure that you get a written opinion from a US patent attorney that you are not infringing any valid claims. If you do not, and infringement is found, you may find yourself having to pay triple damages for 'willful infringement'.

WHAT CAN BE PATENTED?

There are basically only two categories of subject matter that can be patented – *products* and *processes*. Products are broadly anything having physical reality, including machines, manufactured articles, chemical compounds, compositions comprising a mixture of substances, and even living organisms. A process may be a process for manufacturing an article or synthesizing a compound, or may be a method of using or testing a product. However, a patent for a process for making something, for example a chemical compound, also covers the direct product of that process. A patent claiming simply 'the compound of formula X' covers X however it is made, but a process claim to 'a method of production of X by reacting Y and Z' covers X only when made by that process, and not in any other way. A claim to the compound itself covers the compound not only however it is made but also however it is used. Thus a claim to a compound invented as a dyestuff will also cover the compound when used as a pharmaceutical.

There are also some types of subject matter for which the grant of patents is specifically excluded, and these exclusions vary from country to country. For example, some countries do not grant patents on any plants or animals, whereas in Europe only specific plant and animal varieties are excluded, and in the USA there is no such restriction. Similarly, the USA allows patents for methods of surgical or medical treatment or diagnosis, whereas most other countries do not. Nevertheless, the invention that a known drug may be used for a new indication may usually be protected in these countries by patents having a different form of claim. Generally, patents will not be granted in any country for aesthetic creations, mathematical and scientific theories, and discoveries without any practical application.

Pharmaceutical inventions

Within the pharmaceutical field, patentable inventions may include not only new chemical compounds of known structure, but also, for example, biopolymers and mixtures the structure of which has not been fully elucidated. Isolated DNA sequences and genes are also patentable as chemical compounds, although in some countries the scope of protection given by the patent is limited to the disclosed use. Even if a chemical compound is already known, it may be possible to patent variants, such as new optical isomers and crystal forms of the compound, as well as new galenic formulations, mixtures with other active ingredients, manufacturing and purification processes, assay processes, etc.

If a known compound, not previously known to have any pharmaceutical use, is found to be useful as a drug, this invention may be protected by claiming a pharmaceutical composition containing the compound, or, in Europe, the use of the compound as a pharmaceutical. Such claims will cover all pharmaceutical uses of the compound, not only the one found by the inventor. If the invention is that a known drug has a new and unexpected indication, such an invention may be protected in the USA by a 'method of medical treatment' claim ('method of treating a human suffering from disease Y by administering an effective amount of a compound X'), or in Europe by a use claim ('use of compound X for the treatment of disease Y').

REQUIREMENTS FOR PATENTABILITY

For an invention in any of the above categories to be patentable, it must meet three basic criteria:

- It must be *novel*
- It must involve an *inventive step* (must not be obvious)
- It must be *industrially applicable* (must have utility).

Novelty

The first and clearest requirement is that nothing can be patentable which is not new. If a patent were to be granted for something already known, then the grant of a patent in respect of this information would violate the fundamental principle that a patent cannot deprive the public of rights that it already has. There are, however, different definitions of 'novelty'. The most straightforward is that of 'absolute novelty' applied in Europe, Japan, China, and the majority of other countries, which provides that an invention is new if it is not part of the 'state of the art', the state of the art being defined as everything that was available to the public by written or oral publication, use or any other way, in any country in the world, before the priority date of the invention. For example, if it could be proved that the invention had been described before that date in a public lecture given in the Mongolian language in Ulan Bator, a European patent application for the invention would lack novelty even if no European had heard or understood the lecture.

A few countries still have the system of 'local novelty', under which a disclosure of the invention before the priority date destroys novelty only if it is available within that country. Rather more countries, including the USA, have an intermediate 'mixed novelty' system, according to which a later patent application is invalidated by written publication anywhere in the world, but by oral publication or use of the invention only in the home country. Thus a US patent would not be invalidated by the lecture in Ulan Bator, but would be by an account of it published in a newspaper there. Similarly, prior use in a country outside the USA would not invalidate a US patent if there was no written description, whereas a European patent would be invalidated by prior use anywhere in the world, so long as the use made the invention available to the public – for example the sale of a chemical compound that could be analysed.

Novelty in the USA

A more basic difference between the USA and all other countries is that all countries other than the USA have a 'first-to-file' system, whereby if two persons make the same invention the first one to file a patent application gets the patent. The present US system is 'first-to-invent', so that irrespective of who files the first application, the person who can prove the earlier invention date gets the patent. A consequence of this is that in most countries, prior art is what is published before the first filing date (the priority date). In the USA, however, prior art is what is published before the invention date. Since by definition an inventor cannot publish his or her invention before it is invented, self-publication cannot normally be prior art. However, if an invention has been published, by the inventor or by another person, after the invention date, a US patent application for the invention is regarded as lacking novelty unless it is filed within 12 months of the date of publication. This means that an inventor may publish the invention and still obtain a valid US patent so long as a US application is filed within this 12-month period. In the past, many US inventors, particularly those working in universities, sought to take advantage of this so-called grace period, only to find that by so doing they had destroyed their chances of getting any protection in other countries. Now most US inventors are aware of the dangers, and unless they are interested only in obtaining a US patent, they will adhere to the first-to-file principle and file an application before publishing their results. Following passage of the America Invents Act in September 2011, the US system will change to first-to-file on March 16 2013.

Inventive step (non-obviousness)

Whereas the concept of novelty is (or should be) an objective matter, the question of whether or not something involves an inventive step is intrinsically much more difficult, as subjective judgement is involved. The basic principle to remember is that the reason for requiring the presence of an inventive step is that ordinary workers in that field should remain free to apply their normal skills to making minor variations of old products.

Thus the person to whom the invention must be non-obvious in order to be patentable is the 'person skilled in the art', i.e. a worker who is competent but lacks imagination or inventive capability. In the days when the majority of patents were for simple mechanical devices, the person skilled in the art was usually described as an 'ordinary workman'. However, for complex inventions in pharmaceutical chemistry and biotechnology, the 'person skilled in the art' may be considered to be a team of highly qualified scientists.

It is a legal fiction to suppose that such a team could be competent but non-inventive, considering that its members would, if employed in industry, be expected by their company to make inventions, and if academic scientists, would be expected by their university to produce original scientific work, which amounts to much the same thing. The point is that obviousness should be judged by a person with qualifications and imagination that are average for those in the field. It is tempting for a party attacking a patent on the ground of obviousness to use an expert witness with the highest possible qualifications, but it is not very helpful to have a Nobel laureate testify that something is obvious. It may be obvious to a genius, but the real question is whether it is obvious to the normal worker in the field.

It is often very easy to reconstruct an invention with the benefit of hindsight, as a series of logical steps from the prior art, but it does not necessarily follow that the invention was obvious, especially if there is evidence that the invention was commercially successful, or satisfied a need. The question 'If the invention was so obvious, why did no one do it before?' is usually a relevant one to ask.

Industrial applicability (utility)

In Europe it is a requirement that the invention should be capable of industrial application, which is broadly defined and includes making or using the invention in any kind of industry, including agriculture. In the USA, patentable inventions are defined as any new and useful process, machine, manufacture or composition of matter, or any new and useful improvement thereof. The US requirement that the invention be useful has generally been applied no more strictly than the corresponding European requirement, but recently US examination guidelines have been tightened up so as to make more difficult the patenting of DNA sequences for which no real function is known, and the courts both in the USA and the UK have held such patents invalid.

PATENT ISSUES IN DRUG DISCOVERY

The strategies that should be used to obtain patent protection for a compound in development are described later in this chapter. However, some patent issues need to be considered at an earlier stage. Here we consider issues that concern the selection of a compound as a development candidate.

The two questions that need to be answered before significant sums are invested in development activities are:

- What sort of protection can we get for this compound?
- What patent rights of others could prevent us from marketing this compound?

These are two completely different issues. As explained above, it is perfectly possible to have strong patent protection for one's own invention, yet still to be blocked by earlier dominating patent rights owned by someone else. The 'patent situation' for a compound should attempt to give the answers to both questions.

THE STATE OF THE ART

The answers to the two basic questions depend upon the *state of the art* – patent jargon for all material relating to the technical field that has been published at the relevant date. The state of the art (sometimes called the *prior art*) includes not only published scientific papers, but also, for example, what is in textbooks, manufacturers' brochures, newspaper articles, web pages on the Internet and oral presentations at conferences. It also includes patent documents, which may be either granted patents or published patent applications which have not been examined as of the date of publication.

The requirements that a patentable invention must be *novel* and must have an *inventive step* mean that nothing can be patented that is already part of the state of the art, and that anything that is very close to the state of the art may be very difficult to patent.

PATENT DOCUMENTS AS STATE OF THE ART

A granted patent is not only a description, which, like any kind of prior publication, is part of the state of the art. It also contains *claims* defining the scope of protection. Published patent applications also contain claims, but these are often much broader than the claims (if any) that will finally be granted.

Patent documents in the state of the art are therefore important in answering the second basic question, which concerns *freedom to operate*. Granted patents may be invalidated by a court, but as a rule they have a presumption of validity which is hard to challenge. Patent applications do not give exclusionary rights, but may act as a warning flag for rights that may be granted in the future.

EVALUATION BY THE SCIENTIST

The first person to evaluate the patent situation of a possible lead compound must be the research scientist responsible for the project. He or she should be aware of the work being published in the area, and should know who are the main players in the field, what journals and other information sources contain relevant information, and what competitor companies are likely to be filing relevant patent applications. To the extent that the chemical structure of the lead compound is a matter of choice, the research chemist should try to steer away from the known state of the art.

Where the research is in a field in which a number of competitors are active, it is clear that the closer you are to the competition, the closer you are to the prior art, and the more difficult it will be to obtain patent protection. Research managers are sometimes struck by what seems like a great idea – ask the patent department to check where there are gaps in the competitors' patent protection, and then try to work in these gaps. This is actually a very bad idea if the intention is to produce something innovative. Research must drive patenting, not the other way around, and the initial work should be done before the patent situation is checked.

EVALUATION BY THE PATENT PROFESSIONAL

A professional evaluation of the patent situation of a new chemical entity (NCE) needs to be made at about the same time that the filing of a patent application is being considered. The timing of this will depend upon the patent policy of the company or organization owning the invention, but will usually be at the time the compound is ready to enter the development process, i.e. at the time of transition of the compound to 'drug candidate' status.

The patent situation must be established on the basis of a search of the scientific and patent literature. Ideally, the search should be carried out by a professional patent searcher and evaluated by a patent attorney or patent agent. However, it is becoming more and more easy for a patent attorney or a scientist to carry out searches online, and while these are unlikely to be as complete as those done by a professional searcher, such a 'quick and dirty' search may be all that is required at this early stage. At some stage after a patent application has been filed, searches will be carried out in the major patent offices, and these can be used to supplement the search made at the time of filing.

More complete 'freedom to operate' searches must be made at later stages, for example to ensure that the proposed manufacturing process and the chosen pharmaceutical formulation are also free from third-party patent rights.

SOURCES OF INFORMATION

For patent literature there are now a number of databases available online which allow full-text searching by keywords. One, available on the website of the US Patent and Trademark Office (www.uspto.gov), contains fully searchable texts of all US patents since 1976, as well as image files of all US patents back to 1790. A similar database (Esp@cenet) available through the home page of the European Patent Office (www.epo.org) allows searching of European patent applications and PCT applications. For Japan, the database JAPIO, available through the website of the Japanese Patent Office (www.jpo.go.jp), gives English-language abstracts of all Japanese early-published applications from 1976 onwards. Use of these databases is free.

Other databases, maintained by commercial firms which charge user access fees, add value by high-quality abstracts and additional indexing possibilities, and downloading and printing information from these may be quicker and easier than it is from public domain Internet databases.

Chemical Abstracts (CA), published by the Ohio State University, abstracts both patents and scientific literature in the chemical field. The information retrieval system is based on a CA registry number allocated to every published chemical compound; once this has been identified, abstracts of all patents or literature articles mentioning the compound can be listed, and printed out if required.

Derwent Publications Ltd provides a wide range of abstracting and information retrieval systems for both scientific and patent literature. The latter includes the WPI (World Patent Index) database, covering all patents in the major countries issued since 1974. Searches can be made on the basis of keywords, or of partial structures of chemical compounds. Derwent also has a database covering all publications and patents in the field of biotechnology since 1982.

RESULTS OF THE EVALUATION – NCES

If the search shows that the compound lacks novelty, that is, it has already been published, then the best course is to pick a different one for development. Even though it may be possible to obtain some form of secondary patent protection, for example the use of the compound as a medicament if it was previously known for a non-pharmaceutical use, most companies will not invest in the development of a compound unless it will be possible to patent the compound itself.

If the NCE appears to be novel but the search shows that very similar compounds are known, so that the compound may lack an inventive step, the best advice is to go ahead anyway. If the compound proves to have superior properties compared to the known product, these can be used to establish the inventive step. If it does not, it will drop out of development whatever the patent situation.

If the NCE, despite being apparently novel and inventive, appears to be covered by a third-party patent, the advice would be to go ahead only if the third-party patent appears to be invalid or will have expired before your product can reach the market, or if you are sure that you will be able to obtain a licence on acceptable terms.

PATENTING OF RESEARCH TOOLS

In addition to patent issues relating to the compound itself, research tools may also be covered by patents. By 'research tool' is meant anything that contributes to the discovery or development of a drug, without being part of the final product. Examples include genes, cell lines, reagents, markers, assays, screening methods, animal models, etc.

A company whose business it is to sell drugs is not usually interested in patenting research tools, but it is the business of many biotech companies to develop and commercialize such tools, and these companies will naturally wish to obtain patent protection for them. For pharmaceutical companies, such research tool patents and applications raise issues of freedom to operate, particularly if they contain *'reach-through'* claims purporting to cover drugs found by using the patented tools.

Some scientists may believe that research activities, in contrast to the manufacture and sale of a product, cannot be patent infringement. This is not the case. If I have invented a process that is useful in research and have a valid patent for it, I can enforce that patent against anyone using the process without my permission. I can make money from my patent by granting licences for a flat fee, or a fee based on the extent to which the process is used; or by selling kits for carrying out the process or reagents for use in the process (for example the enzymes used in the polymerase chain reaction (PCR) process). What I am *not* entitled to do is to charge a royalty on the sale of drugs developed with the help of my process. I can patent an electric drill, but I should not expect to get a royalty on everything it bores a hole in.

Although some patents have been granted containing claims that would be infringed, for example, by the sale of a drug active in a patented assay, such patents have been successfully challenged in the courts, both in the USA and the UK. Similarly, patents claiming all drugs acting by a newly discovered mechanism have been held invalid as claiming 'not an invention but a research programme'. It is probably an acceptable risk to ignore patents of these types, although some risk of litigation is unavoidable.

Should other types of research tool patents be the subject of a freedom to operate search at an early stage of product development? Probably not. There are simply too many of them, and if no research project could be started without clearance on the basis of such a search, nothing would ever get done. At least for a large company, it is an acceptable business risk to go ahead and assume that if problems arise they can be dealt with at a later stage, normally by taking a licence under any relevant patent.

OBTAINING PATENT PROTECTION FOR A DEVELOPMENT COMPOUND

Filing a patent application

When to file

Given that in most countries the first to file an application gets the patent, it would seem to make sense to file as early as possible as soon as an invention is made. It is not quite as simple as this, however. For one thing, the earlier a patent is filed the earlier it will expire, and particularly in the pharmaceutical field, the last year or two of patent life for a major product can be worth hundreds of millions of dollars. For another, a patent application filed at a very early stage may lack sufficient enabling disclosure to support claims of the desired scope. Too much delay, however, and another party may have filed an earlier application or published a paper that destroys the novelty of the invention.

For pharmaceutical inventions, the decision when to make a first filing will depend on a number of factors, including the intensity of competition in the relevant field. As a general rule, however, it is generally best to wait at least until one or more lead compounds within the scope have shown clear activity in a validated in vitro assay, or in an animal model, i.e. close to the point at which a drug candidate (see Chapter 4) is identified.

Where to file

Normally a single filing in one country will be made, which, under the Paris Convention for the Protection of Industrial Property, can form the basis for a claim to priority in other countries. Some national laws, such as those of the USA and France, require that, for reasons of national security, an application for any invention made in that country must first be filed in that country (unless special permission is obtained). The UK now limits this requirement to certain categories of inventions, but it may be safer to file all UK-originating inventions in the UK first. Other countries, for example Switzerland, are less paranoid, and allow a first filing to be made in any country.

The Paris Convention, now adhered to by the great majority of countries, provides that a later application filed for the same invention in another Convention country within 12 months of the first filing in a Convention country may claim the priority of the original application. This means that the first filing date (the *priority date*) is treated for prior art purposes as if it were the filing date of the later application, so that a publication of the invention before the later application but after the priority date does not invalidate claims for the same invention in the later application. If it were not for the Paris Convention, it would be necessary to make simultaneous filings in all the countries of interest at a very early stage, which would be extremely wasteful of time and money. Instead, a single priority filing may be made and a decision taken before the end of the priority year on what to do with the application.

During the priority year, work on the invention will normally continue, and for example further compounds will be made and tested, new formulations compounded, or new process conditions tried. All this material can be used in preparing the patent applications to be filed abroad, and, where possible, a subsequent application in respect of the country of first filing. It is also possible to file new patent applications for further developments made during the priority year, and then at the foreign filing stage to combine these into a single application. The advantage of this is that the new developments will then have an earlier priority date (the date of filing of the new application) than they otherwise would have (the date of filing of the foreign text).

The foreign filing decision

There are four options to be considered:

- Abandon
- Abandon and refile
- Obtain a patent in the country of first filing only
- File corresponding applications in one or more foreign countries.

Abandonment

If there is no commercial interest in the invention at all, or if a search has shown that it lacks novelty, one can simply do nothing. Sooner or later a fee must be paid or some action taken to keep the application in being, and when this is not done the application will lapse. It is best not to withdraw the application explicitly, as such a positive abandonment is usually irrevocable and applicants have been known to change their minds.

If the applicant wants to ensure that he retains freedom to operate and that no one else can patent the invention, he should have it published, either by continuing an application in his home country long enough for it to issue as a published application (see below) or by sending it to a journal such as *Research Disclosure*, in which any disclosure may be rapidly published for a reasonable fee.

Refiling

It frequently happens that by the time the foreign filing decision must be taken it is not yet possible to decide whether or not to invest time and money in foreign patenting. Commercial interest may be low but could increase later, more testing may have to be done, or the inventors may not have done any more work on the invention since the first application was filed. In such cases the best solution is to start from the beginning again. The existing application is abandoned, a new application is filed, and the 12-month countdown starts all over again. In this case it is essential to meet the requirements of the Paris Convention that the first application be explicitly abandoned before the second application is filed.

Of course, refiling always entails a loss of priority, usually of 8–10 months, and if someone else has published the invention or filed a patent application for it during this time, the refiled application cannot lead to a valid patent. Consequently, in a field where competitors are known to be active refiling may involve an unacceptable risk, and, naturally, if there has been any known publication of the invention since the priority date, abandonment and refiling is ruled out. Such publication most frequently arises from the inventor himself. Most inventors know that they should not publish inventions before a patent application is filed; it is not so generally realized that publication within the priority year can also be very damaging.

Home-country patenting

If the applicant is an individual or a small company having no commercial interests or prospects of licensing outside the home country (which will usually be the country in which the first filing is made), the expense of foreign filing would be wasted, and the applicant will wish only to obtain a patent in the home country. Even where the applicant is a larger company that would normally file any commercially interesting case in several countries, individual applications may be of such low interest that protection in the home country is all that is needed. This option is, of course, more attractive if the home country is a large market such as the USA, rather than a small country such as Switzerland.

Foreign filing

Finally, if an invention appears likely to be commercially important, the decision may be to file corresponding applications in a number of other countries. For the pharmaceutical industry one can assume that the costs of patent protection would be small compared with the value of protection for any compound that actually reaches the market, but at the time when a foreign filing decision must be taken, it is usually impossible to estimate the chance that the product in question will progress that far. Accordingly, one must rely upon some rule of thumb such that if the product is being developed further, foreign filing should be carried out as a matter of course. High patenting costs are a necessary part of the high research overheads of the pharmaceutical industry.

Procedures on foreign filing

National filings

It is possible to file patent applications (in the local language) in the national patent offices of each selected country individually. This involves a large outlay of money at a relatively early stage, and also means that all necessary translations must be prepared in good time before the end of the priority year. It is also very labour-intensive, as the application must be prosecuted separately before each national patent office. Fortunately, there are ways to simplify the procedure.

Regional patent offices

One is that there are certain regional patent offices by which patents in a number of countries can be granted based on a single application filed and prosecuted in one patent office. By far the most important of these is the European Patent Office, which as of April 2012 grants patents for a total of 37 countries. These are all the 27 current EU states plus Albania, Croatia, Iceland, Liechtenstein, Macedonia, Monaco, Norway, San Marino, Switzerland and Turkey. The European application can be filed in English, French or German, and translations into other languages are required only at the time of grant. Once the European patent is granted, opposition to the patent may be filed by any other party within 9 months of the date of grant. If the opposition is wholly or partly successful, the patent is invalidated or limited in scope for all of the designated countries.

Although the European Patent Convention provides for a central filing, grant and opposition procedure, once the European patent is granted it is treated as if it were a bundle of national patents in the designated contracting states, so that, for example, the European patent may be invalidated by the courts in one country without directly affecting its validity in other countries. Proposals have repeatedly been made by the European Commission for a single unitary patent to cover all EU countries, just as a single US patent covers all 50 states, but little real progress has been made in this direction.

Other regional patent offices are the Eurasian Patent Office (Russia and certain former Soviet countries), and ones for English-speaking and French-speaking African countries.

Patent cooperation treaty (PCT)

The PCT allows rights to be established in a large number of countries (144 as of April 2012) by a single international application. Search and optional preliminary examination are carried out before the application goes to the national or regional patent offices. This system gives the maximum flexibility and allows the costs associated with translations, etc., to be significantly postponed. There are now very few economically significant countries that are not members of the PCT, of which the most important is Taiwan. An initial international phase, in which a search and possibly also a preliminary examination is carried out, is followed after 18 months by a national phase, in which selected national or regional patent offices conclude the examination process and grant (or refuse) the patent. The PCT procedure is described in more detail in Box 19.1.

Selection of countries

In deciding the list of countries in which patent protection should be obtained, the main criteria are the strength of patent protection in the country and the size of the market. Now that most countries have joined the World Trade Organization and are obliged by the TRIPs (Trade-Related Aspects of Intellectual Property Rights) agreement to introduce strong patent protection, the most important criterion has become market size. There is no point in filing patents in a country if the size of the market does not justify the costs, no matter how strong its patent laws may be. Nevertheless, for a new chemical entity that may become a market product, filing in 40–60 countries is normal practice. To avoid long discussions each time a decision must be taken, the use of standard filing lists to cover most situations makes a lot of sense.

Maintenance of patents

In nearly all countries, periodic (usually annual) renewal fees must be paid to keep a patent in force. These generally increase steeply towards the end of the patent term, thus encouraging patent owners who are not making commercial use of their patents to make the invention available to the public earlier than would otherwise be the case. To save costs, pharmaceutical patents should be abandoned as soon as they no longer provide protection for a compound that is on the market or is being developed. Maintaining a collection of patents that are not being used is an expensive luxury.

Extension of patent term

The standard patent term provided in the TRIPs agreement is at least 20 years from the filing date. However, because it takes a long time to bring a drug to market, the effective term (the term during which a drug is sold with patent protection) is much less than this. To compensate for these regulatory delays, a number of countries, including EU

Box 19.1 **PCT procedure**

International phase

Filing

An international application can be filed by any national or resident of a PCT country, at a national or regional patent office competent to act for that applicant, or at the International Bureau (World Intellectual Property Office, or WIPO) in Geneva. A single filing fee can give rights in all Contracting States.

International publication and search report

The PCT application is published 18 months from the first priority date, and the search report drawn up by the International Searching Authority (selected from one of a number of patent offices including the USPTO and the EPO) is published at the same time or as soon as possible afterwards. At the same time, a Written Opinion on Patentability is drawn up, indicating on the basis of the search report whether or not the invention appears to be new and non-obvious. If no further steps are taken, this will be issued as the International Preliminary Report on Patentability (IPRP).

International preliminary examination

If the applicant wishes to contest the findings of the Written Opinion, he may within 22 months from the priority date file a *Demand for International Preliminary Examination*, pay a fee and respond to the Written Opinion, possibly also making amendments. This will then be taken into account in the final form of the IPRP.

National phase

After 30 months from the priority date the application may be sent to any of the national or regional patent offices, translated into the local language as necessary. The individual patent offices may rely on the international search and examination reports to any extent they choose in deciding whether or not to grant a patent. This varies from offices which usually ignore the IPRP altogether (e.g. the USPTO), to those which will grant a patent without further examination only if the IPRP is positive (e.g. Turkey), to Singapore, which will automatically grant a patent on any PCT application with an IPRP, whether it is positive or negative. Singapore very sensibly puts the burden on the applicant, who, if he wishes to enforce the patent, would have to prove to the court that the negative IPRP was incorrect.

states, the USA, Switzerland and Japan, allow for patent term extensions of up to 5 years for pharmaceutical (and sometimes agricultural) products. In the USA, patent term extension is one part of the Hatch–Waxman Act, in which the interests of the innovative companies are balanced against those of the generic companies. The former get a longer patent term, the latter are allowed carry out testing for FDA approval during the patent term, so that they can come on the market as soon as patent protection expires. In Europe, extension is provided by means of a separate form of intellectual property right known as a Supplementary Protection Certificate (SPC).

Enforcement of patent rights

Governments grant patents, but do not enforce them. The patent owner must take action against infringement by suing an infringer in the civil courts. If successful, the patentee can obtain an injunction to restrain further infringement, as well as other remedies such as damages and costs. Usually the alleged infringer will counterclaim that the patent is invalid, and if the patentee loses the case the patent may be revoked. This risk, as well as the high cost of litigation, must be weighed against the benefit gained if the infringer is forced out of the market. As an alternative to litigation, the patentee may choose to exploit the patent by granting exclusive or non-exclusive licences for royalties or other forms of compensation, or in exchange for a cross-licence.

Although the procedure for obtaining a patent has been harmonized to a large extent by the PCT and other means, the procedure for enforcement, as well as the cost and the chance of success, varies enormously from one country to another. In the USA, patent cases are heard at first instance in the Federal District Courts, in which the judges are not specialized in intellectual property law and in which many cases are decided by jury verdicts. At the appeal stage, however, the Court of Appeal for the Federal Circuit is a specialized and technically competent court. In England (a separate jurisdiction from Scotland), on the other hand, patent cases are heard either in the Patents County Court or, more usually, in the Patents Court, which is part of the High Court. Both of these are specialized courts with technically literate judges, but appeals from them go to the general Court of Appeal, where the majority of the judges are not patent experts. Which of these two systems gives the fairest results is a matter of debate.

In both the USA and the English systems issues of patent validity are dealt with by the same court that deals with the issue of infringement, and this is also the case in the majority of European and Asian countries. In Germany, Japan, China and Korea, however, these issues are kept separate, and a patent may be invalidated only by a special court or by a branch of the patent office.

It is a problem in many parts of the world that even if the country has a good patent law on paper, enforcement of patent rights may be very difficult for a number of reasons, ranging from lack of experienced judges to inefficiency and even corruption.

Other forms of intellectual property

A *trademark* is a word, design, shape or colour used to distinguish the goods of the trademark owner from those of another manufacturer. Unlike patents, registered trademarks may be renewed at the end of their term and may be kept alive indefinitely, although they may be liable to cancellation if they are not used. Thus, once a patent for a drug has expired a competitor will be able to sell a generic version, but must sell it under the International Non-proprietary Name (INN) or his own trademark, not that of the originator.

Additional forms of IP include *copyright* (e.g. for the text of advertisements and package inserts), and *Internet domain names*, which may, for example, incorporate the name of a product and may be a useful marketing tool.

FURTHER READING

Dutfield G. Intellectual property rights and the life science industries. Aldershot: Ashgate Press; 2003.

Grubb P, Thomsen P. Patents for chemicals, pharmaceuticals and biotechnology: fundamentals of global law, practice and strategy. 5th edn. Oxford: Oxford University Press; 2010.

Kleemann A, Engel J. Pharmaceutical substances: syntheses, patents, applications. New York: Thieme Medical; 2001.

Old F. Inventions, patents, brands and designs. Sydney: Patent Press; 1993.

Reid B. A practical guide to patent law. London: Sweet & Maxwell; 1999.

Rosenstock J. The law of chemical and pharmaceutical invention: patent and nonpatent protection. New York: Aspen Publishers; 1998.

USEFUL WEBSITES

Patent offices

EPO http://www.epo.org

UK http://www.patent.gov.uk or www.ukpats.org.uk

USA http://www.uspto.gov

Japan http://www.jpo.go.jp

WIPO http://www.wipo.int

Professional organizations

Chartered Institute of Patent Attorneys: http://www.cipa.org.uk

European Patents Institute: http://www.patentepi.com

American Intellectual Property Law Association: http://www.aipla.org

Lists of links

http://www.epo.co.at/online/index.htm

http://portico.bl.uk/collections/patents/html

Chapter 20

Regulatory affairs

I Hägglöf, Å Holmgren

INTRODUCTION

This chapter introduces the reader to the role of the regulatory affairs (RA) department of a pharmaceutical company, outlining the process of getting a drug approved, and emphasizing the importance of interactions of regulatory affairs with other functions within the company, and with the external regulatory authorities.

To keep this chapter to a reasonable size the typical examples given refer to the first registration of a new chemical compound. The same way of reasoning also applies, however, to any subsequent change to the approval of products. Depending on the magnitude of the change, the new documentation that needs to be compiled, submitted and approved by health authorities is variable, ranging from a few pages of pharmaceutical data (e.g. for an update to product stability information) to a complete new application for a new clinical use in a new patient group in a new pharmaceutical form.

It needs also to be said that, as every drug substance and every project is unique, the views expressed represent the opinion of the authors and are not necessarily shared by others active in the field.

BRIEF HISTORY OF PHARMACEUTICAL REGULATION

Control of pharmaceutical products has been the task of authorized institutions for thousands of years, and this was the case even in ancient Greece and Egypt.

From the Middle Ages, control of drug quality, composition purity and quantification was achieved by reference to authoritative lists of drugs, their preparation and their uses. These developed into official pharmacopoeias, of which the earliest was probably the New Compound Dispensatory of 1498 issued by the Florentine guild of physicians and pharmacists.

The pharmacopoeias were local rules, applicable in a particular city or district. During the 19th century national pharmacopoeias replaced local ones, and since the early 1960s regional pharmacopoeias have successively replaced national ones. Now work is ongoing to harmonize – or at least mutually recognize – interchangeable use of the US Pharmacopeia, the European Pharmacopoeia and the Japanese Pharmacopoeia.

As described in Chapter 1, the development of experimental pharmacology and chemistry began during the second half of the 19th century, revealing that the effect of the main botanical drugs was due to chemical substances in the plants used. The next step, synthetic chemistry, made it possible to produce active chemical compounds. Other important scientific developments, e.g. biochemistry, bacteriology and serology during the early 20th century, accelerated the development of the pharmaceutical industry into what it is today (see Drews, 1999).

Lack of adequate drug control systems or methods to investigate the safety of new chemical compounds became a great risk as prefabricated drug products were broadly and freely distributed. In the USA the fight against patent medicines led to the passing of the US Pure Food and Drugs Act against misbranding as long ago as 1906. The Act required improved declaration of contents, prohibited false or misleading statements, and required content and purity to comply with labelled information. A couple of decades later, the US Food and Drug Administration (FDA) was established to control US pharmaceutical products.

Safety regulations in the USA were, however, not enough to prevent the sale of a paediatric *sulfanilamide* elixir containing the toxic solvent diethylene glycol. In 1937, 107 people, both adults and children, died as a result of ingesting the elixir, and in 1938 the Food Drug and Cosmetics Act was passed, requiring for the first time approval by the FDA before marketing of a new drug product.

The *thalidomide* disaster further demonstrated the lack of adequate drug control. Thalidomide (Neurosedyn®, Contergan®) was launched during the last years of the 1950s as a non-toxic treatment for a variety of conditions, such as colds, anxiety, depression, infections, etc., both alone and in combination with a number of other compounds, such as analgesics and sedatives.

The reason why the compound was regarded as harmless was the lack of acute toxicity after high single doses. After repeated long-term administration, however, signs of neuropathy developed, with symptoms of numbness, paraesthesia and ataxia. But the overwhelming effects were the gross malformation in infants born to mothers who had taken thalidomide in pregnancy: their limbs were partially or totally missing, a previously extremely rare malformation called *phocomelia* (seal limb). Altogether around 12 000 infants were born with the defect in those few years. Thalidomide was withdrawn from the market in 1961/62.

This catastrophe became a strong driver to develop animal test methods to assess drug safety before testing compounds in humans. Also it forced national authorities to strengthen the requirements for control procedures before marketing of pharmaceutical products (Cartwright and Matthews, 1991).

Another blow hit Japan between 1959 and 1971. The SMON (*subacute myelo-optical neuropathy*) disaster was blamed on the frequent Japanese use of the intestinal antiseptic *clioquinol* (Entero-Vioform®, Enteroform® or Vioform®). The product had been sold without restrictions since early 1900, and it was assumed that it would not be absorbed, but after repeated use neurological symptoms appeared, characterized by paraesthesia, numbness and weakness of the extremities, and even blindness. SMON affected about 10 000 Japanese, compared to some 100 cases in the rest of the world (Meade, 1975).

These tragedies had a strong impact on governmental regulatory control of pharmaceutical products. In 1962 the FDA required evidence of efficacy as well as safety as a condition for registration, and formal approval was required for patients to be included in clinical trials of new drugs.

In Europe, the UK Medicines Act 1968 made safety assessment of new drug products compulsory. The Swedish Drug Ordinance of 1962 defined the medicinal product and required a clear benefit–risk ratio to be documented before approval for marketing. All European countries established similar controls during the 1960s.

In Japan, the Pharmaceutical Affairs Law enacted in 1943 was revised in 1961, 1979 and 2005 to establish the current drug regulatory system, with the Ministry of Health and Welfare assessing drugs for quality, safety and efficacy.

The 1960s and 1970s saw a rapid increase in laws, regulations and guidelines for reporting and evaluating the risks versus the benefits of new medicinal products. At the time the industry was becoming more international and seeking new global markets, but the registration of medicines remained a national responsibility.

Although different regulatory systems were based on the same key principles, the detailed technical requirements diverged over time, often for traditional rather than scientific reasons, to such an extent that industry found it necessary to duplicate tests in different countries to obtain global regulatory approval for new products. This was a waste of time, money and animals' lives, and it became clear that harmonization of regulatory requirements was needed.

European (EEC) efforts to harmonize requirements for drug approval began 1965, and a common European approach grew with the expansion of the European Union (EU) to 15 countries, and then 27. The EU harmonization principles have also been adopted by Norway and Iceland. This successful European harmonization process gave impetus to discussions about harmonization on a broader international scale (Cartwright and Matthews, 1994).

INTERNATIONAL HARMONIZATION

The harmonization process started in 1990, when representatives of the regulatory authorities and industry associations of Europe, Japan and the USA (representing the majority of the global pharmaceutical industry) met, ostensibly to plan an International Conference on Harmonization (ICH). The meeting actually went much further, suggesting *terms of reference* for ICH, and setting up an ICH Steering Committee representing the three regions.

The task of ICH was '… increased international harmonization, aimed at ensuring that good quality, safe and effective medicines are developed and registered in the most efficient and cost-effective manner. These activities are pursued in the interest of the consumer and public health, to prevent unnecessary duplication of clinical trials in humans and to minimize the use of animal testing without compromising the regulatory obligations of safety and effectiveness' (Tokyo, October 1990).

ICH has remained a very active organization, with substantial representation at both authority and industry level from the EU, the USA and Japan. The input of other nations is provided through World Health Organization representatives, as well as representatives from Switzerland and Canada.

ICH conferences, held every 2 years, have become a forum for open discussion and follow-up of the topics decided. The important achievements so far are the scientific guidelines agreed and implemented in the national/regional drug legislation, not only in the ICH territories

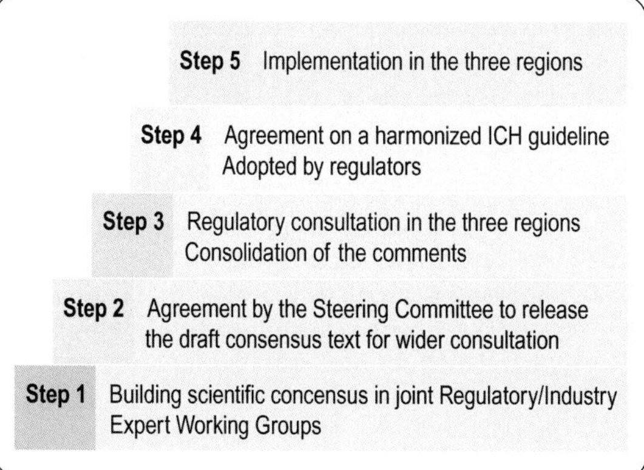
Step 5 Implementation in the three regions
Step 4 Agreement on a harmonized ICH guideline Adopted by regulators
Step 3 Regulatory consultation in the three regions Consolidation of the comments
Step 2 Agreement by the Steering Committee to release the draft consensus text for wider consultation
Step 1 Building scientific concensus in joint Regulatory/Industry Expert Working Groups

Fig. 20.1 Five steps in the ICH process for harmonization of technical issues.

but also in other countries around the world. So far some 50 guidelines have reached ICH approval and regional implementation, i.e. steps 4 and 5 (Figure 20.1). For a complete list of ICH guidelines and their status, see the ICH website (website reference 1).

The process described in Figure 20.1 is very open, and the fact that health authorities and the pharmaceutical industry collaborate from the start increases the efficiency of work and ensures mutual understanding across regions and functions; this is a major factor in the success of ICH.

ROLES AND RESPONSIBILITIES OF REGULATORY AUTHORITY AND COMPANY

The basic division of responsibilities for drug products is that the health authority is protecting public health and safety, and the pharmaceutical company is responsible for all aspects of the drug product. The regulatory approval of a pharmaceutical product permits marketing and is a contract between the regulatory authority and the pharmaceutical company. The conditions of the approval are set out in the dossier and condensed in the prescribing information. Any change that is planned must be forwarded to the regulatory authority for information and, in most cases, new approval before being implemented.

To protect the public health, regulatory authorities also develop regulations and guidelines for companies to follow in order to achieve a balance between the possible risks and therapeutic advantages to patients. The authorities' work is partly financed by fees paid by pharmaceutical companies. Fees may be reduced, under certain conditions, to stimulate research. This may be driven, e.g., by company size or size of target patient groups.

The regulatory authority:

- approves clinical trial applications
- gives procedural and scientific advice to companies during drug development
- approves for marketing drugs that have been scientifically evaluated to provide evidence of a satisfactory benefit/risk ratio
- monitors the safety of the marketed product, based on (a) reports of adverse reactions from healthcare providers, and (b) from compiled and evaluated safety information from the company that owns the product
- can withdraw the licence for marketing in serious cases of non-compliance (e.g. failure on inspections, failure of adequate additional warnings in prescribing information after clinical adverse reactions are reported, or failure of the company to consider serious findings in animal studies).

The company:

- owns the documentation that forms the basis for assessment, is responsible for its accuracy and correctness, for keeping it up to date, and for ensuring that it complies with standards set by current scientific development and the regulatory authorities
- collects, compiles and evaluates safety data, and submits reports to the regulatory authorities at regular intervals – and takes rapid action in serious cases. This might involve the withdrawal of the entire product or of a product batch (e.g. tablets containing the wrong drug or the wrong dose), or a request to the regulatory authority for a change in prescribing information
- has a right to appeal and to correct cases of non-compliance.

The role of the regulatory affairs department

The regulatory affairs (RA) department of a pharmaceutical company is responsible for obtaining approval for new pharmaceutical products and ensuring that approval is maintained for as long as the company wants to keep the product on the market. It serves as the interface between the regulatory authority and the project team, and is the channel of communication with the regulatory authority as the project proceeds, aiming to ensure that the project plan correctly anticipates what the regulatory authority will require before approving the product. It is the responsibility of RA to keep abreast of current legislation, guidelines and other regulatory intelligence. Such rules and guidelines often allow some flexibility, and the regulatory authorities expect companies to take responsibility for deciding how they should be interpreted. The RA department plays an important role in giving advice to the project team on how best to interpret the rules. During the development process sound working relations with authorities are essential, e.g. to discuss such issues as divergence from guidelines, the clinical study programme, and formulation development.

Most companies assess and prioritize new projects based on an intended Target Product Profile (TPP). The RA professional plays a key role in advising on what will be realistic prescribing information ('label') for the intended product. As a member of the project team RA also contributes to designing of the development programme. The RA department reviews all documentation from a regulatory perspective, ensuring that it is clear, consistent and complete, and that its conclusions are explicit. The department also drafts the core prescribing information that is the basis for global approval, and will later provide the platform for marketing. The documentation includes clinical trials applications, as well as regulatory submissions for new products and for changes to approved products. The latter is a major task and accounts for about half of the work of the RA department.

An important proactive task of the RA is to provide input when legislative changes are being discussed and proposed. In the ICH environment there is a greater possibility to exert influence at an early stage.

THE DRUG DEVELOPMENT PROCESS

An overview of the process of drug development is given in Chapters 14–18 and summarized in Figure 20.2. As already emphasized, this sequential approach, designed to minimize risk by allowing each study to start only when earlier studies have been successfully completed, is giving way to a partly parallel approach in order to save development time.

All studies in the non-clinical area – chemistry, pharmacology, pharmacokinetics, pharmaceutical development and toxicology – aim to establish indicators of safety and efficacy sufficient to allow studies and use in man. According to ICH nomenclature, documentation of chemical and pharmaceutical development relates to *quality* assessment, animal studies relate to *safety* assessment, and studies in humans relate to *efficacy*.

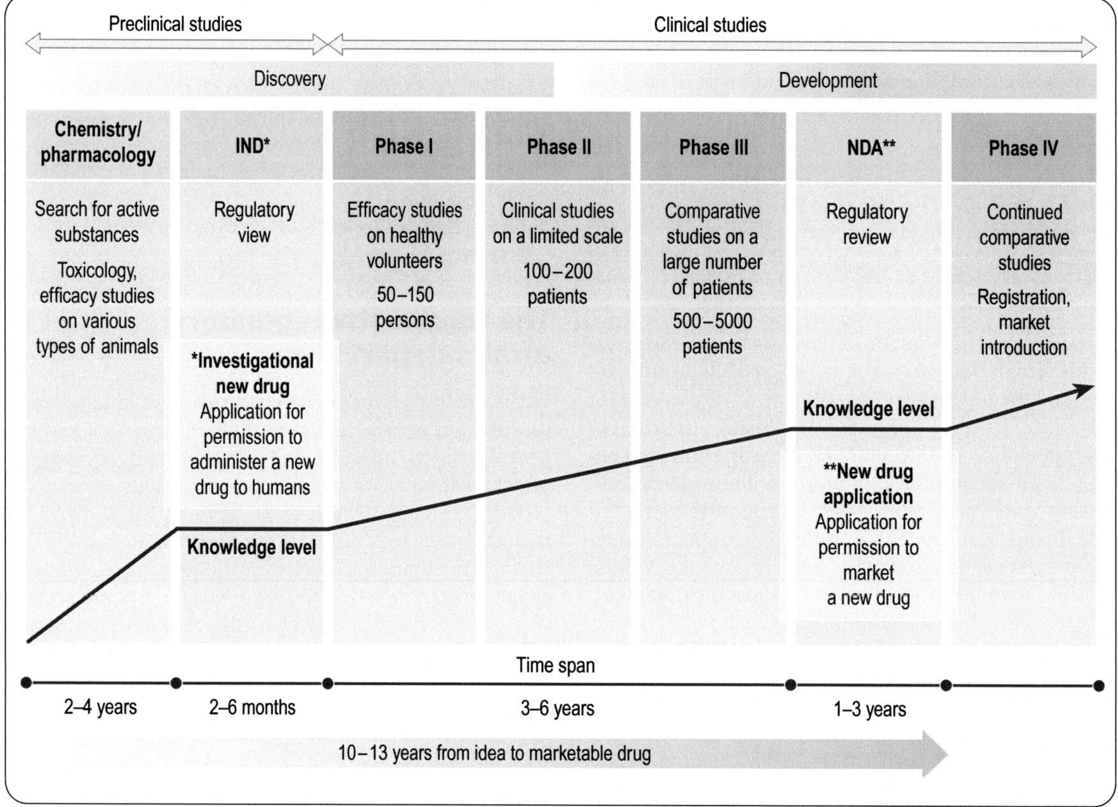

Fig. 20.2 The drug development process.

Quality assessment (chemistry and pharmaceutical development)

The *quality module* of a submission documents purity and assay for the drug substance, and purity data for all the inactive ingredients. The formulation must fulfil requirements for consistent quality and allow storage, and the container must be shown to be fit for its purpose. These aspects of a pharmaceutical product have to be kept under control throughout the development process, as toxicology and pharmacology results are reliable only for substances of comparable purity. Large-scale production, improved synthetic route, different raw material supply, etc., may produce a substance somewhat different from the first laboratory-scale batches. Any substantial change must be known and documented.

The formulation of a product is a challenge. For initial human studies, simple i.v. and oral solutions are needed for straightforward results, whereas for the clinical programme in patients, bioequivalent formulations are essential for comparison of results across studies, and so it is preferable to have access to the final formulation already during Phase II.

If the formulation intended for marketing cannot be completed until late in the clinical phase, bioequivalence studies showing comparable results with the preliminary and final market formulations will be necessary to support the use of results with the preliminary formulation. There may even be situations when clinical studies must be repeated.

The analytical methods used and their validation must be described. Manufacturing processes and their validation are also required to demonstrate interbatch uniformity. However, full-scale validation may be submitted when sales production has eventually started.

Studies on the stability of both substance and products under real-life conditions are required, covering the full time of intended storage. Preliminary stability data are sufficient for the start of clinical studies. The allowable storage time can be increased as data are gathered and submitted. Even marketing authorizations can be approved on less than real-time storage information, but there is a requirement to submit final data when available.

Inactive ingredients as well as active substances need to be documented, unless they are well known and already documented. Even then it may become necessary to perform new animal studies to support novel uses of commonly used additives.

Although the quality module of the documentation is the smallest, the details of requirements and the many changes needed during development and maintenance of a product make it the most resource intensive module from a regulatory perspective. Also, legislation differs most in this area, so it will often be necessary to adapt the documentation for the intended regional submission. RA professionals, however, try to convince regulatory authorities not to create local rules to avoid, as far as possible, different interpretations and duplicate work.

As previously said, all changes to the originally submitted dossier must be made known to the approving regulatory authority. Since the majority of changes are made in the quality section, very small changes take lots of resources for the company as well as for the authority. The US legislation has allowed the submission of annual reports collecting those changes that have no impact on quality. This possibility has also been introduced in EU in 2010 with the purpose of saving time and resources.

Safety assessment (pharmacology and toxicology)

Next we consider how to design and integrate pharmacological and toxicological studies in order to produce adequate documentation for the first tests in humans. ICH guidelines define the information needed from animal studies in terms of doses and time of exposure, to allow clinical studies, first in healthy subjects and later in patients. The principles and methodology of animal studies are described in Chapters 11 and 15. The questions discussed here are *when* and *why* these animal studies are required for regulatory purposes.

Primary pharmacology

The primary pharmacodynamic studies provide the first evidence that the compound has the pharmacological effects required to give therapeutic benefit. It is a clear regulatory advantage to use established models and to be able at least to establish a theory for the mechanism of action. This will not always be possible and is not a firm requirement, but proof of efficacy and safety is helped by a plausible mechanistic explanation of the drug's effects, and this knowledge will also become a very powerful tool for marketing. For example, understanding the mechanism of action of proton pump inhibitors, such as *omeprazole* (see Chapter 4), was important in explaining their long duration of action, allowing once-daily dosage of compounds despite their short plasma half-life.

General pharmacology

General pharmacology[1] studies investigate effects other than the primary therapeutic effects. Safety pharmacology studies (see Chapter 15), which must conform to good laboratory practice (GLP) standards, are focused on identifying the effects on physiological functions that in a clinical setting are unwanted or harmful.

[1]There are a number of widely used terms with similar meanings, e.g. secondary pharmacology, safety pharmacology, high-dose pharmacology, regulatory pharmacology and pharmacodynamic safety.

Although the study design will depend on the properties and intended use of the compound, general pharmacology studies are normally of short duration (i.e. acute, rather than chronic, effects are investigated), and the dosage is increased until clear adverse effects occur. The studies also include comparisons with known compounds whose pharmacological properties or clinical uses are similar.

When required, e.g. when pharmacodynamic effects occur only after prolonged treatment, or when effects seen with repeated administration give rise to safety concerns, the duration of a safety pharmacology study needs to be prolonged. The route of administration should, whenever possible, be the route intended for clinical use.

There are cases when a secondary pharmacological effect has, eventually, been developed into a new indication. *Lidocaine*, for example, was developed as a local anaesthetic agent and its cardiac effects after overdose were considered a hazard. Later that cardiac effect was exploited as a treatment for ventricular arrhythmia.

All relevant safety pharmacology studies must be completed before studies can be undertaken in patients. Complementary studies may still be needed to clarify unexpected findings in later development stages.

Pharmacokinetics: absorption, distribution, metabolism and excretion (ADME)

Preliminary pharmacokinetic tests to assess the absorption, plasma levels and half-life (i.e. exposure information) are performed in rodents in parallel with the preliminary pharmacology and toxicology studies (see Chapter 10).

Studies in humans normally start with limited short-term data, and only if the results are acceptable are detailed animal and human ADME studies performed.

Plasma concentrations observed in animals are used to predict the concentrations that may be efficacious/tolerated in humans, under the assumption that similar biological effects should be produced at similar plasma levels across species. This is a reasonable assumption provided the *in vitro* target affinity is similar.

Investigations during the toxicology programme give the bulk of the pharmacokinetic information due to the long duration of drug exposure and the wide range of doses tested in several relevant species. They also give data about tissue distribution and possible accumulation in the body, including placental transfer and exposure of the fetus, as well as excretion in milk.

Metabolic pathways differ considerably between species, often quantitatively but sometimes also qualitatively. Active metabolites can influence study results, in particular after repeated use. A toxic metabolite with a long half-life may accumulate in the body and disturb results. The characterization and evaluation of metabolites are long processes, and are generally the last studies to be completed in a development programme.

Toxicology

The principles and methodology of toxicological assessment of new compounds are described in Chapter 15. Here we consider the regulatory aspects.

In contrast to the pharmacological studies, toxicological studies generally follow standard protocols that do not depend on the compound characteristics. Active comparators are not used, but the drug substance is compared at various dose levels to a vehicle control, given, if possible, via the intended route of administration.

Single and repeated-dose studies

The acute toxicity of a new compound must be evaluated prior to the first human exposure.

This information is obtained from dose escalation studies or dose-ranging studies of short duration. Lethality is no longer an ethically accepted endpoint. The toxicology requirements for the first exploratory studies in man are described in the ICH guidline M3 which reached step 5 in June 2009 (see website reference 1). Table 20.1 shows the duration of repeated-dose studies recommended by ICH, to support clinical trials and therapeutic use for different periods.

Genotoxicity

Preliminary genotoxicity evaluation of mutations and chromosomal damage (see Chapter 15) is needed before the drug is given to humans. If results from those studies are ambiguous or positive, further testing is required. The entire standard battery of tests needs to be completed before Phase II (see Chapter 17).

Carcinogenicity

The objective of carcinogenicity studies is to identify any tumorigenic potential in animals, and they are required only when the expected duration of therapy, whether continuous or intermittent, is at least 6 months. Examples include treatments for conditions such as allergic rhinitis, anxiety or depression.

Carcinogenicity studies are also required when there is particular reason for concern, such as chemical similarities to known carcinogens, pathophysiological findings in animal toxicity studies, or positive genotoxicity results. Compounds found to be genotoxic by *in vitro* as well as *in vivo* tests are presumed to be trans-species carcinogens with hazards to humans.

Carcinogenicity studies normally run for the lifespan of the test animals. They are performed quite late in the development programme and are not necessarily completed when the application for marketing authorization is submitted. Indeed, for products for which there is a great medical need in the treatment of certain serious diseases, the regulatory authority may agree that submission of carcinogenicity data can be delayed until after marketing approval is granted.

Table 20.1 Duration of repeated-dose toxicity studies

Recommended minimum duration of repeated-dose toxicity studies				
Maximum duration of clinical trials	**To support clinical trials**		**To support marketing**	
	Rodents	*Non-rodents*	*Rodents*	*Non-rodents*
Up to 2 weeks	2 weeks[a]	2 weeks	1 month	1 month
>2 weeks to 1 month	Same as the clinical trial[b]	Same as the clinical trial [b]	3 months	3 months
>1 month to 3 months			6 months	3 months
>3 months to 6 months			6 months[c]	9 months[cd]
>6 months	6 months[bc]	9 months[bcd]		

[a]In the USA, as an alternative to 2-week studies, single-dose toxicity studies with extended examination can support single-dose human trials.
[b]Data from 3-month studies in rodents and non-rodents may be sufficient to start clinical trials longer than 3 months provided longer-term data are made available before extension of the clinical trial.
[c]If paediatric patients are the target population, long-term toxicity studies in juvenile animals may be required.
[d]6 months' studies are acceptable in non-rodents in certain cases, e.g. intermittent treatment of migraine, chronic treatment to prevent recurrence of cancer, indications for which life expectancy is short, animals cannot tolerate the treatment.

Reproductive and developmental toxicity

These studies (see Chapter 15) are intended to reveal effects on male or female fertility, embryonic and fetal development, and peri- and postnatal development.

An evaluation of effects on the male reproductive system is performed in the repeated-dose toxicity studies, and this histopathological assessment is considered more sensitive in detecting toxic effects than are fertility studies. Men can therefore be included in Phase I–II trials before the male fertility studies are performed in animals.

Women may enter early studies before reproductive toxicity testing is completed, provided they are permanently sterilized or menopausal, and provided repeated-dose toxicity tests of adequate duration have been performed, including the evaluation of female reproductive organs.

For women of childbearing potential there is concern regarding unintentional fetal exposure, and there are regional differences (Box 20.1) in the regulations about including fertile women in clinical trials.

Local tolerance and other toxicity studies

The purpose of local tolerance studies is to ascertain whether medicinal products (both active substances and excipients) are tolerated at sites in the body that may come into contact with the product in clinical use. This could mean, for example, ocular, dermal or parenteral administration. Other studies may also be needed. These might be studies on immunotoxicity, antigenicity studies on metabolites or impurities, and so on. The drug substance and the intended use will determine the relevance of other studies.

Box 20.1 **Requirement for reproduction toxicity related to clinical studies in fertile women**

EU:	Embryo/fetal development studies are required before Phase I, and female fertility should be completed before Phase III
USA:	Careful monitoring and pregnancy testing may allow fertile women to take part before reproduction toxicity is available. Female fertility and embryo/fetal assessment to be completed before Phase III
Japan:	Embryo/fetal development studies are required before Phase I, and female fertility should be completed before Phase III.

Efficacy assessment (studies in man)

When the preclinical testing is sufficient to start studies in man, the RA department compiles a clinical trials submission, which is sent to the regulatory authority and the ethics committee (see Regulatory procedures, below).

The clinical studies, described in detail in Chapter 17, are classified according to Table 20.2.

Human pharmacology

Human pharmacology studies refer to the earliest human exposure in volunteers, as well as any pharmacological studies in patients and volunteers throughout the development of the drug.

Table 20.2 ICH classification of clinical studies

Type of study	Study objectives	Traditional terminology
Human pharmacology	Assess tolerance; describe or define pharmacokinetics/pharmacodynamics; explore drug metabolism and drug interactions; estimate activity	Phase I
Therapeutic exploratory	Explore use for the targeted indication; estimate dosage for subsequent studies; provide basis for confirmatory study design, endpoints, methodologies	Phase II
Therapeutic confirmatory	Demonstrate or confirm efficacy; establish safety profile; provide an adequate basis for assessing benefit–risk relationship to support licensing (drug approval); establish dose–response relationship	Phase III (a and b)
Therapeutic use	Refine understanding of benefit–risk relationship in general or special populations and/or environments; identify less common adverse reactions; refine dosing recommendations	Phase IV

The first study of a new drug substance in humans has essentially three objectives:

- To investigate *tolerability* over a range of doses and, if possible, see the symptoms of adverse effects
- To obtain information on *pharmacokinetics*, and to measure bioavailability and plasma concentration/effect relations
- To examine the *pharmacodynamic activity* over a range of doses and obtain a dose–response relationship, provided a relevant effect can be measured in healthy volunteers.

Further human pharmacology studies are performed to document pharmacodynamic and pharmacokinetic effects. Examples of the data needed to support an application for trials in patients are the complete pharmacokinetic evaluation and the performance of bioavailability/bioequivalence studies during the development of new formulations or drug-delivery systems. Information is also obtained on the possible influence of food on absorption, and that of other concomitant medications, i.e. drug interaction. Exploration of metabolic pattern is also performed early in the clinical development process.

Special patient populations need particular attention because they may be unduly sensitive or resistant to treatment regimens acceptable to the normal adult population studied. One obvious category is patients with renal or hepatic impairment, who may be unable to metabolize or excrete the drug effectively enough to avoid accumulation. The metabolic pattern and elimination route are important predictors for such patients, who are not included in clinical trials until late in development.

Gender differences may also occur, and may be detected by the inclusion of women at the dose-finding stage of clinical trials.

An interaction is an alteration in the pharmacodynamic or the pharmacokinetic properties of a drug caused by factors such as concomitant drug treatment, diet, social habits (e.g. tobacco or alcohol), age, gender, ethnic origin and time of administration.

Interaction studies can be performed in healthy volunteers looking at possible metabolism changes when co-administering compounds that share the same enzymatic metabolic pathway. Also, changed pharmacokinetic behaviour can be investigated in combinations of drugs that are expected to be used together. Generally, such human volunteer studies are performed when clinical findings require clarification or if the company wishes to avoid standard warning texts which would otherwise apply to the drug class.

Therapeutic exploratory studies

After relevant information in healthy volunteers has been obtained, safety conclusions from combined animal and human exposure will be assessed internally. If these are favourable, initial patient studies can begin. To obtain the most reliable results, the patient population should be as homogeneous as possible – similar age, no other diseases than the one to be studied – and the design should, when ethically justified, be placebo controlled. For ethical reasons only a limited number of closely monitored patients take part in these studies. Their importance lies in the assumption that any placebo effect in the group treated with active drug should be eliminated by comparison with blinded inactive treatment. They are used primarily to establish efficacy measured against no treatment.

Studies in special populations: elderly, children, ethnic differences

Clinically significant differences in pharmacokinetics between the elderly and the young are due to several factors related to aging, such as impaired renal function, which can increase the variability in drug response, as well as increasing the likelihood of unwanted effects and drug interactions. Bearing in mind that the elderly are the largest group of consumers, this category should be studied as early as possible in clinical trials.

Clinical trials in children

Studies in children require experience from adult human studies and information on the pharmacokinetic profile of the substance. Because of the difficulties, and the often small commercial return, companies have seldom considered it worthwhile to test drugs in children and to seek regulatory approval for marketing drugs for use in children. Nevertheless, drugs are often prescribed 'off-label' for children, on the basis of clinical experience suggesting that they are safe and effective. Such off-label prescribing is undesirable, as clinical experience is less satisfactory than formal trials data as a guide to efficacy and safety, and because it leaves the clinician, rather than the pharmaceutical company, liable for any harm that may result. Recently, requirements to include a paediatric population early have forced the development of new guidance as to how to include children in clinical development. Market exclusivity prolongation has been successfully tried for some years in the USA, and in July 2003 the Federal Food Drug and Cosmetics Act was amended to request paediatric studies in a new submission unless omission is justified. In September of 2007, the Paediatric Research Equity Act replaced the 2003 Act and an assessment was made to evaluate the quality of the studies submitted. The results were positive and between September 2007 and June 2010 more than 250 clinical trials comprising more than 100 000 children have been performed. (see website reference 2).

In Europe the European Commission adopted the Paediatric Regulation in February 2007 (see website reference 3). This stipulates that no marketing approval will be granted unless there is an agreed paediatric investigation plan in place or, alternatively, there is a waiver from the requirement because of the low risk that the product will be considered for use in children. The paediatric studies may, with the agreement of the regulatory authority, be performed after approval for other populations. For new compounds or for products with a Supplementary Protection Certificate (see p. 300), paediatric applications will be given a longer market exclusivity period, and off-patent products will be given a special paediatric use marketing authorization (PUMA); funds will be available for paediatric research in these products.

To further encourage paediatric research, authority scientific advice is free. Paediatric clinical data from the EU and elsewhere are collected in a common European database to avoid repetition of trials with unnecessary exposure in children. The US FDA and the EMA in Europe exchange information on paediatric clinical research.

Ethnic differences

In order for clinical data to be accepted globally, the risk of ethnic differences must be assessed. ICH Efficacy guideline E5 defines a bridging data package that would allow extrapolation of foreign clinical data to the population in the new region. A limited programme may suffice to confirm comparable effects in different ethnic groups.

Ethnic differences may be genetic in origin, as in the example described in Chapter 17, or related to differences in environment, culture or medical practice.

Therapeutic confirmatory studies

The therapeutic confirmatory phase is intended to confirm efficacy results from controlled exploratory efficacy studies, but now in a more realistic clinical environment and with a broader population.

In order to convincingly document that the product is efficacious, there are some 'golden rules' to be aware of in terms of the need for statistical power, replication of the results, etc. Further, for a product intended for long-term use, its performance must usually be investigated during long-term exposure. All these aspects will, however, be influenced by what alternative treatments there are, the intended target patient population, the rarity and severity of the disease as well as other factors, and must be evaluated case by case.

Clinical safety profile

An equally important function of this largest and longest section of the clinical documentation is to capture all adverse event information to enable evaluation of the relative benefit–risk ratio of the new compound, and also to detect rare adverse reactions. To document clinical safety, the ICH E1 guideline on products intended for chronic use stipulates that a minimum of 100 patients be treated for at least 1 year, and 300–600 treated for at least 6 months. In reality, however, several thousand patients usually form the database for safety evaluation for marketing approval.

Not until several similar studies can be analysed together can a real estimate be made of the clinical safety of the product.

The collected clinical database should be analysed across a sensible selection of variables, such as sex, age, race, exposure (dose and duration), as well as concomitant diseases and concomitant pharmacotherapy This type of integrated data analysis is a rational and scientific way to obtain necessary information about the benefits and risks of new compounds, and has been required for FDA submissions for many years, though it is not yet a firm requirement in the EU or Japan.

To further emphasize the accountability for the product by the pharmaceutical company a more proactive legislation for risk evaluation has been introduced in USA and EU. The term Risk Evaluation and Mitigation Strategy

(REMS) in the USA is matched by Risk Management System in EU.

The difference from the established method of reporting adverse reactions that have occurred is that any possible or potential risks for a patient being harmed should be foreseen or identified early and mitigation/minimization activities be planned in advance. The risk management document is generally part of the regulatory approval and follows the product's entire lifecycle. The true risk profile will develop along with the increased knowledge base. The goal is at any time to be able to demonstrate how and why the treatment benefits outweigh the risks (see website references 4 and 5).

Regulatory aspects of novel types of therapy

As emphasized in earlier chapters, the therapeutic scene is moving increasingly towards biological and biopharmaceutical treatments, as well as various innovative, so-called advanced therapies. There are also broadening definitions of what constitutes medical devices. The regulatory framework established to ensure the quality, safety and efficacy of conventional synthetic drugs is not entirely appropriate for many biopharmaceutical products, and even less so for the many gene- and cell-based products currently in development. Recombinant proteins have been in use since 1982 and the regulatory process for such biopharmaceuticals is by now well established, hence this chapter will mainly focus on these. The EU also has, for example, new legislation in force since December 2008 specifically on Advanced Therapy Medicinal Products (ATMP), meaning somatic cell therapy, gene therapy and tissue engineering. This involves requirements for the applicant, as part of a marketing authorization, to establish a risk management system. In addition to the standard requirements in terms of safety follow-up for an approved product, this system should also include an evaluation of the product's effectiveness (see website reference 6). In the USA, there are a number of FDA guidelines relating to cellular and gene therapies. The regulatory framework for even newer therapeutic modalities relating, for example, to nanotechnologies is not yet clearly defined, and the regulatory authorities face a difficult task in keeping up with the rapid pace of technological change.

Biopharmaceuticals

Compared with synthetic compounds, biopharmaceuticals are by their nature more heterogeneous, and their production methods are very diverse, including complex fermentation and recombinant techniques, as well as production via the use of transgenic animals and plants, thereby posing new challenges for quality control. This has necessarily led to a fairly pragmatic regulatory framework. Quality, safety and efficacy requirements have to be no less stringent, but procedures and standards are flexible and generally established on a case-by-case basis. Consequently, achieving regulatory approval can often be a greater challenge for the pharmaceutical company, but there are also opportunities to succeed with novel and relatively quick development programmes.

Published guidelines on the development of conventional drugs need to be considered to determine what parts are relevant for a particular biopharmaceutical product. In addition, there are, to date, seven ICH guidelines dealing exclusively with biopharmaceuticals, as well as numerous FDA and CHMP guidance documents. These mostly deal with quality aspects and, in some cases, preclinical safety aspects. The definition of what is included in the term 'biopharmaceutical' varies somewhat between documents, and therefore needs to be checked. The active substances include proteins and peptides, their derivatives, and products of which they are components. Examples include (but are not limited to) cytokines, recombinant plasma factors, growth factors, fusion proteins, enzymes, hormones and monoclonal antibodies (see also Chapters 12 and 13).

Quality considerations

A unique and critically important feature for biopharmaceuticals is the need to ensure and document viral safety aspects. Furthermore, there must be preparedness for potentially new hazards, such as infective prions. Therefore strict control of the origin of starting materials and expression systems is essential. The current battery of ICH quality guidance documents in this area reflects these points of particular attention (ICH Q5A-E, and Q6B).

At the time when biopharmaceuticals first appeared, the ability to analyse and exactly characterize the end-product was not possible the way it was with small molecules. Therefore, their efficacy and safety depended critically on the manufacturing process itself, and emphasis was placed on 'process control' rather than 'product control'.

Since then, much experience and confidence has been gained. Bioanalytical technologies for characterizing large molecules have improved dramatically and so has the field of bioassays, which are normally required to be included in such characterizations, e.g. to determine the 'potency' of a product. As a result, the quality aspects of biopharmaceuticals are no longer as fundamentally different from those of synthetic products as they used to be. The quality documentation will still typically be more extensive than it is for a small-molecule product.

Today the concept of 'comparability' has been established and approaches for demonstrating product comparability after process changes have been outlined by regulatory authorities. Further, the increased understanding of these products has in more recent times allowed the approval of generic versions also of biopharmaceuticals, so-called follow-on biologics or biosimilars. A legal framework was established first in the EU, in 2004, and the first such approvals (somatropin products) were seen in 2006.

Approvals are so far slightly behind in the USA since there was actually not a regulatory pathway for biosimilars until such provisions were signed into law in March 2010 (see website reference 7). The FDA is, at the time of writing, working on details of how to implement these provisions to approve biosimilars. Also, in Japan, the authorities have published 'Guidelines for the Quality, Safety and Efficacy Assurance of Follow-on Biologics', the most recent version being in March 2009.

Safety considerations

The expectations in terms of performing and documenting a non-clinical safety evaluation for biotechnology-derived pharmaceuticals are well outlined in the ICH guidance document S6. This guideline was revised in 2011 driven by scientific advances and experience gained since publication of the original guidance. It indicates a flexible, case-by-case and science-based approach, but also points out that a product needs to be sufficiently characterized to allow the appropriate design of a preclinical safety evaluation.

Generally, all toxicity studies must be performed according to GLP. However, for biopharmaceuticals it is recognized that some specialized tests may not be able to comply fully with GLP. The guidance further comments that the standard toxicity testing designs in the commonly used species (e.g. rats and dogs) are often not relevant.

To make it relevant, a safety evaluation should include a species in which the test material is pharmacologically active. Further, in certain justified cases one relevant species may suffice, at least for the long-term studies. If no relevant species at all can be identified, the use of transgenic animals expressing the human receptor or the use of homologous proteins should be considered.

Other factors of particular relevance with biopharmaceuticals are potential immunogenicity and immunotoxicity. Long-term studies may be difficult to perform, depending on the possible formation of neutralizing antibodies in the selected species. For products intended for chronic use, the duration of long-term toxicity studies must, however, always be scientifically justified. Regulatory guidance also states that standard carcinogenicity studies are generally inappropriate, but that product-specific assessments of potential risks may still be needed, and that a variety of approaches may be necessary to accomplish this.

In 2006 disastrous clinical trial events took place with an antibody (TGN 1412), where healthy volunteers suffered life-threatening adverse effects. These effects had not been anticipated by the company or the authority reviewing the clinical trial application. The events triggered intense discussions on risk identification and mitigation for so-called first-in-human clinical trials, and in particular for any medicinal product which might be considered 'high-risk'. Since then, specific guidelines for such clinical trial applications have been issued by the regulatory authorities.

Efficacy considerations

The need to establish efficacy is in principle the same for biopharmaceuticals as for conventional drugs, but there are significant differences in practice. The establishment of a dose–response relationship can be irrelevant, as there may be an 'all-or-none-effect' at extremely low levels. Also, to determine a maximum tolerated dose (MTD) in humans may be impractical, as many biopharmaceuticals will not evoke any dose-limiting side effects. Measuring pharmacokinetic properties may be difficult, particularly if the substance is an endogenous mediator. Biopharmaceuticals may also have very long half-lives compared to small molecules, often in the range of weeks rather than hours.

For any biopharmaceutical intended for chronic or repeated use, there will be extra emphasis on demonstrating long-term efficacy. This is because the medical use of proteins is associated with potential immunogenicity and the possible development of neutralizing antibodies, such that the intended effect may decrease or even disappear with time. Repeated assessment of immunogenicity may be needed, particularly after any process changes.

To date, biopharmaceuticals have typically been developed for serious diseases, and certain types of treatments, such as cytotoxic agents or immunomodulators, cannot be given to healthy volunteers. In such cases, the initial dose-escalation studies will have to be carried out in a patient population rather than in normal volunteers.

Regulatory procedural considerations

In the EU, only the centralized procedure can be used for biopharmaceuticals as well as biosimilars (see Regulatory procedures, below). In the USA, biopharmaceuticals are in most cases approved by review of Biologics License Applications (BLA), rather than New Drug Applications (NDA).

Personalized therapies

It is recognized that an individual's genetic makeup influences the effect of drugs. Incorporating this principle into therapeutic practice is still at a relatively early stage, although the concept moves rapidly towards everyday reality, and it presents a challenge for regulatory authorities who are seeking ways to incorporate personalized medicine (pharmacogenomics) into the regulatory process. How a drug product can or should be co-developed with the necessary genomic biomarkers and/or assays is not yet clear. Another regulatory uncertainty has been how the generation of these kinds of data will translate into label language for the approved product. Already in 2005 the FDA issued guidance on a specific procedure for 'Pharmacogenomic Data Submissions' to try and alleviate potential industry concerns and instead promote scientific progress and the gaining of experience in the field. In the EU there is, at the time of writing, draft guidance published on the use of pharmacogenetic methodologies in the pharmacokinetic evaluation of medicinal products.

However, still today, there are relatively few approved products to learn from.

Orphan drugs

Orphan medicines are those intended to diagnose, prevent or treat rare diseases, in the EU further specified as life-threatening or chronically debilitating conditions. The concept also includes therapies that are unlikely to be developed under normal market conditions, where the company can show that a return on research investment will not be possible. To qualify for orphan drug status, there should be no satisfactory treatment available or, alternatively, the intended new treatment should be assumed to be of significant benefit (see website references 8 and 9)

To qualify as an orphan indication, the prevalence of the condition must be fewer than 5 in 10 000 individuals in the EU, fewer than 50 000 affected in Japan, or fewer than 200 000 affected in the USA. Financial and scientific assistance is made available for products intended for use in a given indication that obtain orphan status. Examples of financial benefits are a reduction in or exemption from fees, as well as funding provided by regulatory authorities to meet part of the development costs in some instances. Specialist groups within the regulatory authorities provide scientific help and advice on the execution of studies. Compromises may be needed owing to the scarcity of patients, although the normal requirements to demonstrate safety and efficacy still apply.

The most important benefit stimulating orphan drug development is, however, market exclusivity for 7–10 years for the product, for the designated medical use. In the EU the centralized procedure (see Regulatory procedures, below) is the compulsory procedure for orphan drugs.

The orphan drug incentives are fairly recent. In the USA the legislation dates from 1983, in Japan from 1995, and in the EU from 2000. The US experience has shown very good results; a review of the first 25 years of the Orphan Drug Act resulted in 326 marketing approvals, the majority of which are intended to treat rare cancers or metabolic/endocrinological disorders.

Environmental considerations

Environmental evaluation of the finished pharmaceutical products is required in the USA and EU, the main concern being contamination of the environment by the compound or its metabolites. The environmental impact of the manufacturing process is a separate issue that is regulated elsewhere.

The US requirement for environmental assessment (EA) applies in all cases where action is needed to minimize environmental effects. An Environmental Assessment Report is then required, and the FDA will develop an Environmental Impact Statement to direct necessary action. Drug products for human or animal use can, however, be excluded from this requirement under certain conditions (see website reference 10, p. 301), for example if the estimated concentration in the aquatic environment of the active substance is below 1 part per billion, or if the substance occurs naturally. In Europe a corresponding general guideline was implemented in December 2006 for human medicinal products (see website reference 11).

REGULATORY PROCEDURES

Clinical trials

It is evident that clinical trials can pose unknown risks to humans: the earlier in the development process, the greater the risk. *Regulatory* and *ethical* approvals are based on independent evaluations, and both are required before investigations in humans can begin.

The ethical basis for all clinical research is the Declaration of Helsinki (see website reference 12, p. 301), which states that the primary obligation for the treating physician is to care for the patient. It also says that clinical research may be performed provided the goal is to improve treatment. Furthermore, the subject must be informed about the potential benefits and risks, and must consent to participate. The guardians of patients who for any reason cannot give informed consent (e.g. small children) can agree on participation.

Regulatory authorities are concerned mainly with the scientific basis of the intended study protocol and of course the safety of subjects/patients involved. Regulatory authorities require all results of clinical trials approved by them to be reported back.

All clinical research in humans should be performed according to the internationally agreed Code of Good Clinical Practice, as described in the ICH guideline E6 (see website reference 1, p. 301).

Europe

Until recently, the regulatory requirements to start and conduct clinical studies in Europe have varied widely between countries, ranging from little or no regulation to a requirement for complete assessment by the health authority of the intended study protocol and all supporting documentation.

The efforts to harmonize EU procedures led to the development of a Clinical Trial Directive implemented in May 2004 (see website reference 13, p. 301). One benefit is that both regulatory authorities and ethics committees must respond within 60 days of receiving clinical trials applications and the requirements for information to be submitted are being defined and published in a set of guidelines. Much of the information submitted to the regulatory authority and ethics committee is the same. In spite of the Clinical Trial Directive, however, some national differences in format and information requirements have remained, and upon submission of identical clinical trial protocols in several countries the national reviews may reach different conclusions. Therefore, at the time of writing, there is a pilot Voluntary Harmonization Procedure (VHP) available for applications involving at least three EU member states. This comprises two steps, where in the first round one coordinator on the regulatory authority side manages national comments on the application and provides the applicant with a consolidated list of comments or questions. In the second step the usual national applications for the clinical trial are submitted but national approval should then be gained very rapidly without any further requests for change.

USA

An Investigational New Drug (IND) application must be submitted to the FDA before a new drug is given to humans. The application is relatively simple (see website reference 14, p. 301), and to encourage early human studies it is no longer necessary to submit complete pharmacology study reports. The toxicology safety evaluation can be based on draft and unaudited reports, provided the data are sufficient for the FDA to make a reliable assessment. Complete study reports must be available in later clinical development phases.

Unless the FDA has questions, or even places the product on 'clinical hold', the IND is considered opened 30 days after it was submitted and from then on information (study protocol) is added to it for every new study planned. New scientific information must be submitted whenever changes are made, e.g. dose increases, new patient categories or new indications. The IND process requires an annual update report describing project progress and additional data obtained during the year.

Approval from Institutional Review Board (IRB) is needed for every institution where a clinical study is to be performed.

Japan

Traditionally, because of differences in medical culture, in treatment traditions and the possibility of significant racial differences, clinical trials in Japan have not been useful for drug applications in the Western world. Also, for a product to be approved for the Japanese market, repetition of clinical studies in Japan was necessary, often delaying the availability of products in Japan.

With the introduction of international standards under the auspices of ICH, data from Japanese patients are increasingly becoming acceptable in other countries. The guideline on bridging studies to compensate for ethnic differences (ICH E5; see website reference 1, p. 301) may allow Japanese studies to become part of global development.

The requirements for beginning a clinical study in Japan are similar to those in the USA or Europe. Scientific summary information is generally acceptable, and ethics committee approval is necessary.

Application for marketing authorization

The application for marketing authorization (MAA in Europe, NDA in the USA, JNDA in Japan) is compiled and submitted as soon as the drug development programme has been completed and judged satisfactory by the company. Different authorities have differing requirements as to the level of detail and the format of submissions, and it is the task of the RA department to collate all the data as efficiently as possible to satisfy these varying requirements with a minimum of redrafting.

The US FDA in general requires raw data to be submitted, allowing them to make their own analysis, and thus they request the most complete data of all authorities. European authorities require a condensed dossier containing critical evaluations of the data, allowing a rapid review based on conclusions drawn by named scientific experts. These may be internal or external, and are selected by the applicant.

Japanese authorities have traditionally focused predominantly on data generated in Japan; studies performed elsewhere being supportive only.

Below, the procedures adopted in these three regions are described in more detail.

Europe

Several procedures are available for marketing authorization in the EU (Figure 20.3, see website reference 13):

- *National procedure,* in which the application is evaluated by one regulatory authority. This procedure is allowed for products intended for that country only. Also, it is the first step in a mutual recognition procedure.
- *Mutual recognition,* in which a marketing approval application is assessed by one national authority, the Reference Member State (RMS), which subsequently defends the approval and evaluation in order to gain mutual recognition of the assessment from other European authorities. The pharmaceutical company may select countries of interest. These, the Concerned Member States, have 90 days to recognize the initial assessment. The Mutual Recognition procedure is used for harmonization and conversion of nationally approved products. After mutual recognition the final marketing authorizations are given as national decisions, but the scientific assessment is quicker and requires fewer resources from all national authorities. In the

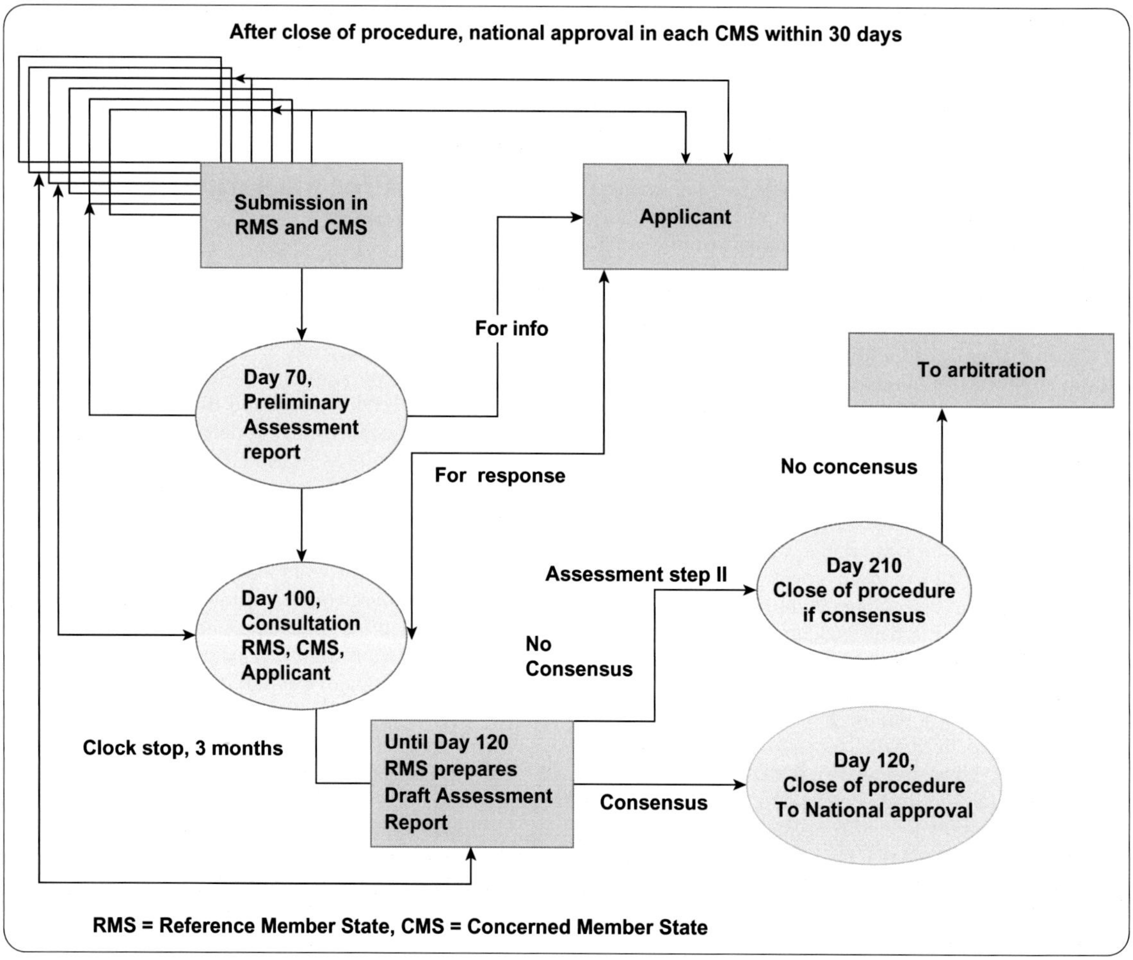

Fig. 20.3 One of the submission processes for marketing approval in EU, the Decentralized Procedure.

case of non-agreement, referral to EMA for arbitration is done as a last resort. But before arbitration is considered, the Coordination Group for Mutual Recognition and Decentralised Procedures (CMDh/CMDv) will try to resolve outstanding issues. This is a group composed of expert members from European regulatory authorities. The worst outcome of an arbitration would be that the marketing authorizations obtained are withdrawn in all EU countries, including the RMS.

- *Decentralized procedure* is similar to the Mutual Recognition Procedure. It is a modernization the aim of which is to share the work among authorities earlier in the process, with the possibility of a decision being reached before 120 days have passed from receipt of a valid submission. It is the procedure of choice for a new chemical entity that for any reason is not submitted to follow the centralized procedure.
- *Centralized procedure* is a 'federal' procedure carried out by the EMA, with scientists selected from CHMP to perform the review, the approval body being the European Commission. This procedure is mandatory for biotechnological products, biosimilars, orphan drugs as well as products intended to treat diabetes, AIDS, cancer, neurodegenerative disorders, autoimmune diseases and viral diseases.
- The centralized procedure starts with the nomination of one CHMP member to act as *rapporteur*, who selects and leads the assessment team. A selected *co-rapporteur* and team make a parallel review. The European Commission approves the application based on a CHMP recommendation, which in turn is based on the assessment reports by the two

rapporteur teams. Products approved in this way can be marketed in all EU countries with the same prescribing information, packs and labels.

CHMP is prepared to give scientific advice to companies in situations where published guidance on the European position is not available, or when the company needs to discuss a possible deviation from guidelines. Such advice, as well as advice from national regulatory authorities, may be very valuable at any stage of the development programme, and may later be incorporated in new guidelines. Providing advice requires considerable effort from CHMP specialists, and fees have to be paid by the pharmaceutical company.

USA

The FDA is more willing than other large authorities to take an active part in planning the drug development process. Some meetings between the FDA and the sponsoring company are more or less compulsory. One such example is the so-called end-of-Phase II meeting. This is in most cases a critically important meeting for the company in which clinical data up until that point is presented to the FDA together with a proposed remaining phase III programme and the company's target label. The purpose is to gain FDA feedback on the appropriateness of the intended NDA package and whether, in particular, the clinical data are likely to enable approval of a desirable product label. It is important that the advice from the FDA is followed. At the same time, these discussions may make it possible in special cases to deviate from guidelines by prior agreement with the FDA. Furthermore, these discussion meetings ensure that the authority is already familiar with the project when the dossier is submitted.

The review time for the FDA has decreased substantially in the last few years (see Chapter 22). Standard reviews should be completed within 10 months, and priority reviews of those products with a strong medical need within 6 months.

The assessment result is usually communicated either as an approval or as a complete response letter. The latter is in essence a request for additional information or data before approval.

Japan

Also in Japan the regulatory authority is today available for consultation, allowing scientific discussion and feedback during the development phase. These meetings tend to follow a similar pattern to those in the USA and EU and have made it much easier to address potential problems well before submission for marketing approval is made.

These changes have meant shorter review times and a more transparent process. The review in Japan is performed by an Evaluation Centre, and the ultimate decision is made by the MHLW based on the Evaluation Centre's report.

It is worth mentioning that health authorities, in particular in the ICH regions, have well-established communications and often assist and consult each other.

The common technical document

Following the good progress made by ICH in creating scientific guidelines applicable in the three large regions, discussions on standardizing document formats began in 1997. The aim was to define a standard format, called the Common Technical Document (CTD), for the application for a new drug product. It was realized from the outset that harmonization of *content* could not be achieved, owing to the fundamental differences in data requirements and work processes between different regulatory authorities. Adopting a common *format* would, nonetheless, be a worthwhile step forward.

The guideline was adopted by the three ICH regions in November 2000 and subsequently implemented, and it has generally been accepted in most other countries. This saves much time and effort in reformatting documents for submission to different regulatory authorities. The structure of the CTD (see website reference 1, p. 301) is summarized in Figure 20.4.

Module 1 (not part of the CTD) contains regional information such as the application form, the suggested prescribing information, the application fee, and also other information that is not considered relevant in all territories, such as environmental assessment (required in the USA and Europe, but not in Japan). Certificates of different regional needs are also to be found in Module 1, as well as patent information not yet requested in the EU.

Module 2 comprises a very brief general introduction, followed by summary information relating to quality, safety (i.e. non-clinical studies) and efficacy (i.e. clinical studies). Quality issues (purity, manufacturing process, stability, etc.) are summarized in a single document of a maximum 40 pages. The non-clinical and clinical summaries each consist of a separate *overview* (maximum 30 pages) and *summaries of individual studies*. The overviews in each area are similar to the previous EU Expert Reports in that they present critical evaluations of the programme performed. Detailed guidelines (see website references 1, 13 and 14), based on existing US, European and Japanese requirements, are available to indicate what tabulated information needs to be included in these summaries, and how the written summaries should be drafted. The non-clinical section has been fairly non-controversial. The guidance is very similar to the previous US summary, with clear instructions on how to sort the studies regarding animals, doses, durations of treatment and routes of administration.

The clinical summary is similar to what was required by the FDA, incorporating many features taken from the

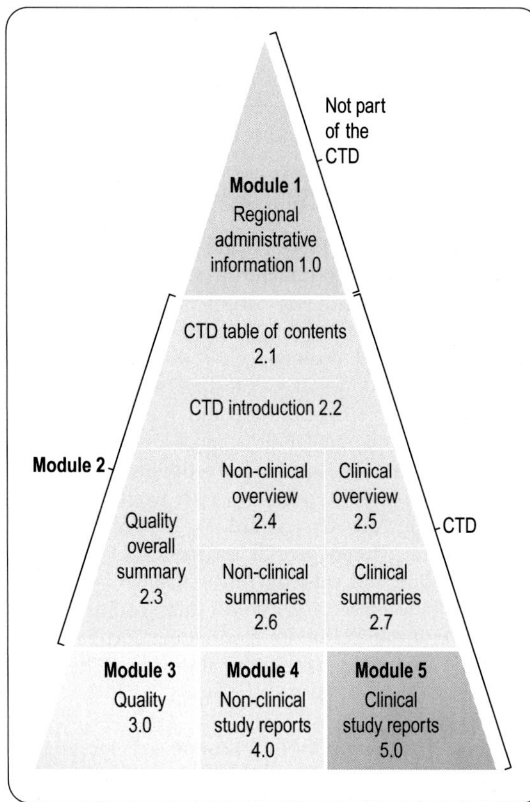

Fig. 20.4 Diagrammatic representation of the organization of the Common Technical Document (CTD).

Integrated Summaries of Efficacy (ISE) and Safety (ISS). ISE will generally fit in the clinical summary document. The ISS document has proved very useful in drawing conclusions from the clinical studies by sensible pooling and integration, but is too large (often more than 400 pages in itself) to be accepted in the EU and Japan. This problem may be resolved by including the ISS as a separate report in Module 5.

Modules 3–5 comprise the individual study reports. Most reports are eligible for use in all three regions, possibly with the exception at present of Module 3, Quality, which may need regional content.

There is a gradual shift to fully electronic submissions – known as e-CTD – in place of the large quantities of paper which have comprised an application for marketing approval. As this gets fully implemented experimental data will be lodged mainly in databases, allowing the information to be exchanged between pharmaceutical companies and regulatory authorities much more easily. Guidelines on the structure and interface between databases in the industry setting and those at the authorities are available.

ADMINISTRATIVE RULES

Patent protection and data exclusivity

Supplementary protection certificate

During the 1980s, the time taken to develop and obtain marketing approval for a new drug increased so much that the period of market exclusivity established by the original patent could be too short to allow the company to recoup its R&D costs. To overcome this problem (see Chapter 19), the EU Council in 1992 introduced rules allowing companies to apply for a Supplementary Protection Certificate (SPC), matching similar legislation in the USA and Japan. This can prolong market protection by a maximum of 5 years to give an overall period of exclusivity of up to 15 years.

The application for an SPC has to be submitted within 6 months of first approval anywhere in Europe, within or outside the EU, and from then on the clock starts. It is thus strategically important to obtain first approval in a financially important market for best revenue.

Data exclusivity

Data exclusivity should not be confused with patent protection. It is a means to protect the originators data, meaning that generic products cannot be approved by referring to the original product documentation until the exclusivity period has ended. For a new chemical entity the protection may be up to 10 years, depending on region. The generation of paediatric data may extend it even further, between 6 and 12 months.

Pricing of pharmaceutical products – 'the fourth hurdle'

The 'fourth hurdle' or 'market access' are expressions for the ever growing demand for cost-effectiveness in pharmaceutical prescribing. Payers, whether health insurance companies or publicly funded institutions, now require more stringent justification for the normally high price of a new pharmaceutical product. This means that, if not in the original application, studies have to demonstrate that the clinical benefit of a new compound is commensurate with the suggested price, compared to the previous therapy of choice in the country of application.

To address this concern, studies in a clinical trials programme from Phase II onwards now normally include health economic measures (see Chapter 18). In the USA, certainly, it is advantageous to have a statement of health economic benefit approved in the package insert, to justify reimbursement. Reference pricing systems are also being implemented in Europe. A favourable benefit–risk evaluation is no longer sufficient: value for money must also be demonstrated in order to have a commercially successful product (see also Chapter 21).

LIST OF ABBREVIATIONS

CHMP	Committee for Medicinal Products for Human Use, the new name to replace CPMP early 2004
CTD	Common Technical Document
CMDh/ CMDv	Coordination Group for Human/Veterinary Medicinal Products for Mutual Recognition and Decentralised Procedure (EU)
EC	Ethics Committee (EU), known as Institutional Review Board (IRB) in USA
eCTD	Electronic Common Technical Document
EMA	European Medicines Agency
ERA	Environmental Risk Assessment (EU)
EU	European Union
FDA	Food and Drug Administration; the US Regulatory Authority
GCP	Good clinical practice
GLP	Good laboratory practice
GMP	Good manufacturing practice
ICH	International Conference on Harmonization
IND	Investigational New Drug application (US)
IRB	Institutional Review Board (US), equivalent to Ethics Committee in Europe
ISS	Integrated Summary of Safety (US)
JNDA	Japanese New Drug Application
MAA	Marketing Authorization Application (EU), equivalent to NDA in USA
MHLW	Ministry of Health, Labor and Welfare (Jpn)
MTD	Maximum tolerated dose
NDA	New Drug Application (USA)
NTA	Notice to Applicants; EU set of pharmaceutical regulations, directives and guidelines
SPC	Supplementary Protection Certificate
WHO	World Health Organization

REFERENCES

Cartwright AC, Matthews BR. Pharmaceutical product licensing requirements for Europe. London: Ellis Horwood; 1991.

Cartwright AC, Matthews BR, editors. International pharmaceutical product registration. London: Taylor and Francis; 1994.

Drews J. In quest of tomorrow's medicines. New York: Springer-Verlag; 1999.

Meade TW. Subacute myelo-optic neuropathy and clioquinol. An epidemiological case-history for diagnosis. British Journal of Preventive and Social Medicine 1975;29:157–69.

WEBSITE REFERENCES

1. http://www.ich.org/
2. http://www.fda.gov/Drugs/DevelopmentApprovalProcess/DevelopmentResources/ucm049867.htm
3. http://ec.europa.eu/health/files/eudralex/vol-1/reg_2006_1902/reg_2006_1902_en.pdf
4. http://www.fda.gov/downloads/Drugs/GuidanceCompliance RegulatoryInformation/Guidances/UCM184128.pdf
5. http://www.ema.europa.eu/docs/en_GB/document_library/Regulatory_and_procedural_guideline/2009/10/WC500004888.pdf
6. http://www.ema.europa.eu/docs/en_GB/document_library/Regulatory_and_procedural_guideline/2009/10/WC500006326.pdf
7. http://www.fda.gov/Drugs/GuidanceComplianceRegulatory Information/ucm215031.htm
8. http://www.ema.europa.eu/ema/index.jsp?curl=pages/special_topics/general/general_content_000034.jsp&murl=menus/special_topics/special_topics.jsp&mid=WC0b01ac058002d4eb
9. http://www.fda.gov/ForIndustry/DevelopingProductsforRare DiseasesConditions/default.htm
10. http://www.fda.gov/downloads/Drugs/GuidanceCompliance RegulatoryInformation/Guidances/ucm070561
11. http://www.ema.europa.eu/docs/en_GB/document_library/Scientific_guideline/2009/10/WC500003978.pdf
12. http://www.wma.net/en/30publications/10policies/b3/index.html
13. http://ec.europa.eu/health/documents//eudralex/index_en.htm
14. http:/www.fda.gov

Chapter **21**

The role of pharmaceutical marketing

V M Lawton

INTRODUCTION

This chapter puts pharmaceutical marketing into the context of the complete life-cycle of a medicine. It describes the old role of marketing and contrasts that with its continually evolving function in a rapidly changing environment and its involvement in the drug development process. It examines the move from the product-centric focus of the 20th century to the customer-centric focus of the 21st century.

Pharmaceutical marketing increased strongly in the 10–15 years following the Second World War, during which time thousands of new molecules entered the market 'overwhelming' physicians with new scientific facts to learn in order to safely and appropriately prescribe these breakthroughs to their patients. There was a great dependence on the pharmaceutical companies' marketing departments and their professional sales representatives to give the full information necessary to support the prescribing decision.

Evidence-based marketing is based on data and research, with rigorous examination of all plans and follow-up to verify the success of programmes. Marketing is a general term used to describe all the various activities involved in transferring goods and services from producers to consumers. In addition to the functions commonly associated with it, such as advertising and sales promotion, marketing also encompasses product development, packaging, distribution channels, pricing and many other functions. It is intended to focus all of a company's activities upon discovering and satisfying customer needs.

Management guru Peter F. Drucker claimed that marketing 'is so basic it cannot be considered a separate function. … It is the whole business seen from the point of view of its final result, that is, from the customer's point of view.' Marketing is the source of many important new ideas in management thought and practice – such as flexible manufacturing systems, flat organizational structures and an increased emphasis on service – all of which are designed to make businesses more responsive to customer needs and preferences.

A modern definition of marketing could be:

> *'A flexible customer focused business planning function, including a wide variety of activities, aimed at achieving profitable sales'.*

HISTORY OF PHARMACEUTICAL MARKETING

There are not many accessible records of the types of marketing practised in the first known drugstore, which was opened by Arab pharmacists in Baghdad in 754, (http://en.wikipedia.org/wiki/Pharmaceutical_industry-cite_note-1) and the many more that were operating throughout the medieval Islamic world and eventually in medieval Europe. By the 19th century, many of the drug stores in Europe and North America had developed into larger pharmaceutical companies with large commercial functions. These companies produced a wide range of medicines and marketed them to doctors and pharmacists for use with their patients.

In the background, during the 19th century in the USA, there were the purveyors of tonics, salves and cure-alls, the travelling medicine shows. These salesmen specialized in selling sugared water or potions such as *Hostetter's Celebrated Stomach Bitters* (with an alcoholic content of 44%, which undoubtedly contributed to its popularity). In the late 1800s, Joseph Myers, the first '*snake oil*' marketer, from Pugnacity, Nebraska, visited some Indians harvesting their

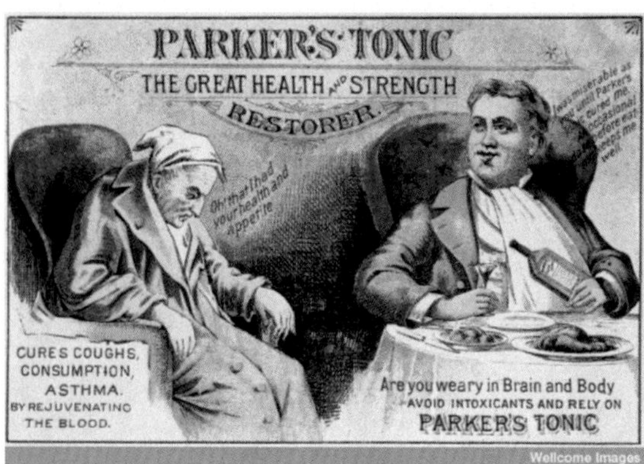

Fig. 21.1 Picture of old style advertising.
Reproduced with kind permission of the Wellcome Trust.

'medicine plant', used as a tonic against venomous stings and bites. He took the plant, *Echinacea purpurea*, around the country and it turned out to be a powerful antidote to rattlesnake bites. However, most of this unregulated marketing was for ineffective and often dangerous 'medicines' (Figure 21.1).

Medical innovation accelerated in the 1950s and early 1960s with more than 4500 new medicines arriving on the market during the decade beginning in 1951. By 1961 around 70% of expenditure on drugs in the USA was on these newly arrived compounds. Pharmaceutical companies marketed the products vigorously and competitively. The tools of marketing used included advertising, mailings and visits to physicians by increasing numbers of professional sales representatives.

Back in 1954, Bill Frohlich, an advertising executive, and David Dubow, a visionary, set out to create a new kind of information company that could enable organizations to make informed, strategic decisions about the marketplace. They called their venture Intercontinental Marketing Services (IMS), and they introduced it at an opportune time, when pharmaceutical executives had few data to consult when in the throes of strategic or tactical planning. By 1957, IMS had published its first European syndicated research study, an audit of pharmaceutical sales within the West German market. Its utility and popularity prompted IMS to expand into new geographies – Great Britain, France, Italy, Spain and Japan among them. Subsequent acquisitions in South Africa, Australia and New Zealand strengthened the IMS position, and by 1969 IMS, with an annual revenue of $5 million, had established the gold standard in pharmaceutical market research in Europe and Asia. IMS remains the largest supplier of data on drug use to the pharmaceutical industry, providers, such as HMOs and health authorities, and payers, such as governments.

The medical associations were unable to keep the doctors adequately informed about the vast array of new drugs. It fell, by default, upon the pharmaceutical industry to fill the knowledge gap. This rush of innovative medicines and promotion activity was named the 'therapeutic jungle' by Goodman and Gilman in their famous textbook (Goodman and Gilman, 1960). Studies in the 1950s revealed that physicians consistently rated pharmaceutical sales representatives as the most important source in learning about new drugs. The much valued 'detail men' enjoyed lengthy, in-depth discussions with physicians. They were seen as a valuable resource to the prescriber. This continued throughout the following decades.

A large increase in the number of drugs available necessitated appropriate education of physicians. Again, the industry gladly assumed this responsibility. In the USA, objections about the nature and quality of medical information that was being communicated using marketing tools (Podolsky and Greene, 2008) caused controversy in medical journals and Congress. The Kefauver–Harris Drug Control Act of 1962 imposed controls on the pharmaceutical industry that required that drug companies disclose to doctors the side effects of their products, allowed their products to be sold as generic drugs after having held the patent on them for a certain period of time, and obliged them to prove on demand that their products were, in fact, effective and safe. Senator Kefauver also focused attention on the form and content of general pharmaceutical marketing and the postgraduate pharmaceutical education of the nation's physicians. A call from the American Medical Association (AMA) and the likes of Kefauver led to the establishment of formal Continued Medical Education (CME) programmes, to ensure physicians were kept objectively apprised of new development in medicines. Although the thrust of the change was to provide medical education to physicians from the medical community, the newly respectable CME process also attracted the interest and funding of the pharmaceutical industry. Over time the majority of CME around the world has been provided by the industry (Ferrer, 1975).

The marketing of medicines continued to grow strongly throughout the 1970s and 1980s. Marketing techniques, perceived as 'excessive' and 'extravagant', came to the attention of the committee chaired by Senator Edward Kennedy in the early 1990s. This resulted in increased regulation of industry's marketing practices, much of it self-regulation (see Todd and Johnson, 1992); *http://www.efpia.org/Content/Default.asp?PageID=296flags*).

The size of pharmaceutical sales forces increased dramatically during the 1990s, as major pharmaceutical companies, following the dictum that 'more is better', bombarded doctors' surgeries with its representatives. Seen as a competitive necessity, sales forces were increased to match or top the therapeutic competitor, increasing frequency of visits to physicians and widening coverage to all potential customers. This was also a period of great success in the discovery of many new 'blockbuster' products that addressed many unmet clinical needs. In many countries representatives were given targets to call on eight to 10 doctors per day, detailing three to four products in the same visit. In an average call on the doctor of less than 10 minutes, much of the information was delivered by rote with little time for interaction and assessment of the point of view of the customer. By the 2000s there was one representative for every six doctors. The time available for representatives to see an individual doctor plummeted and many practices refused to see representatives at all. With shorter time to spend with doctors, the calls were seen as less valuable to the physician. Information gathered in a 2004 survey by Harris Interactive and IMS Health (Nickum and Kelly, 2005) indicated that fewer than 40% of responding physicians felt the pharmaceutical industry was trustworthy. Often, they were inclined to mistrust promotion in general. They granted reps less time and many closed their doors completely, turning to alternative forms of promotion, such as e-detailing, peer-to-peer interaction, and the Internet.

Something had to give. Fewer 'blockbusters' were hitting the market, regulation was tightening its grip and the downturn in the global economy was putting pressure on public expenditure to cut costs. The size of the drug industry's US sales force had declined by 10% to about 92 000 in 2009, from a peak of 102 000 in 2005 (Fierce Pharma, 2009). This picture was mirrored around the world's pharmaceutical markets. ZS Associates, a sales strategy consulting firm, predicted another drop in the USA – this time of 20% – to as low as 70 000 by 2015. It is of interest, therefore, that the USA pharmaceutical giant Merck ran a pilot programme in 2008 under which regions cut sales staff by up to one-quarter and continued to deliver results similar to those in other, uncut regions. A critical cornerstone of the marketing of pharmaceuticals, the professional representative, is now under threat, at least in its former guise.

PRODUCT LIFE CYCLE

It is important to see the marketing process in the context of the complete product life cycle, from basic research to genericization at the end of the product patent. A typical product life cycle can be illustrated from discovery to decline as follows (William and McCarthy, 1997) (Figure 21.2).

The product's life cycle period usually consists of five major steps or phases:

- Product development
- Introduction
- Growth
- Maturity
- Decline.

Product development phase

The product development phase begins when a company finds and develops a new product idea. This involves translating various pieces of information and incorporating them into a new product. A product undergoes several changes and developments during this stage. With pharmaceutical products, this depends on efficacy and safety. Pricing strategy must be developed at this stage in time for launch. In a number of markets for pharmaceuticals, price approval must be achieved from payers (usually government agencies). **Marketing plans**, based on market research and product strengths, for the launch and development of the product, are established and approved within the organization. Research on expectations of customers from new products should form a significant part of the marketing strategy. Knowledge, gained through market research, will also help to segment customers according to their potential for early adoption of a product. Production capacity is geared up to meet anticipated market demands.

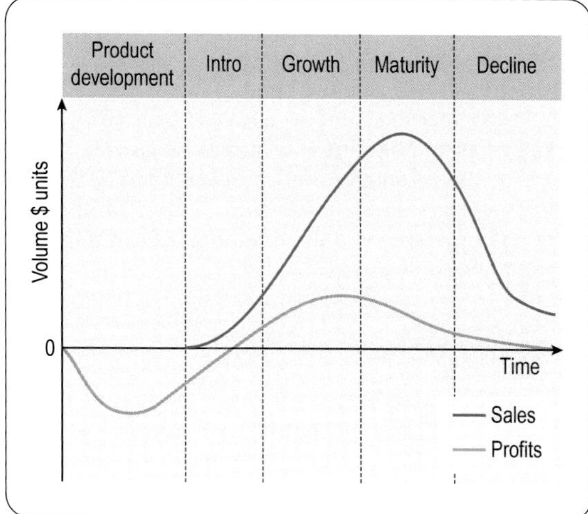

Fig. 21.2 General product life cycle graph.

Introduction phase

The introduction phase of a product includes the product launch phase, where the goal is to achieve maximum impact in the shortest possible time, to establish the product in the market. Marketing promotional spend is highest at this phase of the life cycle. Manufacturing and supply chains (distribution) must be firmly established during this phase. It is vital that the new product is available in all outlets (e.g. pharmacies) to meet the early demand.

Growth phase

The growth phase is the time the when the market accepts the new entry and when its market share grows. The maturity of the market determines the speed and potential for a new entry. A well-established market hosts competitors who will seek to undermine the new product and protect its own market share. If the new product is highly innovative relative to the market, or the market itself is relatively new, its growth will be more rapid.

Marketing becomes more targeted and reduces in volume when the product is well into its growth. Other aspects of the promotion and product offering will be released in stages during this period. A focus on the efficiency and profitability of the product comes in the latter stage of the growth period.

Maturity phase

The maturity phase comes when the market no longer grows, as the customers are satisfied with the choices available to them. At this point the market will stabilize, with little or no expansion. New product entries or product developments can result in displacement of market share towards the newcomer, at the expense of an incumbent product. This corresponds to the most profitable stage for a product if, with little more than maintenance marketing, it can achieve a profitable return. A product's branding and positioning synonymous with the quality and reliability demanded by the customer will enable it to enjoy a longer maturity phase. The achievement of the image of 'gold standard' for a product is the goal. In pharmaceutical markets around the world, the length of the maturity phase is longer in some than in others, depending on the propensity of physicians to switch to new medicines. For example, French doctors are generally early adopters of new medicines, where British doctors are slow.

Decline phase

The decline phase usually comes with increased competition, reduced market share and loss of sales and profitability. Companies, realizing the cost involved in defending against a new product entry, will tend to reduce marketing to occasional reminders, rather than the full-out promotion required to match the challenge. With pharmaceutical products, this stage is generally realized at the end of the patent life of a medicine. Those companies with a strong R&D function will focus resources on the discovery and development of new products.

PHARMACEUTICAL PRODUCT LIFE CYCLE (Figure 21.3)

As soon as a promising molecule is found, the company applies for patents (see Chapter 19). A patent gives the company intellectual property rights over the invention for

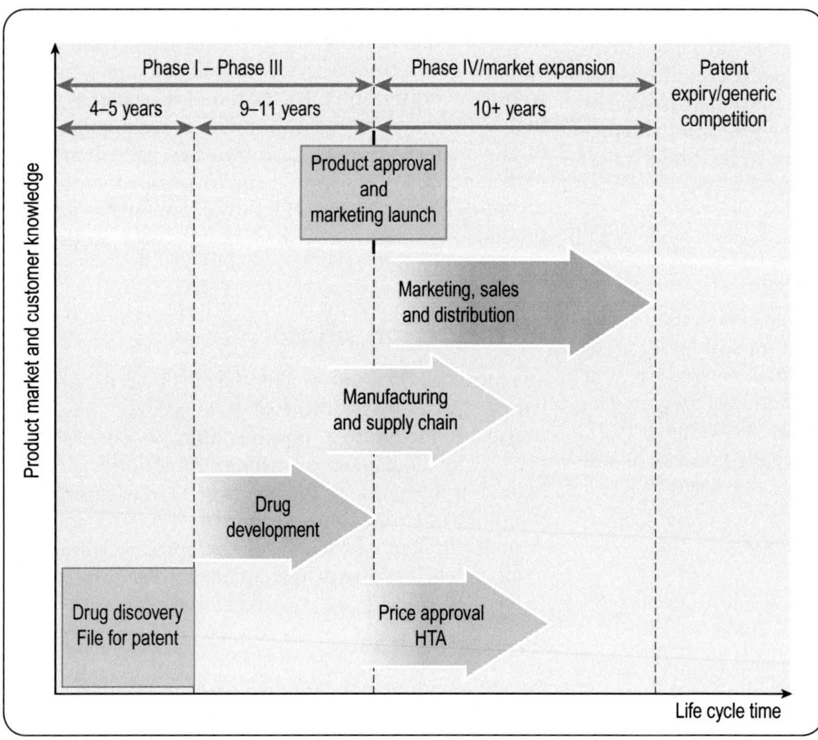

Fig. 21.3 Pharmaceutical life cycle graph.

around 20 years. This means that the company owns the idea and can legally stop other companies from profiting by copying it. Sales and profits will enable the manufacturer to reinvest in R&D:

- For a pharmaceutical product the majority of patent time could be over before the medicine even hits the market
- Once it is produced it takes some time for the medicine to build up sales and so achieve market share; in its early years the company needs to persuade doctors to prescribe and use the medicine
- Once the medicine has become established then it enters a period of maturity; this is the period when most profits are made
- Finally as the medicine loses patent protection, copies (generic products) enter the market at a lower cost; therefore, sales of the original medicine decline rapidly.

The duration and trend of product life cycles vary among different products and therapeutic classes. In an area of unmet clinical need, the entry of a new efficacious product can result in rapid uptake. Others, entering into a relatively mature market, will experience a slower uptake and more gradual growth later in the life cycle, especially if experience and further research results in newer indications for use (Grabowski et al., 2002).

TRADITIONAL PHARMACEUTICAL MARKETING

Clinical studies

Pharmaceutical marketing depends on the results from clinical studies. These pre-marketing clinical trials are conducted in three phases before the product can be submitted to the medicines regulator for approval of its licence to be used to treat appropriate patients. The marketing planner or product manager will follow the development and results from these studies, interact with the R&D function and will develop plans accordingly. The three phases (described in detail in Chapter 17) are as follows.

Phase I trials are the first stage of testing in human subjects.

Phase II trials are performed on larger groups (20–300) and are designed to assess how well the drug works, as well as to continue Phase I safety assessments in a larger group of volunteers and patients.

Phase III studies are randomized controlled multicentre trials on large patient groups (300–3000 or more depending upon the disease/medical condition studied) and are aimed at being the definitive assessment of how effective the drug is, in comparison with current 'gold standard' treatment.

Marketing will be closely involved in the identification of the gold standard, through its own research. It is common practice that certain Phase III trials will continue while the regulatory submission is pending at the appropriate regulatory agency. This allows patients to continue to receive possibly life-saving drugs until the drug can be obtained by purchase. Other reasons for performing trials at this stage include attempts by the sponsor at 'label expansion' (to show the drug works for additional types of patients/diseases beyond the original use for which the drug would have been approved for marketing), to obtain additional safety data, or to support marketing claims for the drug.

Phase IV studies are done in a wider population after launch, to determine if a drug or treatment is safe over time, or to see if a treatment or medication can be used in other circumstances. Phase IV clinical trials are done after a drug has gone through Phases I, II and III, has been approved by the Regulator and is on the market.

Phase IV is one of the fastest-growing area of clinical research today, at an annual growth rate of 23%. A changing regulatory environment, growing concerns about the safety of new medicines, and various uses for large-scale, real-world data on marketed drugs' safety and efficacy are primary drivers of the growth seen in the Phase IV research environment. Post-marketing research is an important element of commercialization that enables companies to expand existing markets, enter new markets, develop and deliver messaging that directly compares their products with the competition. Additionally, payer groups and regulators are both demanding more post-marketing data from drug companies.

Advantages of Phase IV research include the development of data in particular patient populations, enhanced relationship with customers and development of advocacy among healthcare providers and patients. These studies help to open new communication channels with healthcare providers and to create awareness among patients. Phase IV data can also be valuable in the preparation of a health economics and HTA file, to demonstrate cost effectiveness.

Identifying the market

At the stage when it appears that the drug is likely to be approved for marketing, the product manager performs market research to identify the characteristics of the market. The therapeutic areas into which the new product will enter are fully assessed, using data from standard sources to which the company subscribes, often IMS (Intercontinental Marketing Services). These data are generally historic and do not indicate what could happen nor do they contain much interpretation. The product manager must begin to construct a story to describe the market, its dynamics, key elements and potential. This is the time to generate extensive hypotheses regarding the market and its potential. Although these hypotheses can be tested, they are not extensively validated. Therefore the level of confidence in the data generated at this stage would not normally enable the marketer to generate a reliable plan for entry to the market, but will start to indicate what needs to be done to generate more qualitative and quantitative data.

When the product label is further developed and tested, further **market research**, using **focus groups** (*a form of qualitative research in which a group of people are asked about their perceptions, opinions, beliefs and attitudes towards a new concept and the reasons for current behaviour*) of physicians to examine their current prescribing practice and rationale for this behaviour. These data are extensively validated with more qualitative research. The identification of the target audiences for the new medicines is critical by this stage.

Traditionally, for the most part, the pharmaceutical industry has viewed each physician customer in terms of his/her current performance (market share for a given product) and potential market value. Each company uses basically the same data inputs and metrics, so tactical implementation across the industry is similar from company to company.

The product

Features, attributes, benefits, limitations (FABL)

A product manager is assigned a product before its launch and is expected to develop a marketing plan for the product that will include the development of information about the existing market and a full understanding of the product's characteristics. This begins with **Features**, such as the specific mechanism of action, the molecular form, the tablet shape or colour. Closely aligned to this are the product **Attributes**, usually concrete things that reside in the product including how it functions. These are characteristics by which a product can be identified and differentiated. For example, these can include the speed of onset of action, absence of common side effects, such as drowsiness, or a once per day therapy rather than multiple doses. Then come the **Benefits** of the new product. Benefits are intrinsic to the customer and are usually abstract. A product attribute expressed in terms of what the doctor or patient gets from the product rather than its physical characteristics or features. A once per day therapy can lessen the intrusion of medicine taking on patient's lives. Lack of drowsiness means the patient complies with the need to take the medicine for the duration of the illness and is able to function effectively during their working day. The benefits may also accrue to the physician as patient compliance indicates that the patient is feeling well, thanks to the actions of the doctor. It is critically important for the pharmaceutical marketer to maintain balance in promotional material. The **Limitations** of the product, where they could lead to the medicine being given to a patient for whose condition the medicine is not specifically indicated, must be clearly indicated in all materials and discussions with the doctor. The potential risk of adverse reactions of a medicine must also be clearly addressed in marketing interactions with medical professionals.

The analysis of the product in this way enables the marketer to produce a benefit ladder, beginning with the product features and attributes and moving to the various benefits from the point of view of the customer. Emotional benefits for the customer in terms of how they will feel by introducing the right patient to the right treatment are at the top of the ladder. It is also important for the product manager to construct a benefit ladder for competitive products in order to differentiate.

Armed with these data and the limited quantitative data, the product manager defines the market, identifies the target audience and their behaviour patterns in prescribing and assesses what must be done to effect a change of behaviour and the prescription of the new medicine once launched. A key classification of a target physician is his or her position in the **Adoption Pattern** of innovative new products. There are three broad classifications generally used:

- Early adopters/innovators: those who normally are quick to use a new product when it is available
- Majority: most fall into this category. There are the **early majority** and the **late majority**, defined by their relative speed of adoption. Some are already satisfied and have no need for a new product. Some wait for others to try first, preferring to wait until unforeseen problems arise and are resolved. Improved products (innovative therapies) may move this group to prescribe earlier
- Laggards/conservatives: this group is the slowest adopter, invariably waiting for others to gain the early experience. They wait for something compelling to occur, such as additional evidence to support the new product, or a new indication for which they do not currently have a suitable treatment.

Assessing the competition

It is critical for a product marketer to understand the competition and learn how to out-manoeuvre them. Market research is the starting point. A complete analysis of the competitive market through product sales, investment levels and resource allocation helps the marketer to develop the marketing plan for his own product. But it is important to understand the reason for these behaviours and critically evaluate their importance and success.

A comprehensive review of competitor's activities and rationale for them is also necessary. Tools are available to facilitate this in the U.S., for example, PhRMA (the industry association), publish a New Medicines Database that tracks potential new medicines in various stages of development. The database includes medicines currently in clinical trials or at the FDA for evaluation (http://www.phrma.org/newmeds/). However, it is not just a desk bound exercise for a group of bright young marketers. Hypotheses, thus formed, must be tested against the customer perception of them.

The appearance of promotional aids, such as 'detail aids', printed glossies containing key messages, desktop branded reminder items (e.g. calendars), or 'door openers' (pens, stick-it pads, etc.) to get past the 'dragon on the door' (receptionist), are common, but do they work? In the pharmaceutical industry, for many years, marketing has been a little like the arms war. Rep numbers are doubled or tripled because that's what the competition is doing. Identical looking detail pieces, clinical study papers wrapped in a shiny folder with the key promotional messages and product label printed on it, appear from all competitors. Regulations known as 'medical-legal control' are in place, internally and at a national level, to ensure that promotional messages are accurately stated, balanced and backed by well referenced evidence, such as clinical trial data and the approved product label.

Are promotional activities being focused on key leverage points and appropriate behavioural objectives? Before embracing what seems to be a good idea from the competition, the marketer needs to understand how this is perceived by the customer. New qualitative research needs to be conducted to gain this insight. One of the principal aims of successful marketing is to differentiate one product from another. It would, therefore, seem to be counter-intuitive for an assessment of competitor behaviour to conclude that copying the idea of a competitor is somehow going to automatically enable you to out-compete them. Much of traditional pharmaceutical marketing implementation has been outsourced to agencies. These organizations are briefed about the product, the market into which it will enter and the key therapeutic messages the company wishes to convey. The companies retain the preparation and maintenance of the marketing plan and, in general, leave the creative, behavioural side of the preparation to the agency. It is not, therefore, surprising that a formulaic approach to marketing delivery is the norm.

A classic example of this effect came in the 1990s with Direct to Consumer advertising (DTC). This form of direct marketing, in the printed media, television and radio, is legally permitted in only a few countries, such as the USA and New Zealand. Its original conception, for the first time, was to talk directly to patients about the sorts of medication that they should request from their physician. Anyone glued to breakfast television in the USA will be bombarded with attractive messages about what you could feel like if you took a particular medicine. These messages always contain a balance about contraindications and possible adverse reactions. Patients are encouraged to consult their physician. This concept was original and seems to have been effective in a number of cases (Kaiser Family Foundation, 2001) with increased sales volumes. Then practically every major company jumped on the bandwagon and competed for prime-time slots and the most attractive actors to play the role of patient. The appearance of these messages is practically identical and one washes over another. Probably the only people to pay them much attention, because of the volume and sameness, are the pharmaceutical marketers and the advertising agencies that are competing for the business. As for the physicians, little attention was paid to their reaction to this visual-media-informed patient.

In assessing how successful DTC has been, early data from the USA (Kaiser Family Foundation, 2001) observed, on average, a 10% increase in DTC advertising of drugs within a therapeutic drug class resulted in a 1% increase in sales of the drugs in that class. Applying this result to the 25 largest drug classes in 2000, the study found that every $1 the pharmaceutical industry spent on DTC advertising in that year yielded an additional $4.20 in drug sales. DTC advertising was responsible for 12% of the increase in prescription drugs sales, or an additional $2.6 billion, in 2000. DTC advertising did not appear to affect the relative market share of individual drugs within their drug class. In the decade to 2005 in the USA, spend on DTC practically tripled to around $4.2 billion (Donohue et al., 2007). This level of expenditure and impact on prescriptions has caused a great deal of controversy driven by traditional industry critics. However, some benefits have accrued, including the increased interaction between physicians and patients. In surveys, more than half of physicians agree that DTC educates patients about diseases and treatments. Many physicians, however, believe that DTC encourages patients to make unwarranted requests for medication.

From a marketing point of view, new concepts like DTC can prove helpful. Sales increase and patients become a new and legitimate customer. The cost of entry, particularly in financially difficult times can be prohibitive for all but a few key players. For those who are in this group, it becomes imperative that they stay there, as it is still a viable if costly segment. The naysayers are successfully containing DTC to the USA and New Zealand. The clarion calls for a moratorium and greater FDA regulation have still been avoided by those who market in this way. Will the investment in this type of marketing continue to pass the test of cost effectiveness and revenue opportunity? Competitive marketing demands a continuous critical assessment of all expenditure according to rigorous ROI (return on investment) criteria.

DTC advertising expenditure decreased by more than 20% from 2007 to 2009. Economic pressures and the global financial meltdown have resulted in a tighter budgetary situation for the pharmaceutical industry. These pressures have been strongly affected by rapidly disappearing blockbuster drugs and decreasing R&D productivity.

e-Marketing

e-Marketing is a process, using the internet and other electronic media, of marketing a brand or concept by directly connecting to the businesses of customers.

In pharmaceuticals, electronic marketing has been experimented with since the late 1990s. As a branch of DTC, it has been limited to only a couple of markets, the USA and New Zealand, because local laws elsewhere do not permit DTC communication about medicines. Some companies have created websites for physician-only access with some success, in terms of usage, but difficult to assess in terms of product uptake. Electronic detailing of physicians, that is use of digital technology: the Internet and video conferencing, has been used in some markets for a number of years. There are two types of e-detailing: interactive (virtual) and video. Some physicians find this type of interaction convenient, but the uptake has not been rapid or widespread, nor has its impact been accurately measured in terms of utility.

While e-Marketing has promise and theoretically great reach, the pharmaceutical industry in general has done little more than dabble in it. It is estimated to occupy around 1–3% of DTC budgets. Anecdotally staff recruited for their e-Marketing expertise have not integrated well into the highly regulated media market of the pharmaceutical industry.

CME

Continuing Medical Education is a long established means for medical professionals to maintain and update competence and learn about new and developing areas of their field, such as therapeutic advances. These activities may take place as live events, written publications, online programmes, audio, video, or other electronic media (see http://www.accme.org/dir_docs/doc_upload/9c795f02-c470-4ba3-a491-d288be965eff_uploaddocument.pdf). Content for these programmes is developed, reviewed, and delivered by a faculty who are experts in their individual clinical areas.

Funding of these programmes has been largely provided by the pharmaceutical industry, often through Medical Education and Communications Companies or MECCs. A number of large pharmaceutical companies have withdrawn from using these sorts of third-party agencies in the USA, due to the controversy concerning their objectivity. The Swedish health system puts a cap of 50% on the level of contribution to costs of the pharmaceutical industry.

This type of activity is beneficial to the medical community and provides, if only through networking, an opportunity to interact with the physicians. The regulation of content of these programmes is tight and generally well controlled, but a strong voice of discontent about the involvement of the industry continues to be sounded. The fact is that a key stakeholder in the medical decision-making process wants and benefits from these programmes, as long as they are balanced, approved and helpful. If the pharmaceutical industry wants to continue with the funding and involvement, then it should be seen as a legitimate part of the marketing template.

Key opinion leaders

Key opinion leaders (KOL), or 'thought leaders', are respected individuals in a particular therapeutic area, such as prominent medical school faculty, who influence physicians through their professional status. Pharmaceutical companies generally engage key opinion leaders early in the drug development process to provide advocacy and key marketing feedback. These individuals are identified by a number of means, reputation, citations, peer review and even social network analysis.

Pharmaceutical companies will work with KOLs from the early stage of drug development. The goal is to gain early input from these experts into the likely success and acceptability of these new compounds in the future market. Marketing personnel and the company's medical function work closely on identifying the best KOLs for each stage of drug development. The KOL has a network which, it is hoped, will also get to know about a new product and its advantages early in the launch phase. The KOL can perform a number of roles, in scientific development, as a member of the product advisory board and an advisor on specific aspects of the product positioning.

The marketing manager is charged with maintaining and coordinating the company's relationship with the KOL. Special care is taken by the company of the level of payment given to a KOL and all payments have to be declared to the medical association which regulates the individual, whatever the country of origin. KOLs can be divided into different categories. *Global, national* and *local* categorizations are applied, depending on their level of influence. Relationships between the company and a particular opinion leader can continue throughout the life cycle of a medicine, or product franchise, for example rheumatology, cardiovascular disease.

PRICING

Pharmaceutical pricing is one of the most complex elements of marketing strategy. There is no one answer as to how members of the industry determine their pricing strategy. Elements to consider are whether there is ***freedom of pricing at launch,*** such as in the USA, the UK and Germany, or ***regulated price setting*** as in France, Italy and Spain.

Freedom of pricing

The criteria for price setting are many and varied, including consideration of the market dynamics. Pricing of established therapies, the ability, or otherwise to change prices at a later stage than the product launch, the value added by the new product to the market and the perception of its affordability, are just some of the considerations. A vital concern of the company is the recovery of the costs of bringing the product to the market, estimated at an average of $1.3 billion for primary care medicines.

The marketing team, health economic analysts, financial function and global considerations are all part of the pricing plan. Cost-effectiveness analyses and calculations of benefit to the market are all factored into the equation. When a global strategy is proposed, market research is conducted along with pricing sensitivity analyses.

Regulated pricing

In the majority of markets where the government are also the payers, there is a formal process after the medical approval of a drug for negotiating a reimbursement price with the industry. The prices for multinational companies are set globally and the goal is to achieve the same or closely similar prices in all markets.

However, in matters of health and its perceived *affordability* each nation retains its sovereignty. Bodies such as the OECD gather and compare data from each of its 33 member states. The reports it issues highlight trends in pharmaceutical pricing and give each country easy access to the different approaches each regulator uses.

Different approaches abound throughout the regulated markets and include:

- **Therapeutic reference pricing,** where medicines to treat the same medical condition are placed in groups or 'clusters' with a single common reimbursed price. Underpinning this economic measure is an implicit assumption that the products included in the cluster have an equivalent effect on a typical patient with this disease
- **Price-volume** agreements, where discounts could be negotiated on volume commitments
- **Pay for performance** models, where rebates could be achieved if the efficacy is not as expected
- **Capitation** models where the expenditure is capped at a certain level.

There are a myriad of different approaches across the nations. The goal of these systems is generally cost containment at the government level. From a marketing point of view, the Global Brand Manager must be familiar with and sensitive to the variety of pricing variables. At the local level, a product manager needs to be aware of the concerns of the payer and plan discussions with key stakeholders in advance of product launch. Increasingly, the onus will be on the marketer to prove the value of the medicine to the market.

Prices with which a product goes to market rarely grow during the product life cycle in all but a few markets. However, there are frequent interventions to enforce price reductions, usually affecting the whole industry, in regulated markets over the marketed life of a medicine.

HEALTH TECHNOLOGY ASSESSMENT (HTA)

Health technology assessment (HTA) is a multidisciplinary activity that systematically examines the safety, clinical efficacy and effectiveness, cost, cost-effectiveness, organizational implications, social consequences and legal and ethical considerations of the application of a health technology – usually a drug, medical device or clinical/surgical procedure (see http://www.medicine.ox.ac.uk/bandolier/painres/download/whatis/What_is_health_tech.pdf).

The development of HTAs over the 20 years prior to 2010 has been relatively strong. Before that, in the '70s *outcomes research* assessed the effectiveness of various interventions. The Cochrane Collaboration is an international organization of 100 000 volunteers that aims to help people make well-informed decisions about health by preparing, maintaining and ensuring the accessibility of systematic reviews of the benefits and risks of healthcare interventions (http://www.cochrane.org/). INAHTA (International Network of Agencies for Health Technology Assessment) is a non-profit organization that was established in 1993 and has now grown to 50 member agencies from 26 countries including North and Latin America, Europe, Asia, Australia and New Zealand. All members are non-profit-making organizations producing HTAs and are linked to regional or national government. Three main forces have driven the recent developments of HTA: concerns about the adoption of unproven technologies, rising costs and an inexorable rise in consumer expectations. The HTA approach has been to encourage the provision of research information on the cost effectiveness of health technologies, including medicines.

NICE, the National Institute for Health and Clinical Excellence was established in the UK in 1999, primarily to help the NHS to eliminate inequality in the delivery of certain treatments, including the more modern and effective drugs, based upon where a patient lived. This became known as the 'postcode lottery'. Over time, NICE also developed a strong reputation internationally for the development of clinical guidelines. In terms of the entry of new medicines and the assessment of existing treatments, NICE's activities and influence attracted the attention of the global pharmaceutical industry. In the UK, NICE drew up and announced lists of medicines and other technologies it planned to evaluate. A number of health authorities used the impending reviews to caution practitioners to wait for the results of the evaluations before using the treatments. This became known, particularly in the pharmaceutical industry, as 'NICE blight'. The phenomenon was magnified in importance by the length of time taken to conduct reviews and the time between announcement that a review was to take place and it taking place.

A NICE review includes the formation of a team of experts from around the country, each of whom contributes to the analysis. Data for these reviews are gathered from a number of sources including the involved pharmaceutical company. These reports involve a number of functions within a company, usually led by a health economics expert. The marketing and medical functions are also involved and, in a global company, head office personnel will join the team before the final submission, as the results could have a material impact on the successful uptake of a medicine throughout the world. The importance of the launch period of a medicine, the first 6 months, has been well documented by IMS (IMS, 2008b). Delays in the HTA review, having been announced, inevitably affect uptake in certain areas.

HTA bodies abound throughout the world. Their influence is growing and they are increasingly relied upon by governments and health services. The methodology used by these agencies is not consistent. Different governments use HTAs in different ways, including for politically motivated cost-containment ends. For the pharmaceutical company, the uncertainty caused by the addition of these assessments requires a new approach to the cost effectiveness and value calculations to ensure an expeditious entry into a market. New expertise has been incorporated into many organizations with the employment of health economists. Marketing managers and their teams have started to understand the importance of HTA in the life cycle of a new medicine. The added value and cost effectiveness of medicines are now a critical part of the marketing mix. It is clear that, in one form or another, HTAs are here to stay.

NEW PRODUCT LAUNCH

The marketing plan is finalized and approved, the strategy and positioning are established, the price is set, the target audiences are finalized and segmented according to the key drivers in their decision-making process. It is now time to focus on the product launch.

Registration

When the medicine has been medically approved, there are formalities, different in each market concerning the registration and pricing approval.

Manufacturing and distribution

Product must be made for shipment, often through wholesalers, to retail outlets. Sufficient stock must be available to match the anticipated demand. Samples for distribution to physicians by reps will be made ready for launch.

Resource allocation

This is planned to ensure the product has the largest ***share of voice*** compared to the competition when launched. That is in terms of numbers and types of sales force (specialist and GP) according to the target audiences, and medical media coverage with advertising. In addition representative materials, including detail aids, leave behind brochures and samples.

Launch meeting

Sales representatives will have been trained in the therapeutic area, but the launch meeting will normally be their first sight of the approved product label. The positioning of the product and key messages will be revealed with the first promotional tools they will be given. The overall strategy will be revealed and training will take place. The training of reps includes practice in using promotional materials, such as detail aids, in order to communicate the key messages. Sometimes practising physicians are brought into the meeting to rehearse the first presentations (***details***) with the reps. Each rep must attain a high level of understanding, technical knowledge and balanced delivery before he or she is allowed to visit doctors.

Media launch

Marketing will work with public affairs to develop a media release campaign. What can be communicated is strictly limited in most markets by local regulation and limitations in direct to consumer (DTC) rules. It is a matter of public interest to know that a new medicine is available, even though the information given about the new medicine is rather limited.

Target audience

The launch preparations completed, it is time for the product to enter the market. The bright, enthusiastic sales force will go optimistically forward. In general, the maturity of the market and level of satisfaction with currently available therapy will determine the level of interest of the target audiences.

It is important to cover the highest potential doctors in the early stages with the most resource. The *innovators* and *early adopters* prescribe first and more than the others. The proportion varies by therapy area and by country, making around 5% and 10% of total prescriptions respectively.

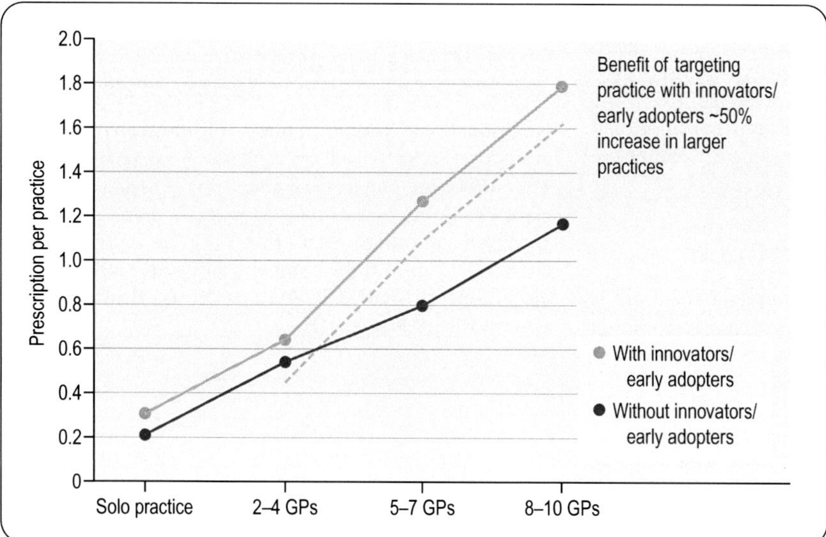

Fig. 21.4 Innovators graph.
Reproduced with kind permission of IMS Health Consulting.

In a study from IMS covering launches from 2000 to 2005, an analysis of the effect of *innovators, early adopters* and *early majority* revealed these groups as being responsible for more than half of all prescriptions in the first 6 months from launch. After the first 6 months the late majority and conservative prescribers start to use the product. From this period on, the number of prescriptions begins to resemble that of the physicians in each of the groups (IMS, 2009).

Another advantage of early focus on innovators is their influence on others in their group practice. In this case, prescribing per practice is higher than for equivalent-sized practices that lack an innovator prescriber (Figure 21.4).

The influence of innovators and early adopters on group prescribing

Patients driving launch success

Three types of patients make up the early uptake of medicines:

- *New patients*, who have not received previous drug therapy (e.g. Viagra; Gardasil)
- *Switch patients*, who have received another drug therapy
- *Add-on patients*, who have the new therapy added to their current treatment.

The success with which these types of patient are captured will determine the success of the launch and subsequent market share growth. An excellent launch tends to come as a result of the level of success in achieving switch patients. In most treatment areas there are a cohort of patients who are not responding well to existing therapy, or who suffer side effects from the treatment. The role of marketing in helping doctors to identify pools of existing patients is important, even before launch of the new product.

Early penetration of the market by targeting the right type of physicians and the right type of patients is predictive of continued success in the post-launch period, according to the IMS launch excellence study (IMS, 2009). A key predictor of success is the size of the dynamic market (new prescriptions, switches, plus any add on prescriptions) that a launch captures.

An excellent launch requires:

- That the right stakeholders be addressed in the right sequence
- Winning leading market share
- Outperformance of the competition in prescriber-focused promotion.

The first 6 months

IMS studies of launch excellence (IMS, 2008b; IMS, 2009) illustrate clearly that in a global product launch, the first 6 months are critical. Those that achieve launch excellence, according to the criteria above, continue to do well through the following stage of the life cycle. Those that do not achieve launch excellence rarely recover. Fewer than 20% of launches significantly improve their uptake trajectory between 6 and 18 months on the market after an unsuccessful early launch period.

Decline in prescriber decision-making power

A significant trend which represents a major challenge to traditional pharmaceutical marketing is the observed ongoing decline in the impact and predictability of the relationship between prescriber-focused promotional investment and launch market share achievement, in the early years of launch.

Implementing the market plan

Once the product has been successfully launched and is gaining market share, the role of marketing is to continue to implement the marketing plan, adjusting strategy as necessary to respond to the competitive challenge.

The process is of necessity dynamic. Results and changes in the market have to be continuously tracked and, as necessary, decisions should be re-evaluated. At the outset, the product manager develops a *market map*, according to the original market definition. Experience in the market will often necessitate the redrawing of parts of the map, according to the opportunity and barriers to entry.

A *customer portrait* developed pre-launch will also need to be re-evaluated with experience in the market. The changing environment is identifying new customers and stakeholders, who are traditionally not engaged in the marketing process, including non-prescribers, e.g. payers and patients (Figure 21.5)

Life cycle management of the product is no longer an automatic process that gradually sorts itself out. It needs to be managed with the same enthusiasm and systematic rigor as a new product launch. The contribution to country growth from launches of products in the previous 3 years indicates a continued decline across the top eight pharmaceutical markets (Figure 21.6).

CHANGING ENVIRONMENT – CHANGING MARKETING

Traditional pharmaceutical marketing has served the pharmaceutical industry well over the past 60 years, but less so as we move on. The development of the market over time has the majority of the industry doing the same things and effectively cancelling each other out. The importance of differentiation from the competition is still high, whether the product or market is weak or strong. How can it be achieved? (See Box 21.1.)

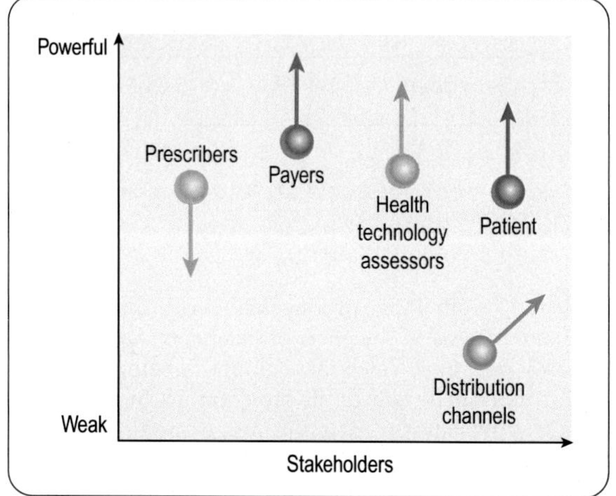

Fig. 21.5 Power shift graph.
Reproduced with kind permission of IMS Health Consulting.

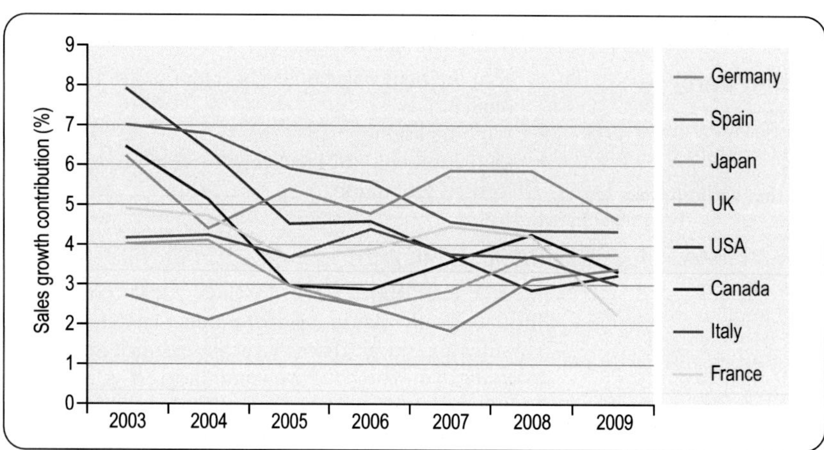

Fig. 21.6 Country launch contribution graph.
Reproduced with kind permission of IMS Health Consulting.

Box 21.1 **Competitive differentiation**

Product status/opportunities

Weak or disappearing:	Strong or emerging:
• Promotional spending and sales force size	• Ethical promotion and regulatory conformity
• Product innovation and differentiation	• Utilisation of medical technology
• Managed care and contracting relationships	• Internet
• DTC	• Marketing sophistication

The philosophy of the 1990s and early 2000s was that 'more is better'. More reps, more physician visits, more samples, more congresses and so on. All the while the old customer, the physician, was closing doors on sales reps, and losing trust in the industry's motives and integrity. Additionally, the physician as **provider** is losing power as the principal source of therapeutic decision making. Within the traditional pharmaceutical marketplace, over 70% of marketing spend is focused on physicians. Does this allocation any longer make sense? Companies are structured and resourced in order to serve this stakeholder, not the other customers who are increasingly vital to the success or otherwise of new medicines.

The key stakeholder

Even more important, a new customer base is appearing, one of whose goals is to contain costs and reduce the rapid uptake of new medicines without any 'perceived' innovative benefit. At the time of introduction, this **payer** may be told of the 'benefit' claimed by the manufacturer. If the communicator of this message is an official of a health department, it is unlikely that they will be able, or motivated, to convince the payer of the claimed benefit. As the **payers** are rapidly taking over as the key stakeholder, it is imperative that the marketer talks directly to them. The pharmaceutical industry has viewed this stakeholder as something of a hindrance in the relationship between them and their 'real' customer, the doctor. It is likely that the feeling may be mutual. Industry has generally failed to understand the perspective and values of the payer, willing to accept an adversarial relationship during pricing and reimbursement discussions.

Values of the stakeholders

Decisions made on whether a new medicine adds value and is worth the investment depend on what the customer values. The value systems of the key stakeholders in the pharmaceutical medicine process need to be considered, to see where they converge or otherwise. A value system has been defined by PWC (2009) as 'the series of activities an entity performs to create value for its customers and thus for the entity itself.' The **pharmaceutical** value proposition 'starts with the raising of capital to fund R&D, concluding with the marketing and resulting sale of the products. In essence, it is about making innovative medicines that command a premium price'.

The **payer**'s value system begins with raising revenue, through taxation or patient contribution. The value created for patients and other stakeholders is by managing administration and provision of healthcare. For the payer, the goal is to have a cost-effective health system and to enhance its reputation with its customers, or voters in the case of governments. It aims to minimize its costs and keep people well. At the time of writing, the UK health department is proposing a system of 'value based pricing' for pharmaceuticals, although no one seems to be able to define what it means.

The **provider**, in this case the physician, wants to provide high quality of care, economically and for as long as necessary. This stakeholder values an assessment of the health of a given population and to know what measures can be taken to manage and prevent illness.

The convergence of these three stakeholders' value systems, says the PWC report, is as follows. 'The value healthcare **payers** generate depends on the policies and practices of the providers used'; whereas **providers** generate value based on the revenues from payers and drugs that pharmaceutical companies provide. As for the pharmaceutical company the value it provides is dependent on access to the patients who depend on the payers and physicians. In this scenario each of the partners is by definition dependent on the others. An antagonistic relationship between these parties is, therefore, counterproductive and can result in each of the stakeholders failing to achieve their goals. A telling conclusion for the pharmaceutical industry is that they must work with payers and providers, to determine what sort of treatments the market ***wants*** to buy.

Innovation

Another conundrum for the pharmaceutical industry is the acceptance from the stakeholders of their definition of innovation. Where a patient, previously uncontrolled on one statin, for example, may be well controlled by a later entry from the same class, the payer may not accept this as innovative. They are unwilling to accept the fact that some patients may prefer the newer medicine if it means paying a premium to obtain it. With the aid of HTA (health technology assessment), the payer may use statistical data to 'disprove' the cost effectiveness of the new statin and block its reimbursement. The pharmaceutical company will find it difficult to recoup the cost of R&D associated with bringing the drug to the market. The PWC report (2009) addresses this problem by suggesting that the industry should start to talk to the key stakeholders, payers, providers and patients during Phase II of the development process. It is at this stage, they suggest, that pricing plans should start to be tested with stakeholders, rather than waiting until well into Phase III/launch. It is possible to do this, but the real test of whether a medicine is a real advance comes in the larger patient pool after launch. Post-marketing follow-up of patients and Phase IV research can help to give all stakeholders reassurance about the value added by a new medicine. It was in the 1990s, after the launch of simvastatin, that the 6-year-long 4S (Scandinavian Simvastatin Survival Study Group, 1994) study showed that treatment with this statin significantly reduced the risk of morbidity and mortality in at-risk groups, thus fundamentally changing an important aspect of medical practice. At Phase II, it would have been difficult to predict this. With today's HTA intervention, it is difficult to see if the product would have been recommended at all for use in treatment.

R&D present and future

It has been said that the primary care managed 'blockbuster' has had its day. Undoubtedly R&D productivity is going through a slow period. Fewer breakthrough treatments are appearing (IMS, 2008a) as, in Germany 'only seven truly innovative medicines were launched in 2007', from 27 product launches.

More targeted treatment solutions are being sought for people with specific disease subtypes. This will require reinvention at every step of the R&D value chain. Therapies developed using advances in molecular sciences, genomics and proteomics could be the medicines of the future.

Big pharmaceutical companies are changing research focus to include biologicals and protein-based compounds (http://www.phrma.org/files/Biotech%202006.pdf). Partnerships between big pharma and biotech companies are forming to extend their reach and to use exciting technologies such as allosteric modulation to reach targets which have been elusive through traditional research routes. The possible demise of the traditional discovery approach may be exaggerated, but it highlights the need to rethink and revise R&D.

Products of the future

Generic versions of previous 'blockbuster' molecules, supported by strong clinical evidence, are appearing all the time, giving payers and providers choice without jeopardizing patient care. This is clearly the future of the majority of primary care treatment. But if a sensible dialogue and partnership is the goal for all stakeholders in the process, generics should not only provide care, but should also allow *headroom for innovation*.

It would seem reasonable that a shift in emphasis from primary to secondary care research will happen. It would also seem reasonable that the pharmaceutical industry will need to think beyond just drugs and start to consider complete care packages surrounding their medical discoveries, such as diagnostic tests and delivery and monitoring devices.

Marketers will need to learn new specialties and prepare for more complex interactions with different providers. Traditional sales forces will not be the model for this type of marketing. Specialist medicines are around 30% more expensive to bring to market. They treat smaller populations and will, therefore, demand high prices to recoup the development cost. The debate with payers, already somewhat stressed, will become much more important. The skills of a marketer and seller will of necessity stretch far beyond those needed for primary care medicines. The structure and scope of the marketing and sales functions will have to be tailored to the special characteristics of these therapies.

THE FUTURE OF MARKETING

If the industry and the key stakeholders are to work more effectively together, an appreciation of each other's value systems and goals is imperative. The industry needs to win back the respect of its customers for its pivotal role in the global healthcare of the future.

The excess of over-enthusiastic marketing and sales personnel in the 'more is better' days of pharmaceutical promotion has been well documented and continues to grab the headlines. Regulation and sanctions have improved the situation significantly, but there is still lingering suspicion between the industry and its customers.

The most effective way to change this is greater transparency and earlier dialogue throughout the drug discovery and development process. Marketing personnel are a vital interface with the customer groups and it is important that they are developed further in the new technologies and value systems upon which the customer relies. Although they will not be the group who conduct the HTA reports from the company, they must be fully cognizant of the process and be able to discuss it in depth with customers.

Pharmaceutical marketing must advance beyond simplistic messages and valueless giveaways to have the aim of adding value in all interactions with customers. Mass marketing will give way to more focused interactions to communicate clearly the value of the medicines in specific patient groups.

The new way of marketing

Marketing must focus on the benefits of new medicines from the point of view of each of the customers. The past has been largely dominated by a focus on product attributes and an insistence on their intrinsic value. At one point, a breakthrough medicine almost sold itself. All that was necessary was a well-documented list of attributes and features. That is no longer the case.

It seems as if the provider physician is not going to be the most important decision maker in the process anymore. Specialist groups of key account managers should be developed to discuss the benefits and advantages of the new medicine with health authorities.

Payers should be involved much earlier in the research and development process, possibly even before research begins, to get the customer view of what medicines are needed from their point of view. Price and value added must be topics of conversation in an open and transparent manner, to ensure full understanding.

The future of marketing is in flux. As Peter Drucker said, 'Marketing is the whole business seen from the customer's point of view. Marketing and innovation produce results; all the rest are costs. Marketing is the distinguishing, unique function of the business.' (Tales from the marketing wars, 2006). This is a great responsibility and an exciting opportunity for the pharmaceutical industry. It is in the interests of all stakeholders that it succeeds.

REFERENCES

Donohue JM, Cevasco M, Rosenthal MB. A decade of direct-to-consumer advertising of prescription drugs. New England Journal of Medicine 2007;357:673–81.

Ferrer JM. How are the costs of continuing medical education to be defrayed? Bulletins of the New York Academy of Medicine 1975;51:785–8.

Fierce Pharma. Sales force cuts have only just begun – FiercePharma. Available online at: http://www.fiercepharma.com/story/sales-force-cuts-have-only-just-begun/2009-01-20#ixzz15RcrOVn0; 2009.

Goodman LS, Gilman A. The pharmacological basis of therapeutics: a textbook of pharmacology, toxicology, and therapeutics for physicians and medical students. 2nd ed. New York: Macmillan; 1960.

Grabowski H, Vernon J, DiMasi J. Returns on research and development for 1990s new drug introductions, pharmacoeconomics, 2002. Adapted by IBM Consulting Services. Available online at: http://www.aei.org/docLib/20040625_Helms.pdf; 2002.

IMS. Intelligence. 360: global pharmaceutical perspectives 2007, March 2008. Norwalk, Connecticut: IMS Health, 2008a.

IMS. Launch excellence 2008, study of 3000 launches across 8 markets from 2000–7. Norwalk, Connecticut: IMS Health, 2008b.

IMS. Achieving global launch excellence, January 2009. Norwalk, Connecticut: IMS Health, 2009.

Kaiser Family Foundation. Understanding the effects of direct-to-consumer prescription drug advertising, November 2001. Available online at: www.kff.org/content/2001/3197/DTC%20Ad%20Survey.pdf; 2001.

Nickum C, Kelly T. Missing the mark(et). PharmExecutive.com, Sep 1, 2005; 2005.

Pharmaceutical Research and Manufacturers of America (PhRMA). New Medicines Database and Medicines in Development: Biotechnology (http://www.phrma.org/newmeds/).

Podolsky SH, Greene JA. A historical perspective of pharmaceutical promotion and physician education. JAMA 2008;300:831–3, doi:300/7/831 [pii]10.1001/jama.300.7.831.

Price Waterhouse Cooper. Pharma 2020, which path will you take? Available online at: http://www.pwc.com/gx/en/pharma-life-sciences/pharma-2020/pharma-2020-vision-path.jhtml; 2009.

Scandinavian Simvastatin Survival Study Group. Randomized trial of cholesterol lowering in 4444 patients with coronary heart disease: the Scandinavian Simvastatin Survival Study (4S). Lancet 1994;344:1383–9. PMID 7968073.

Todd JS, Johnson KH. American Medical Association Council on Ethical and Judicial Affairs. Annotated guidelines on gifts to physicians from industry. Journal of Oklahoma State Medical Association 1992;5:227–31.

Trout, Jack. Tales from the marketing wars: Peter Drucker on marketing (http://www.forbes.com/2006/06/30/jack-trout-on-marketing-cxjt0703drucker.html).

William D, McCarthy JE. Product life cycle: 'essentials of marketing'. Richard D Irwin Company; 1997.

Section 4

Facts and figures

Chapter 22

Drug discovery and development: facts and figures

H P Rang, R G Hill

In this chapter we present summary information about the costs, timelines and success rates of the drug discovery and development operations of major pharmaceutical companies. The information comes from published sources, particularly the websites of the Association for the British Pharmaceutical Industry (www.abpi.org.uk), the European Federation of Pharmaceutical Industries and Associations (www.efpia.eu) and the Pharmaceutical Research and Manufacturers of America (www.phrma.org). Much of this information comes, of course, directly or indirectly from the pharmaceutical companies themselves, who are under no obligation to release more than is legally required. In general, details of the development process are quite well documented, because the regulatory authorities must be notified of projects in clinical development. Discovery research is less well covered, partly because companies are unwilling to divulge detailed information, but also because the discovery phase is much harder to codify and quantify. Development projects focus on a specific compound, and it is fairly straightforward to define the different components, and to measure the cost of carrying out the various studies and support activities that are needed so that the compound can be registered and launched. In the discovery phase, it is often impossible to link particular activities and costs to specific compounds; instead, the focus is often on a therapeutic target, such as diabetes, Parkinson's disease or lung cancer, or on a molecular target, such as a particular receptor or enzyme, where even the therapeutic indication may not yet be determined. The point at which a formal drug discovery project is recognized and 'managed' in the sense of having a specific goal defined and resources assigned to it, varies greatly between companies. A further complication is that, as described in Section 2 of this book, the scientific strategies applied to drug discovery are changing rapidly, so that historic data may not properly represent the current situation. For these reasons, it is very difficult to obtain anything more than crude overall measures of the effectiveness of drug discovery research. There are, for example, few published figures to show what proportion of drug discovery projects succeed in identifying a compound fit to enter development, whether this probability differs between different therapeutic areas, and how it relates to the resources allocated. We attempt to predict some trends and new approaches at the end of this chapter.

As will be seen from the analysis that follows, the most striking aspects of drug discovery and development are that (a) failure is much more common than success, (b) it costs a lot, and (c) it takes a very long time (Figure 22.1). By comparison with other research-based industries, pharmaceutical companies are playing out a kind of slow-motion and very expensive arcade game, with the odds heavily stacked against them, but offering particularly rich rewards.

SPENDING

Worldwide, the R&D spending of the American-based pharmaceutical companies has soared, from roughly $5 billion in 1982 to $40 billion in 1998 and $70 billion in both 2008 and 2009. Figure 22.2 shows total R&D expenditure for US-based companies over the period 1995–2009. The R&D expenditure of the 10 largest pharmaceutical companies in 2009 averaged nearly $5 billion per company over the range of Roche at $8.7 billion to Lilly at $4.13 billion (Carroll, 2010). Marketing and administration costs for these companies are about three times as great as R&D costs. The annual increase in R&D spending in the industry in most cases has exceeded sales growth over the last decade, reflecting the need to increase productivity

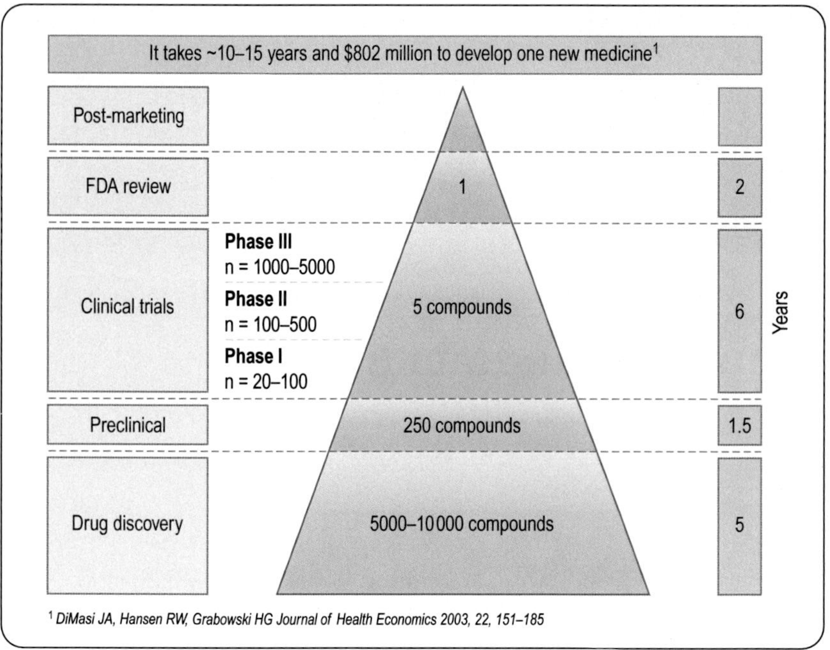

Fig. 22.1 The attrition of compounds through the discovery and development pipeline (PhRMA).
Reproduced, with permission, from DiMasi et al., 2003.

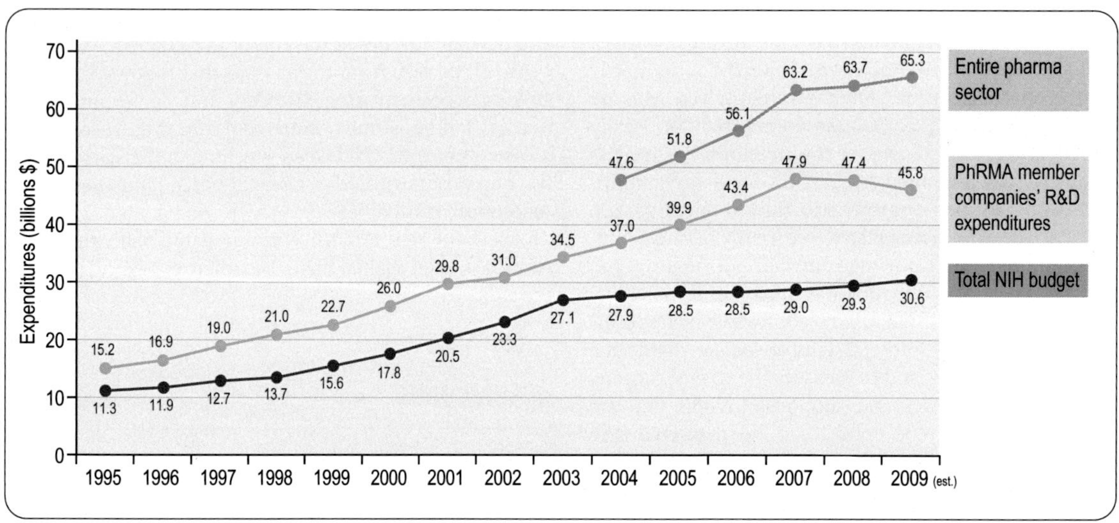

Fig. 22.2 Private vs public spending on R&D in the USA (PhRMA).

(see Kola and Landis, 2004). Today a minimum of 15–20% of sales revenues are reinvested in R&D, a higher percentage than in any other industry (Figure 22.3). The tide may have turned, however, and in 2010 the overall global R&D spend for the industry fell to $68 billion (a 3% reduction from 2009) (Hirschler, 2011). This fall reflects a growing disillusion with the poor returns on money invested in pharmaceutical R&D and some companies (notably Pfizer with a 25% reduction over the next 2 years) have announced plans to make further cuts in their budgets. The overall cost of R&D covers discovery research as well as the various development functions, described in Section 3 of this book. The average distribution of R&D expenditure on these different functions is

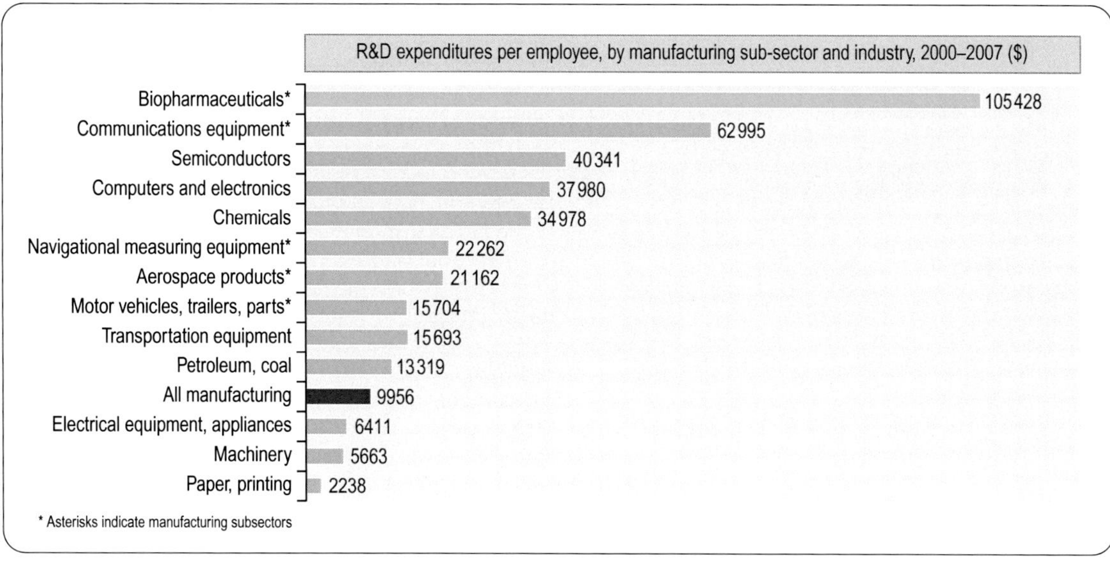

Fig. 22.3 The pharmaceutical industry spends more on R&D than any other industry (PhRMA).

Table 22.1 R&D expenditure by function (2008)

Function	Total R&D costs (%)		
			US
Discovery and preclinical development			27
Clinical development	Phase I & II	21.1	53.6
	Phase III	32.5	
Approval			4.7
Phase IV / pharmacovigilance			14.4

Data from PhRMA Membership Survey 2010 (calculated from 2008 data).

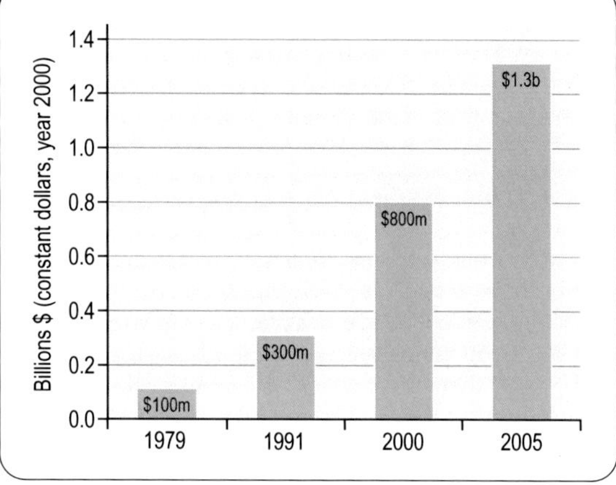

Fig. 22.4 The costs (corrected for inflation) of drug development continue to increase (PhRMA, 2011).

shown in Table 22.1. These proportions represent the overall costs of these different functions and do not necessarily reflect the costs of developing an individual compound. As will be discussed later, the substantial drop-out rate of compounds proceeding through development means that the overall costs cover many failures as well as the few successes. Overall cost of developing a compound to launch and how much this has increased between 1979 and 2005 is shown in Figure 22.4.

Numbers of compounds in clinical development according to therapeutic classes is shown in Figure 22.5, based on a survey of the American research-based pharmaceutical industry, and is dominated by four therapeutic areas, namely:

- Central nervous system disorders (including Alzheimer's disease, schizophrenia, depression, epilepsy and Parkinson's disease)
- Cancer, endocrine and metabolic diseases (including osteoporosis, diabetes and obesity)
- Cardiovascular diseases (including atherosclerosis, coronary disease and heart failure)
- Infectious diseases (including bacterial, viral and other infections such as malaria).

Condition	Number of medicines in development
Alzheimer's and other dementias	98
Arthritis	74
Cancer	878
• Breast cancer	125
• Colorectal cancer	82
• Lung cancer	120
• Leukemia	119
• Skin cancer	86
Cardiovascular disorders	237
Diabetes mellitus	193
HIV/AIDS	81
Mental and behavioral disorders	252
Parkinson's disease	25
Respiratory disorders	334
Rare diseases	303

Fig. 22.5 Numbers of compounds in clinical development for different therapeutic targets (PhRMA, 2011).

The trend in the last decade has been away from cardiovascular disease towards other priority areas, particularly cancer and metabolic disorders, and also a marked increase in research on biopharmaceuticals, whose products are used in all therapeutic areas. There is also a marked increase in the number of drugs being introduced for the treatment of rare or orphan diseases driven by enabling legislation in the USA and EU (see Chapter 20).

How much does it cost to develop a drug?

Estimating the cost of developing a drug is not as straightforward as it might seem, as it depends very much on what is taken into account in the calculation. Factors such as 'opportunity costs' (the loss of income that theoretically results from spending money on drug development rather than investing it somewhere else) and tax credits (contributions from the public purse to encourage drug development in certain areas) make a large difference, and are the source of much controversy. The Tufts Centre for Drug Development Studies estimated the average cost of developing a drug in 2000 to be $802 million, increasing to $897 million in 2003[1] (DiMasi et al., 2003; Figure 22.1), compared with $31.8 million (inflation-adjusted) in 1987, and concluded that the R&D cost of a new drug is increasing at an annual rate of 7.4% above inflation.

Based on different assumptions, even larger figures – $1.1 billion per successful drug launch over the period 1995–2000, and $1.7 billion for 2000–2002 – were calculated by Gilbert et al. (2003).

The fact that more than 70% of R&D costs represents discovery and 'failure' costs, and less than 30% represents direct costs (which, being determined largely by requirements imposed by regulatory authorities, are difficult to reduce), has caused research-based pharmaceutical companies in recent years to focus on improving (a) the efficiency of the discovery process, and (b) the success rate of the compounds entering development (Kola and Landis, 2004). A good recent example of expensive failure of a compound in late-stage clinical development is illustrated by the experience of Pfizer with their cholesterol ester transfer protein (CETP) inhibitor, torcetrapib (Mullard, 2011). This new approach to treating cardiovascular disease by raising levels of the 'good' HDL cholesterol had looked very promising in the laboratory and in early clinical testing, but in late 2006 development was halted when a large Phase III clinical trial revealed that patients treated with the drug had an increased risk of death and heart problems. At the point of termination of their studies Pfizer had already spent $800 million on the project. The impact extended beyond Pfizer, as both Roche (dalcetrapib) and Merck (anacetrapib) had their own compounds acting on this mechanism in clinical development. It was necessary to decide if this was a class effect of the mechanism or whether it was just a compound-specific off-target effect limited to torcetrapib. Intensive comparisons of these agents in collaboration with academic groups and a published full analysis of the torcetrapib clinical trial data allowed the conclusion that this was most likely to be an effect limited to torcetrapib, possibly mediated by aldosterone, and it was not seen with the other two CETP blockers (Mullard, 2011). Roche and Merck were able to restart their clinical trials, but using very large numbers of patients and focusing on clinical outcomes to establish efficacy and safety. The Pfizer experience probably added 4 years to the time needed to complete development of the Merck compound anacetrapib and made this process more expensive (for example the pivotal study that started in 2011 will recruit 30 000 patients) with no guarantee of commercial success. In addition the patent term available to recover development costs and to make any profit is now 4 years shorter (see Chapter 19). It is not unreasonable to estimate that collectively the pharmaceutical industry will have spent more than $3 billion

[1]Quote from a commentary on this analysis (Frank RG (2003) Journal of Health Economics 22: 325): 'These are impressively large numbers, usually associated with a purchase of jet fighters – 40 F16s in fact'.

investigating CETP as a mechanism before we have either a marketed product or the mechanism is abandoned.

SALES REVENUES

Despite the stagnation in compound registrations over the past 25 years, the overall sales of pharmaceuticals have risen steadily. In the period 1999–2004 the top 14 companies showed an average sales growth of 10% per year, whereas in 2004–2009 growth was still impressive but at a lower rate of 6.7% per year. However, the boom years may be behind us and the prediction is that for 2009–2014 the growth will be a modest 1.2% per year (Goodman, 2009). Loss of exclusivity as patents expire is the most important reason for reduced sales growth (Goodman, 2009). The total global sales in 2002 reached $400.6 billion and in 2008 had risen to $808 billion (EFPIA, 2010). In Europe the cost of prescribed drugs accounts for some 17% of overall healthcare costs (EFPIA, 2010).

Profitability

For a drug to make a profit, sales revenue must exceed R&D, manufacture and marketing costs. Grabowski et al. (2002) found that only 34% of new drugs introduced between 1990 and 1994 brought in revenues that exceeded the average R&D cost (Figure 22.6). This quite surprising result, which at first sight might suggest that the industry is extremely bad at doing its sums, needs to be interpreted with caution for various reasons. First, development costs vary widely, depending on the nature of the compound, the route of administration and the target indication, and so a drug may recoup its development cost even though its revenues fall below the average cost. Second, the development money is spent several years before any revenues come in, and sales predictions made at the time development decisions have to be taken are far from reliable. At any stage, the decision whether or not to proceed is based on a calculation of the drug's 'net present value' (NPV) – an amortised estimate of the future sales revenue, minus the future development and marketing costs. If the NPV is positive, and sufficiently large to justify the allocation of development capacity, the project will generally go ahead, even if the money already spent cannot be fully recouped, as terminating it would mean that *none* of the costs would be recouped. At the beginning of a project NPV estimates are extremely unreliable – little more than guesses – so most companies will not pay much attention to them for decision-making purposes until the project is close to launch, when sales revenues become more predictable. Furthermore, unprofitable drugs may make a real contribution to healthcare, and companies may choose to develop them for that reason.

Even though only 34% of registered drugs in the Grabowski et al. (2002) study made a profit, the profits on those that did so more than compensated for the losses on the others, leaving the industry as a whole with a large overall profit during the review period in the early 1990s. The situation is no longer quite so favourable for the industry, partly because of price control measures in healthcare, and partly because of rising R&D costs. In the future there will be more emphasis on the relative efficacy of drugs and it will only be those new agents that have demonstrable superiority over generic competitors that will be able to command high prices (Eichler et al., 2010). It is likely that the pharmaceutical industry will adapt to changed circumstances, although whether historical profit margins can be maintained is uncertain.

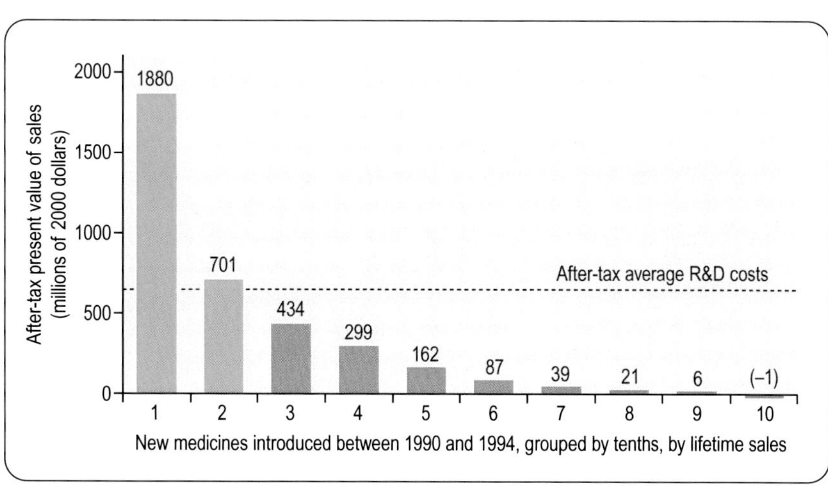

Fig. 22.6 Few drugs are commercially successful (PhRMA, 2011).

Pattern of sales

The distribution of sales (2008 figures) by major pharmaceutical companies according to different therapeutic categories is shown in Table 22.2. Recent changes reflect a substantial increase in sales of anticancer drugs and drugs used to treat psychiatric disorders. The relatively small markets for drugs used to treat bacterial and parasitic infections contrasts sharply with the worldwide prevalence and severity of these diseases, a problem that is currently being addressed at government level in several countries. The USA represents the largest and fastest-growing market for pharmaceuticals (61% of global sales in 2010). Together with Europe (22%) and Japan (5%), these regions account for 88% of global sales. The rest of the established world market accounts for only 10%, with 3% in emerging markets (EFPIA, 2010). The approaching patent cliff (see later) suggests that with the current business model there may be a 5–10% reduction in sales and a 20–30% reduction in net income over 2012–2015 for the 13 largest companies (Munos, 2009). Not all predictions are pessimistic and IMS have recently opined that global drug sales will top $1 trillion in 2014 (Berkrot, 2010). Whilst accepting that growth in USA and other developed markets is slowing, they believe that this will be more than compensated for by growth in developing markets (China is growing at 22–25% per year and Brazil at 12–15% per year).

Table 22.2 Global sales by therapeutic area (Maggon, 2009)

Therapeutic area	$US billions
Arthritis	35
Infectious disease	24
Cancer	70
Cardiovascular disease	105
Central nervous system	118
Diabetes	21
Respiratory disease	25

Blockbuster drugs

The analysis by Grabowski et al. (2002) showed that 70% of the industry's profits came from 20% of the drugs marketed, highlighting the commercial importance of finding 'blockbuster' drugs – defined as those achieving annual sales of $1 billion or more – as these are the ones that actually generate significant profits. A recent analysis of pharmaceutical company pipelines showed that 18 new blockbusters were registered in the period 2001–2006, roughly four per year globally among the 30 or so new compounds that are currently being registered each year. In 2000, a total of 44 marketed drugs achieved sales exceeding $1 billion, compared with 17 in 1995 and 35 in 1999. The contribution of blockbuster drugs to the overall global sales also increased from 18% in 1997 to 45% in 2001, reflecting the fact that sales growth in the blockbuster sector has exceeded that in the market overall. The top 10 best selling drugs in 2010 are shown in Table 22.3 and this

Table 22.3 Global sales of top ten drugs (from IMS, 2011)

Drug	Trade name	Type	Indication	Sales 1998 ($bn)	Sales 2010 ($bn)
Atorvastatin	Lipitor	HMG CoA reductase nhibitor	Cholesterol lowering	1.9	12.7
Clopidogrel	Plavix	Adenosine receptor antagonist	Anti-platelet anticoagulant		8.8
Fluticasone/ salmeterol	Seretide	Steroid/β adrenoceptor agonist	Asthma		8.5
Esomeprazole	Nexium	Proton pump inhibitor	Gastric ulcer		8.3
Quetiapine	Seroquel	Atypical antipsychotic drug	Schizophrenia		6.8
Cerivastatin	Crestor	HMG CoA reductase inhibitor	Cholesterol lowering		6.7
Etanercept	Enbrel	TNF R2 fusion protein	Arthritis/psoriasis		6.2
Infliximab	Remicade	Anti-TNF mab	Arthritis/psoriasis		6.0
Adulimumab	Humira	Anti-TNF mab	Arthritis/psoriasis		5.9
Olanzapine	Zyprexa	Atypical antipsychotic	Schizophrenia	2.37	5.7

Table 22.4 Top 10 drugs worldwide (blockbusters) 2000

Drug	Trade name	Class	Launch year	Sales 2000 (US$bn)	Change since 1999 (%)
Omeprazole	Prilosec	Proton pump inhibitor	89	6.26	5.9
Simvastatin	Zocor	HMGCR inhibitor	91	5.21	17.5
Atorvastatin	Lipitor	HMGCR inhibitor	96	5.03	32.6
Amlodipine	Norvasc	Vasodilator	92	3.36	12.4
Loratadine	Claritin	Non-sedating antihistamine	93	3.01	12.6
Lansoprazole	Prevacid	Proton pump inhibitor	95	2.82	27.0
Epoetin-α	Procrit	Erythropoietic factor	90	2.71	29.4
Celecoxib	Celebrex	Cyclooxygenase 2 inhibitor	98	2.61	77.7
Fluoxetine	Prozac	SSRI	87	2.5	–0.6
Olanzapine	Zyprexa	Atypical antipsychotic	96	2.37	26.6

should be compared with the top 10 best selling drugs in 2000 shown in Table 22.4. Only atorvastatin and olanzapine appear in both tables as many of the other drugs have become generics in the interim and have, therefore, lost much of their sales revenue due to competition. It is also noteworthy that there was only one biological in the top 10 in 2000 whereas in 2010 there were three. Munos (2009) analysed the peak sales achieved by 329 recently introduced drugs and calculated that the probability of a new product achieving blockbuster status was only 21%, even though companies take a drug into clinical development only if they believe it has blockbuster potential.

The spate of pharmaceutical company mergers in the last decade has also been driven partly by the need for companies to remain in blockbuster territory despite the low rate of new drug introductions and the difficulty of predicting sales. By merging, companies are able to increase the number of compounds registered and thus reduce the risk that the pipeline will contain no blockbusters. This may have a negative effect on R&D performance and creativity, however (Kneller, 2010; LaMattina, 2011)

TIMELINES

One important factor that determines profitability is the time taken to develop and launch a new drug, in particular the time between patent approval and launch, which will determine the length of time during which competitors are barred from introducing cheap generic copies of the drug. A drug that is moderately successful by today's standards might achieve sales of about $400 million/year, so each week's delay in development, by reducing the competition-free sales window, will cost the company roughly $8 million.

Despite increasing expenditure on R&D costs and decreased output, the mean development time from first synthesis or isolation (i.e. excluding discovery research preceding synthesis of the development compound) to first launch was over 14 years in 1999, having increased somewhat over the preceding decade. Half of this time was taken up by discovery and preclinical development and half by clinical studies. A further 2 years was required for FDA review and approval. The long FDA review times during the 1980s have since come down substantially (Reichert, 2003), mainly because user fees and fast-track procedures for certain types of drug were introduced. Current estimates of time taken for R&D leading to a new marketed product are in the region of 10 years with a further 2 or 3 years need for preparation and submission of the regulatory package and its approval (EFPIA, 2010).

There are, of course, wide variations in development times between individual projects, although historically there has been little consistent difference between different therapeutic areas (with the exception of anti-infective drugs, for which development times are somewhat shorter, and anticancer drugs, for which they have been longer by about 2 years). During the 1990s, most biopharmaceuticals were recombinant versions of human hormones, and their clinical development was generally quicker than that of small molecules. More recently, biopharmaceuticals have become more diverse and many monoclonal antibodies have been developed, and these have generally encountered more problems in development because their therapeutic and unwanted effects are unpredictable, and so clinical development times for biopharmaceuticals have tended to increase.

Table 22.5 Discovery timelines

	Target identification and validation	Screening	Lead optimization	Total discovery	Preclinical development	Total to clinic
McKinsey (1997)						
	10–36	1–3	7–14	18–53	8–16	26–69
2000 predicted	6–17	1	5–9	12–27	7–15	19–42
Andersen (1997)						
	10–24	6–24	24–36	40–84	6–30	46–114
2000 predicted	5–8	1–12	12–18	18–38	5–8	23–46

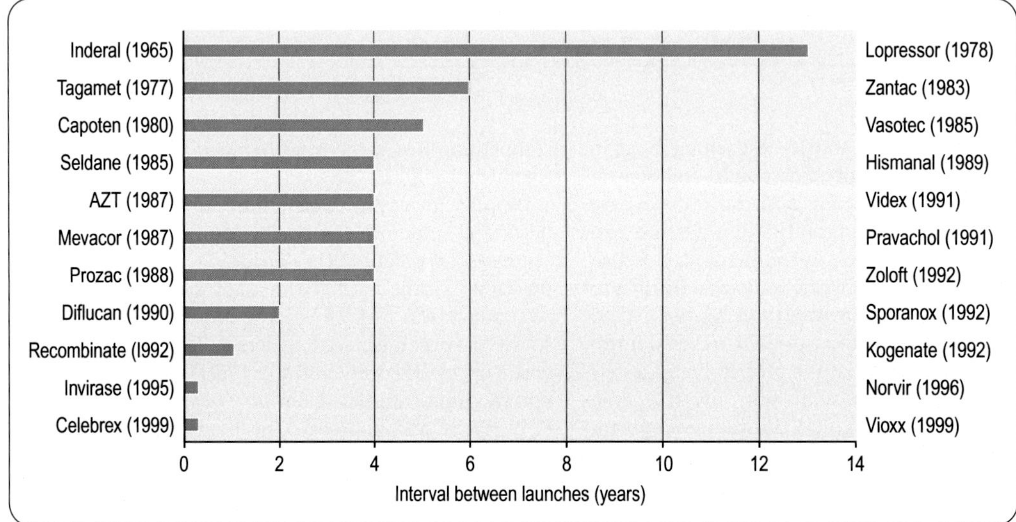

Fig. 22.7 Period of exclusivity is shrinking (PhRMA, 2011).

Information about the time taken for discovery – from the start of a project to the identification of a development compound – is sparse in the public literature. Management consultants McKinsey and Arthur Andersen estimate that in 1995, the time taken from the start of the discovery project to the start of clinical studies was extremely variable, ranging from 21 to 103 months (Table 22.5). Both studies predicted a reduction in discovery time by the year 2000 to 46 months or less, owing to improved discovery technologies. Although solid data are lacking, few believe that such a dramatic improvement has actually occurred.

Intensifying competition in the pharmaceutical marketplace also is demonstrated by the shrinking period of exclusivity during which the first drug in a therapeutic class is the sole drug in that class, thereby reducing the time a premium can be charged to recover the R&D expenditure. For example, cimetidine (Tagamet), an ulcer drug introduced in 1977, had an exclusivity period of 6 years before another drug in the same class, ranitidine (Zantac), was introduced. In contrast, celecoxib (Celebrex), the first selective cyclooxygenase-2 inhibitor (COX-2), which had a significant advantage over established non-steroidal anti-inflammatory drugs, was on the market only 3 months before a second, very similar, drug, rofecoxib (Vioxx), was approved (Figure 22.7). (Vioxx was withdrawn in 2004, because it was found to increase the risk of heart attacks: other COX-2 inhibitors were subsequently withdrawn or given restricted labels.)

Loss of patent protection opens up the competition to generic products (the same compound being manufactured and sold at a much lower price by companies that

Table 22.6 Selected drugs facing patent expiry in the USA 2010–2012 (from Harrison, 2011)

Branded drug (INN drug name; company)	Indication	Worldwide 2009 sales (billion)*	Expected patent expiry
Aricept (donepezil; Eisai/Pfizer)	Alzheimer's-type dementia	¥303.8 (US$3.61)	Nov 2010
Lipitor (atorvastatin; Pfizer)	High cholesterol	US$11.43	2011
Zyprexa (olanzapine; Eli Lilly & Company)	Schizophrenia, bipolar 1 disorder	US$4.92	2011
Lexapro (escitalopram; Forest Laboratories/Lundbeck)	Depression and anxiety	DKK 7.77 (US$1.37)	2012
Actos (pioglitazone; Takeda)	Type 2 diabetes	¥334.5 (US$3.98)°	2012
Plavix (clopidogrel; Sanofi-Aventis/ Bristol-Myers Aquibb)	Clot-related cardiovascular events	US$6.15	2012
Lovenox (enoxaparin; Sanofi-Aventis)	Acute deep vein thrombosis	€3.04($4.03)	2012
Seroquel (quetiapine; AstraZeneca)	Schizophrenia, bipolar disorder, major depressive disorder	US$4.87	2012

*Data from company annual reports. ° Europe and the Americas. INN, international nonproprietary name.

have not invested in the R&D underlying the original discovery), and the sales revenue from the branded compound generally falls sharply. Over the period 2010–2014 drugs generating combined revenues of $78 billion (Harrison, 2011) will lose patent protection (Table 22.6). Half of the revenue erosion is predicted to be in 2011 as Lipitor (atorvastatin) loses patent protection. This drug (see Table 22.3) earned >$12 billion for Pfizer in 2010 and accounts for more than 20% of their total revenues. The loss of patent protection and the introduction of low-priced generic atorvastatin will not only affect Pfizer, as other drugs with longer patent life in the statin class will now face significant competition on price as well as on efficacy. These global figures vary from year to year as individual high-revenue drugs drop out of patent protection, and the revenue swings for an individual company are of course much more extreme than the global average, so maintaining a steady pipeline of new products and timing their introduction to compensate for losses as products become open to generic competition is a key part of a company's commercial strategy.

PIPELINES AND ATTRITION RATES

As we have already seen, the number of new chemical entities registered as pharmaceuticals each year has declined over the last decade or at best has stayed flat, and various analyses (Drews, 2003a,b; Kola and Landis, 2004; Munos, 2009) have pointed to a serious 'innovation deficit'. According to these calculations, to sustain a revenue growth rate of 10% – considered to be a healthy level – the 10 largest pharmaceutical companies each needed to launch on average 3.1 new compounds each year, compared to 1.8 launches per company actually achieved in 2000 – a rate insufficient to maintain even zero growth. As mergers increase the size of companies and their annual revenues these numbers increase proportionally (e.g. in 2003 Pfizer had revenues of $45 billion and to sustain this level of income it would need to generate nine NCEs per year (Kola and Landis, 2004)). A recent survey indicated that the top 10 pharmaceutical companies are producing 1.17 NCEs per year if based in the USA and 0.83 NCEs per year if based in Europe – a considerable shortfall (Pammolli et al., 2011). Goodman (2009) concluded that most pharmaceutical companies are not replacing the products they lose from patent expiry sufficiently quickly and can only remain competitive by rigorous cost-cutting initiatives. The large numbers of layoffs in the industry in the last 2 years would support his conclusion.

The number of clinical trials being carried out in each therapeutic area (Figure 22.5) provides a measure of potential future launches. The figures shown may somewhat overestimate the numbers, because official notification of the start of clinical projects is obligatory, but projects may be terminated or put on hold without formal notification. Estimates of the number of active preclinical projects are even more unreliable, as companies are under no obligation to reveal this information, and the definition of what constitutes a project is variable. The number of clinical trials appears large in relation to the number of new compounds registered in each year, partly because each trial usually lasts for more than 1 year, and partly because many trials (i.e. different indications, different dosage forms) are generally performed with each compound, including previously registered compounds as well as new ones.

The fact that in any year there are more Phase II than Phase I clinical projects in progress reflects the longer duration of Phase II studies, which more than offsets the effect of attrition during Phase I. The number of Phase III projects is smaller, despite their longer duration, because of the attrition between Phase II and Phase III.

High attrition rates – which would horrify managers in most technology-based industries – are a fact of life in pharmaceuticals, and are the main reason why drug discovery and development is so expensive and why drug prices are so high in relation to manufacturing costs. The cumulative attrition based on projects in the mid-1990s, predicts an overall success rate of 20% from the start of clinical development (Phase I). A more recent analysis quoted by the FDA (FDA Report, 2004) suggest a success rate of compounds entering Phase I trials of only 8%, and this can be even lower for particular therapeutic areas (e.g. 5% for oncology (Kola and Landis, 2004)).

The main reasons currently for failure of compounds are summarized in Figure 22.8 (Arrowsmith, 2011). It can be seen that the situation has changed little since Kola and Landis (2004) showed that unsatisfactory pharmacokinetic properties and lack of therapeutic efficacy in patients were the commonest shortcomings in 1991 but that by 2000 the pharmacokinetic issues had largely been addressed. As discussed in Chapter 10, determined efforts have been made to control for pharmacokinetic properties in the discovery phase, and this appears to have reduced the failure rate during development. Accurate prediction of therapeutic efficacy in the discovery phase remains a problem, however, particularly in disease areas, such as psychiatric disorders, where animal models are unsatisfactory. The analysis in Figure 22.8A shows that large numbers of drugs with novel mechanisms of action are failing in areas of high medical need such as cancer and neurodegeneration. In Figure 22.8B it can be seen that 66% of failures are due to lack of clinical efficacy regardless of therapeutic target and 21% due to inadequate safety (Arrowsmith, 2011). It has been estimated that in a typical research project 20–30% of the time is spent fine-tuning molecules to fit the available animal models of disease perfectly even though in many cases these models are not predictive of clinical efficacy (Bennani, 2011). It is especially concerning that drugs are still failing due to lack of efficacy in Phase III clinical trials (see Figure 22.9) and that, although increasing numbers of compounds are reaching Phase I and II clinical evaluation, the number of active Phase III compounds has not increased between 1997 and 2007. It has been suggested that the remedy is to make Phase II trials more rigorous on the grounds that Phase II failures are less disruptive and less costly than Phase III failures (Arrowsmith, 2011). Even having reached the registration phase, 23% of compounds subsequently fail to become marketed products (Kola and Landis, 2004). The problem of lack of predictability of long-term

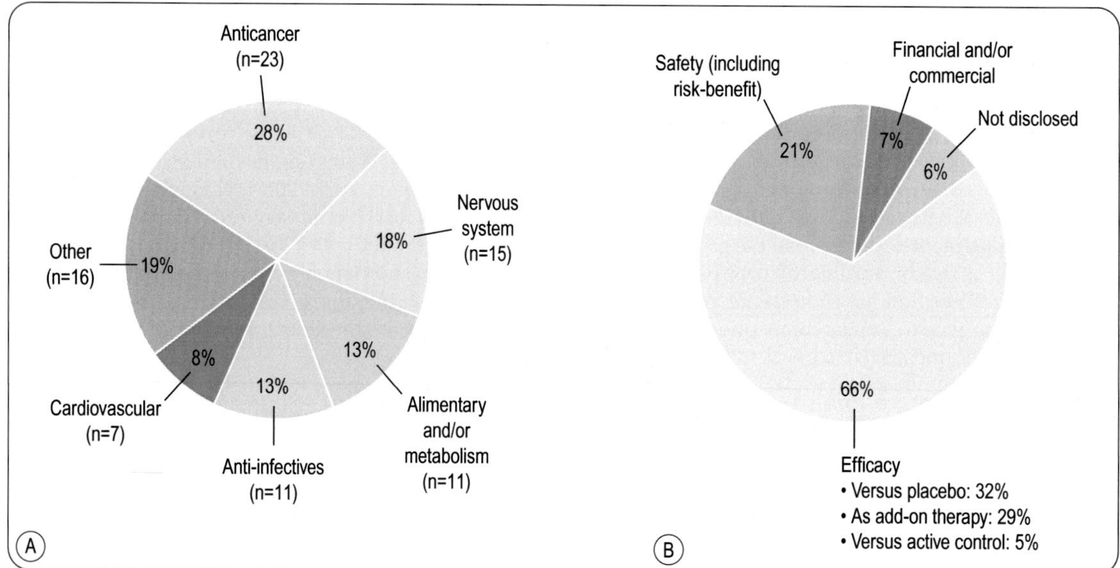

Fig. 22.8 Reasons for compound failure in development.
Reproduced, with permission, from Arrowsmith, 2011.

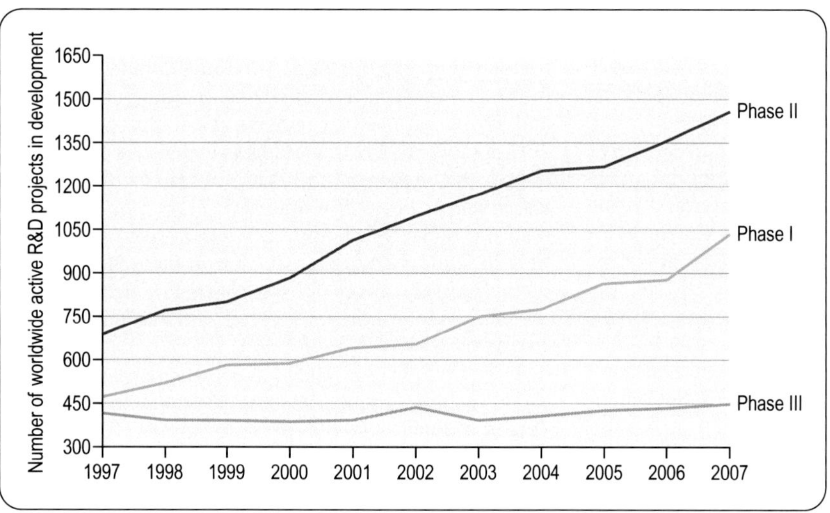

Fig. 22.9 Numbers of compounds in Phase III trials is not increasing year on year (Parexel Handbook data).

toxicity such that compounds need to be withdrawn after launch is still largely intractable.

BIOTECHNOLOGY-DERIVED MEDICINES

An increasing share of research and development projects is devoted to the investigation of therapies using biotechnology-derived molecules (see Chapters 12 and 13). The first such product was recombinant human insulin (Humulin), introduced by Lilly in 1982. From 1991 to 2003, 79 out of 469 (17%) new molecules registered were biopharmaceuticals. Recently (2002–2008) the proportion was around 30% – partly reflecting reduced numbers of small molecules registered in recent years – and this is predicted to increase to about 50% over the next few years. In 2002 an estimated 371 biopharmaceuticals were in clinical development (PhRMA Survey, 2002), with strong emphasis on new cancer therapies (178 preparations) and infectious diseases, including AIDS (68 preparations). One growth area is monoclonal antibodies (MAbs). The first agent in this class, adulimumab, was approved by the FDA in 2002, but between then and 2010 an additional six were registered with three under review. In 2010 there were seven in Phase III and 81 in Phase I or II clinical trials (Nelson et al., 2010). Overall biologicals have had a higher probability of success than small molecules with 24% of agents entering Phase I trials becoming marketed products (Kola and Landis, 2004).

Many biotechnology-based projects originate not in mainstream pharmaceutical companies, but in specialized small biotechnology companies, which generally lack the money and experience to undertake development projects. This has resulted in increased in-licensing activities, whereby a large company licenses in and develops the substance, for which it pays fees, milestone payments and, eventually, royalties to the biotechnology company.

RECENT INTRODUCTIONS

An analysis of the 58 new substances approved by the FDA in the period 2001–2002 showed that about half of the new synthetic compounds were directed at receptor targets (mostly GPCRs, and some steroid receptors), all of which had been identified pharmacologically many years earlier, as had the transporter and enzyme targets. Only a minority of the new compounds were 'first-in-class' drugs. In 2006 only about 30% of the drugs approved by the FDA were new chemical compounds the rest being modified formulations or new uses for existing drugs (Austin, 2006). The 20% of compounds directed at infectious agents in 2002 were also mainly 'follow-up' compounds, directed at familiar targets, and so it is clear that during the 1990s, when these drugs were being discovered and developed, the industry was operating quite conservatively (DiMasi and Faden, 2011). Although, as described in Section 2, many new technologies are being applied in the hope of improving the speed and efficiency of drug discovery, drug targets and therapeutic approaches had not really changed. You are more likely to produce blockbusters, it was argued, by following the routes that produced blockbusters in the past than by trying new approaches with the aim of being 'first-in-class' (DiMasi and Faden, 2011). In a survey of 259 drugs registered by the FDA between 1999 and 2008

(Swinney and Anthony, 2011) it was found that only 75 of the 259 were first-in-class agents with novel mechanisms of action. Of the small molecule drugs in the survey target-based screening had produced 17 with 28 being discovered by using phenotypic disease model screening. Thus, even though the industry is becoming more centred on molecular target-based screening, this is not the source of the majority of new drugs. One worrying trend is the reduction in effort across the industry in the search for new drugs to treat psychiatric and neurological disorders, as, although this is the most difficult research area, the medical need for drugs has never been higher (Abbott, 2010; Kaitin and Milne, 2011).

Biopharmaceuticals registered between 1999 and 2008 include several protein mediators produced by recombinant methods and a number of monoclonal antibodies. Vaccines are also strongly represented. Of the 75 first-in-class drugs registered by the FDA in this period, 50 (67%) were small molecules and 25 (33%) were biologicals. Judging from the portfolio of new biotechnology products currently undergoing clinical evaluation, the trend towards biopharmaceuticals is set to continue, with cancer and inflammation/autoimmune diseases as the main therapeutic targets. A milestone was reached in 2012 when a biological became the world's top selling drug as a consequence of patent expiry for the previous top sellers (Hirschler, 2012).

Some new drug introductions are aimed at small patient populations sometimes coupled with a biomarker to identify sensitive groups of patients who will benefit, and, as a consequence, these drugs are hyper-expensive (Hunter and Wilson, 2011). One recent example is a new treatment for multiple sclerosis from Novartis where a course of treatment will cost $48 000 in the USA (Von Schaper and Kresge, 2011). It is not clear whether such treatments will be affordable (Hunter and Wilson, 2011) or whether they will be beneficial to the profitability of the industry in the long term.

PREDICTING THE FUTURE?

Many models have been proposed as the ideal way to discover drugs, but there is now general cynicism and the intrinsic cyclical nature of drug discovery is likely to have been the real reason for swings from failure to success rather than the approach taken by the industry. Predicting the future, especially the facts and figures is therefore a dangerous game! A number of factors have become apparent in the recent past that will change our world in ways which we probably could not have guessed at 5 years ago. The belief that drug discovery could be industrialized is clearly a mistaken one. Access to larger numbers of molecular targets, larger numbers of drug like compounds and faster screening technology has not led to more registered drugs. Similarly our knowledge of human genome has not yet paid off. We are learning more about disease processes day by day, but much of this knowledge is difficult to translate into drug discovery. More and more senior figures in the pharmaceutical industry are standing up in public and saying we need to reinvent the industry (Bennani, 2011; Paul et al., 2010). It seems inevitable (as mentioned above) that if we cannot close the gap between drugs losing patent protection and new product introductions then the industry will shrink. We have seen for the first time in living memory a reduction in the R&D spending of the industry driven by the realization that spending more on R&D year on year did not work (Hirschler, 2011). The driver now is to reduce costs where possible, get the investment right and only invest where probability of success is high (Kola and Landis, 2004; Paul et al., 2010). This is coupled with a need to streamline development (FDA, 2011) and kill drugs that are not clearly an improvement over what we already have as early as is feasible (Paul et al., 2010; Figure 22.10). Some companies are seeing the need to empower creative talent and admit that drug discovery is as much an art as a science (Bennani, 2011; Douglas et al., 2010; Paul et al., 2010). The crucial reorganization may already have happened with much of the creative part of drug discovery moving over to the biotech sector or to academic centres for drug discovery (Kotz, 2011; Stephens et al., 2011). This in turn is leading to more partnerships between different pharmaceutical companies, and between pharmaceutical companies, biotech and academia. It is interesting to note that the academic contribution to drug discovery may have been underestimated in the past (Stephens et al., 2011).

The economics of our business will have shifted geographically by 2015 (IMS, 2011) with the US share of the global market declining from 41% in 2010 to 31% in 2015. At that time the US and EU combined are likely to reflect only 44% of global spending on medicines. This in turn is driving where investment in R&D and manufacturing facilities is being made. It is already evident that cuts in R&D spending in the UK and USA are paralled by an increase in spending in Asia, especially in China (see Zang, 2011). The other important shift that is happening is from proprietary medicines to generics and in 2015 it is likely that a major growth area will be generics which will account for 39% of the total drug spend compared with 27% in 2010 (IMS, 2011). We are thus victims of our own success as the blockbusters of 2005 become the generics of 2015. Around 50% of the new drugs that will drive profitability in 2015 will be biologicals and the majority of these will be monoclonal antibodies (IMS, 2011).

Our world will look very different 5 years from now with an increasingly complex social, legal, scientific and political environment. The pharmaceutical industry will continue to be important and governments will have to ensure that a fair reward for innovation (see Aronson et al., 2012) is still achievable but how this will be done is at present unclear.

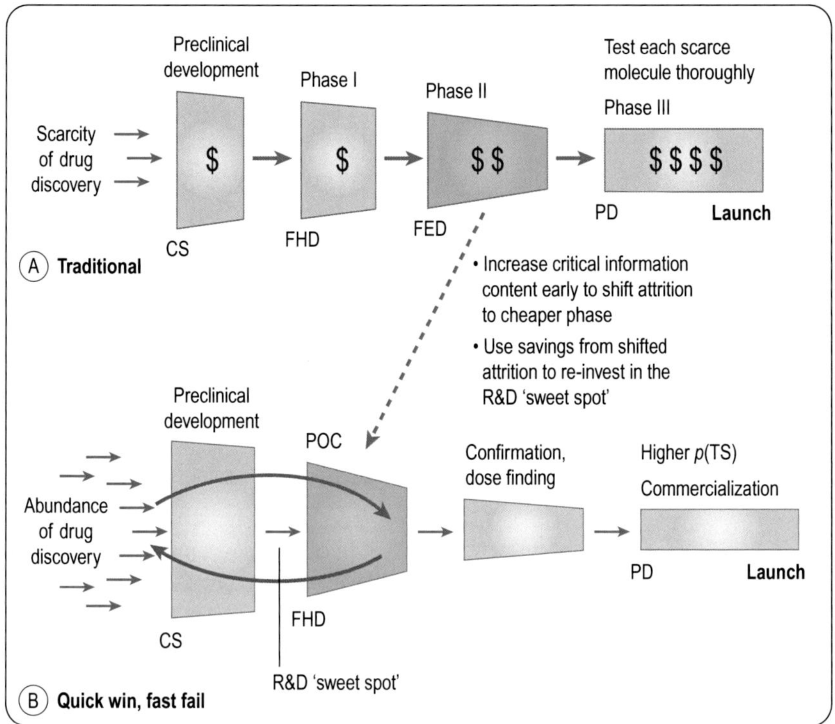

Fig. 22.10 The quick win/fast fail model for drug development.
Reproduced, with permission, from Paul et al., 2010.

REFERENCES

Abbott A. The drug deadlock. Nature 2010;468:178–9.

Arthur Andersen Consultants. Report on innovation and productivity; 1997.

Aronson JK, Ferner RE, Hughes DA. Defining rewardable innovation in drug therapy. Nature Rev Drug Discov 2012;11:253–4.

Arrowsmith J. Phase III and submission failures: 2007–10. Nature Reviews. Drug Discovery 2011;10:1.

Association of the British Pharmaceutical Industry (website: www.abpi.org.uk).

Austin DH. Research and development in the pharmaceutical industry. Congressional Budget Office Study; 2006. p. 55.

Bennani YL. Drug discovery in the next decade: innovation needed ASAP. Drug Discovery Today – in press; 2011.

Berkrot B. Global drug sales to top $1 trillion in 2014: IMS. Reuters Business and Financial News Apr 20th 2010; 2010.

Carroll J. Top 15 Pharma R&D budgets. FiercePharma 12th August 2010 (www.fiercepharma.com/node/35385/print); 2010.

DiMasi JA, Hansen RW, Grabowski HG. The price of innovation: new estimates of drug development costs. Journal of Health Economics 2003;22:151–85.

DiMasi JA, Faden LB. Competitiveness in follow-on drug R&D: a race or imitation? Nature Reviews. Drug Discovery 2011;10:23–7.

Douglas FL, Narayanan VK, Mitchell L, et al. The case for entrepreneurship in R&D in the pharmaceutical industry. Nature Reviews. Drug Discovery 2010;9:683–9.

Drews J. Strategic trends in the drug industry. Drug Discovery Today 2003a;8:411–20.

Drews J. In quest of tomorrow's medicines. 2nd ed. New York: Springer-Verlag; 2003b.

EFPIA. The pharmaceutical industry in figures. Brussels: European Federation of Pharmaceutical Industries and Associations; 2010. p. 40.

Eichler H-G, Bioechl-Daum B, Abadie E, et al. Relative efficacy of drugs: an emerging issue between regulatory agencies and third-party payers. Nature Reviews. Drug Discovery 2010;9:277–91.

FDA. Report. Challenge and opportunity on the critical path to new medical products. (www.fda.gov/oc/initiatives/criticalpath/whitepaper.html); 2004.

FDA. Advancing regulatory science at FDA: a strategic plan, 2011. p. 34

Gilbert J, Hnaske P, Singh A. Rebuilding big pharma's business model. InVivo, the Business & Medicine Report,

21(10). Norwalk, Conn: Windhover Information; 2003. 21(10).

Goodman M. Pharmaceutical industry financial performance. Nature Reviews. Drug Discovery 2009;8:927–8.

Grabowski H, Vernon J, DiMasi JA. Returns on research and development for 1990s new drug introductions. Pharmacoeconomics 2002;20:11–29.

Harrison C. The patent cliff steepens. Nature Rev Drug Discov 2011;10: 12–3.

Hirschler B. Drug R&D spending fell in 2010 and heading lower. Reuters Business and Financial News 30th June 2011 (www.reuters.com/assets/print?aid=USL6E7HO1BL20110626); 2011.

Hirschler B. Abbott drug tops sales as Lipitor, Plavix era ends. Reuters Business and Financial News April 11th 2012 (www.reuters.com/assets/print?aid=USL6E8FA3WO20120411); 2012.

Hunter D, Wilson J. Hyper-expensive treatments. Background paper for Forward Look 2011. London: Nuffield Council on Bioethics; 2011. p. 23.

IMS. The global use of medicines: outlook through 2015. IMS Institute for Healthcare Informatics; 2011. p27.

Kaitin K, Milne CP. A dearth of new meds. Scientific American 2011 August:16.

Kneller R. The importance of new companies for drug discovery: origins of a decade of new drugs. Nature Reviews. Drug Discovery 2010;9:867–82.

Kola I, Landis J. Can the pharmaceutical industry reduce attrition rates? Nature Reviews. Drug Discovery 2004;3:711–6.

Kotz J. Small (molecule) thinking in academia. SciBX 2011;4; doi:10,1038/scibx.2011.617.

LaMattina JL. The impact of mergers on pharmaceutical R&D. Nature Reviews. Drug Discovery 2011;10:559–60.

McKinsey. Report. Raising innovation to new heights in pharmaceutical R&D; 1997.

Maggon K. Global Pharmaceutical Market Intelligence Monograph http://knol.google.com/k/global-pharmaceutical-market-intelligence-monograph; 2009.

Mullard A. Learning lessons from Pfizer's $800 million failure. Nature Reviews. Drug Discovery 2011;10: 163–4.

Munos B. Lessons from 60 years of pharmaceutical innovation. Nature Reviews. Drug Discovery 2009;8: 959–68.

Nelson AL, Dhimolea E, Reichert JM. Development trends for human monoclonal antibody therapeutics. Nature Reviews. Drug Discovery 2010;9:767–74.

Pammolli F, Magazzini L, Riccaboni M. The productivity crisis in pharmaceutical R&D. Nature Reviews. Drug Discovery 2011;10:428–38.

Paul SM, Mytelka DS, Dunwiddie CT, et al. How to improve R&D productivity: the pharmaceutical industry's grand challenge. Nature Reviews. Drug Discovery 2010;9: 203–14.

PhRMA Survey. Biotechnology medicines in development. (www.phrma.org/newmedicines/surveys.cfm); 2002.

Pharmaceutical Research and Manufacturers of America, 2011. (www.phrma.com).

Reichert JM. Trends in development and approval times for new therapeutics in the United States. Nature Reviews. Drug Discovery 2003;2:695–702.

Stephens AJ, Jensen JJ, Wyller K, et al. The role of public sector research in the discovery of drugs and vaccines. New England Journal of Medicine 2011;364:535–41.

Swinney DC, Anthony J. How were new medicines discovered? Nature Reviews. Drug Discovery 2011;10: 507–19.

Von Schaper E, Kresge N. Novartis $48,000 pill spurs price increases for MS drugs. Bloomberg Business Week March 23rd 2011 (www.businessweek.com/news/2011-03-21/novartis-s-48-000-pill-spurs-u-s-price); 2011.

Zang J. Moving from made in China to discovered in China. Lecture at Academy of Medical Sciences 2011, May 2011.

Index

NB: Page numbers in *italics* refer to boxes, figures and tables.

A

D

E

M

N

O

U

V

W

X

Y

Z